Advances in Biomedical Imaging

Advances in Biomedical Imaging

Edited by **Ned Wolf**

hayle
medical

New York

Published by Hayle Medical,
30 West, 37th Street, Suite 612,
New York, NY 10018, USA
www.haylemedical.com

Advances in Biomedical Imaging
Edited by Ned Wolf

International Standard Book Number: 978-1-63241-402-1 (Hardback)

The publisher's policy is to use permanent paper from mills that operate a sustainable forestry policy. Furthermore, the publisher ensures that the text paper and cover boards used have met acceptable environmental accreditation standards.

Trademark Notice: Registered trademark of products or corporate names are used only for explanation and identification without intent to infringe.

Printed in the United States of America.

Contents

Preface

The purpose of the book is to provide a glimpse into the dynamics and to present opinions and studies of some of the scientists engaged in the development of new ideas in the field from very different standpoints. This book will prove useful to students and researchers owing to its high content quality.

Biomedical imaging is an essential part of the medical world. It refers to the method and practice of scanning and visually presenting the interior of human body for examination and medical purposes. Biomedical imaging has enabled doctors and researchers to diagnose many diseases which were previously unknown. It uses technologies like Ultrasound, X-ray, radiology, etc; to examine the deformities in the internal organs of human body. This book provides comprehensive insights into the field of biomedical imaging. Those interested in this field will find this book useful. It will serve as a valuable source of reference for graduates and post-graduates as this book contains extensive case studies, theories and practical applications.

At the end, I would like to appreciate all the efforts made by the authors in completing their chapters professionally. I express my deepest gratitude to all of them for contributing to this book by sharing their valuable works. A special thanks to my family and friends for their constant support in this journey.

Editor

Measurement of Intervertebral Cervical Motion by Means of Dynamic X-Ray Image Processing and Data Interpolation

Paolo Bifulco, Mario Cesarelli, Maria Romano, Antonio Fratini, and Mario Sansone

Department of Electrical Engineering and Information Technologies (DIETI), University of Naples "Federico II," Via Claudio 21, 80125 Naples, Italy

Correspondence should be addressed to Mario Cesarelli; cesarell@unina.it

Academic Editor: J. C. Chen

Accurate measurement of intervertebral kinematics of the cervical spine can support the diagnosis of widespread diseases related to neck pain, such as chronic whiplash dysfunction, arthritis, and segmental degeneration. The natural inaccessibility of the spine, its complex anatomy, and the small range of motion only permit concise measurement in vivo. Low dose X-ray fluoroscopy allows time-continuous screening of cervical spine during patient's spontaneous motion. To obtain accurate motion measurements, each vertebra was tracked by means of image processing along a sequence of radiographic images. To obtain a time-continuous representation of motion and to reduce noise in the experimental data, smoothing spline interpolation was used. Estimation of intervertebral motion for cervical segments was obtained by processing patient's fluoroscopic sequence; intervertebral angle and displacement and the instantaneous centre of rotation were computed. The RMS value of fitting errors resulted in about 0.2 degree for rotation and 0.2 mm for displacements.

1. Introduction

Neck pain is a common musculoskeletal problem experienced by the vast majority of the population [1, 2]. Alterations of cervical spine mechanics that compromise the stabilizing mechanisms of the cervical spine (such those originated by chronic whiplash dysfunction [3], arthritis [4, 5], and segmental degeneration [6]) can be possible causes of neck pain.

Detection of spinal instability (degenerative or traumatic) is based on accurate measurement of intervertebral kinematic [7]. In particular, forward displacement of the vertebrae greater than 3.5 mm and angle between adjacent endplates greater than 11 degree is regarded as a sign of instability [8] and indication for surgery.

Quantitative measurements of segmental kinematics also find use in the evaluation of cervical arthroplasty, assessment of disc prosthesis, postsurgery followup, and so forth [9–11].

In spite of their paramount importance in clinical application, accurate measurement of the intervertebral kinematic are hindered by the natural inaccessibility of the spine, the complexity of its anatomy, and physiology and the extremely small range of motion achieved at segmental level.

Although most of the injuries and degenerative pathologies of the cervical spine are associated with reduced mobility and pain, there is no gold standard for the measurement of the kinematics of the cervical spine, not even for the measurement of its range of motion as a whole. Many techniques were proposed to measure spine kinematics [12–15]. These techniques include those radiological (functional radiography, cine-radiography, stereo radiography, TC, MRI, etc.), those based on external markers motion tracking (electrogoniometers, inclinometers, electromagnetic markers, optical skin markers, etc.), those ultrasonic, and those invasive (e.g., insertion of rigid markers in the vertebra bones in the context of a surgical operation).

The simpler and less invasive methods (e.g., external goniometers, optical markers, etc.) can only provide appropriate information about the entire cervical range of motion, but they are unable to accurately assess intervertebral motion (relatively large errors are associated with the sliding between skin markers and bones). Despite patient's radiation exposure, the radiological methods are currently preferred for many diagnoses. In particular, functional radiography is the clinical standard to detect segmental instability and decide whether to perform a surgery. Intervertebral kinematics measurements are currently based on functional flexion-extension radiography [16–18]. However, this method involves the use of few, end-of-range spinal positions, while in-between intervertebral motion is disregarded.

It is worth mentioning that some authors suggested that disc degeneration may lead to abnormal location of intervertebral center of rotation while maintaining intervertebral translation and rotation within a normal range [16, 19, 20]. Other studies [21, 22] supported that the center of rotation is the most sensitive and specific measurement for detecting damage of intervertebral disc and facet joints.

Because of the indirect methodology and the physician manual selection on radiographies, intervertebral kinematic measurements suffer from large inaccuracy. This is particularly true for the estimation of center of rotation because small errors in vertebra location result in much larger errors on the estimation of the center of rotation.

This study proposes a methodology for measuring the cervical intervertebral kinematics based on the processing of dynamic X-ray images able to provide objective measurements and a continuous description of spontaneous patient motion.

X-ray fluoroscopy can allow time-continuous screening of cervical vertebrae during spontaneous neck flexion extension. Fluoroscopy is based on high-gain image intensifiers to strongly reduce the X-ray radiation dose and allow prolonged recording, but it produces images with a much poorer SNR than conventional radiography. The position and orientation of each cervical vertebra were estimated frame by frame of the fluoroscopy sequence by means of an opportune time-varying image processing. The intervertebral kinematics was then estimated by combining the trajectories of two adjacent vertebrae. Clinically, relevant concise measurements were also computed as well as the trajectories of the instantaneous centre of rotation. Motion data were interpolated and filtered with nonfitting splines to obtain a time-continuous description of the joint kinematics. Approximation error analysis was also performed.

2. Materials and Methods

A 9-inche digital fluoroscopy device (Stenoscop, GE Medical Systems) was used for in vivo measurement. The X-ray tube parameters were adjusted for each subject; on average, they were set to 1 mAs and 50 kVp; the acquisition frame rate was set to 4 frame/sec; the focus-plane length was about 1 m. Digital radiological frames were acquired directly from the fluoroscopy device. Each image is memorized as raw image format (uncompressed), it is formed by 576 pixels, and luminance is encoded with 256 levels of gray, and the pixel size is 0.45 by 0.45 mm. The C-arm was set in horizontal

position and the subject was put in, with his neck as close as possible to the image intensifier. Subjects were fastened to an adjustable-height chair by apposite belts in order to obtain shoulder stabilization. Subjects were instructed to spontaneously perform the maximum possible flexion-extension movement of their neck. Before recording, the subject became familiar with the assigned task in order to perform it correctly and enough slowly. The entire flexion-extension movement was performed in about 30 seconds. A calibration phantom was used to test for geometrical distortions and to measure image noise at different gray-levels.

Since vertebra registration is mainly based on matching of bones edges (a derivation operation is required on the images), noise reduction of the fluoroscopic images is of paramount importance.

In fluoroscopy, the numbers of X-ray photons are strongly reduced to keep patient's radiation dose acceptably low. The limited availability of photons per pixel generates the so-called quantum noise. Quantum noise is by far the most dominant noise in fluoroscopic images [23]. Quantum noise is a signal-dependent Poisson-distributed noise source [24], and its strength varies over the image depending on the local grey-level intensity. This noise cannot be considered space invariant, additive, Gaussian, and white.

An accurate noise model [25], considering Poisson's distribution, was held to quantitatively measure the fluoroscopic image noise. Preliminary, the relationship between noise variance and mean pixel intensity relative to the fluoroscopy device setup was estimated. Then, the fluoroscopy sequences were preprocessed by using an edge-preserving, adaptive average filter that incorporate the information of noise variance versus grey intensity [26]. By holding this information, noise suppression can be exclusively performed by averaging the only local data that have high probability to be included in the noise statistics. Filter operates both in space and time, preserving edges and motion [26].

Vertebra tracking was achieved by image template matching [27, 28]. Cervical vertebrae were assumed to be rigid and the analysis was limited to the sagittal plane [29, 30] (see Figure 1).

A template of each cervical vertebra was chosen by selecting portion of the vertebra projection that does not superimpose with adjacent vertebra along with the whole the patient's motion. In particular, the cervical vertebra template included the anterior vertebral body cortex and the spino-laminar junction particularly visible on the radiographic projection of spinous process (the area of the facet joints was excluded). The inclusion of the posterior process in the template (in contrast with lumbar spine tracking [26], where only the vertebral body was considered) makes the error in vertebra positioning lower.

Vertebra tracking was achieved by matching the preselected vertebra template opportunely displaced and rotated on each of the image of the fluoroscopic sequence [31, 32].

The template matching was based on a particular image similarity index (GNCC), which combines the normalized cross-correlations of the horizontal and vertical gradients

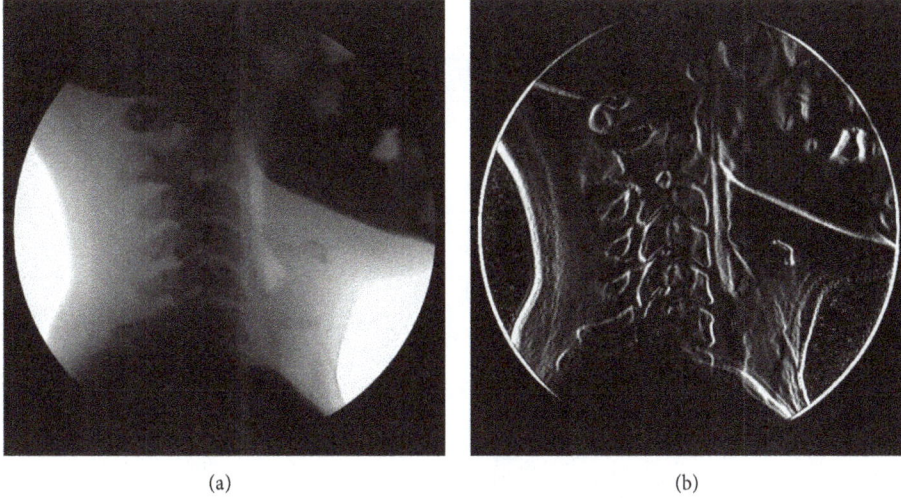

FIGURE 1: A prefiltered image of a fluoroscopic sequence (a) and the correspondent gradient image (b).

of the fluoroscopic image. The GNCC index was obtained according to the following formula:

$$
\begin{aligned}
&\text{GNCC}\,(i, j) \\
&= \frac{1}{2} \cdot \frac{\sum_{(x,y)\in T} g_x\,(i + x, j + y) \cdot t_x\,(x, y)}{\sqrt{\sum_{(x,y)\in T} g_x^2\,(i + x, j + y)} \cdot \sqrt{\sum_{(x,y)\in T} t_x^2\,(x, y)}} \\
&\quad + \frac{1}{2} \cdot \frac{\sum_{(x,y)\in T} g_y\,(i + x, j + y) \cdot t_y\,(x, y)}{\sqrt{\sum_{(x,y)\in T} g_y^2\,(i + x, j + y)} \cdot \sqrt{\sum_{(x,y)\in T} t_y^2\,(x, y)}},
\end{aligned}
\tag{1}
$$

where g_x and g_y are the components of the gradient vector in the horizontal and vertical directions of a generic fluoroscopic image and t_x and t_y are the components of the gradient vector relative to the template; the summations are extended to the only pixels, of coordinates (x, y), belonging to the template. It is worth noting that this expression for the cross-correlation index not only takes into account the product of the gradient magnitudes but also performs a scalar product between the gradient vectors. This improves accuracy of vertebra location with respect to the simple normalized cross-correlation image matching.

Since each vertebra can be spatially translated and rotated in between two fluoroscopic images, the maximum of the GNCC index was searched in the three parameter spaces: x-displacement, y-displacement, and rotation angle. This was obtained by progressively rotating the template with 0.1 degree increments and repeatedly computing the GNCC index. The coordinates of the global maximum of the GNCC index estimate the template displacement, while the angle corresponding to that maximum is held as the template rotation. Furthermore, 2D cubic interpolation of the GNCC function provided a subpixel accuracy for the vertebra displacement.

At the end of the vertebra tracking procedure, the estimated x- and y-displacements and angles of rotation of a selected vertebra are available for all the frames of the fluoroscopic sequence. These three parameters, over

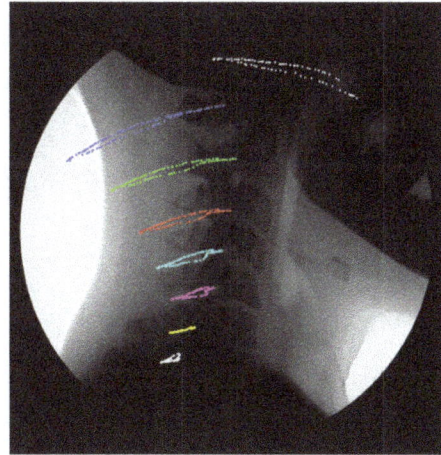

FIGURE 2: Absolute trajectories of vertebrae during flexion-extension.

time, completely describe the planar, rigid motion (i.e., the trajectory) of each cervical vertebra (see Figure 2).

From these data, the intervertebral description of motion was obtained, that is, the trajectory of the upper vertebra with respect to the lower vertebra considered motionless.

In particular, the intervertebral angle of rotation α_{IV} was given by

$$
\alpha_{IV} = \alpha_{UV} - \alpha_{LV}
\tag{2}
$$

and the intervertebral displacements (x_{IV}, y_{IV}) were given by

$$
\begin{pmatrix} x_{IV} \\ y_{IV} \end{pmatrix} = \begin{pmatrix} \cos(-\alpha_{LV}) & -\sin(-\alpha_{LV}) \\ \sin(-\alpha_{LV}) & \cos(-\alpha_{LV}) \end{pmatrix} \cdot \begin{pmatrix} x_{UV} - x_{LV} \\ y_{UV} - y_{LV} \end{pmatrix},
\tag{3}
$$

where α_{UV} is the angle of rotation of the upper vertebra, α_{LV} is the rotation of the lower vertebra, (x_{UV}, y_{UV}) are the x- and y-displacements of the upper vertebra, and (x_{LV}, y_{LV}) are the x- and y-displacements of the lower vertebra.

The intervertebral discrete-time data were interpolated by quintic nonfitting spline (similarly to [33]) providing both

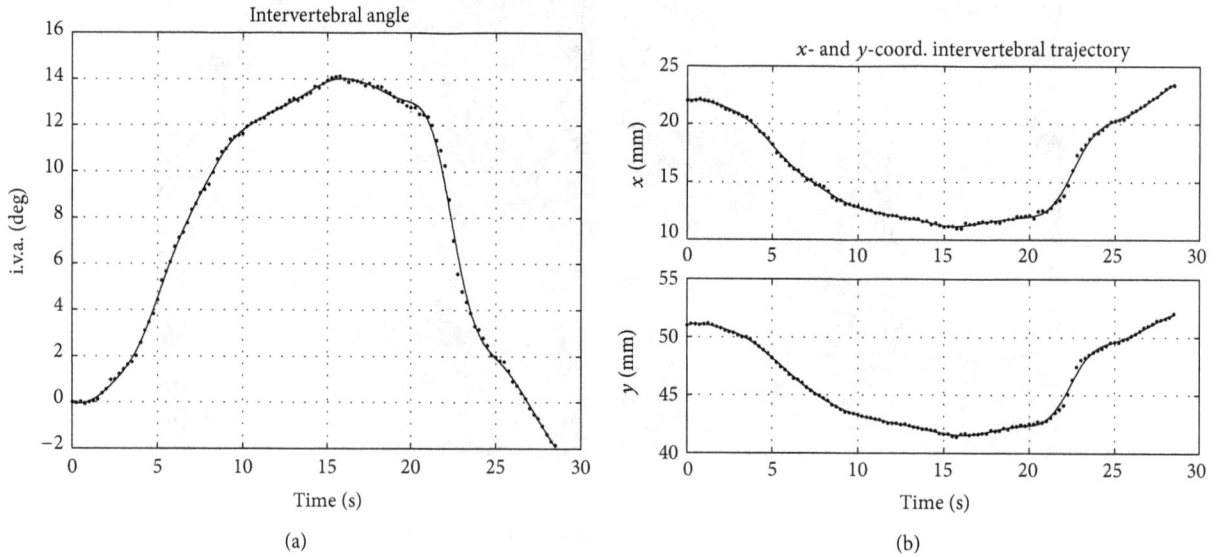

FIGURE 3: Segment C5-C6. (a) Intervertebral angle measurements (dots) and spline interpolation (cont. line). (b) Intervertebral displacements.

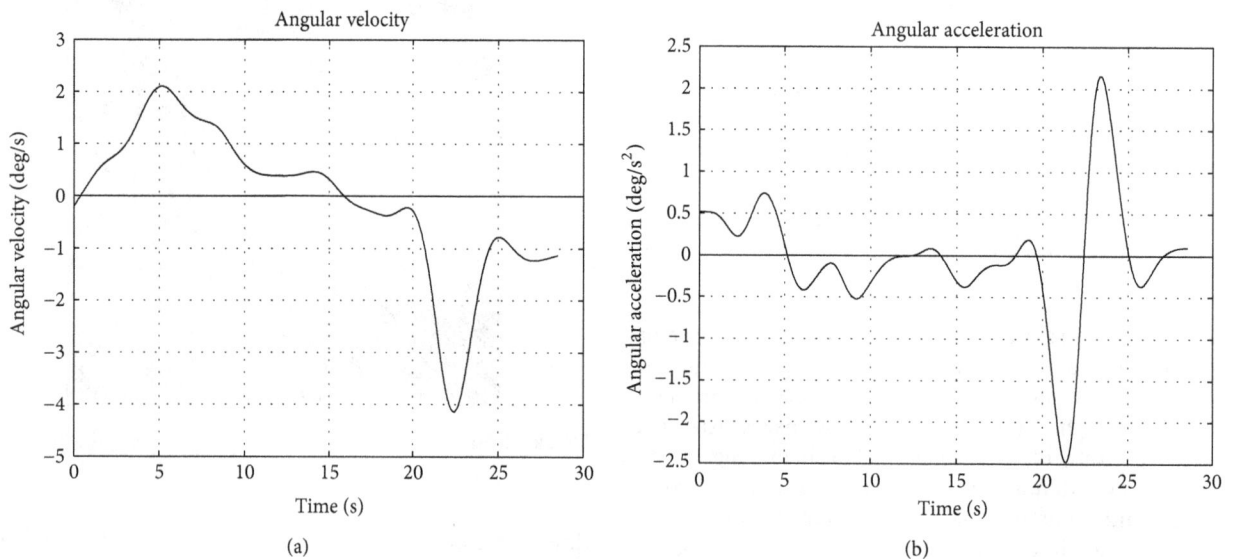

FIGURE 4: Intervertebral angular velocity (a) and acceleration (b) computed by deriving the polynomial spline approximation of the rotation.

a continuous-time description of motion and a low-pass filtering of the experimental data. The intervertebral discrete-time kinematic signals can be considered as a summation of the true kinematic signal (i.e., intervertebral motion) and noise (i.e., measurement error). Since true intervertebral motion can be only gradual and smooth, it is band-limited. On the contrary, measurement errors depend on several factors (e.g., imperfections in the algorithms, computation approximation, and quantization errors) and they can be considered as additive, Gaussian, and white (i.e., band-unlimited). Therefore, the lower frequency part of the signals is associated with the motion signal, while the remaining (high-frequency content) is exclusively related to noise.

Fitting errors (i.e., residuals) of the spline interpolation were analyzed as they represent a quantitative index of

the precision of the measurement made. The change-sign and Box-Pierce tests for whiteness were performed to ensure that the measurement errors were uncorrelated (i.e., representative of random noise and not motion).

Instantaneous centre of rotations (ICRs) were also computed but only for absolute angular velocities greater than 1 degree per second.

3. Results

Once the absolute cinematic is computed (see Figure 2), the intervertebral measurements were computed. As an example, the intervertebral kinematics of the segment C5-C6 is presented in Figure 3.

(a)

(b)

(c)

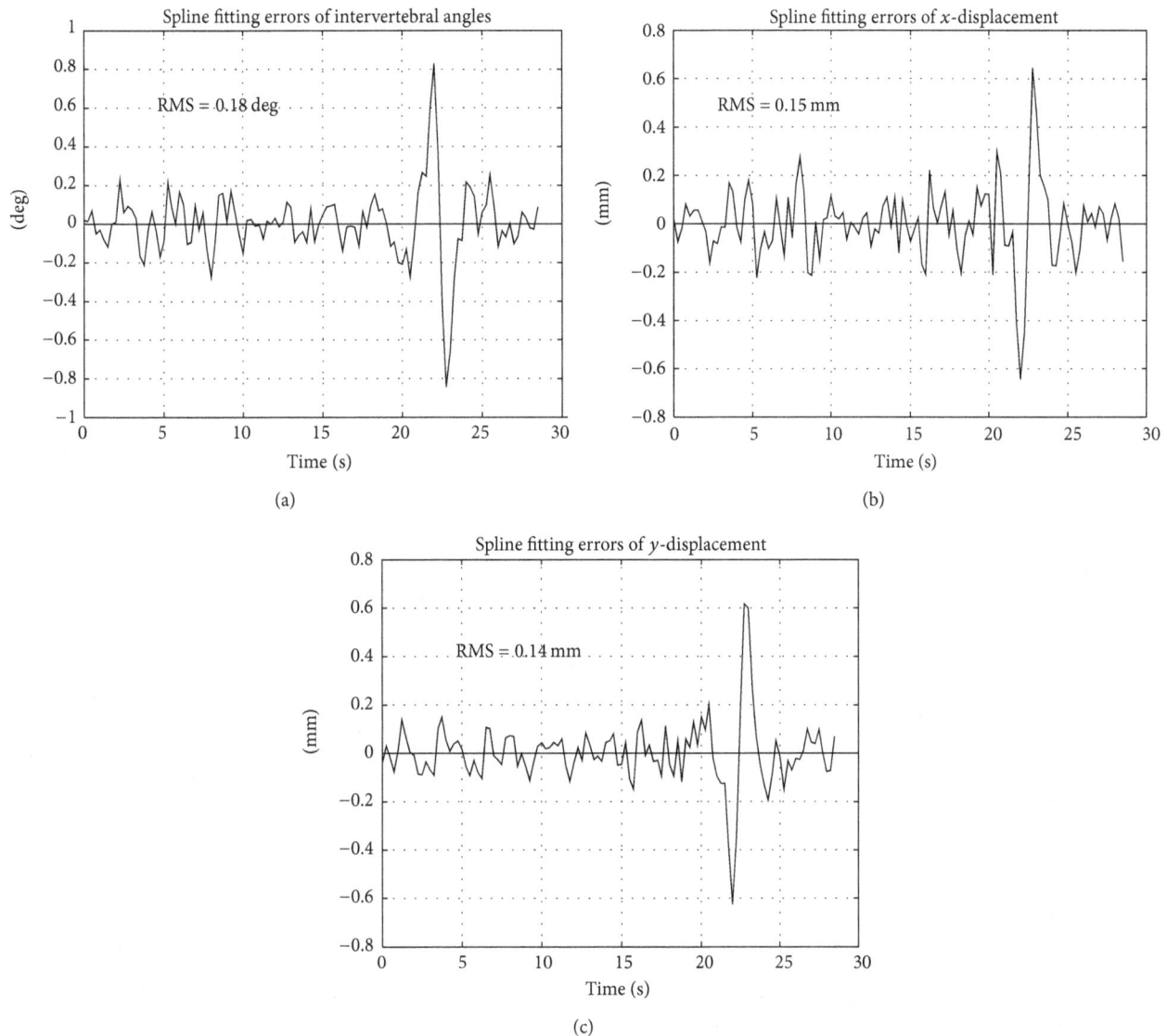

FIGURE 5: Fitting errors of spline interpolation: (a) intervertebral angle; (b) intervertebral x-displacement, and (c) y-displacement.

Discrete measurements are depicted as dots, while the spline polynomial interpolations are shown as continuous lines.

The extension phase develops in the time interval 3–9 s, while the flexion mainly at 21–24 s. Angular and linear velocities and acceleration were analytically calculated from the coefficients of the interpolating polynomial (Figure 4). Angle and displacement measurements can be considered as a superposition of the true kinematic signal (i.e., intervertebral motion) and noise (i.e., measurement error). The true kinematic signal can be considered band-limited (motion can only be gradual and smooth). Conversely, measurement error depends on several factors and can be generally considered as additive and white (i.e., uncorrelated, band-unlimited). Therefore, the lower frequency part of the signals (spline interpolated) is mainly associated with motion, while the remaining is associated with noise.

Figure 5 represents the spline fitting errors (i.e., residual of the interpolation) for the intervertebral angle and the displacements. The whiteness test of the measurement errors was verified (with a significance level of 0.05) for spline smoothing parameters, $P > 0.95$. However, a larger error in correspondence of the flexion is visible, where the angular velocity resulted about in double of that corresponding to extension.

RMS values of the residuals resulted in 0.18 degree for the intervertebral angle and 0.15 mm and 0.14 mm for the intervertebral x- and y-displacements, respectively.

As an example, trajectories of the instantaneous centers of rotation of the segment C5-C6 are represented in Figure 6 superimposed on a schematic profile of the vertebrae.

During flexion (time interval 21–24 s), the ICRs move somewhat anteriorly, while in extension (3–9 s), move posteriorly. ICR trajectories result placed in the same location,

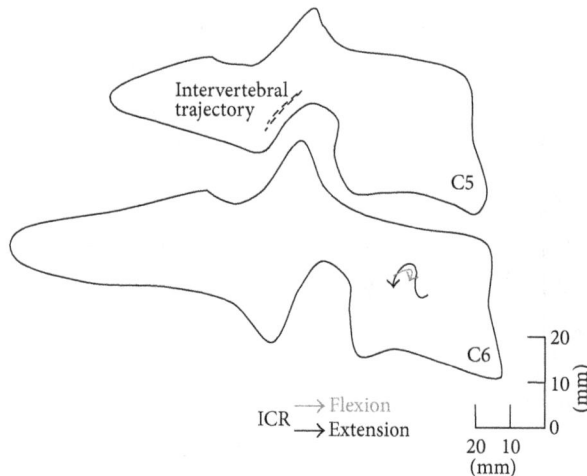

FIGURE 6: ICR trajectories during flexion and extension.

they found in previous studies [20] for the finite centers of rotation (i.e., computed between two extremes of motion).

4. Discussion

Intervertebral kinematics closely relates to the condition of the soft tissue (disk, ligaments, etc.) intended to constrain segmental motion to maintain stability. Despite its importance, intervertebral kinematics is difficult to measure in vivo: direct measurements are not clinically viable, and little errors in estimation of vertebrae positioning may cause large relative errors in intervertebral measures. By means of fluoroscopy, it is possible to describe the whole progress of intervertebral motion in the plane of view. Template matching techniques can provide estimation of vertebra position in each frame. Then, spline interpolation provides both noise reduction and continuous representation of motion. Analysis of the measurement error shows their uncorrelation.

It is worth to underline that the sampling frequency (i.e., the frame rate) has to respect Nyquist's theorem. Therefore, the movements of the patients should be enough slowly and smooth. At the moment, this technique seems inadequate to measure intervertebral kinematics (e.g., disk deformations) during vibrations [34, 35] and rapid mechanical stress or shock (as in case of car accidents, which are common cause of cervical whiplash). In these cases, the hypothesis that the high frequency components of the measured kinematics are exclusively related to noise is not fulfilled.

Previous studies [22] pointed out that the intervertebral centre of rotation is much more sensible to mild degeneration of disk and ligament. Most of the literature presents the finite centre of rotation (easier to compute) that represents only an approximation of the ICR. ICR trajectories can provide better understanding of the segmental motion in vivo.

Accurate measurement of intervertebral kinematics can offer an objective diagnostic tool to evaluate mechanical alteration of cervical segments and also can support evaluation and settings of different prostheses even during the implantation.

Acknowledgments

This study was partially supported by "DRIVEr Monitoring: Technologies, Methodologies, and IN-vehicle INnovative systems for a safe and ecocompatible driving" DRIVE IN2 project—funded by the Italian National Program Piano Operativo Nazionale Ricerca e Competitività 2007/13—and by "QUantitative Assessment of Muscle Treatments" QUAM project—funded by Italian Ministry of Economic Development.

References

[1] R. Fejer, K. O. Kyvik, and J. Hartvigsen, "The prevalence of neck pain in the world population: a systematic critical review of the literature," *European Spine Journal*, vol. 15, no. 6, pp. 834–848, 2006.

[2] P. Côté, J. D. Cassidy, and L. Carroll, "The epidemiology of neck pain: what we have learned from our population-based studies," *The Journal of the Canadian Chiropractic Association*, vol. 47, no. 4, pp. 284–290, 2003.

[3] E. Kristjansson, G. Leivseth, P. Brinckmann, and W. Frobin, "Increased sagittal plane segmental motion in the lower cervical spine in women with chronic whiplash-associated disorders, grades I-II: a case-control study using a new measurement protocol," *Spine*, vol. 28, no. 19, pp. 2215–2221, 2003.

[4] S. Imagama, Y. Oishi, Y. Miura et al., "Predictors of aggravation of cervical spine instability in rheumatoid arthritis patients: the large joint index," *Journal of Orthopaedic Science*, vol. 15, no. 4, pp. 540–546, 2010.

[5] R. Takatori, D. Tokunaga, H. Hase et al., "Three-dimensional morphology and kinematics of the craniovertebral junction in rheumatoid arthritis," *Spine*, vol. 35, no. 23, pp. E1278–E1284, 2010.

[6] T. F. Boselie, P. C. Willems, H. van Mameren, R. de Bie, E. C. Benzel, and H. van Santbrink, "Arthroplasty versus fusion in single-level cervical degenerative disc disease," *Cochrane Database of Systematic Reviews*, vol. 9, Article ID CD009173, 2012.

[7] M. M. Panjabi, C. Lydon, A. Vasavada, D. Grob, J. J. Crisco III, and J. Dvorak, "On the understanding of clinical instability," *Spine*, vol. 19, no. 23, pp. 2642–2650, 1994.

[8] A. A. White III, R. M. Johnson, M. M. Panjabi, and W. O. Southwick, "Biomechanical analysis of clinical stability in the cervical spine," *Clinical Orthopaedics and Related Research*, vol. 109, pp. 85–96, 1975.

[9] A. Nabhan, W. I. Steudel, A. Nabhan, D. Pape, and B. Ishak, "Segmental kinematics and adjacent level degeneration following disc replacement versus fusion: RCT with three years of follow-up," *Journal of Long-Term Effects of Medical Implants*, vol. 17, no. 3, pp. 229–236, 2007.

[10] R. C. Sasso and N. M. Best, "Cervical kinematics after fusion and bryan disc arthroplasty," *Journal of Spinal Disorders and Techniques*, vol. 21, no. 1, pp. 19–22, 2008.

[11] A. Nabhan, B. Ishak, W. I. Steudel, S. Ramadhan, and O. Steimer, "Assessment of adjacent-segment mobility after cervical disc replacement versus fusion: RCT with 1 year's results," *European Spine Journal*, vol. 20, no. 6, pp. 934–941, 2011.

[12] J. Chen, A. B. Solinger, J. F. Poncet, and C. A. Lantz, "Meta-analysis of normative cervical motion," *Spine*, vol. 24, no. 15, pp. 1571–1578, 1999.

[13] K. Jordan, "Assessment of published reliability studies for cervical spine range-of-motion measurement tools," *Journal of Manipulative and Physiological Therapeutics*, vol. 23, no. 3, pp. 180–195, 2000.

[14] F. Antonaci, S. Ghirmai, G. Bono, and G. Nappi, "Current methods for cervical spine movement evaluation: a review," *Clinical and Experimental Rheumatology*, vol. 18, no. 2, supplement 19, pp. S45–S52, 2000.

[15] T. Prushansky and Z. Dvir, "Cervical motion testing: methodology and clinical implications," *Journal of Manipulative and Physiological Therapeutics*, vol. 31, no. 7, pp. 503–508, 2008.

[16] J. Dimnet, A. Pasquet, M. H. Krag, and M. M. Panjabi, "Cervical spine motion in the sagittal plane: kinematic and geometric parameters," *Journal of Biomechanics*, vol. 15, no. 12, pp. 959–969, 1982.

[17] A. Leone, G. Guglielmi, V. N. Cassar-Pullicino, and L. Bonomo, "Lumbar intervertebral instability: a review," *Radiology*, vol. 245, no. 1, pp. 62–77, 2007.

[18] T. Maeda, T. Ueta, E. Mori et al., "Soft-tissue damage and segmental instability in adult patients with cervical spinal cord injury without major bone injury," *Spine*, vol. 37, no. 25, pp. E1560–E1566, 2012.

[19] S.-W. Lee, E. R. C. Draper, and S. P. F. Hughes, "Instantaneous center of rotation and instability of the cervical spine: a clinical study," *Spine*, vol. 22, no. 6, pp. 641–648, 1997.

[20] H. van Mameren, H. Sanches, J. Beursgens, and J. Drukker, "Cervical spine motion in the sagittal plane II: position of segmental averaged instantaneous centers of rotation—a cineradiographic study," *Spine*, vol. 17, no. 5, pp. 467–474, 1992.

[21] T. Brown, C. A. Reitman, L. Nguyen, and J. A. Hipp, "Intervertebral motion after incremental damage to the posterior structures of the cervical spine," *Spine*, vol. 30, no. 17, pp. E503–508, 2005.

[22] H. Hwang, J. A. Hipp, P. Ben-Galim, and C. A. Reitman, "Threshold cervical range-of-motion necessary to detect abnormal intervertebral motion in cervical spine radiographs," *Spine*, vol. 33, no. 8, pp. E261–E267, 2008.

[23] M. J. Tapiovaara, "SNR and noise measurements for medical imaging: II. Application to fluoroscopic x-ray equipment," *Physics in Medicine and Biology*, vol. 38, no. 12, pp. 1761–1788, 1993.

[24] L. C. Chan, K. A. Katsaggelos, and V. A. Sahakian, "Image sequence filtering in quantum limited noise with applications to low-dose fluoroscopy," *IEEE Transactions on Medical Imaging*, vol. 12, no. 3, pp. 610–621, 1993.

[25] M. Cesarelli, P. Bifulco, T. Cerciello, M. Romano, and L. Paura, "X-ray fluoroscopy noise modeling for filter design," *International Journal of Computer Assisted Radiology and Surgery*, vol. 8, no. 2, pp. 269–278, 2013.

[26] T. Cerciello, P. Bifulco, M. Cesarelli, and A. Fratini, "A comparison of denoising methods for X-ray fluoroscopic images," *Biomedical Signal Processing and Control*, vol. 7, no. 6, pp. 550–559, 2012.

[27] G. P. Penney, J. Weese, J. A. Little, P. Desmedt, D. L. G. Hill, and D. J. Hawkes, "A comparison of similarity measures for use in 2-D-3-D medical image registration," *IEEE Transactions on Medical Imaging*, vol. 17, no. 4, pp. 586–595, 1998.

[28] J. Wu, M. Kim, J. Peters, H. Chung, and S. S. Samant, "Evaluation of similarity measures for use in the intensity-based rigid 2D-3D registration for patient positioning in radiotherapy," *Medical Physics*, vol. 36, no. 12, pp. 5391–5403, 2009.

[29] P. Bifulco, M. Sansone, M. Cesarelli, R. Allen, and M. Bracale, "Estimation of out-of-plane vertebra rotations on radiographic projections using CT data: a simulation study," *Medical Engineering and Physics*, vol. 24, no. 4, pp. 295–300, 2002.

[30] P. Bifulco, M. Cesarelli, R. Allen, M. Romano, A. Fratini, and G. Pasquariello, "2D-3D registration of CT vertebra volume to fluoroscopy projection: a calibration model assessment," *EURASIP Journal on Advances in Signal Processing*, vol. 2010, Article ID 806094, 2010.

[31] P. Bifulco, M. Cesarelli, R. Allen, M. Sansone, and M. Bracale, "Automatic recognition of vertebral landmarks in fluoroscopic sequences for analysis of intervertebral kinematics," *Medical and Biological Engineering and Computing*, vol. 39, no. 1, pp. 65–75, 2001.

[32] T. Cerciello, M. Romano, P. Bifulco, M. Cesarelli, and R. Allen, "Advanced template matching method for estimation of intervertebral kinematics of lumbar spine," *Medical Engineering and Physics*, vol. 33, no. 10, pp. 1293–1302, 2011.

[33] P. Bifulco, M. Cesarelli, T. Cerciello, and M. Romano, "A continuous description of intervertebral motion by means of spline interpolation of kinematic data extracted by videofluoroscopy," *Journal of Biomechanics*, vol. 45, no. 4, pp. 634–641, 2012.

[34] A. Fratini, A. la Gatta, P. Bifulco, M. Romano, and M. Cesarelli, "Muscle motion and EMG activity in vibration treatment," *Medical Engineering and Physics*, vol. 31, no. 9, pp. 1166–1172, 2009.

[35] M. Cesarelli, A. Fratini, P. Bifulco, A. la Gatta, M. Romano, and G. Pasquariello, "Analysis and modelling of muscles motion during whole body vibration," *EURASIP Journal on Advances in Signal Processing*, vol. 2010, Article ID 972353, 2010.

A Comparison of Hyperelastic Warping of PET Images with Tagged MRI for the Analysis of Cardiac Deformation

Alexander I. Veress,[1] **Gregory Klein,**[2] **and Grant T. Gullberg**[3,4]

[1] *Department of Mechanical Engineering, University of Washington, Seattle Washington, Stevens Way, P.O. Box 352600, Seattle, WA 98195, USA*
[2] *Synarc Inc., Newark, CA 94560, USA*
[3] *Lawrence Berkeley National Laboratory, Berkeley, CA 94720, USA*
[4] *Department of Radiology, University of California San Francisco, San Francisco, CA 94143, USA*

Correspondence should be addressed to Alexander I. Veress; averess@uw.edu

Academic Editor: Koon-Pong Wong

The objectives of the following research were to evaluate the utility of a deformable image registration technique known as hyperelastic warping for the measurement of local strains in the left ventricle through the analysis of clinical, gated PET image datasets. Two normal human male subjects were sequentially imaged with PET and tagged MRI imaging. Strain predictions were made for systolic contraction using warping analyses of the PET images and HARP based strain analyses of the MRI images. Coefficient of determination R^2 values were computed for the comparison of circumferential and radial strain predictions produced by each methodology. There was good correspondence between the methodologies, with R^2 values of 0.78 for the radial strains of both hearts and from an $R^2 = 0.81$ and $R^2 = 0.83$ for the circumferential strains. The strain predictions were not statistically different ($P \leq 0.01$). A series of sensitivity results indicated that the methodology was relatively insensitive to alterations in image intensity, random image noise, and alterations in fiber structure. This study demonstrated that warping was able to provide strain predictions of systolic contraction of the LV consistent with those provided by tagged MRI Warping.

1. Introduction

Diagnostic imaging technologies play a vital role in reducing the morbidity and mortality associated with heart failure, cardiac ischemia, and infarction. The assessment of regional left ventricular (LV) function is currently used as a major diagnostic and prognostic indicator in patients with cardiovascular disease [1–4]. Single photon emission computed tomography (SPECT) and positron emission tomography (PET) are commonly used for evaluation of cardiovascular disease and can allow for not only evaluation of perfusion, but with gated acquisitions these nuclear images can also be used to evaluate global cardiac function measures like ejection fraction (EF) and regional function measures such as wall motion and myocardial wall thickening. Local wall motion and thickening remain the most common methods used for evaluation of LV regional wall function in the clinical setting.

They are, however, indirect measures of cardiac function. Deformation in the form of wall strain represents a direct measurement of tissue elongation and contraction. These measures provide more information on the functional health of cardiac tissue than regional wall motion [5–8], allowing for earlier and more exact diagnoses to be made.

There has been growing interest in the use of deformable image registration methods for automated segmentation [9, 10] and deformation measurement of the left ventricle directly from low resolution SPECT images [11–13]. It has been suggested that these types of models can provide accurate quantitative measures of cardiac function (EF, deformation, strain) [11–13] in order to evaluate cardiac function.

Hyperelastic warping is a deformable image registration method that can determine deformations directly from the analysis of clinical medical imaging modalities such as MRI [14, 15], ultrasound [16], and microPET imaging [17].

The objective of the following study was to perform an initial comparison of strain predictions provided by hyperelastic warping of clinical PET images with strain predictions provided by the analysis of tagged MRI images from the same individuals. The point strain predictions were compared in numerous locations throughout the LV walls. Additionally, a series of studies were conducted to evaluate the sensitivity of the warping analysis to changes in image intensity level, the addition of noise to the images, and changes in the assumed underlying LV fiber structure.

2. Materials and Methods

2.1. Hyperelastic Warping. In hyperelastic warping, the FE representation of the LV is deformed during the registration process. The forces responsible for the registration deformation are derived from the differences in image intensity of two volumetric image data sets. The first of these image data sets is the reference image, known as the template (T). This is the starting point in the analysis and represents the geometry upon which the FE model is based upon. The forces responsible for deforming the FE model are functions of the differences in image intensity between the template image and one or more target images (S).

2.1.1. Local Image Registration. A brief description of the theory underlying hyperelastic warping image registration follows. The deformation map of the registration of the FE model representation of the template image with the target image is defined as $\varphi(X) = x = X + u(X)$, where x represents the current (deformed) coordinates corresponding to X, the undeformed coordinates, and $u(X)$ is the displacement field. $F(X)$ is the deformation gradient which is a function of this deformation map:

$$F(X) = \frac{\partial \varphi(X)}{\partial X}. \qquad (1)$$

The image based forces responsible local registration of the discretized template image (T) with a target image (S) [18, 19] is defined by an energy term as follows:

$$U(X, \varphi) = \frac{\psi}{2}(T(X) - S(\varphi))^2, \qquad (2)$$

where ψ is a penalty parameter that enforces alignment of the template model with the target image.

Hyperelastic warping is the process in which an energy functional is minimized. This energy functional consists of the total hyperelastic strain energy W from the material model and the image based term (2). The total energy takes the form:

$$E(\varphi) = \int_\beta W(X, C) \frac{dv}{J} - \int_\beta U(T(X), S(\varphi)) \frac{dv}{J}, \qquad (3)$$

where $J = \det(F)$ is the Jacobian and $C = F^T F$ is the left Cauchy-Green deformation tensor. The first term in (3) is the hyperelastic strain energy which serves to regularize the registration process. The first variation of this term gives the weak form of the momentum equations for nonlinear solid mechanics [20], while the first variation of the functional U in (3) gives rise to the following image-based force term:

$$DU(X, \varphi) \cdot \eta = -\psi \left[(T(X) - S(\varphi)) \frac{\partial S(\varphi)}{\partial \varphi} \cdot \eta \right]. \qquad (4)$$

This term drives the discretized template deformation based on the pointwise differences in image intensity (force magnitude) and the gradients (force direction). Complete details of this formulation can be found in the following work [21, 22] as well as its application to the analysis of cardiac imaging [14, 17, 23, 24].

Hyperelastic warping assumes that a hyperelastic material model defines the behavior of the material depicted in the images. In this manner, the FE model serves a dual purpose: first it is a discretized representation of the template image used in the generation of the warping forces described previously. It also represents the LV depicted in the images due to the realistic constitutive model and material property definitions defined in the LV model. For this work, the LV was defined as a transversely isotropic material [17, 24–26] in order to define the passive mechanics of the LV. Details of the passive material model and its implementation in the warping algorithm may be found in the following [21]. Transversely isotropic constitutive models are commonly used in modeling the left ventricle [27].

2.2. Active Contraction Constitutive Model. In order to register the LV from the end-diastolic starting point to the end-systolic state, a physiologically realistic "time varying elastance" active contraction model [28, 29] constitutive model was utilized to contract the template FE model. The total Cauchy stress tensor **T** in the fiber direction (unit vector **a**) is defined as the sum of the active stress tensor $T^{(a)}$ (**a** ⊗ **a**) and the passive stress tensor generated by the passive material model **T**$^{(p)}$ as follows:

$$\mathbf{T} = \mathbf{T}^{(p)} + T^{(a)}(\mathbf{a} \otimes \mathbf{a}). \qquad (5)$$

The active fiber stress tensor $T^{(a)}$ is defined as

$$T^{(a)} = T_{\max} \frac{Ca_0^2}{Ca_0^2 + ECa_{50}^2} C_t, \qquad (6)$$

where $T_{\max}$ is the intracellular calcium concentration and C_t governs the shape of the activation curve [29] and is based on literature values. The length dependent calcium sensitivity ECa_{50} is governed by the following equation:

$$ECa_{50} = \frac{(Ca_0)_{\max}}{\sqrt{\exp[B(l - l_0)] - 1}}, \qquad (7)$$

where $(Ca_0)_{\max} = 4.35\,\mu$M is the peak intracellular calcium concentration, $B = 4.75\,\mu$m^{-1} governs the shape of the peak isometric tension-sarcomere length relation, $l_0 = 1.58\,\mu$m is the sarcomere length at which no active tension develops, and l is the sarcomere length which is the product of the fiber stretch $\tilde{\lambda}$ and the unloaded length $l_r = 2.04\,\mu$m.

2.2.1. Subject Specific Active Contraction. Rather than rely on literature values for the active contraction, a subject specific active contraction methodology was developed and applied to globally align the LV model with end-systolic image. The amount of active contraction applied to the models was governed by the amount of intensity mismatch in the images themselves. These element based image intensity differences were averaged over the entire LV mesh. This average difference in image intensity was used to define C_t in

$$\mathbf{T}^{(a)} = \mathbf{T}_{\max} \frac{\mathrm{Ca}_0^2}{\mathrm{Ca}_0^2 + E\mathrm{Ca}_{50}^2} \lambda_a C_t. \qquad (8)$$

The average image intensity difference given in (9) was used to define the shape of the active contraction curve for all of the elements representing the LV wall. λ_a is a penalty parameter that enforces alignment of the template model with the target image as follows:

$$C_t = \frac{1}{\text{numelems}} \sum_{i=1}^{\text{numelems}} \left(\mathbf{T}(X,\varphi) - S(X,\varphi)\right), \qquad (9)$$

where numelems is the number of elements comprising the LV. This formulation using the average difference in image intensities was used rather than the local differences in image intensities such as is applied in warping forces, in order to produce a uniform transmural contractile stress $\mathbf{T}^{(a)}$. In this manner, the warping contractile forces are controlled by the overall registration of the model to the target image producing subject specific contraction.

2.3. Image Data Sets. Two 3D test cases were used for this initial evaluation of hyperelastic warping for determining systolic deformations using PET images. Two, mid-twenty, male volunteers were sequentially imaged, with PET and tagged MRI. The gated PET data were acquired on a CTI/Siemens ECAT EXACT HR scanner in list mode format using ^{18}F-fluorodeoxyglucose ([18]FDG). Acquisition of emission data was begun approximately 40 minutes after injection of the isotope to allow clearance from the blood pool, and acquisition continued for 20 to 60 minutes. A retrospective respiratory and cardiac double gating procedure was used to reconstruct the images into 40 msec intervals. To simplify the analysis, data from only the end-expiration portion of the respiratory cycle were used. Images were reconstructed into $256 \times 256 \times 47$ voxel volumes using filtered backprojection. The resulting images were resampled into standard short axis orientations with dimensions $100 \times 100 \times 42$ voxels ($1.5 \times 1.5 \times 3.5$ mm). The left ventricle was the principal feature in the resulting field of view. A 10–30 minute transmission scan was acquired prior to injection of the isotope. This scan was combined with a 60 min blank scan to correct for the effects of attenuation. A normalization file was then used to correct the emission, transmission, and blank data on a bin-by-bin basis.

A 1.5 T Siemens scanner was used to obtain the MRI tagged data of the same patients. Spatial modulation of

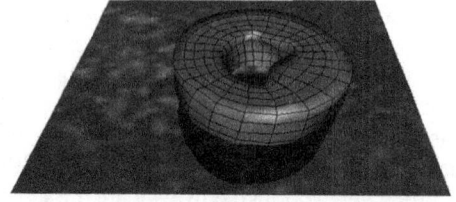

FIGURE 1: Finite element mesh of Heart 1 at the end-systolic state of the analysis superimposed on the end-systolic PET image. The FE LV model has 3366 nodes and 2712 elements.

magnetization (SPAMM) was used to create the tags and acquire data in short-axis planes with each image slice being synchronized to the R wave of the EKG signal, and sequential images were acquired at 40 ms intervals. Image data were formatted into 256×256 pixel matrices with a 378 FOV and 10 mm slice separation. The MRI image data sets were manually coregistered to the corresponding PET images using rigid body rotations and translations of the images. Complete details of both the PET and MRI image acquisition may be found in [30].

2.4. Strain Analyses

2.4.1. Tagged MRI Strain Analysis. The tagged MRI image data sets were analyzed using the commercially available harmonic phase (HARP) software package (Diagnosoft HARP, http://www.diagnosoft.com). Each short axis slice of the image data sets was analyzed using 2D HARP analysis. Epicardial, midwall, endocardial, circumferential, and radial strain measurements were determined for 4 regions (anterior, posterior, septal, and lateral), resulting in 12 radial and 12 circumferential strain measurements per image slice.

2.4.2. Warping Strain Analysis. The FE based warping models were given subject specific geometries for the two hearts using methodology described previously [17, 31]. Briefly, the 3D finite element meshes were created using surfaces based upon semiautomatic segmentation of the end-diastolic PET images (template). Each FE mesh had 3366 nodes and 2712 elements (Figure 1). The models were assigned realistic material properties [26, 32] using the material model components described previously. The fiber distributions used in the FE models were defined as $-82°$ epicardial to $80°$ endocardial [33]. The end-diastolic PET image data set was used as the template image, and the end-systolic PET image was used as the target image for each case. These time points were chosen in order to match the tagged MRI data used in the HARP analyses.

The analysis was run from a time of zero to a time of 1. These times do not represent the actual time over the cardiac cycle, rather they represent the end-points of the analysis time over which the analysis of the images is made. The time allows for control of the application of the active contraction stresses (8) as well as control over the local warping forces in (4) during the analysis. For the global alignment phase, the active contraction warping was applied using a linearly increasing

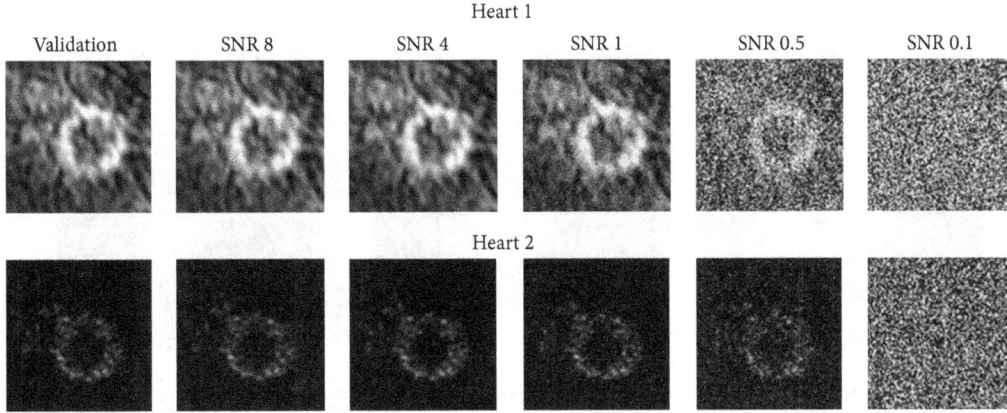

FIGURE 2: Mid ventricular slices of the image data sets used in the validation and SNR 8-SNR 0.1 analyses. The image data sets with an SNR of 0.1 demonstrate that there remains little or no image information of the LV in the images.

penalty ψ_a in (8) through 2/3 of the analysis (6.7 seconds) after which it was held constant until the end of the analysis. The warping penalty ψ in (9) and (11) was defined as linearly increasing over the course of the entire analysis [17, 31].

2.4.3. Comparison of the Registration Results. Qualitative assessment of the registration between the warping epi- and endocardial surfaces and the tagged MRI image data sets was performed. The surfaces were superimposed upon both the PET and tagged MRI image data sets using the WarpLab software (http://www.mrl.sci.utah.edu/software/warplab). WarpLab is a freely distributed finite element postprocessing program that was designed to simultaneously display the FE models and the corresponding images, allowing for the visual evaluation of the deformation and registration results.

A quantitative assessment of the methodologies was made by comparing the warping radial and circumferential strain predictions with the HARP based strain measurements for the same locations. The comparisons were made using the point strains at each location for each methodology without any averaging being made. The coefficient of determination (R^2) between the two measurements was determined by correlating the strains determined by MRI with the strains predicted by warping. A Bland-Altman analysis was conducted on these strain predictions to assess the amount of agreement between the methodologies as well as to identify possible bias in the warping predictions. A regression analysis was performed on the Bland-Altman error data in order to identify trends in the warping predictions. The percent root mean squared errors (%RMSE) was used to compare the tagged MRI strain data with the strains predicted by hyperelastic warping using the tagged MRI data as the Gold Standard (10). The %RMSE was calculated as follows:

$$\%\text{RMSE} = \sqrt{\frac{1}{N_{\text{nodes}}} \sum_{i=1}^{N_{\text{nodes}}} \frac{\left(\varepsilon_{\text{tagged}} - \varepsilon_{\text{Warp}}\right)^2}{\left(\varepsilon_{\text{tagged}}\right)^2}}.$$

(10)

Here, $\varepsilon_{\text{tagged}}$ represented the strain value in the tagged analysis, $\varepsilon_{\text{warp}}$ was the predicted strain value for the node corresponding to this location in the warping analysis, and N_{nodes} was the total number of nodes in the elements representing the myocardial wall. Additionally, paired student's t-tests were used to assess statistical differences in the means of the strain predictions.

2.5. Sensitivity Studies

2.5.1. Sensitivity to the Addition of Gaussian Image Noise. A series of sensitivity studies were conducted in order to evaluate the sensitivity of the strain predictions from warping to the addition of noise to the images being analyzed using methodology demonstrated in our previous studies [24, 34]. An independent additive noise model [35] was used to modify the original template and target images. The intensities of the original template and target images were considered true images $s(i, j)$, where i and j represent pixel coordinates. Random noise $n(i, j)$ was added to the true images to create the noisy image $I(i, j)$:

$$I(i, j) = s(i, j) + n(i, j).$$

(11)

The noise was defined by the standard deviation (σ_n) of a zero mean normal probability distribution for noise image intensities [35], and σ_i was the standard deviations of the image intensities for the template and target images. The signal to noise ratio (SNR) was defined as

$$\text{SNR} = \frac{\sigma_i}{\sigma_n}.$$

(12)

Images having SNR values of 8, 4, 1, 0.5, and 0.1 were evaluated (Figure 2). Coefficients of determination and %RMSE were determined for the warping analysis of these images.

2.5.2. Sensitivity to Changes in Image Intensity. The intensities of nuclear based images represent the relative uptake of the

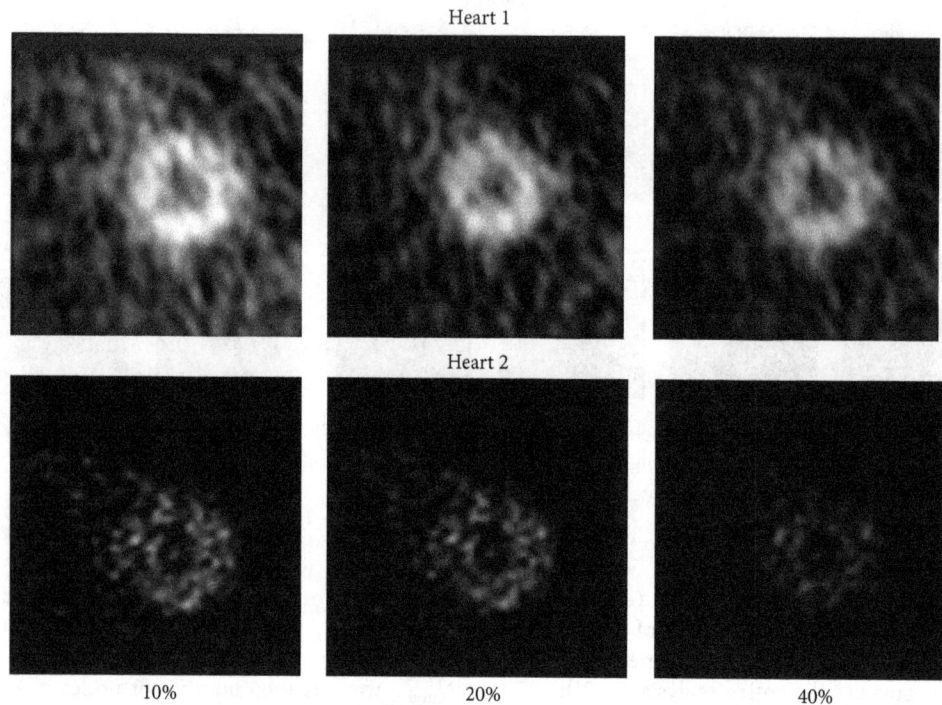

FIGURE 3: Mid ventricular slices of the images used in the image intensity sensitivity studies. These images represent the 10%, 20%, and 40% reductions in voxel intensity.

tracer, in this case ^{18}FDG, by the tissue. As the relative uptake of tracer can vary widely for nuclear imaging studies, a series of studies were carried out to determine how changes in the image intensities of the images would affect the warping strain distributions. The intensities (counts) of the template and the target image data sets were both reduced by 10%, 20%, and by 40% (Figure 3). Each case was analyzed using hyperelastic warping, and the strains were compared.

2.5.3. Relative Contribution of the Active Contraction Component. The active contractile component of warping is responsible for the global alignment of the LV model with the target image. In order to determine the contribution of the active contraction component of hyperelastic warping to the overall accuracy of the strain predictions, the validation study was repeated with the active contraction component being turned off. No other warping parameters were altered. Strains were again compared with the validation study.

2.5.4. Effect of Changes in Fiber Distribution. Currently, it is extremely difficult to determine the fiber distribution of the LV for a living human subject or animal model noninvasively. Therefore, it is valuable to determine the relative sensitivity of warping to variations in the transmural fiber distribution, given that the fiber distribution used in the models will likely be based upon literature values. In order to study the effects of changes in the fiber distribution, the baseline transmural

inclination angles of −82, 0, 80 (epi-, mid-, endocardial wall) used in the validation study were increased and decreased by 5%. This resulted in distributions of −86, 0, 84 and −78, 0, 76. The warping analyses were then repeated for each of these cases. Only the fiber distributions were altered with no other analysis parameters being changed. The circumferential and radial strains were compared with the tagged MRI strains as described previously.

2.5.5. Effect of Fiber Distribution on the Active Contraction Component. The effect of changes in the fiber distribution on the active contraction component alone was made by evaluating the SNR 0.1 image data sets while altering the model fiber distributions. The SNR 0.1 images contain virtually no image information being completely made up of Guassian noise (Figure 2, far right panel). The differences in image intensities, in this case random noise will, on the element basis, create small image based forces. The lack of coherent image gradients means that these image based forces will be randomly oriented and will not contribute to changing the configuration of the FE LV model leaving only the active contraction to alter the LV model. Using these models, the effect of changes in the fiber distribution on the active contraction component alone was evaluated by increasing and decreasing the inclination angles for the SNR 0.1 analysis by 5% as described previously. The strain predictions from these cases were compared with the validation study and the SNR 0.1 analysis with the normal fiber distribution.

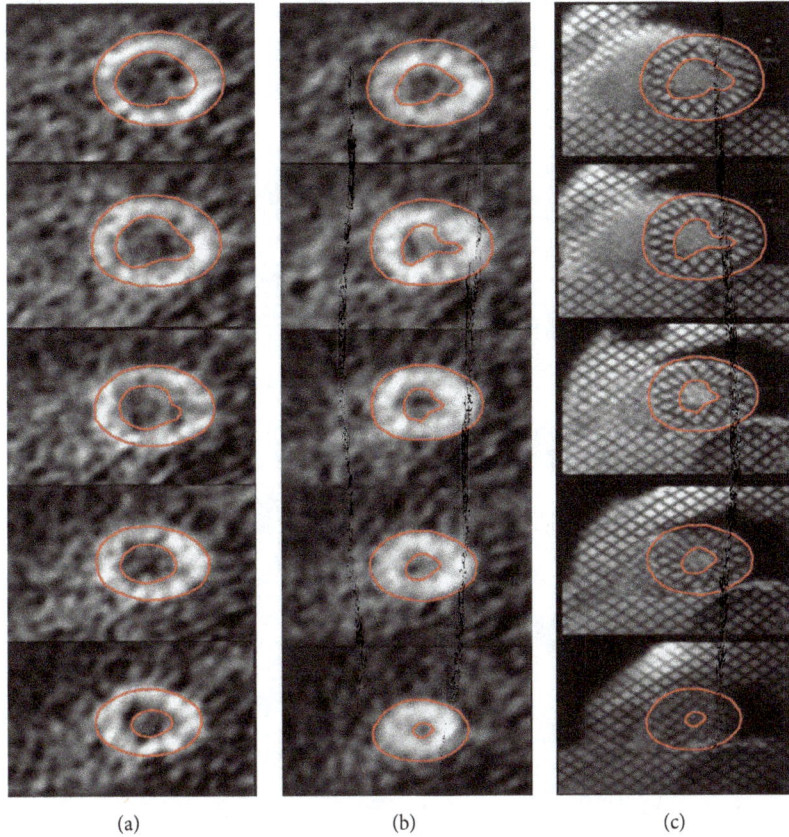

(a)   (b)   (c)

FIGURE 4: Registration comparison Heart 1. Warping analysis of Heart 1 indicates that excellent image registration was achieved on this image data set. The epi- and endocardial surfaces of the warping model correspond with those surfaces in the higher resolution MRI images on the right (c). (a) End-diastolic images (template) used in the warping analysis, (b) the end-systolic PET (target) images, and (c) the corresponding end-systolic tagged MRI images. Every fourth slice is displayed.

3. Results

3.1. Comparison of Registration Results. The visual comparison of the registered warping epi- and endocardial surfaces with the end-systolic tagged MRI images indicated that the analyses achieved excellent image registration for both hearts. The model epi- and endocardial surfaces for both models show very good correspondence with these surfaces in the tagged MRI images (Figures 4(c) and 5(c)). The FE model epi- and endocardial surfaces are displayed with the PET images used in the analysis (Figures 4(a), 4(b), 5(a), and 5(b)).

The comparison of the warping strain predictions with the results of tagged MRI analysis indicated good agreement between the analysis methods (Figure 6) with R^2 values of 0.78 to 0.83. Bland-Altman analyses (Figure 7) of these results indicated that the warping strain predictions were lower than the tagged MRI analysis for both the radial and circumferential directions. In the radial direction there appears to be a tendency towards greater underestimation at higher strain values. The average strain results were not statistically different ($P \leq 0.01$).

3.2. Sensitivity Studies. The results of the sensitivity studies (Tables 1 and 2) indicate that alterations in fiber distribution,

moderate decreases in image intensity, and the addition of noise down to an SNR 4 for Heart 1 and SNR 1 for Heart 2 had little effect on the warping predicted strains. The results indicated that there was little change in the R^2 values and the %RMSE for these cases. The error values for the SNR 1 case of Heart 1 and SNR 0.5 for Heart 2 displayed a marked degradation of the strain predictions resulting in large increases in the error measures and decreases in the R^2 values from the addition of image noise. SNR cases below these values showed improvement in the error measures.

The removal of the active contraction from the analysis led to regions of severe misregistration of the FE models with the end-systolic images. There were several locations of misregistration on the epicardial surfaces for each short axis slice. An example of this is given in Figure 8. The endocardial surfaces of the model simply did not register the corresponding surfaces shown in the end-systolic tagged MRI images. The effect upon the strain predictions were also pronounced with increases in the %RMSE as well as a degradation in the R^2 values for both hearts (Tables 1 and 2).

The effect of changes in the fiber distribution on the strain predictions was significant when active contraction was the only loading on the FE models. The error measures (%RMSE) increased in magnitude in the circumferential direction for

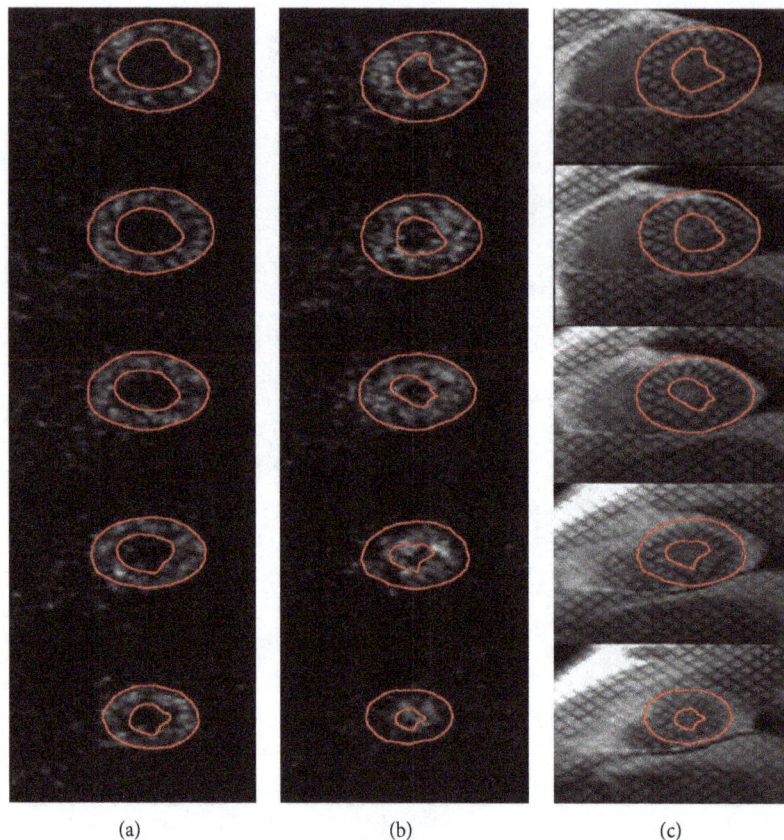

(a) (a)
(b)
(c)

FIGURE 5: Registration comparison Heart 2. Warping analysis of Heart 2 also shows that excellent registration was achieved on this data set. (a) End-diastolic images used in the warping analysis, (b) the end-systolic PET images, and (c) the corresponding end-systolic tagged MRI images.

TABLE 1: Sensitivity results for Heart 1. The sensitivity study results for the Heart 1 analyses indicate that warping was relatively insensitive to image noise, moderate decreases in image intensity, and changes in fiber orientation. An SNR level of 1 (bold) caused severe degradation of the registration results with large increases in %RMSE and a reduction of the R^2 values. The lack of active contraction in the analysis also resulted in degradation of the error measures.

	Cir. strain		Radial strain	
	%RMSE	R^2	%RMSE	R^2
Validation study	0.098	0.813	0.138	0.780
SNR 8	0.109	0.813	0.122	0.780
SNR 4	0.109	0.811	0.133	0.798
SNR 1	**0.236**	**0.220**	**0.196**	**0.210**
SNR 0.5	0.280	0.770	0.439	0.790
SNR 0.1	0.131	0.786	0.145	0.750
Reduction in fiber angle (+5%)	0.105	0.813	0.143	0.796
Increase in fiber angle (−5%)	0.116	0.810	0.122	0.800
10% reduction in intensity	0.117	0.820	0.116	0.780
20% reduction in intensity	0.116	0.810	0.139	0.800
40% reduction in intensity	0.129	0.783	0.139	0.790
No active contraction	0.181	0.770	0.191	0.750

TABLE 2: Sensitivity results for Heart 2. The results of Heart 2 analyses show similar trends to those seen in the Heart 1 analyses. An SNR level of 0.5 (bold) caused severe degradation of the registration results also with large increases in %RMSE and a reduction of the R^2 values.

	Cir. strain		Radial strain	
	%RMSE	R^2	%RMSE	R^2
Validation study	0.093	0.830	0.113	0.780
SNR 8	0.095	0.824	0.113	0.773
SNR 4	0.099	0.820	0.113	0.773
SNR 1	0.099	0.821	0.113	0.804
SNR 0.5	**0.329**	**0.094**	**0.412**	**0.080**
SNR 0.1	0.114	0.790	0.124	0.770
Reduction in fiber angle (+5%)	0.092	0.830	0.110	0.780
Increase in fiber angle (−5%)	0.092	0.840	0.100	0.790
10% reduction in intensity	0.092	0.850	0.100	0.800
20% reduction in intensity	0.095	0.840	0.100	0.790
40% reduction in intensity	0.096	0.830	0.110	0.790
No active contraction	0.156	0.638	0.214	0.612

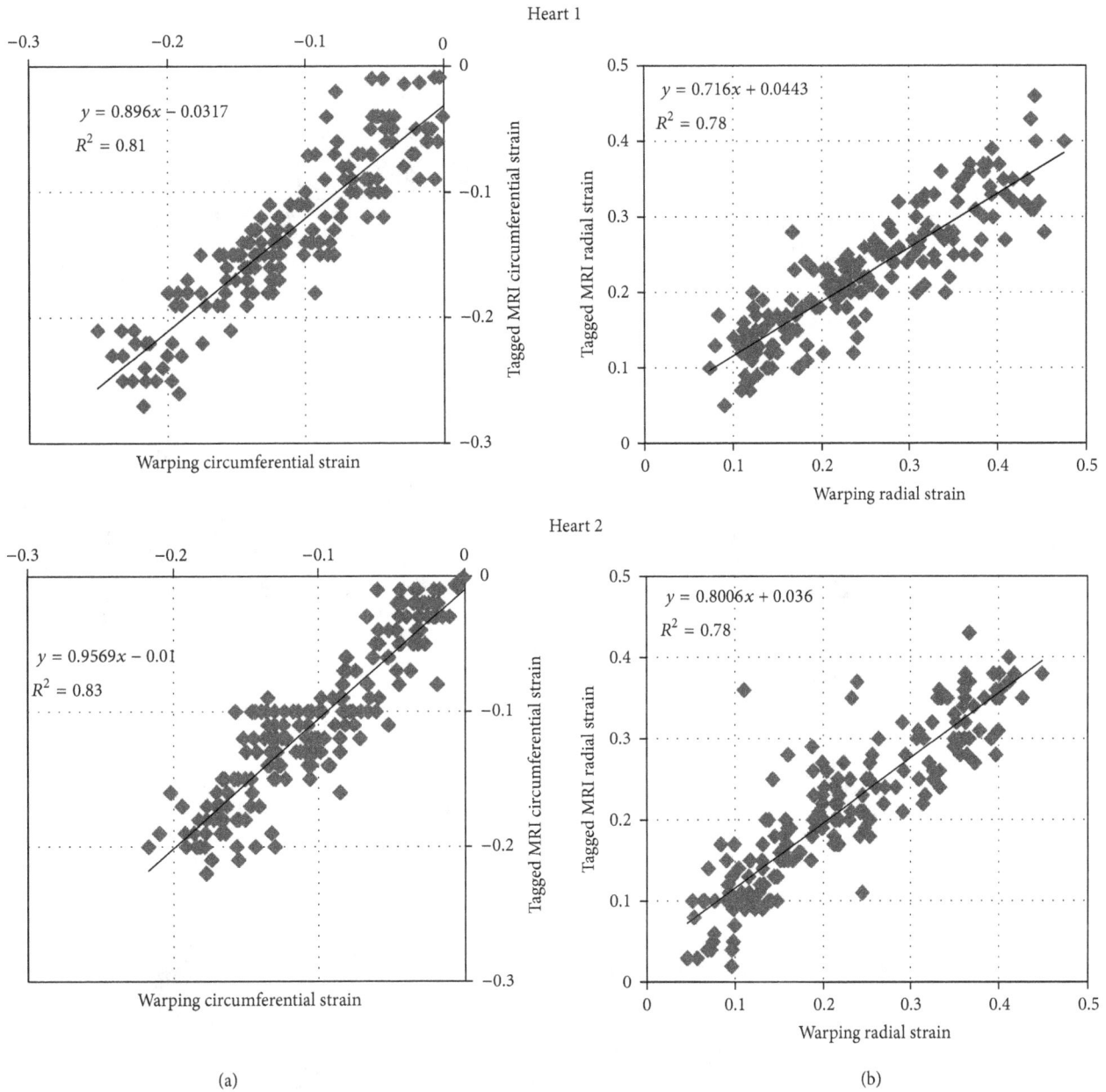

FIGURE 6: The comparisons of strains for tagged MRI analysis and the warping analysis show relatively good agreement with the comparisons of the circumferential strains (a) having R^2 values of 0.81 for Heart 1 and 0.83 for Heart 2. The comparisons of the radial strains (b) had R^2 values of 0.78 for both hearts.

Heart 1 with changes in fiber distribution. However, the %RMSE showed little change for the radial direction for Heart 1 compared with the normal fiber SNR 0.1 results (Table 3). The R^2 values for Heart 1 cases showed slight decreases for both of these strain measures. In contrast, the active contraction fiber distribution analysis for Heart 2 showed increased %RMSE for both the circumferential and radial directions compared with the normal fiber SNR 0.1 case. The R^2 values also showed large decreases in value.

4. Discussion

The qualitative and quantitative evaluations of this initial validation study indicated that warping analysis of clinical PET images can provide point strain predictions consistent with those determined by tagged MRI analysis. The results show distinct trends in the comparison of the strain methodologies. The warping strain estimates showed a slight tendency towards underestimation for the circumferential

Heart 1

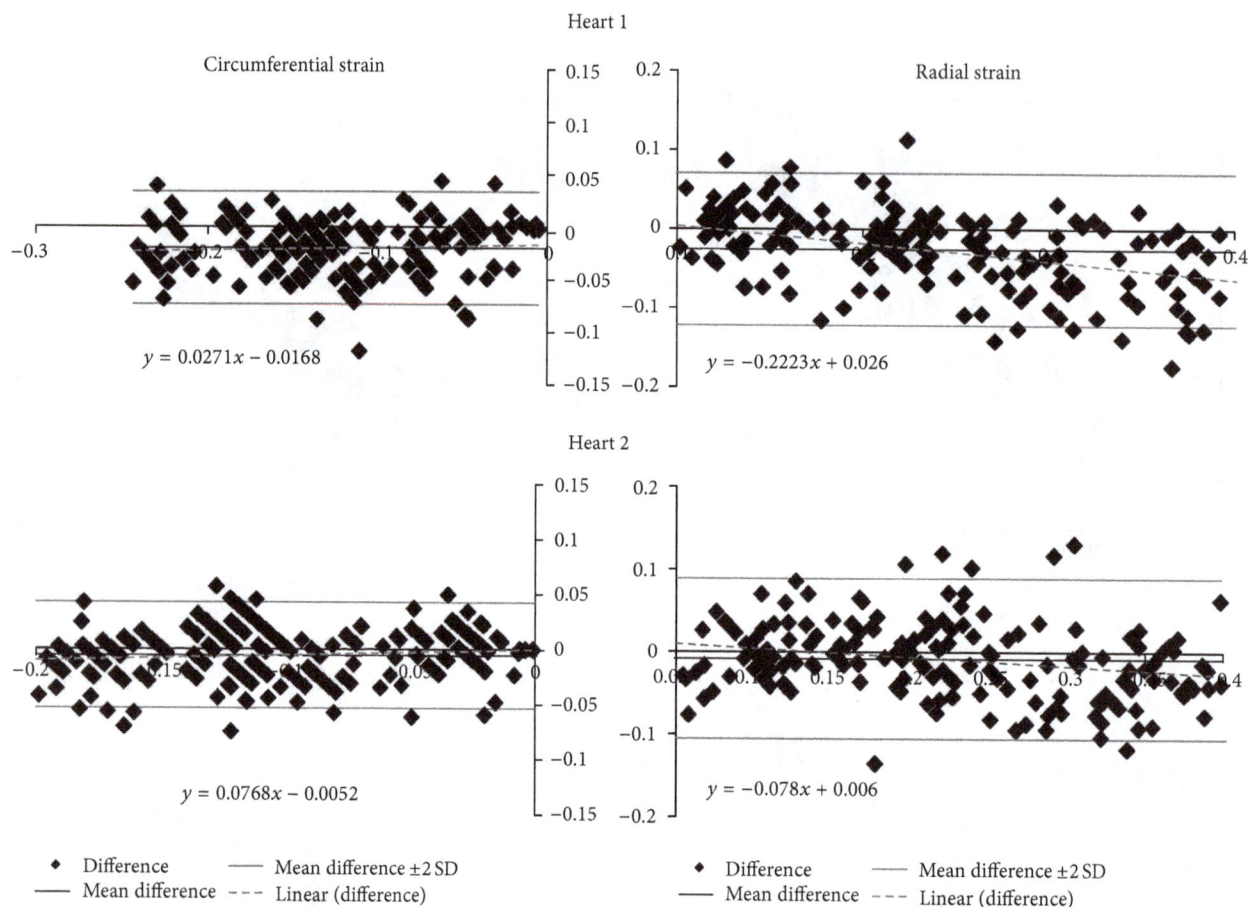

Circumferential strain

$y = 0.0271x - 0.0168$

Radial strain

$y = -0.2223x + 0.026$

Heart 2

$y = 0.0768x - 0.0052$

$y = -0.078x + 0.006$

◆ Difference ——— Mean difference ±2 SD
——— Mean difference - - - Linear (difference)

◆ Difference ——— Mean difference ±2 SD
——— Mean difference - - - Linear (difference)

FIGURE 7: The Bland-Altman analysis comparing the warping strain results with those of the tagged MRI analysis. The warping strain predictions underestimated the strain results compared with the tagged MRI strain predictions. Warping showed little bias in the circumferential direction for both hearts with the linear regression analysis (dashed lines) showing relatively flat slopes in the circumferential strain.

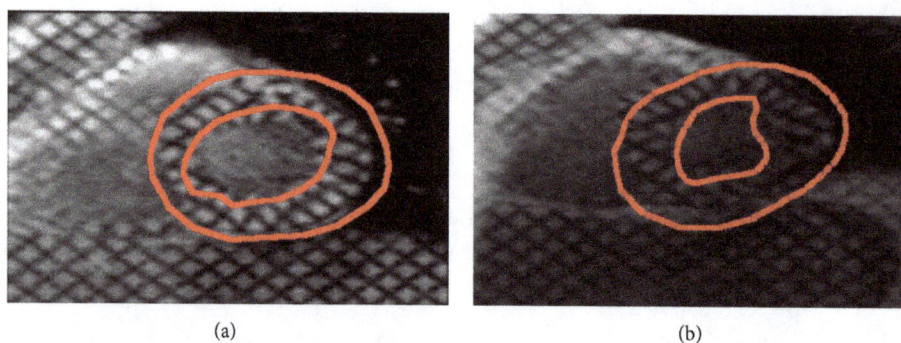

(a)

(b)

FIGURE 8: Illustrating misregistration of images when active contraction is not used. Heart 1 (a) shows anterior-lateral as well as septal misregistration for the epicardial surface. Heart 2 (b) shows posterior-lateral and septal misregistration for the epicardial surface.

direction compared with the tagged MRI analysis results as indicated by the slope of the regression lines being less than 1.0 in Figure 6. This tendency was more pronounced for the radial direction predictions where the amount of underestimation increased as indicated by the slopes of

the regression lines being smaller than the values for the circumferential direction.

The radial strain results were not surprising as there are only two to three tags across the wall (Figures 4(c) and 5(c)). Two to three tags provide a relatively low resolution for the

TABLE 3: Effect of changes in fiber distribution on the active contraction component alone for Hearts 1 and 2. Changes in inclination angle had a direct effect upon the strain predictions for the SNR 0.1 cases, particularly in the circumferential direction strain predictions.

	Cir. strain		Radial strain	
	%RMSE	R^2	%RMSE	R^2
Heart 1				
Validation study	0.098	0.813	0.138	0.780
SNR 0.1 normal fiber	0.131	0.786	0.145	0.750
SNR 0.1 + 5% IA	0.212	0.745	0.144	0.735
SNR 0.1 − 5% IA	0.160	0.753	0.142	0.737
Heart 2				
Validation study	0.093	0.830	0.113	0.780
SNR 0.1 normal fiber	0.114	0.790	0.124	0.770
SNR 0.1 + 5% IA	0.156	0.630	0.214	0.600
SNR 0.1 − 5% IA	0.247	0.302	0.331	0.500

IA: inclination angle.

prediction of the radial strains, and this tends to homogenize the radial strain results (Figures 6 and 7). In the warping analysis there are 10 sample points spread transmurally across the wall where the images are sampled. These are spaced approximately 0.5–1.5 mm apart depending upon where in the mesh the elements are located thus providing a substantially higher spatial resolution.

The sensitivity studies indicate that warping was relatively insensitive to changes in the fiber distribution as well as being insensitive to modest decreases in image intensities. The addition of moderate amounts of additive noise also showed little effect upon the predicted strains. However, a SNR level of 1 for Heart 1 and 0.5 for Heart 2 produced large increases in %RMSE. These errors resulted from noise induced distortions of the finite element meshes. However, as more noise was introduced (lower SNR values), the error measures improved due to the decrease and elimination of the intensity gradients in the images. These high SNR cases resulted in the magnitude of the image forces being decreased, but more importantly, the forces become randomly oriented leaving the active contraction as the primary loading on the models. These results also suggest that using a realistic material model can provide a reasonable strain distribution within regions where little image intensity information is available. The extreme example of this situation was the SNR 0.1 cases where no image information depicting the LV was left in the images.

The analysis of the SNR 0.1 image data sets allowed for the evaluation of the active contraction component without any other loading on the models. As expected, the effects of the fiber distribution were pronounced in these cases (Table 3) as all of the loading responsible for LV deformation is transmitted along the fibers. These results were in contrast to the sensitivity study where the fiber distribution was altered for the analysis of the validation image data sets. These studies indicated that alterations in fiber distribution produced little change in the error measures (Tables 1 and 2). Taken together, these results suggest that the active contraction forces only provide enough contraction to approximately align the LV

model with the end-systolic image data set, and it is local warping forces that produce the deformations necessary for registration of the FE model with the target image.

The work presented in this paper is the first time point strain predictions were evaluated using clinical PET images compared with clinical tagged MRI image data sets. The results are consistent with previous warping studies. For example, warping analysis of cine-MRI images of the LV compared well with tagged MRI image analysis [36] for regional strains (average septal, lateral, posterior, and anterior) in the same patient. A comparison of warping strain predictions for the medial collateral ligament (MCL) undergoing flexion based upon the analysis of cine MRI images showed excellent agreement with strain surface marker measurements [15]. A previous, nonclinical, validation study for the use of warping with cardiac microPET imaging indicated that warping analysis strain predictions showed excellent agreement with the LV strains predicted by a forward finite element model that was used to create a set of synthetic target microPET image data sets used in the analysis [17].

Limitations. Obtaining deformation information from nuclear based images presents problems that are unique to these imaging modalities. PET and SPECT images are based upon the uptake in tissue of nuclear tracers imaged over relatively long periods of time (up to 60 minutes for these studies) resulting in average geometric or spatial representations of the myocardium. Patient movement, gating errors during PET acquisition and changes in heart rate during this time span could all contribute to uncompensated blurring that might affect surface representations. Furthermore, the images themselves have relatively low spatial resolutions compared with other modalities such as the tagged MRI images used for comparison in the present study. One might expect that the geometries portrayed in the images and the relatively low spatial resolution of PET would compromise the image registration. Resolution and distortions due to motion issues would then manifest in the inability of the warping methodology to produce registered models that correspond to the geometry portrayed in the higher resolution MRI images. However, the present study demonstrated that warping could produce good image registration (Figures 4 and 5) without the introduction of obvious artifacts that would have had a negative effect upon the strain predictions.

Another possible source of error in the analysis of clinical PET images is that the relative uptake of tracer documented in the images will vary from patient to patient. In the present study, the histograms for the images (Figure 9) indicate that the dynamic range of the images of Heart 1 was far greater than that of Heart 2. The images of Heart 1 had a substantially higher mean intensity value as well as a greater standard deviation for the full 3D image data set than those of Heart 2. These differences in dynamic range did not appear to affect warping strain predictions compared to the tagged MRI analysis. PET based image intensity distributions may also vary over the cardiac cycle. The template image of Heart 1 had a mean intensity value of 91.2 for the histogram compared with the mean intensity histogram value in the target of 86.4 (Figure 10). This represents a 6% drop in the average intensity.

Count: 270000   Min: 0
Mean: 86.364   Max: 255
StdDev: 46.042

(a)

Count: 250000   Min: 0
Mean: 12.893   Max: 255
StdDev: 21.496

(b)

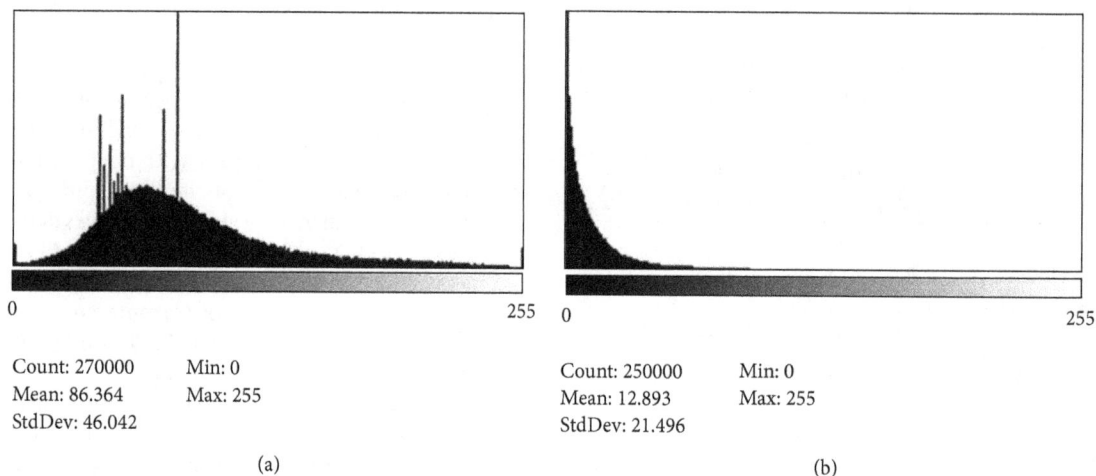

FIGURE 9: The two PET image data sets analyzed in the present study represent very different intensity distributions (full volumetric image sets). The histogram for Heart 1 (a) has a higher mean intensity value and standard deviation than those of Heart 2 (b) image data set.

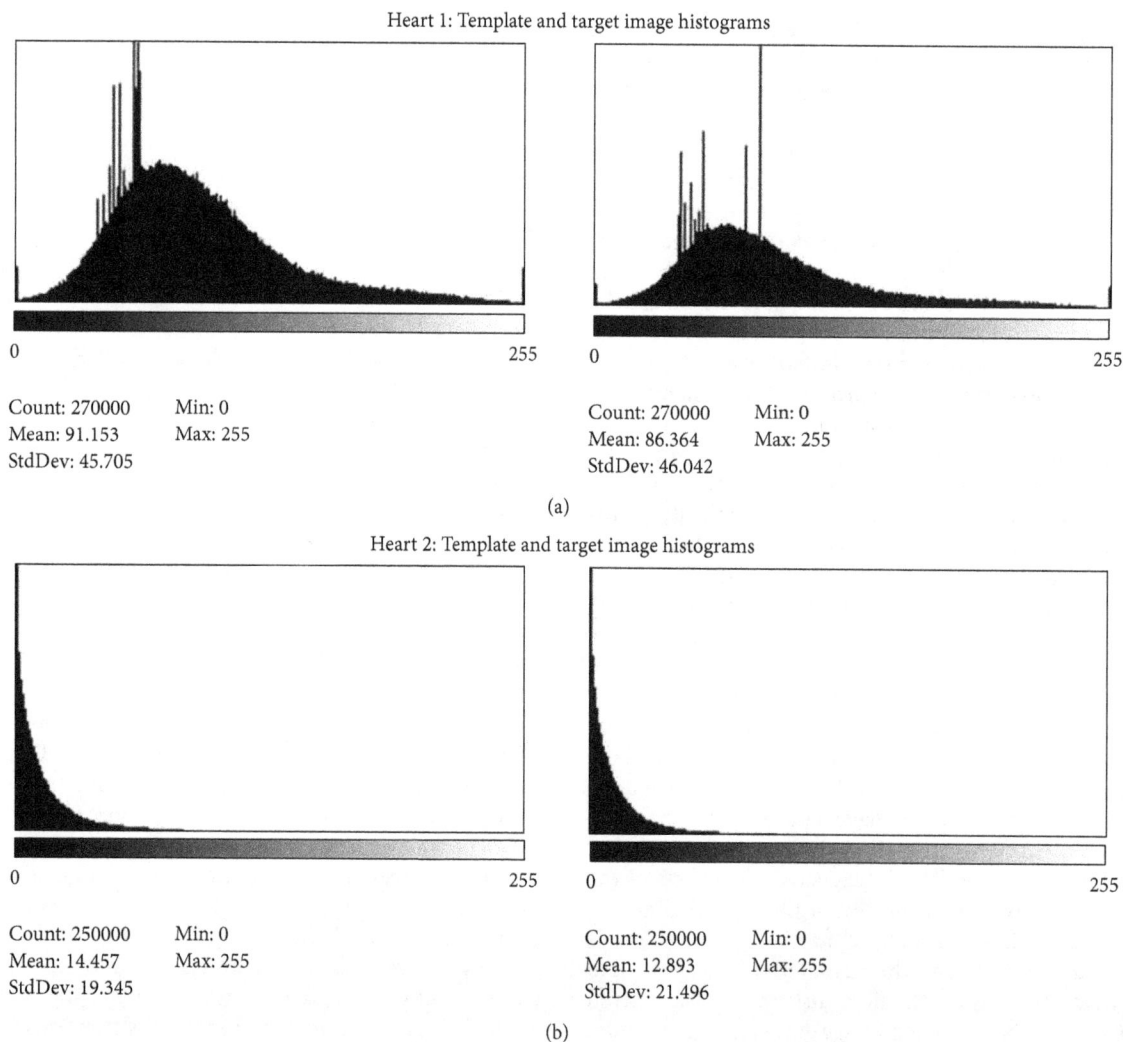

Heart 1: Template and target image histograms

Count: 270000   Min: 0
Mean: 91.153   Max: 255
StdDev: 45.705

Count: 270000   Min: 0
Mean: 86.364   Max: 255
StdDev: 46.042

(a)

Heart 2: Template and target image histograms

Count: 250000   Min: 0
Mean: 14.457   Max: 255
StdDev: 19.345

Count: 250000   Min: 0
Mean: 12.893   Max: 255
StdDev: 21.496

(b)

FIGURE 10: The mean image intensity of the template images in both Heart 1 (a) and Heart 2 (b) had higher mean intensity values than the final target image data sets.

In contrast, the images of Heart 2 had mean image intensity values of 14.5 in the template image and 12.9 for the target image, so an approximately 10% decrease in image intensity. The analysis results do not show any effect of the change in image intensity over the cardiac cycle. These results confirm those of our previous work [17] where intensity differences between the template and target image data sets did not affect the strain predictions. These results support the idea that systolic contraction "brightening" due to partial volume effects may have little or no effect on the strain predictions.

Warping can produce 3D Greene-Lagrange strain fields, rather than just the in-plane strain predictions as was provided by the tagged MRI analysis used in the present study. One of the primary limitations of 2D, in-plane, analysis methods is that it neglects to account for the effects of through plane motion of the heart. In a given image plane, the tissue seen and being analyzed at the reference configuration (end-diastole) is not the same tissue that is seen in this same image plane at end of the analysis (end-systole). As the base moves toward the apex, the tissue moves through the image plane. Through plane motion likely contributed to the differences in the strain predictions between the two methods.

One of the primary limitations of the present study was that only two image data sets were available for analysis. A larger number of image data sets would have allowed for greater confidence in the results. However, even with just the two image data sets, the results suggest that the point strain predictions made from the warping analyses were consistent with those obtained using tagged MRI analysis.

Another limitation was that the registration analyses were made on images of normal hearts. The analysis of cardiac PET images with perfusion defects from ischemia or infarction has direct clinical relevance for the use of this technology. This being the case, a possible problem with hyperelastic warping would be that the active contraction component could cause an underestimation of the strains within regions having moderate perfusion defects. This would be the case where the average intensity difference in the images (12), that drives the active contraction component of warping, would be the primary loading on the elements within the defect rather than the forces derived from the local differences in image intensity (11). This issue can be addressed in two ways. First, the active contraction penalty value used to approximately register the model with the target images was the minimum that provided reasonable alignment as subjectively judged by the user. Therefore, this methodology will likely be adequate for slight to moderate perfusion defects. Second, the analysis of images that contain one or more low perfusion regions will likely require use of additional methods in order to obtain accurate strain predictions within these segments. This would involve the identification of the elements that are within the perfusion defect(s) in order to alter the analysis parameters. Software has been developed that can be used to directly identify the elements that lie within a perfusion defect [37]. The material properties of these elements can then be altered, such that no active contraction is applied within these regions.

The noise component added to the images for the SNR analyses did not represent the type of noise found in PET imaging. The noise found in reconstructed PET data does not have a Gaussian distribution [38]. Additionally, the additive noise model that was applied to the validation PET images was overly simplistic, as there are numerous sources for noise in PET imaging, including the noise associated with the numerous corrections that are applied (randoms, attenuation, etc.) as well as the noise associated with the image reconstruction process itself (e.g., filter back projection). Each of these sources of noise introduces its own noise distribution to the overall noise in the images. It would have been difficult in the present study to reproduce the complex processes associated with the noise generation found in PET imaging.

5. Conclusions

The present study has indicated that hyperelastic warping was able to provide reasonable strain predictions through the analysis of clinical PET images depicting systolic contraction that were consistent with those obtained using the HARP analysis of tagged MRI images. The sensitivity studies indicated that the methodology was relatively insensitive to moderate alterations in image intensity and image noise as well as alterations in the assumed fiber structure. Warping analysis of PET images appears to be able to provide a relatively robust method to obtain estimates of wall strains in the human LV.

Conflict of Interests

The authors do not have any formal relationships with Diagnosoft, Inc. or the Musculoskeletal Research Laboratories, the developer of WarpLab software.

Acknowledgments

The authors would like to acknowledge these sources of funding: NIH Grant nos. R03 EB008450, R01 EB07219, and R01 EB000121, the Director, Office of Science, Office of Biological and Environmental Research, and Biological Systems Science Division of the US Department of Energy under Contract no. DE-AC02-05CH11231.

References

[1] K. G. Morris, S. T. Palmeri, and R. M. Califf, "Value of radionuclide angiography for predicting specific cardiac events after acute myocardial infarction," *American Journal of Cardiology*, vol. 55, no. 4, pp. 318–324, 1985.

[2] L. J. Shaw, S. K. Heinle, S. Borges-Neto, K. Kesler, R. E. Coleman, and R. H. Jones, "Prognosis by measurements of left ventricular function during exercise," *Journal of Nuclear Medicine*, vol. 39, no. 1, pp. 140–146, 1998.

[3] H. D. White, R. M. Norris, and M. A. Brown, "Left ventricular end-systolic volume as the major determinant of survival after recovery from myocardial infarction," *Circulation*, vol. 76, no. 1, pp. 44–51, 1987.

[4] S. H. Johnson, C. Bigelow, K. L. Lee, D. B. Pryor, and R. H. Jones, "Prediction of death and myocardial infarction by radionuclide angiocardiography in patients with suspected coronary artery

disease," *American Journal of Cardiology*, vol. 67, no. 11, pp. 919–926, 1991.

[5] H. Fujimoto, H. Honma, T. Ohno, K. Mizuno, and S. Kumita, "Longitudinal doppler strain measurement for assessment of damaged and/or hibernating myocardium by dobutamine stress echocardiography in patients with old myocardial infarction," *Journal of Cardiology*, vol. 55, no. 3, pp. 309–316, 2010.

[6] C. Schneider, K. Jaquet, S. Geidel et al., "Regional diastolic and systolic function by strain rate imaging for the detection of intramural viability during dobutamine stress echocardiography in a porcine model of myocardial infarction," *Echocardiography*, vol. 27, no. 5, pp. 552–562, 2010.

[7] F. Weidemann, C. Dommke, B. Bijnens et al., "Defining the transmurality of a chronic myocardial infarction by ultrasonic strain-rate imaging: Implications for identifying intramural viability—an experimental study," *Circulation*, vol. 107, no. 6, pp. 883–888, 2003.

[8] J. Garot, J. A. C. Lima, B. L. Gerber et al., "Spatially resolved imaging of myocardial function with strain-encoded MR: comparison with delayed contrast-enhanced MR imaging after myocardial infarction," *Radiology*, vol. 233, no. 2, pp. 596–602, 2004.

[9] J. Montagnat, M. Sermesant, H. Delingette, G. Malandain, and N. Ayache, "Anisotropic filtering for model-based segmentation of 4D cylindrical echocardiographic images," *Pattern Recognition Letters*, vol. 24, no. 4-5, pp. 815–825, 2003.

[10] M. Sermesant, Y. Coudiere, H. Delingette, and N. Ayache, "Progress towards an electro-mechanical model of the heart for cardiac image analysis," in *Proceedings of the IEEE International Symposium on Biomedical Imaging (ISBI '02)*, 2002.

[11] M. Sermesant, C. Forest, X. Pennec, H. Delingette, and N. Ayache, "Deformable biomechanical models: application to 4D cardiac image analysis," *Medical Image Analysis*, vol. 7, no. 4, pp. 475–488, 2003.

[12] A. Sitek, G. J. Klein, G. T. Gullberg, and R. H. Huesman, "Deformable model of the heart with fiber structure," *IEEE Transactions on Nuclear Science*, vol. 49, no. 3, pp. 789–793, 2002.

[13] S. M. Choi, Y. K. Lee, and M. H. Kim, "Quantitative analysis of gated SPECT images using an efficient physical deformation model," *Computers in Biology and Medicine*, vol. 34, no. 1, pp. 15–33, 2004.

[14] N. S. Phatak, S. A. Maas, A. I. Veress, N. A. Pack, E. V. R. Di Bella, and J. A. Weiss, "Strain measurement in the left ventricle during systole with deformable image registration," *Medical Image Analysis*, vol. 13, no. 2, pp. 354–361, 2009.

[15] N. S. Phatak, Q. Sun, S. E. Kim et al., "Noninvasive determination of ligament strain with deformable image registration," *Annals of Biomedical Engineering*, vol. 35, no. 7, pp. 1175–1187, 2007.

[16] A. I. Veress, J. A. Weiss, G. T. Gullberg, D. G. Vince, and R. D. Rabbitt, "Strain measurement in coronary arteries using intravascular ultrasound and deformable images," *Journal of Biomechanical Engineering*, vol. 124, no. 6, pp. 734–741, 2002.

[17] A. I. Veress, J. A. Weiss, R. H. Huesman et al., "Measuring regional changes in the diastolic deformation of the left ventricle of SHR rats using microPET technology and hyperelastic warping," *Annals of Biomedical Engineering*, vol. 36, no. 7, pp. 1104–1117, 2008.

[18] G. E. Christensen, R. D. Rabbitti, and M. I. Miller, "3D brain mapping using a deformable neuroanatomy," *Physics in Medicine and Biology*, vol. 39, no. 3, pp. 609–618, 1994.

[19] G. E. Christensen, R. D. Rabbitt, and M. I. Miller, "Deformable templates using large deformation kinematics," *IEEE Transactions on Image Processing*, vol. 5, no. 10, pp. 1435–1447, 1996.

[20] J. E. Marsden and T. J. R. Hughes, *Mathematical Foundations of Elasticity*, Minneola, NY, USA, 1994.

[21] A. I. Veress, N. Phatak, and J. A. Weiss, "Deformable image registration with hyperelastic warping," in *The Handbook of Medical Image Analysis: Segmentation and Registration Models*, vol. 3, Marcel Dekker, New York, NY, USA, 2005.

[22] A. E. Bowden, R. D. Rabbitt, and J. A. Weiss, "Anatomical registration and segmentation by Warping template finite element models," in *Laser-Tissue Interaction IX*, vol. 3254 of *Proceedings of SPIE*, pp. 469–476, January 1998.

[23] J. A. Weiss, R. D. Rabbitt, A. E. Bowden, and B. N. Maker, "Incorporation of medical image data in finite element models to track strain in soft tissues," in *Laser-Tissue Interaction IX*, vol. 3254 of *Proceedings of SPIE*, pp. 477–484, January 1998.

[24] A. I. Veress, G. T. Gullberg, and J. A. Weiss, "Measurement of strain in the left ventricle during diastole with cine-mri and deformable image registration," *Journal of Biomechanical Engineering*, vol. 127, pp. 1195–1207, 2005.

[25] J. A. Weiss, B. N. Maker, and S. Govindjee, "Finite element implementation of incompressible, transversely isotropic hyperelasticity," *Computer Methods in Applied Mechanics and Engineering*, vol. 135, no. 1-2, pp. 107–128, 1996.

[26] A. I. Veress, W. P. Segars, B. M. W. Tsui, and G. T. Gullberg, "Incorporation of a left ventricle finite element model defining infarction into the XCAT imaging phantom," *IEEE Transactions on Medical Imaging*, vol. 30, no. 4, pp. 915–927, 2011.

[27] J. D. Humphrey, *Cardiovascular Solid Mechanics Cells, Tissues and Organs*, Springer, New York, NY, USA, 2002.

[28] J. M. Guccione and A. D. McCulloch, "Mechanics of active contraction in cardiac muscle: part I-constitutive relations for fiber stress that describe deactivation," *Journal of Biomechanical Engineering*, vol. 115, no. 1, pp. 72–81, 1993.

[29] J. M. Guccione and A. D. McCulloch, "Mechanics of active contraction in cardiac muscle: part II-constitutive relations for fiber stress that describe deactivation," *Journal of Biomechanical Engineering*, vol. 115, pp. 82–90, 1993.

[30] G. J. Klein and R. H. Huesman, "Four-dimensional processing of deformable cardiac PET data," *Medical Image Analysis*, vol. 6, no. 1, pp. 29–46, 2002.

[31] A. I. Veress, J. A. Weiss, R. D. Rabbitt, J. N. Lee, and G. T. Gullberg, "Measurement of 3D left ventricular strains during diastole using image warping and untagged MRI images," in *Proceedings of the IEEE Computer in Cardiology*, pp. 165–168, September 2001.

[32] A. I. Veress, W. P. Segars, J. A. Weiss, B. M. W. Tsui, and G. T. Gullberg, "Normal and pathological NCAT image and phantom data based on physiologically realistic left ventricle finite-element models," *IEEE Transactions on Medical Imaging*, vol. 25, no. 12, pp. 1604–1616, 2006.

[33] G. Buckberg, J. I. E. Hoffman, A. Mahajan, S. Saleh, and C. Coghlan, "Cardiac mechanics revisited: the relationship of cardiac architecture to ventricular function," *Circulation*, vol. 118, no. 24, pp. 2571–2587, 2008.

[34] A. I. Veress, J. A. Weiss, G. J. Klein, and G. T. Gullberg, "Quantification of 3D left ventricular deformation using hyperelastic warping: comparisons between MRI and PET imaging," in *Computers in Cardiology 2002*, pp. 709–712, September 2002.

[35] R. C. Gonzalez and R. E. Woods, *Digital Image Processing*, Addison-Wesley, 1992.

[36] N. S. Phatak, S. A. Maas, A. I. Veress, N. A. Pack, E. V. R. Di Bella, and J. A. Weiss, "Strain measurement in the left ventricle during systole with deformable image registration," *Medical Image Analysis*, vol. 13, no. 2, pp. 354–361, 2009.

[37] A. I. Veress, G. Fung, B. M. Tsui, W. P. Segars, and G. T. Gullberg, "Incorporation of perfusion information into a finite element model of the left ventricle," in *Proceedings of the ASME Summer Bioengineering Conference*, Farmington, Pa, USA, June 2011.

[38] C. C. Watson, M. E. Casey, B. Bendriem et al., "Optimizing injected dose in clinical PET by accurately modeling the counting-rate response functions specific to individual patient scans," *Journal of Nuclear Medicine*, vol. 46, no. 11, pp. 1825–1834, 2005.

Microwave Imaging of Human Forearms: Pilot Study and Image Enhancement

Colin Gilmore,[1] **Amer Zakaria,**[2] **Stephen Pistorius,**[3,4] **and Joe LoVetri**[2]

[1] *TRTech Inc., Winnipeg MB, Canada R3T 6A8*
[2] *Department of Electrical and Computer Engineering, University of Manitoba, Winnipeg MB, Canada R3T 5V6*
[3] *Department of Physics and Astronomy, University of Manitoba, Winnipeg MB, Canada R3T 2N2*
[4] *Medical Physics, CancerCare Manitoba, Winnipeg MB, Canada R3E 0V9*

Correspondence should be addressed to Amer Zakaria; zakaria@cc.umanitoba.ca

Academic Editor: Jun Zhao

We present a pilot study using a microwave tomography system in which we image the forearms of 5 adult male and female volunteers between the ages of 30 and 48. Microwave scattering data were collected at 0.8 to 1.2 GHz with 24 transmitting and receiving antennas located in a matching fluid of deionized water and table salt. Inversion of the microwave data was performed with a balanced version of the multiplicative-regularized contrast source inversion algorithm formulated using the finite-element method (FEM-CSI). T1-weighted MRI images of each volunteer's forearm were also collected in the same plane as the microwave scattering experiment. Initial "blind" imaging results from the utilized inversion algorithm show that the image quality is dependent on the thickness of the arm's peripheral adipose tissue layer; thicker layers of adipose tissue lead to poorer overall image quality. Due to the exible nature of the FEM-CSI algorithm used, prior information can be readily incorporated into the microwave imaging inversion process. We show that by introducing prior information into the FEM-CSI algorithm the internal anatomical features of all the arms are resolved, significantly improving the images. The prior information was estimated manually from the blind inversions using an *ad hoc* procedure.

1. Introduction

Microwave imaging (MWI) is an alternative imaging modality that promises several advantages over more established modalities such as X-ray, ultrasound, or MRI. Advantages include low cost, use of safer nonionizing radiation, the ability to image bulk-electrical tissue properties, and the ability to provide functional imaging without the use of contrast agents [1]. Microwave imaging applications have primarily focused on breast cancer [2–7], although extremity (arm and leg) imaging has also received attention [1, 8–12]. While standard X-ray imaging gives reliable indication of bone injury, some researchers have indicated that diagnosing the condition of soft tissue is important for the final outcome of treatment [8], and microwaves may potentially be used to assess the soft tissue component of an injured extremity. Despite the potential advantages of microwaves as an imaging modality, the technology has not yet seen widespread use in clinics outside of research labs (e.g., the largest study involves 400 volunteers [13]).

We believe that the best argument for the use of microwave imaging is that it promises to fill a niche within the medical imaging world, providing a nonionizing, inexpensive imaging modality which is capable of imaging soft tissue contrast. The three most common medical imaging modalities are ultrasound, X-rays (both planar and CT), and magnetic resonance imaging (MRI). Ultrasound is inexpensive and nonionizing but has trouble distinguishing between soft tissues. Planar X-rays are inexpensive and give only a small dose of ionizing radiation but also struggle with imaging soft tissue contrast. X-ray CT is somewhat inexpensive and has good soft tissue contrast imaging capabilities but gives a significant dose of ionizing radiation per scan. (This radiation is particularly important for children: a single abdominal helical CT in young female children results in 1 in 1000 risks of fatal cancer later in life [14].) MRI is nonionizing, offers excellent soft

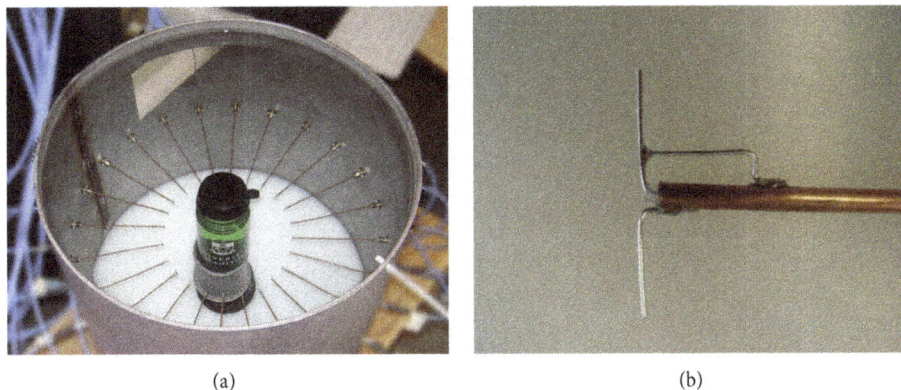

(a)   (b)

FIGURE 1: (a) The MWI system metallic enclosure with a glycerol-/water-based imaging phantom. (b) A dipole antenna with quarter wavelength balun.

tissue contrast imaging, but scanners are expensive to buy and maintain, and a single scan can take over an hour.

Due to the significant differences in permittivity between soft/hard tissues and other bodily fluids [15], its use of non-ionizing radiation, the ability to provide quantitative images, and relatively inexpensive hardware, microwave tomography could become a viable modality in medical imaging. In addition to the aforementioned breast cancer and soft tissue injury imaging, there are also opportunities in cyst fluid identification, screening/monitoring programs for degenerative muscular disorders (e.g., muscular dystrophy), lung carcinomas, stroke identification, and others that to date have not received much attention [16].

Despite this promise, initiating further clinical interest requires experimental images of live tissue, showing that the technology is capable of providing clinically relevant images. However, imaging live humans is more challenging than imaging phantoms as volunteer safety, movement, variations in size, and the presence of complex tissues, not entirely predicted by simplified phantoms, need to be considered. (It has often been noted that the gap between theory and practice is larger in practice than it is in theory.) We argue that the largest barrier to microwave tomography (MWT) is actually the lack of clinical images available to be taken to the clinical professionals who regularly read anatomical images (e.g., radiologists). Once these images have been generated, these professionals can further direct the technology.

In this work, we take a large step towards a general 2D clinical imaging system by presenting (to the best of our knowledge) the first study of microwave limb imaging with multiple individuals (either human or animal). We have elected to image the forearms of 5 human volunteers with varying ages and (importantly) varying levels of adipose tissue. The quantitative microwave images are supplemented with collocated (but not simultaneous) MRI images of the same limb. This study outlines the capabilities and some of the remaining challenges for microwave imaging of human tissues, and provides useful information on *in vivo* permittivity measurement. In addition, an enhancement for the microwave imaging reconstruction quality is introduced by incorporating prior information about the forearm's adipose layer into the inversion algorithm utilized in this work.

The paper is arranged as follows. An overview of the experimental system utilized in our study is outlined in Section 2. The considered problem's mathematical formulation as well as a description of the inversion algorithm is given in Section 3. Methods related to performing various measurements are described in Section 4. The preliminary microwave imaging results of the volunteers along with the MRI scans are presented in Section 5. Enhancements to the MWI results by the use of prior information are shown in Section 6. Finally, the paper is closed by a brief conclusion in Section 7.

2. System Overview

The microwave imaging system consists of a network analyzer (Agilent PNA network analyzer E8363) connected to a 2 × 24 matrix switch (Agilent 87050A-K24). Twenty-four dipole antennas with a quarter wavelength balun are arranged at even intervals of 15° in a circular array at the midpoint height along the inside of a metallic cylinder. This system is similar to a previously described system [17] and has also been presented in [18]. The antennas are located at a radius of 9.4 cm from the center of the chamber. The enclosure has a radius of 22.4 cm and is filled, to a height of 44.4 cm, with the matching fluid. Figure 1(a) shows a photograph of the MWI system metallic enclosure with a tissue-mimicking imaging phantom in the imaging region, while a picture of a single dipole antenna is shown in Figure 1(b). The total volume of fluid in the chamber is approximately 70.0 L. The system is capable of imaging from approximately 800 MHz to 1.2 GHz in a salt/deionized water background.

The experimental apparatus is controlled via a computer workstation which is connected through a local-ethernet device. In-house developed software is used to collect the dataset for each desired image. Data for 20 discrete frequencies are acquired in slightly less than 1 minute. The number of measurements per frequency is 24 × 23.

2.1. Matching Fluid.
In general, biomedical microwave imaging requires the use of a matching fluid [19]. Our system uses a fluid of deionized water and table salt. The salt is added in order to introduce loss into the matching fluid, which reduces

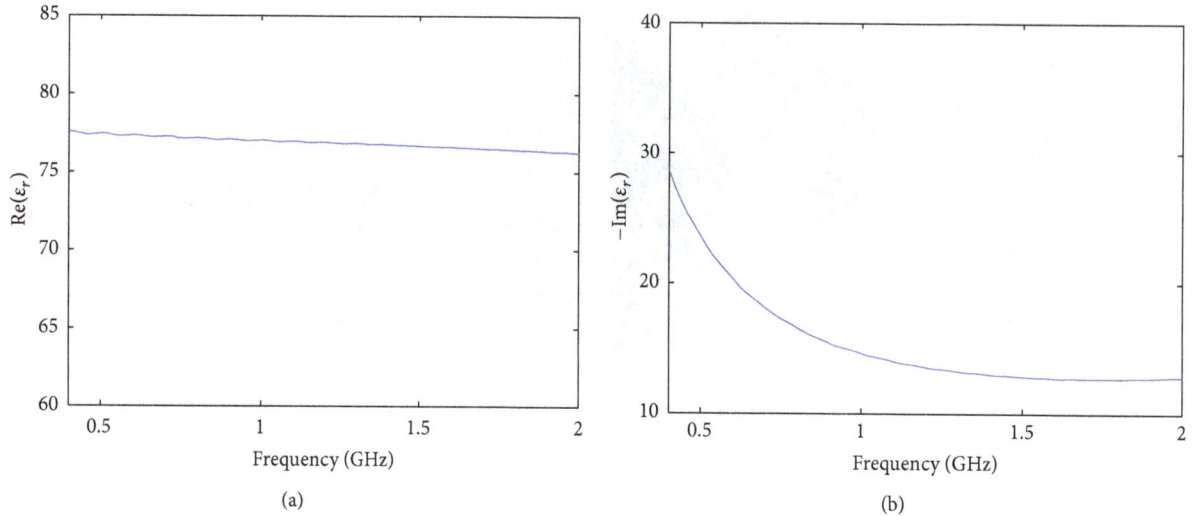

(a)

(b)

FIGURE 2: (a) Real and (b) imaginary components of the complex relative permittivity used in our MWI system as matching fluid.

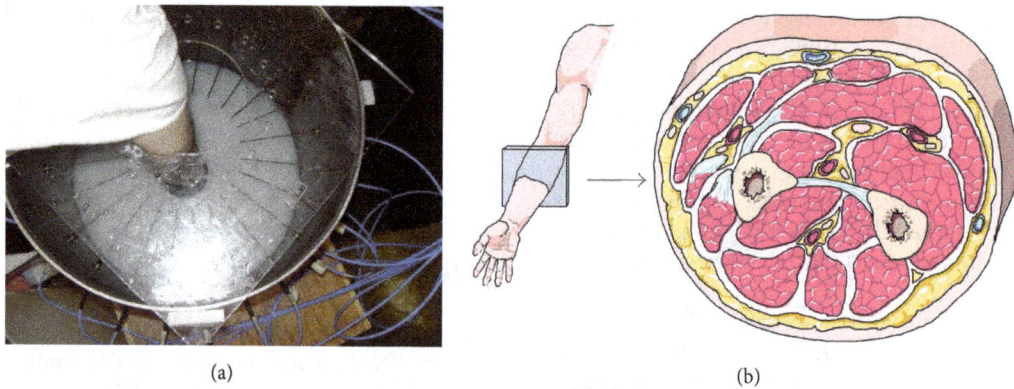

(a)   (b)

FIGURE 3: (a) A volunteer's arm inside the microwave imaging system. (b) Forearm anatomy, with the approximate location of microwave imaging plane.

the modeling error: the mismatch between the assumed computational model and the physical experiment. However, adding too much salt can decrease the signal to noise of the measurement to unacceptable levels. We have previously determined that an appropriate amount of salt is 2.5–4.5 grams per liter [18], and for this study we use approximately 3.1 grams/liter. A plot of matching fluid complex relative permittivity is shown in Figure 2. At a frequency of 1 GHz, the relative permittivity of the matching fluid is $\epsilon_r \approx 77 - j15$.

3. Mathematical Formulation

We consider a two-dimensional (2D) mathematical formulation with the electric field polarized along the longitudinal z-axis of the problem. A time-harmonic field of frequency f is assumed. An object of interest (OI) within an imaging domain $\mathscr{D}$ is immersed in an inhomogeneous background medium contained within an imaging chamber. The space within the imaging chamber Ω is confined by a boundary Γ. The OI and the background medium are assumed to be nonmagnetic with permeability $\mu = \mu_0$, the free space

permeability. At a 2D position vector $\mathbf{r} = x\hat{x} + y\hat{y}$, the OI's relative complex permittivity is given as

$$
\begin{aligned}
\epsilon_r(\mathbf{r}) &= \epsilon_r'(\mathbf{r}) - j\epsilon_r''(\mathbf{r}) \\
&= \epsilon_r'(\mathbf{r}) - \frac{j\sigma_{\text{eff}}(\mathbf{r})}{(2\pi f\epsilon_0)},
\end{aligned}
\tag{1}
$$

where $j^2 = -1$, ϵ_r' and σ_{eff} are, respectively, the real relative permittivity and the effective conductivity of the OI, and ϵ_0 is the permittivity of free space. Note that ϵ_r' and σ_{eff} are frequency dependent. Given the complex relative permittivity of the background as $\epsilon_b(\mathbf{r})$, the contrast of the OI within $\mathscr{D}$ is defined as

$$
\chi(\mathbf{r}) \triangleq \frac{(\epsilon_r(\mathbf{r}) - \epsilon_b(\mathbf{r}))}{\epsilon_b(\mathbf{r})},
\tag{2}
$$

whereas outside $\mathscr{D}$ $\chi = 0$.

The chamber is illuminated successively by one of the T transmitters, producing an incident field $E_t^{\text{inc}}(\mathbf{r})$ defined as the field produced by transmitter t in the presence of the inhomogeneous background medium and in the absence of

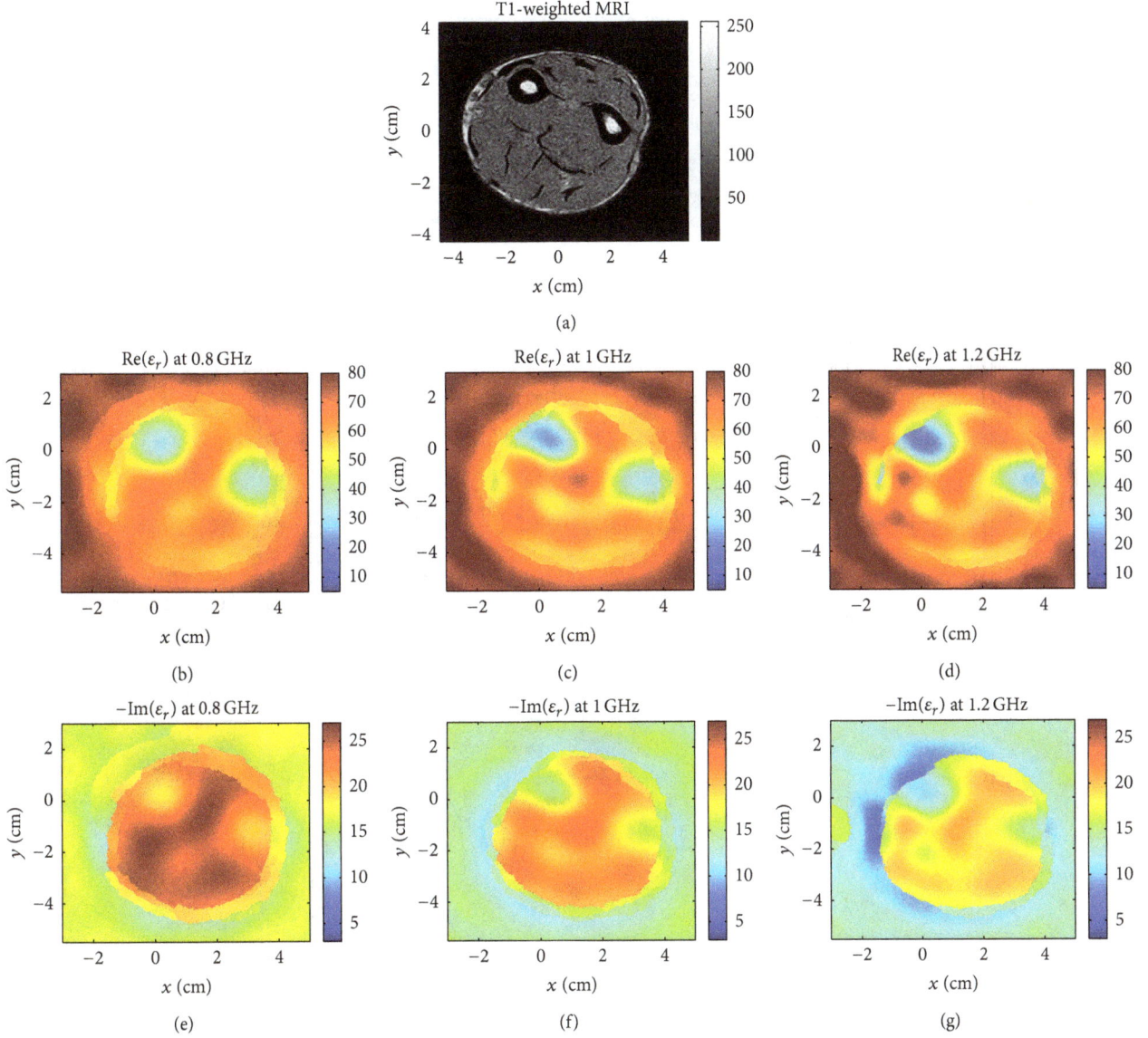

FIGURE 4: Volunteer 1: (a) the T1-weighted MRI image. MWI reconstructions of the relative complex permittivity real and imaginary components at (b), (e) 0.8 GHz, (c), (f) 1 GHz, and (d), (g) 1.2 GHz.

the OI. The transmitters are assumed to be 2D electric point sources (lines sources in 3D) with the incident field produced by transmitter t calculated as

$$E_t^{\text{inc}}(\mathbf{r}) = \frac{1}{j4} H_0^{(2)}\left(k_b |\mathbf{r} - \mathbf{r}_t|\right). \tag{3}$$

Here $H_0^{(2)}$ is the zeroth-order Hankel function of the second kind, $k_b(\mathbf{r}) = 2\pi f \sqrt{\mu_0 \epsilon_0 \epsilon_b(\mathbf{r})}$ is the background medium wavenumber, and $\mathbf{r}_t$ is the location of transmitter t.

In the presence of the OI, the resultant field in the chamber is the total field $E_t^{\text{tot}}(\mathbf{r})$. Both the incident and total fields are measured at R receiver locations positioned on a measurement surface $\mathcal{S}$. The scattered field, due to the difference in electrical properties between the OI and the background

medium, is defined as $E_t^{\text{sct}}(\mathbf{r}) \triangleq E_t^{\text{tot}}(\mathbf{r}) - E_t^{\text{inc}}(\mathbf{r})$ and is governed by the scalar Helmholtz equation

$$\nabla^2 E_t^{\text{sct}}(\mathbf{r}) + k_b^2(\mathbf{r}) E_t^{\text{sct}}(\mathbf{r}) = -k_b^2(\mathbf{r}) w_t(\mathbf{r}), \tag{4}$$

where $w_t(\mathbf{r}) \triangleq \chi(\mathbf{r}) E_t^{\text{tot}}(\mathbf{r})$ is the contrast source.

The boundary-value problem, defined by (4) as well as boundary conditions, is solved using FEM [20]. The discretization of the MWI problem using FEM is detailed in [21].

3.1. Inversion Algorithm.
MWI is associated with an inverse scattering problem, which can be solved using optimization-based algorithms that attempt to minimize a cost functional. The minimization optimizes variables that relate to the properties of the OI. Depending on the algorithm's outcome, MWI

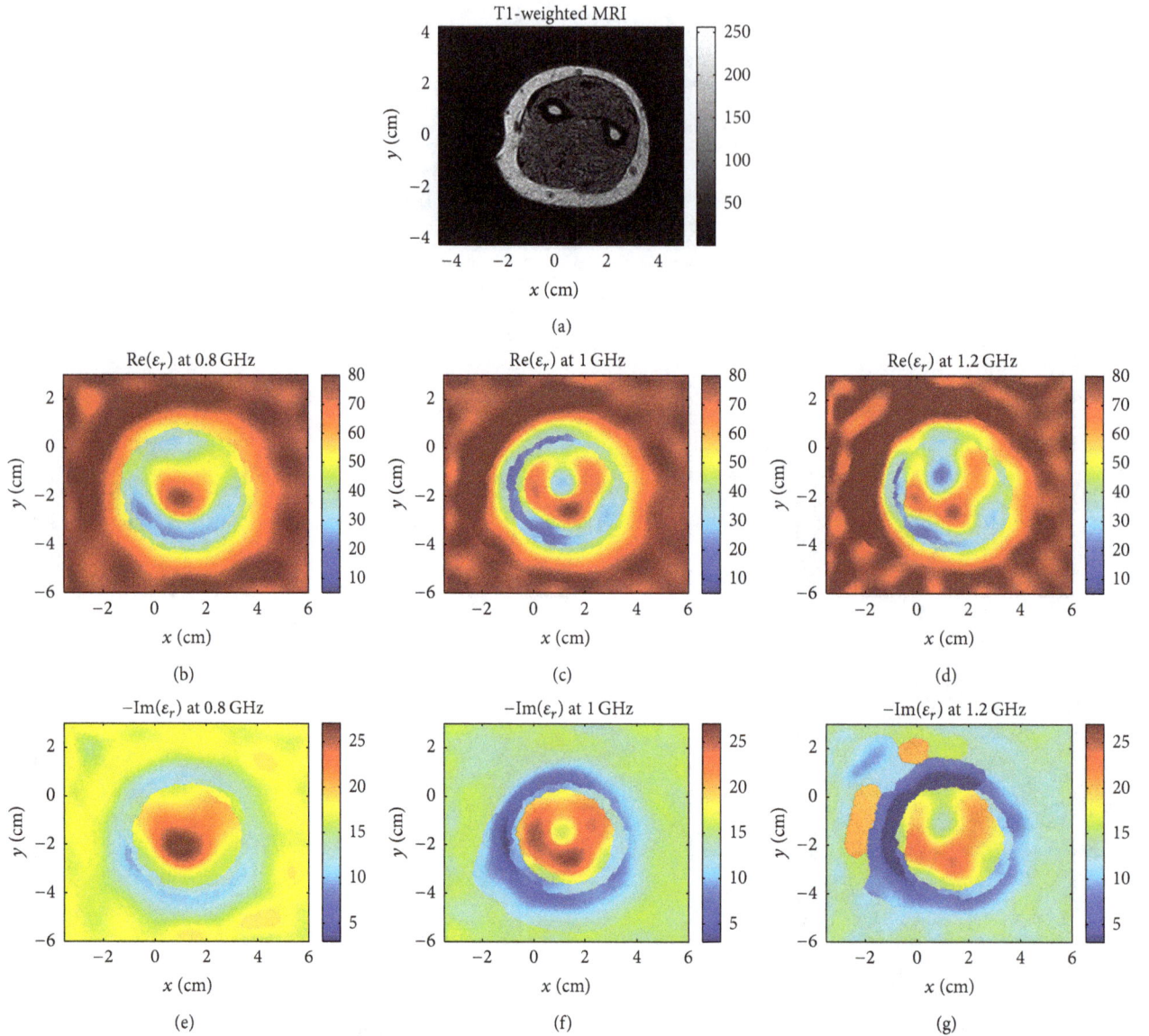

FIGURE 5: Volunteer 2: (a) the T1-weighted MRI image. MWI reconstructions of the relative complex permittivity real and imaginary components at (b), (e) 0.8 GHz, (c), (f) 1 GHz, and (d), (g) 1.2 GHz.

techniques may be generally split into two categories: quantitative (tomographic) techniques and qualitative (radar-based) techniques. Tomographic techniques (e.g., [17, 22–25]) use a limited number of discrete frequencies and provide simultaneous quantitative images of the dielectric constant and effective conductivity at those frequencies. On the other hand, radar techniques (e.g., [26–29]) use a large number of discrete frequencies (or time-domain pulses) and provide a single qualitative image of the "reflectivity" of the OI. We use the quantitative tomographic reconstruction technique in this work.

In this paper, the experimental data are inverted using the contrast source inversion algorithm formulated using the finite-element method (FEM-CSI) [30, 31]. FEM-CSI offers the ability of performing the inversion on an unstructured grid of triangles with varying mesh density; the density of

the mesh elements can be varied so as to decrease the algorithm's computational complexity without compromising the reconstruction quality [32]. In addition, FEM-CSI eases the incorporation of prior information as inhomogeneous background; as will be demonstrated in Section 6, this feature is used to improve the quality of the reconstructions. The FEM-CSI algorithm is implemented in MATLAB and takes approximately 30 minutes per image on a machine with two 2.8 GHz quad-core processors.

The outcome of the inversion algorithm is enhanced by utilizing a balanced multiplicative regularizer [33, 34]. The weighted L_2-norm total variation regularizer has edge-preserving capabilities [35], as well as the ability to correct the imbalance that may exist between the real and imaginary components of the OI's relative permittivity.

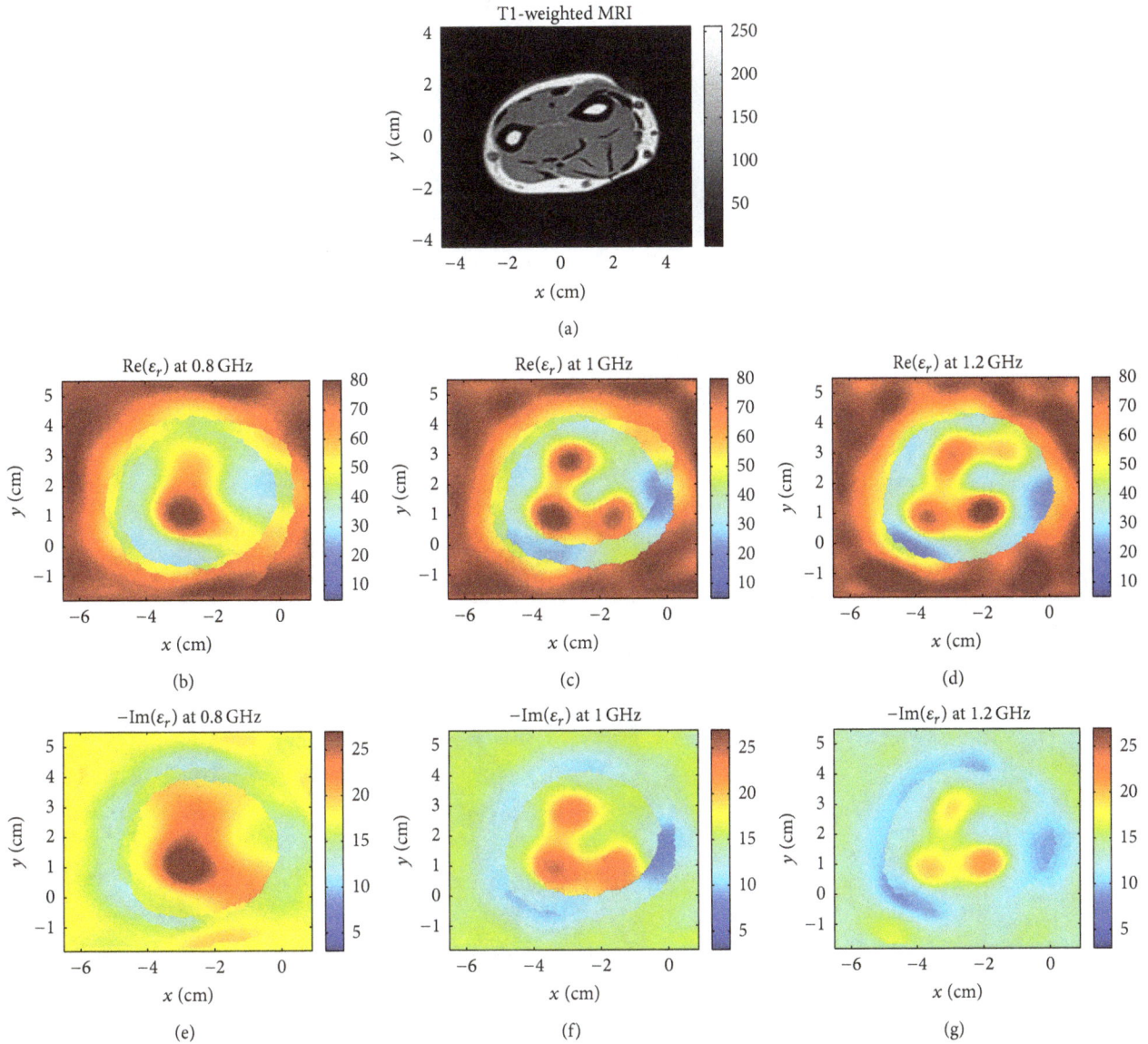

FIGURE 6: Volunteer 3: (a) the T1-weighted MRI image. MWI reconstructions of the relative complex permittivity real and imaginary components at (b), (e) 0.8 GHz, (c), (f) 1 GHz, and (d), (g) 1.2 GHz.

4. Methods

All research was carried out at the University of Manitoba under a University of Manitoba Biomedical Research Ethics Board approved protocol. Volunteer inclusion criteria were that the volunteers were over 18, without implants or tattoos, and not pregnant. Five individuals were used in this pilot study. Each volunteer had one forearm imaged of his/her choice (left/right). The sex, age, and left/right forearm information is listed in Table 1. A Plexiglas lid on the chamber, with a hole in the center, was used to help volunteers keep their arms supported and minimize motion during data collection. Each volunteer was asked to obtain a comfortable position and then hold their arm as still as possible during the data collection. Data collection time was slightly less than 1 minute for all frequencies. A photograph of a volunteer's arm in the imaging system is shown in Figure 3(a). For reference, we

TABLE 1: Volunteer data.

Number	Sex (M/F)	Age (years)	Forearm (left/right)
Volunteer 1	M	32	Right
Volunteer 2	F	30	Right
Volunteer 3	F	48	Left
Volunteer 4	M	47	Right
Volunteer 5	M	42	Left

have included a diagram of the arm's anatomical structure at the approximate spot of the imaging plane in Figure 3(b).

For each volunteer, 23×24 data points (S-parameter measurements) were collected in 100 MHz steps from 0.4 to 2 GHz, although not all frequencies are suitable for imaging. For this imaging system and antennas, we have empirically found that the best imaging frequencies are between 0.8 and

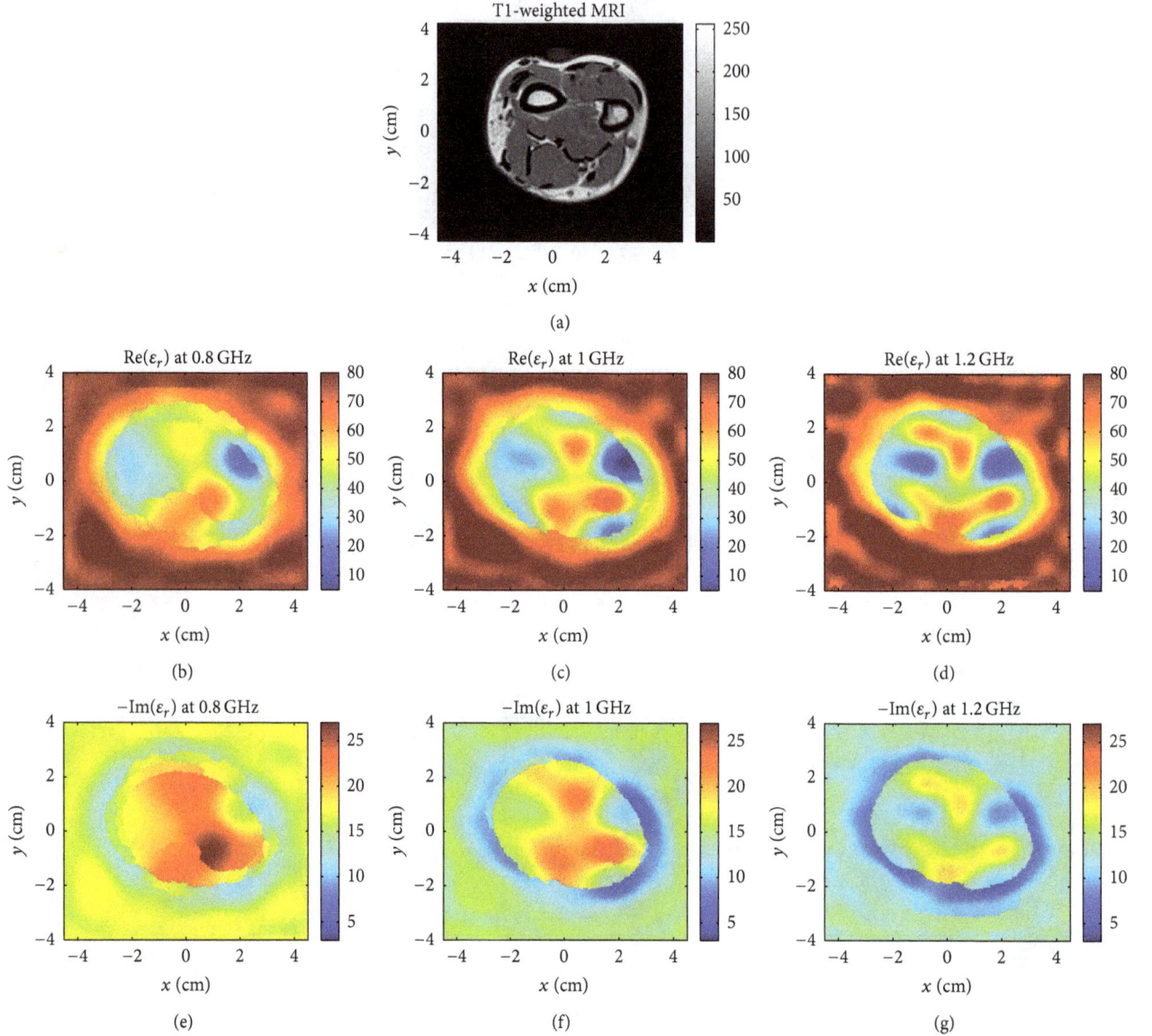

FIGURE 7: Volunteer 4: (a) the T1-weighted MRI image. MWI reconstructions of the relative complex permittivity real and imaginary components at (b), (e) 0.8 GHz, (c), (f) 1 GHz, and (d), (g) 1.2 GHz.

1.2 GHz, mostly due to the antennas radiating efficiently in this range. Prior to imaging of each volunteer, data were also taken of the empty fluid-filled chamber and of a 3.5-inch diameter metallic cylinder centered in the chamber. The empty chamber measurements constitute measurements of the incident field, and the metallic cylinder is used for calibration. Details of the calibration method may be found in [17, 18, 36].

4.1. Noise Metric. To provide an estimate of the signal to noise ratio of the experimental microwave data, we define a noise metric (used previously in [18]) as

$$N = \frac{1}{n_{i,j}} \sum_{(i,j)\text{ pairs}} \frac{\left\| u_{i,j}^{\text{sct}} - u_{j,i}^{\text{sct}} \right\|}{\left\| u_{i,j}^{\text{sct}} \right\|}, \qquad (5)$$

where $u_{i,j}^{\text{sct}}$ is the calibrated scattered field measurement, and the sum is taken over all transmit-receive pairs of i and j, and $n_{i,j}$ is the total number of transmit-receive pairs. We justify this metric since from reciprocity $u_{i,j} = u_{j,i}$ and anything else in the data must be noise. This metric (most importantly) is capable of detecting volunteer movement, as the measurements $u_{i,j}$ and $u_{j,i}$ can be up to 1 minute apart. If the metric is significantly higher for a volunteer than for a stationary phantom target, the volunteer was likely moving enough to create image artifacts, and we recollect the data. The metric also provides a measure of the thermal measurement noise. It does not account for modeling error (the differences between our assumed computational model and physical measurement system). Table 2 presents the noise metric, N, for each inverted data set.

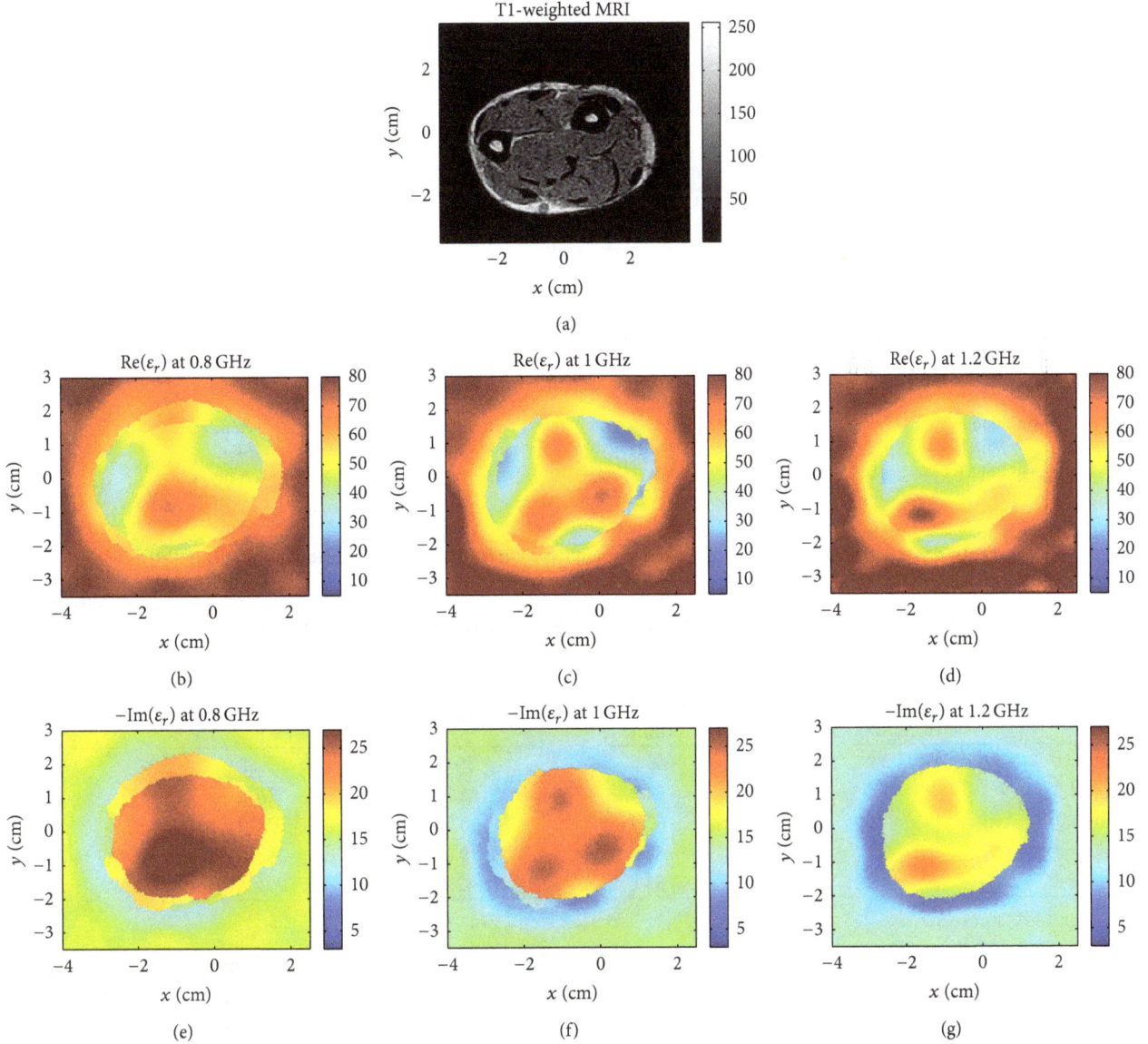

FIGURE 8: Volunteer 5: (a) the T1-weighted MRI image. MWI reconstructions of the relative complex permittivity real and imaginary components at (b), (e) 0.8 GHz, (c), (f) 1 GHz, and (d), (g) 1.2 GHz.

TABLE 2: Noise metric N of experimental data.

	0.8 GHz	1 GHz	1.2 GHz
Volunteer 1	24.7%	21.1%	31.0%
Volunteer 2	15.4%	15.4%	23.7%
Volunteer 3	27.8%	22.6%	30.0%
Volunteer 4	17.6%	18.8%	26.0%
Volunteer 5	22.2%	21.9%	33.0%

4.2. MRI. To provide a baseline of each volunteers anatomy, each volunteer was also imaged with a 0.2 T Esaote E-scan XQ MRI, using a forearm coil. This occurred less than 1 hour after the collection of the microwave data. A standard T1 gradient echo protocol was used to obtain transverse MR images in the same plane as the microwave data. To provide an approximate landmarking location for the transverse plane, a vitamin E capsule was affixed with medical tape to the arm at approximately the same height as the microwave imaging plane. The capsule was not present during microwave imaging.

We have attempted to manually coregister the MRI and microwave images. The axes for each volunteer's images are identical, but we have rotated the microwave data to obtain a similar arm orientation between the two modalities. However, the accuracy of the coregistration is limited since the volunteers arm and body positions were different in the MRI and microwave imaging systems. In the microwave system, volunteers were standing and the arm held vertically with the hand clenched in a fist resting on a pad at the bottom of the chamber. In the MRI system the volunteers were supine and the arm held horizontally, with the forearm resting on the MRI forearm coil and the hand in an open resting position,

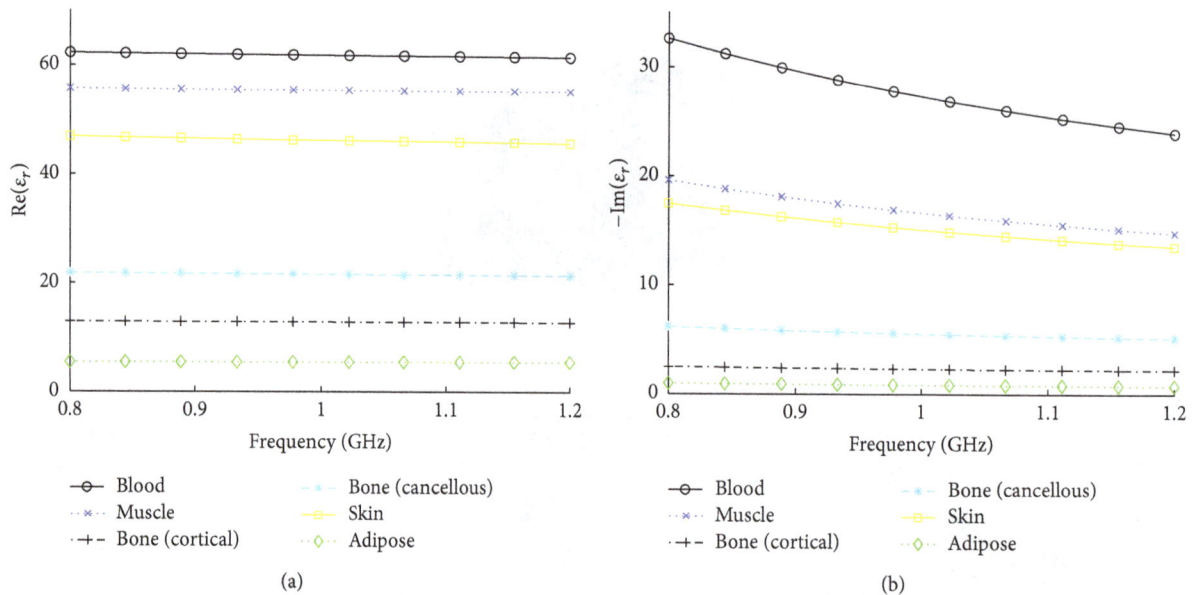

(a)

(b)

FIGURE 9: Relative permittivities of various human tissues from 0.8 to 1.2 GHz using the model in [15].

TABLE 3: Measured results from MRI images and estimates of lowest/highest relative permittivities from MWI in the muscle region at 1 GHz.

	MRI			MWI	
	Max. adipose Thickness (mm)	Arm width (mm)	Ratio	Min/Max of Re(ϵ_r)	Min/Max of $-$Im(ϵ_r)
Volunteer 1	3.9	64.6	16.6	56/68	22/24
Volunteer 2	8.7	53.8	6.2	31/68	22/28
Volunteer 3	7.1	60.9	8.5	33/70	18/28
Volunteer 4	7.0	63.0	9.0	34/60	20/26
Volunteer 5	4.3	53.1	12.3	29/66	23/28

Further, support pads were inserted into the MRI coil, which added varying degrees of compression to the forearm soft tissue. The resultant soft tissue deformations between the two modalities prevent ideal coregistration.

5. Experimental Results

For each volunteer, we present a figure with the MRI image and a series of microwave-based images of the complex relative permittivities at 0.8, 1, and 1.2 GHz. Figures 4 to 8 show the results for all 5 volunteers. All color scales are kept identical for real and imaginary parts of the relative permittivity throughout this work.

In Table 3, we list the maximum thickness of the adipose layer for each volunteer, as measured from the MRI. Table 3 also presents the width of the arm, from a transect taken along the line defined by the center of the two bones for each volunteer, and the ratio of the width to maximum adipose thickness (the width-to-adipose ratio). Furthermore, using the MWI reconstructions we added also to Table 3 our estimates (to the nearest whole number) of the relative permittivities inside the muscle region of the microwave reconstruction for all the 5 volunteers. These estimates were obtained by identifying the muscle in the MRI and then determining the pixels in

the microwave image within the muscle region that had the lowest and highest values. These regions were, in some cases, difficult to select, so the results in Table 3 are estimates only.

5.1. Discussion. As a companion for this discussion, we have included tissue relative permittivities taken from the literature [15, 37] in Figure 9. The measurements from the literature were taken *ex vivo*. However, many *in vivo* tissue relative permittivities are not the same as those measured *ex vivo*, for example, [38, 39]. These differences are due to temperature changes, tissue dehydration, and devascularization of the excised tissues [38]. As our microwave imaging system measures *in vivo*, the relative permittivities presented in Figure 9 should not be taken as the exact expected values, rather as a general guideline.

As can be seen from Figures 4, 5, 6, 7, and 8, the quality of the microwave reconstructions is improved for volunteers with less adipose tissue with the two arm bones being visible in volunteers 1, 4, and 5. This corresponds to the three smallest maximum adipose thicknesses (3.9, 7.0, and 4.3 mm) and the highest width-to-adipose ratios (16.6, 9.0, and 12.3 mm, as taken from the data). For volunteers 2 and 3, which have the thickest adipose tissue and highest width-to-adipose ratios, the two bones are not readily visible in the microwave images,

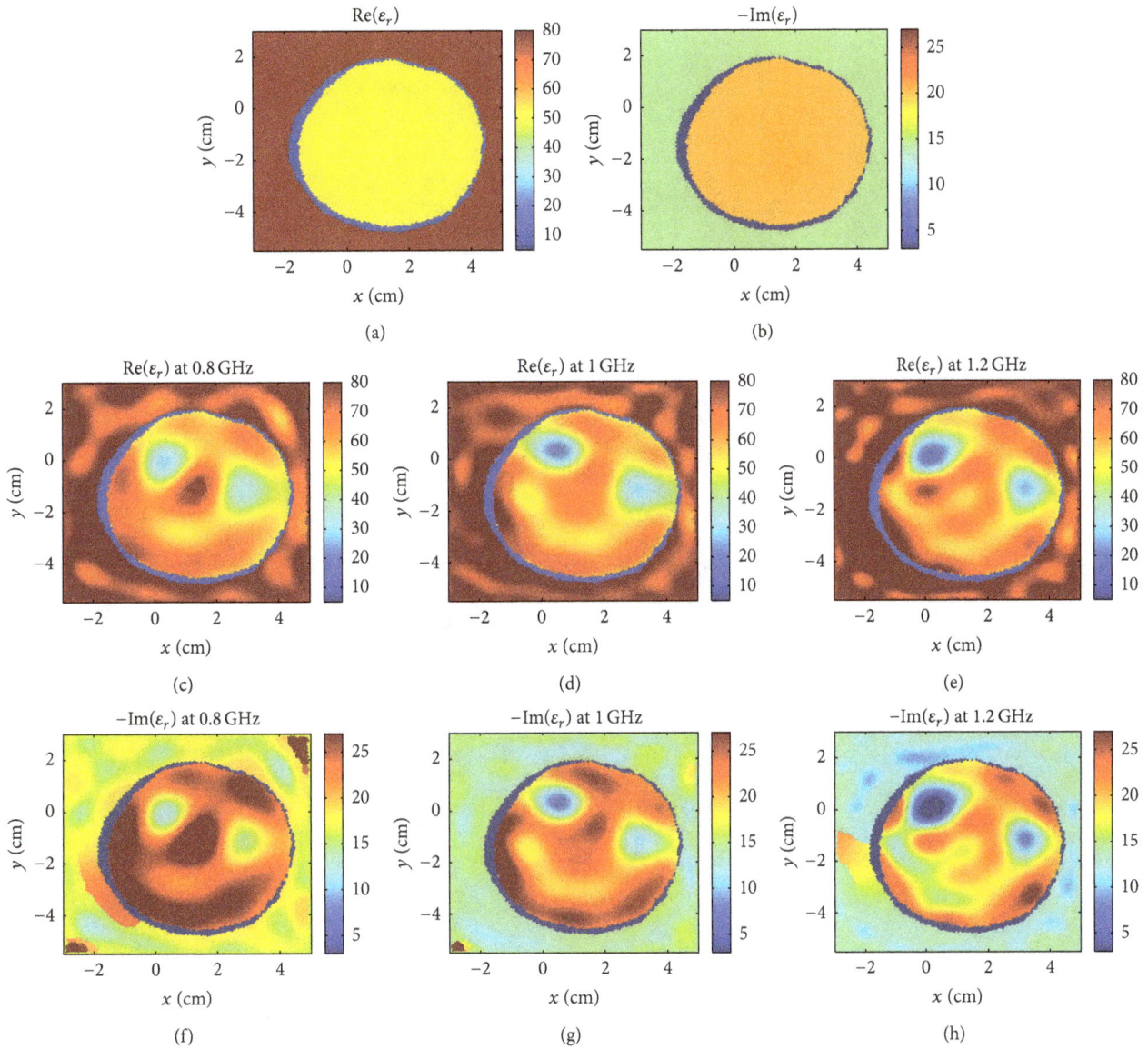

FIGURE 10: Volunteer 1: (a)-(b) prior information. The reconstruction when prior information is used as inhomogeneous background at (c), (f) 0.8 GHz, (d), (g) 1 GHz, and (e), (h) 1.2 GHz.

and in the real part of the permittivity there are significant artifacts inside the arm. For example, in the real part of the 1 GHz reconstructions there are regions with $\epsilon_r \approx 80$, which is not expected inside the arm.

It is clear that the image quality is strongly and inversely dependent on the thickness of the subcutaneous adipose layer. For volunteer 1 (Figure 4), both bones are visible at all three frequencies. The real part of the permittivity of the muscle tissue varies between 56 and 67 (approx.) for all three frequencies, while the average imaginary permittivity of the muscle drops steadily as the frequency increases (approximately 28, 23, and 21 for 0.8, 1, and 1.2 GHz). This agrees with the trends seen in the permittivity values in the literature: from Figure 9, we expect the real part of the permittivity of muscle and blood to be relatively constant across this frequency range, while the imaginary part of the permittivity is expected to decrease as the frequency increases. As noted, we do not expect exact agreement between the literature and measured values because of the differences between *in vivo* and *ex vivo* measurements.

The noise metric results for the experimental data in Table 2 show that image quality differences between volunteers are not due to differences in signal to noise levels, at least with respect to volunteer movement and thermal noise. This is clear because the best images (volunteer 1) have a noise metric higher than the poorest images (volunteer 2) for all 3 frequencies presented. Of course there could still be differences in modeling error between volunteers (e.g., there could be more 3D artifacts from a given volunteer's arm), but this is not quantifiable. We expect that the differences seen in the noise metric between the volunteers are due to minor volunteer movement during the measurement procedure.

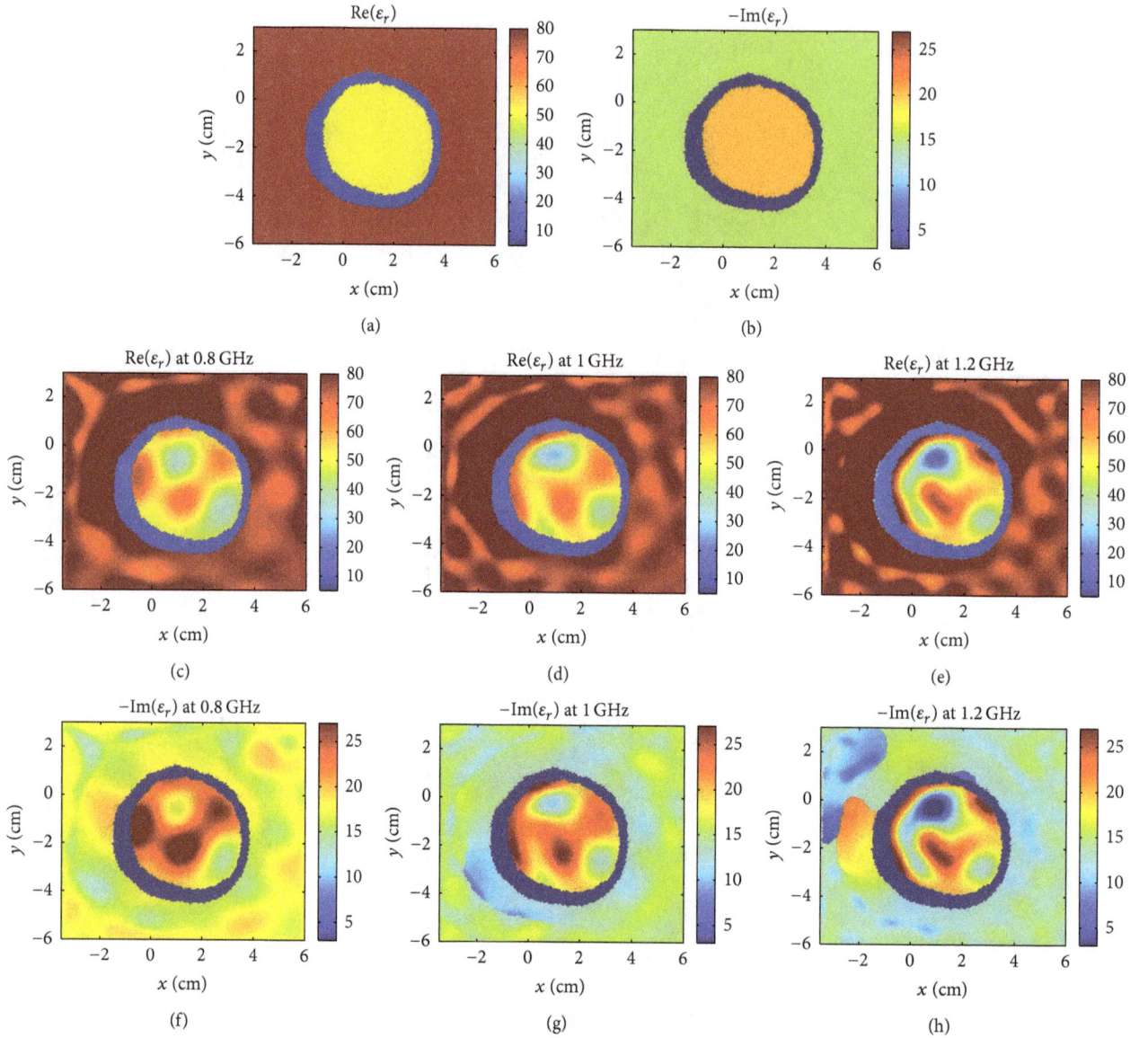

FIGURE 11: Volunteer 2: (a)-(b) prior information. The reconstruction when prior information is used as inhomogeneous background at (c), (f) 0.8 GHz, (d), (g) 1 GHz, and (e), (h) 1.2 GHz.

With respect to limb imaging in the literature, we know of only one other human forearm [40], collected with a 64-antenna system at 2.33 GHz, which we have previously inverted in [41]. Our previous imaging results compare well with our images from volunteer 1 in this study, despite lower frequency and significantly fewer antennas in our system. Although we cannot know for certain, we suspect that the volunteer in [40] had low adipose content in his/her forearm.

Another limb imaging in the literature considers swine limbs [1, 9]. In [9], the swine limb is excised, and qualitatively the 2D images in [9] are similar to our images for volunteers 1, 4, and, 5 in that (a) the bone tissue is readily visible; (b) the exterior of the limb is well-defined; and (c) similar muscle permittivities were found. With respect to the live-swine forearm images in [1], our images are qualitatively better in that (a) the exterior shape of the limb is readily visible and (b) we

seem to see muscle permittivities which more closely match the expected values (we do note that [1] is primarily concerned with functional, not structural, imaging, and this may have affected system design, matching fluid selection, etc.).

Although images are not shown here, we have tried marching-on-frequency inversion with the experimental data, which resulted in no visible improvement in images (we struggled to see any difference by eye). We speculate that the use of a greater frequency range (e.g., 1 GHz to 6 GHz, [42]) would lead to improvements and note that this result is only applicable to our system.

6. Prior Information Incorporation

The use of prior information to enhance the quality of the reconstructions in MWI has been investigated previously in

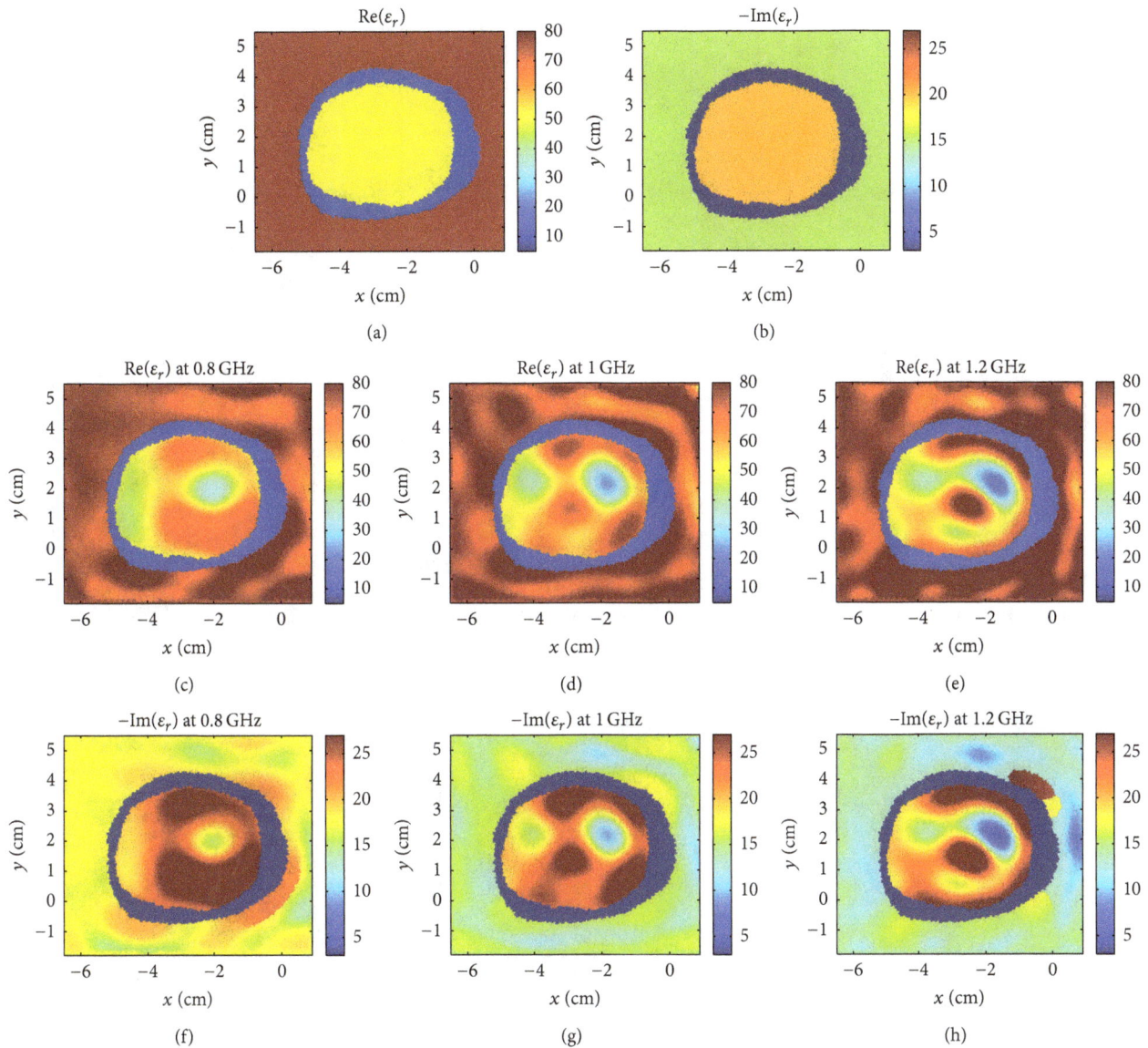

FIGURE 12: Volunteer 3: (a)-(b) prior information. The reconstruction when prior information is used as inhomogeneous background at (c), (f) 0.8 GHz, (d), (g) 1 GHz, and (e), (h) 1.2 GHz.

the literature. We categorize the various methodologies into two groups: the first category uses prior information about the *structure* of the OI being imaged [43, 44], whereas the second incorporates information about the *electrical properties* of the OI [45]. Hybridization of the two categories is also possible. For example, a hybrid technique may incorporate the prior information about the OI structure and properties into the mathematical operator that describes the physics of the inverse scattering problem [31, 46]. In this section, we make novel use of FEM-CSI ability of incorporating estimated prior information as an inhomogeneous background in its forward scattering operator.

6.1. Estimation and Inversion. While incorporating prior information into FEM-CSI is relatively simple, the challenge becomes developing a methodology of accurately estimating

the nonuniform adipose layer. Although non-MWI-based techniques are certainly possible [47, 48], in this paper the estimation of each volunteer's forearm adipose layer from the blind inversion images is done manually. That is, we manually identify three different regions from the blind inversion results: the outer background, a single adipose layer, and an inner muscle region. Due to the *ad hoc* nature of estimating the regions, different people may get different estimates; the estimations used in this paper were obtained by a *trained eye* that has been studying synthetic models of the forearm to understand how the location of the adipose layer can be identified from blind inversion results. Such investigations are best performed using synthetic model and data. Preliminary results using automated procedures have been investigated by our group [49] but are beyond the scope of the paper. In this section, the goal is to show that *substantial* improvements can

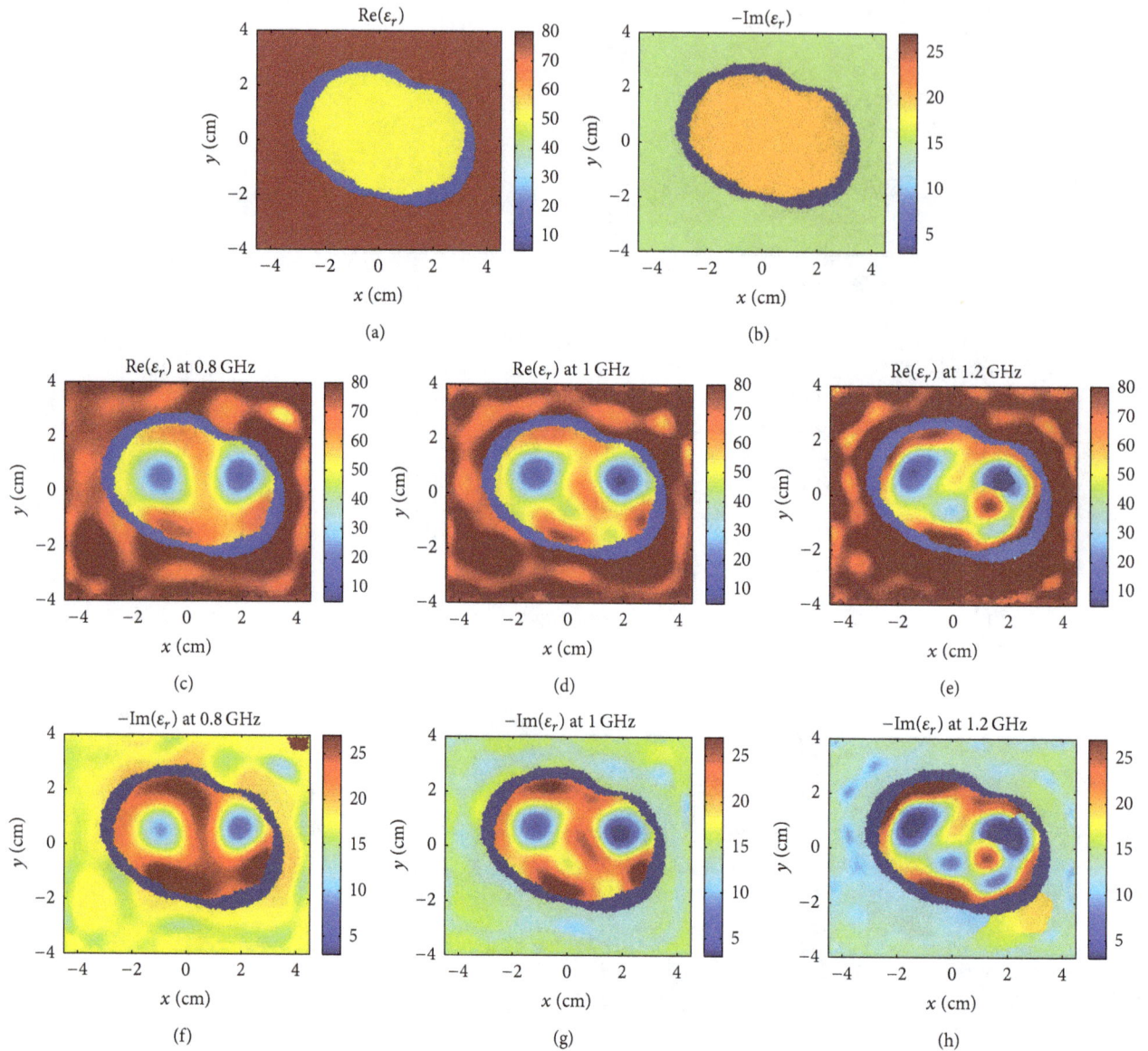

FIGURE 13: Volunteer 4: (a)-(b) prior information. The reconstruction when prior information is used as inhomogeneous background at (c), (f) 0.8 GHz, (d), (g) 1 GHz, and (e), (h) 1.2 GHz.

be obtained even via an *ad hoc* technique of estimating the prior information.

The manual steps which are used to create the inhomogeneous background for each volunteer's forearm can be summarized as follows.

(i) A blind inversion of the experimental dataset is performed at 1 GHz using the balanced MR-FEM-CSI algorithm.

(ii) A nonuniform adipose layer location is estimated within the resulting image using our experience of which the region within the blind result might be adipose. For example, the estimation of the adipose layer is largely obtained from viewing the imaginary part of the blind reconstruction. While the adipose layer was

being estimated, we did not use the associated MRI image.

(iii) The unstructured mesh nodes within the identified layer are assigned the complex relative permittivity of $\epsilon_r = 10 - j1$, which is an estimated value taken from published values of permittivity for adipose tissue [15].

(iv) The nodes outside the adipose layer are assigned the permittivity of the salt-water matching medium.

(v) The nodes enclosed by the adipose layer are assigned a relative permittivity value of $\epsilon_r = 50 - j20$, an estimated value for the muscle.

(vi) The inversion algorithm is rerun using the estimated prior information as a inhomogeneous background.

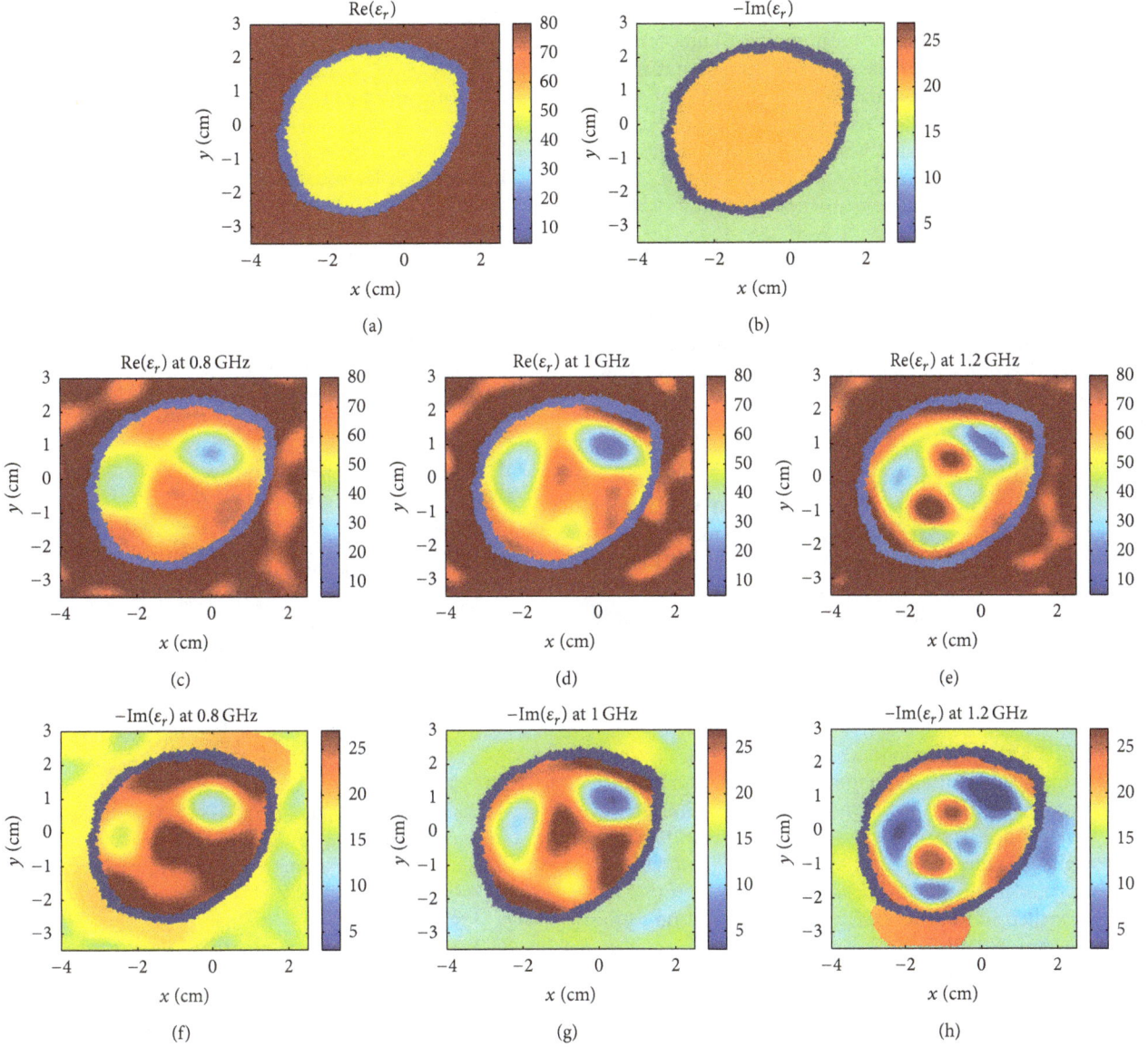

FIGURE 14: Volunteer 5: (a)-(b) prior information. The reconstruction when prior information is used as inhomogeneous background at (c), (f) 0.8 GHz, (d), (g) 1 GHz, and (e), (h) 1.2 GHz.

The same estimated inhomogeneous background is used to invert the data at the three frequencies: 0.8, 1, and 1.2 GHz.

The inversion results at 0.8, 1, and 1.2 GHz are shown in Figures 10, 11, 12, 13, and 14. For each volunteer, the real and imaginary components of the estimated prior information are shown in subfigures (a) and (b) and the inversion results utilizing the prior information as inhomogeneous background in subfigures (c)–(h).

6.2. Discussion. For all volunteers, the use of the adipose layer as inhomogeneous background resulted in a substantially improved reconstruction of the forearms: the two bones can be clearly identified in all figures. The algorithm preserved the adipose layer used as prior information. With respect to

the muscle tissues, the mean of the reconstructed dielectric values is close to values from the blind inversion in Section 5. As for the variations within the muscle regions, we speculate that they are due to the presence of other tissues (e.g., nerves, blood vessels, tendons, and connective tissues) in the forearm; these features can be observed in the MRI image. These improvements are of course only qualitative but clearly show the correct anatomical structure of the forearm. We have undertaken a controlled quantitative study, using synthetic numerical phantoms, of the improvements that are obtained with the use of prior information in the form of a known adipose layer. This study confirms that improvements in image quality are possible, but details are not included herein.

Artifacts, outside the forearms, are visible in the imaginary part reconstruction of several volunteers, for example, Figure 10(f) for volunteer 1 and Figure 11(g) for volunteer 2.

These artifacts may be due to an error in estimating the adipose layer thickness and/or the location of the outer forearm boundary. In addition, the dielectric values used as prior data are *ex vivo* values taken from the literature, which may not be the same as the *in vivo* permittivity values [38]. Furthermore, the reconstruction of the left bone for volunteer 3, Figures 12(c) and 12(d), is not as good as the right bone; again the reason could be an error in the estimation of the adipose layer thickness.

For all the volunteers, the reconstructions at 1.2 GHz are not good compared to the results at 0.8 and 1 GHz. We believe that the reason is due to the higher noise level in the measurements at 1.2 GHz in comparison to the other two frequencies. As shown in Table 2, the calculated noise metric, N, is largest at 1.2 GHz for all the volunteers.

7. Conclusion

To the best of our knowledge, we have presented in this paper the first study of microwave limb imaging with multiple individuals (either human or animal). The use of an MRI image of the same transverse plane of the forearm as the microwave image has allowed us to determine the importance of adipose tissue with respect to the quality of the microwave images. Without the use of prior information, the microwave image quality is good only when the thickness of the adipose tissue is low.

The MWI reconstructions are improved when incorporating prior information as inhomogeneous background in the inversion algorithm; the internal anatomical features of all the volunteers' forearms with varying adipose tissue thickness were resolved. While the estimation of the prior information was performed manually using an *ad hoc* method, it improved the reconstruction results significantly in comparison to the blind inversion.

Supplanting the *ad hoc* technique used to extract prior information from the *blind* inversions of the experimental datasets with automated techniques is a topic for our future work. Preliminary investigations have revealed that it is possible to perform this information extraction automatically using image processing techniques, that is, postprocessing the blind inversion images. Alternative methods may also be possible such as the use of simple calipers to obtain the thickness of the adipose tissue in conjunction with methods to locate the boundary of the arm within the imaging domain, for example, using radar- or laser-based techniques.

Acknowledgments

This work was supported by Western Economic Diversification Canada, Natural Sciences and Engineering Research Council of Canada, and CancerCare Manitoba. The authors thank the University of Manitoba Nano-Systems Fabrication Lab for supplying the deionized water.

References

[1] S. Semenov, J. Kellam, B. Nair et al., "Microwave tomography of extremities: 2. Functional fused imaging of flow reduction and simulated compartment syndrome," *Physics in Medicine and Biology*, vol. 56, no. 7, pp. 2019–2030, 2011.

[2] P. M. Meaney, M. W. Fanning, T. Raynolds et al., "Initial clinical experience with microwave breast imaging in women with normal mammography," *Academic Radiology*, vol. 14, no. 2, pp. 207–218, 2007.

[3] S. P. Poplack, T. D. Tosteson, W. A. Wells et al., "Electromagnetic breast imaging: results of a pilot study in women with abnormal mammograms," *Radiology*, vol. 243, no. 2, pp. 350–359, 2007.

[4] E. C. Fear, P. M. Meaney, and M. A. Stuchly, "Microwaves for breast cancer detection?" *IEEE Potentials*, vol. 22, no. 1, pp. 12–18, 2003.

[5] M. Lazebnik, D. Popovic, L. McCartney et al., "A large-scale study of the ultrawideband microwave dielectric properties of normal, benign and malignant breast tissues obtained from cancer surgeries," *Physics in Medicine and Biology*, vol. 52, no. 20, pp. 6093–6115, 2007.

[6] D. W. Winters, J. D. Shea, P. Kosmas, B. D. Van Veen, and S. C. Hagness, "Three-dimensional microwave breast imaging: dispersive dielectric properties estimation using patient-specific basis functions," *IEEE Transactions on Medical Imaging*, vol. 28, no. 7, pp. 969–981, 2009.

[7] M. Klemm, I. Craddock, J. Leendertz et al., "Clinical trials of a UWB imaging radar for breast cancer," in *Proceedings of the 4th European Conference on Antennas and Propagation (EuCAP '10)*, pp. 1–4, April 2010.

[8] S. Semenov, J. Kellam, Y. Sizov et al., "Microwave tomography of extremities: 1. Dedicated 2D system and physiological signatures," *Physics in Medicine and Biology*, vol. 56, no. 7, pp. 2005–2017, 2011.

[9] S. Y. Semenov, A. E. Bulyshev, A. Abubakar et al., "Microwave-tomographic imaging of the high dielectric-contrast objects using different image-reconstruction approaches," *IEEE Transactions on Microwave Theory and Techniques*, vol. 53, no. 7, pp. 2284–2293, 2005.

[10] S. Semenov, "Microwave tomography: review of the progress towards clinical applications," *Philosophical Transactions of the Royal Society A*, vol. 367, no. 1900, pp. 3021–3042, 2009.

[11] S. Semenov, J. Kellam, P. Althausen et al., "Microwave tomography for functional imaging of extremity soft tissues: feasibility assessment," *Physics in Medicine and Biology*, vol. 52, no. 18, pp. 5705–5719, 2007.

[12] S. Salvador, E. Fear, M. Okoniewski, and J. Matyas, "Exploring joint tissues with microwave imaging," *IEEE Transactions on Microwave Theory and Techniques*, vol. 58, no. 8, pp. 2307–2313, 2010.

[13] T. M. Grzegorczyk, P. M. Meaney, P. M. Kaufman, R. M. di Florio Alexander, and K. D. Paulsen, "Fast 3-D tomographic microwave imaging for breast cancer detection," *IEEE Transactions on Medical Imaging*, vol. 31, no. 8, pp. 1584–1592, 2012.

[14] E. J. Hall, "Lessons we have learned from our children: cancer risk from diagnostic radiology," *Pediatric Radiology*, vol. 32, no. 10, pp. 700–706, 2002.

[15] S. Gabriel, R. W. Lau, and C. Gabriel, "The dielectric properties of biological tissues: III. Parametric models for the dielectric spectrum of tissues," *Physics in Medicine and Biology*, vol. 41, no. 11, pp. 2271–2293, 1996.

[16] C. Kaye, J. LoVetri, A. Zakaria, and M. Osadrahimi, "Feasibility study of microwave tomography for in vivo characteristic of tissue as a diagnostic technique for human disease," in *Proceedings of IEEE International Symposium on Antennas and*

Propagation and USNC/URSI National Radio Science Meeting (AP-S/USNC-URSI '12), July 2012.

[17] C. Gilmore, P. Mojabi, A. Zakaria et al., "A wideband microwave tomography system with a novel frequency selection procedure," *IEEE Transactions on Biomedical Engineering*, vol. 57, no. 4, pp. 894–904, 2010.

[18] C. Gilmore, A. Zakaria, J. LoVetri, and S. Pistorius, "A study of matching fluid loss in a biomedical microwave tomography system," *Medical Physics*, vol. 40, no. 2, Article ID 023101, 14 pages, 2012.

[19] P. M. Meaney, S. A. Pendergrass, M. W. Fanning, D. Li, and K. D. Paulsen, "Importance of using a reduced contrast coupling medium in 2D microwave breast imaging," *Journal of Electromagnetic Waves and Applications*, vol. 17, no. 2, pp. 333–355, 2003.

[20] J. Jin, *The Finite Element Method in Electromagnetics*, John Wiley & Sons, New York, NY, USA, 2002.

[21] A. Zakaria, *The finite-element contrast source inversion method for microwave imaging applications [Ph.D. dissertation]*, University of Manitoba, 2012.

[22] A. Abubakar, P. M. van den Berg, and J. J. Mallorqui, "Imaging of biomedical data using a multiplicative regularized contrast source inversion method," *IEEE Transactions on Microwave Theory and Techniques*, vol. 50, no. 7, pp. 1761–1771, 2002.

[23] T. Rubk, P. M. Meaney, P. Meincke, and K. D. Paulsen, "Nonlinear microwave imaging for breast-cancer screening using Gauss-Newton's method and the CGLS inversion algorithm," *IEEE Transactions on Antennas and Propagation*, vol. 55, no. 8, pp. 2320–2331, 2007.

[24] R. K. Amineh, M. Ravan, A. Trehan, and N. K. Nikolova, "Near-field microwave imaging based on aperture raster scanning with TEM horn antennas," *IEEE Transactions on Antennas and Propagation*, vol. 59, no. 3, pp. 928–940, 2011.

[25] M. Ostadrahimi, P. Mojabi, A. Zakaria, J. LoVetri, and L. Shafai, "Enhancement of Gauss-Newton inversion method for biomedical tissueimaging," *IEEE Transactions on Microwave Theory and Techniques*. Accepted.

[26] M. Klemm, I. J. Craddock, J. A. Leendertz, A. Preece, and R. Benjamin, "Radar-based breast cancer detection using a hemispherical antenna array—experimental results," *IEEE Transactions on Antennas and Propagation*, vol. 57, no. 6, pp. 1692–1704, 2009.

[27] D. Flores-Tapia, M. O'Halloran, and S. Pistorius, "A bimodal reconstruction method for breast cancer imaging," *Progress in Electromagnetics Research*, vol. 118, pp. 461–486, 2011.

[28] D. Kurrant and E. Fear, "Defining regions of interest for microwave imaging using near-field reflection data," *IEEE Microwave Theory and Techniques Society*, vol. 61, no. 5, pp. 2137–2145, 2013.

[29] M. El-Shenawee and E. L. Miller, "Spherical harmonics microwave algorithm for shape and location reconstruction of breast cancer tumor," *IEEE Transactions on Medical Imaging*, vol. 25, no. 10, pp. 1258–1271, 2006.

[30] P. M. van den Berg and R. E. Kleinman, "A contrast source inversion method," *Inverse Problems*, vol. 13, no. 6, pp. 1607–1620, 1997.

[31] A. Zakaria, C. Gilmore, and J. LoVetri, "Finite-element contrast source inversion method for microwave imaging," *Inverse Problems*, vol. 26, no. 11, Article ID 115010, 2010.

[32] A. Zakaria and J. LoVetri, "A study of adaptive meshing in FEM-CSI for microwave tomography," in *Proceedings of the 14th*

International Symposium on Antenna Technology and Applied Electromagnetics and the American Electromagnetics Conference (ANTEM/AMEREM '10), pp. 1–4, Ottawa, Canada, July 2010.

[33] A. Zakaria, C. Gilmore, S. Pistorius, and J. LoVetri, "Balanced multiplicative regularization for the contrast source inversion method," in *Proceedings of the 28th International Review of Progress in Applied Computational Electromagnetics Conference (ACES '12)*, Columbus, Ohio, USA, 2012.

[34] A. Zakaria and J. LoVetri, "Application of multiplicative regularization to the finite-element contrast source inversion method," *IEEE Transactions on Antennas and Propagation*, vol. 59, no. 9, pp. 3495–3498, 2011.

[35] P. M. van den Berg, A. Abubakar, and J. T. Fokkema, "Multiplicative regularization for contrast profile inversion," *Radio Science*, vol. 38, no. 2, 2003.

[36] C. Gilmore, A. Zakaria, P. Mojabi, M. Ostadrahimi, S. Pistorius, and J. LoVetri, "The University of Manitoba microwave imaging repository: a two-dimensional microwave scattering database for testing inversion and calibration algorithms," *IEEE Antennas and Propagation Magazine*, vol. 53, no. 5, pp. 126–133, 2011.

[37] S. Gabriel, R. W. Lau, and C. Gabriel, "The dielectric properties of biological tissues: II. Measurements in the frequency range 10 Hz to 20 GHz," *Physics in Medicine and Biology*, vol. 41, no. 11, pp. 2251–2269, 1996.

[38] R. J. Halter, T. Zhou, P. M. Meaney et al., "The correlation of in vivo and ex vivo tissue dielectric properties to validate electromagnetic breast imaging: initial clinical experience," *Physiological Measurement*, vol. 30, no. 6, pp. S121–S136, 2009.

[39] D. Haemmerich, O. R. Ozkan, J.-Z. Tsai et al., "Changes in electrical resistivity of swine liver after occlusion and postmortem," *Medical and Biological Engineering and Computing*, vol. 40, no. 1, pp. 29–33, 2002.

[40] J. J. Mallorqui, N. Joachimowicz, J. C. Bolomey, and A. P. Broquetas, "Database of "in vivo" measurements for quantitative microwave imaging and reconstruction algorithms available," *IEEE Antennas and Propagation Magazine*, vol. 37, no. 5, pp. 87–89, 1995.

[41] C. Gilmore, P. Mojabi, and J. LoVetri, "Comparison of an enhanced distorted born iterative method and the multiplicative-regularized contrast source inversion method," *IEEE Transactions on Antennas and Propagation*, vol. 57, no. 8, pp. 2341–2351, 2009.

[42] C. Gilmore, A. Abubakar, W. Hu, T. M. Habashy, and P. M. van den Berg, "Microwave biomedical data inversion using the finite-difference contrast source inversion method," *IEEE Transactions on Antennas and Propagation*, vol. 57, no. 5, pp. 1528–1538, 2009.

[43] M. Haynes, J. Stang, and M. Moghaddam, "Microwave breast imaging system prototype with integrated numerical characterization," *International Journal of Biomedical Imaging*, vol. 2012, Article ID 706365, 18 pages, 2012.

[44] A. Golnabi, P. Meaney, S. Geimer, and K. Paulsen, "Comparison of no-prior and soft-prior regularization in biomedical microwave imaging," *Journal of Medical Physics*, vol. 36, no. 3, pp. 159–170, 2011.

[45] A. Fhager and M. Persson, "Using a priori data to improve the reconstruction of small objects in microwave tomography," *IEEE Transactions on Microwave Theory and Techniques*, vol. 55, no. 11, pp. 2454–2462, 2007.

[46] A. Abubakar, W. Hu, P. M. van den Berg, and T. Habashy, "A finite-difference contrast source inversion method," *Inverse Problems*, vol. 24, no. 6, Article ID 065004, 17 pages, 2008.

[47] T. C. Williams, J. Bourqui, T. R. Cameron, M. Okoniewski, and E. C. Fear, "Laser surface estimation for microwave breast imaging systems," *IEEE Transactions on Biomedical Engineering*, vol. 58, no. 5, pp. 1193–1199, 2011.

[48] M. J. Pallone, P. M. Meaney, and K. D. Paulsen, "Surface scanning through a cylindrical tank of coupling fluid for clinical microwave breast imaging exams," *Medical Physics*, vol. 39, no. 6, pp. 3102–3111, 2012.

[49] A. Zakaria, A. Baran, and J. LoVetri, "Estimation and use of prior information in FEM-CSI for biomedical microwave tomography," *IEEE Antennas and Wireless Propagation Letters*, vol. 11, pp. 1606–1609, 2012.

4

SIVIC: Open-Source, Standards-Based Software for DICOM MR Spectroscopy Workflows

Jason C. Crane, Marram P. Olson, and Sarah J. Nelson

Surbeck Laboratory for Advanced Imaging, Department of Radiology and Biomedical Imaging, University of California, San Francisco, CA 94158-2330, USA

Correspondence should be addressed to Jason C. Crane; jason.crane@ucsf.edu

Academic Editor: Li Shen

Quantitative analysis of magnetic resonance spectroscopic imaging (MRSI) data provides maps of metabolic parameters that show promise for improving medical diagnosis and therapeutic monitoring. While anatomical images are routinely reconstructed on the scanner, formatted using the DICOM standard, and interpreted using PACS workstations, this is not the case for MRSI data. The evaluation of MRSI data is made more complex because files are typically encoded with vendor-specific file formats and there is a lack of standardized tools for reconstruction, processing, and visualization. SIVIC is a flexible open-source software framework and application suite that enables a complete scanner-to-PACS workflow for evaluation and interpretation of MRSI data. It supports conversion of vendor-specific formats into the DICOM MR spectroscopy (MRS) standard, provides modular and extensible reconstruction and analysis pipelines, and provides tools to support the unique visualization requirements associated with such data. Workflows are presented which demonstrate the routine use of SIVIC to support the acquisition, analysis, and delivery to PACS of clinical ^{1}H MRSI datasets at UCSF.

1. Introduction

MR spectroscopic imaging (MRSI) is a powerful imaging technique that provides spatially resolved metabolic information. It has been used together with anatomical and functional imaging to improve diagnostic specificity in multiple diseases, and it shows promise for improving treatment planning and the ability to monitor therapeutic response [1–11].

Despite great interest in this technology from the research and clinical communities, the adoption of advanced MRSI methods has been relatively slow, with a relatively limited number of studies having applied such techniques in clinical trials of new therapies. A major limitation in integrating MRSI into these studies has been the lack of commercially available methods for visualization and interpretation of the data. For conventional 3D imaging, the use of the DICOM [12] standard has resulted in a great deal of interoperability between software packages, imaging archives, and data. However, despite the existence of a DICOM standard for encoding MRSI data [13], current datasets are still created with vendor-specific proprietary formats. This results in a low degree of interoperability between imaging devices, picture archiving and communication systems (PACS), and software packages for analyzing the data. This situation is particularly problematic for multicenter collaborations, which require complicated workflows and file format conversions to evaluate data from multiple vendors. As a result, information about variations in metabolic parameters is typically delivered to PACS in the form of static DICOM secondary capture images, which hinders its integration with other types of multimodal imaging data [3]. This hinders the development and validation of postprocessing methodologies as well as the integration of MRSI data into routine radiological workflows.

The open-source software package known as SIVIC (Spectroscopic Imaging, VIsualization, and Computing) [14, 15] was developed at UCSF to address the limitations of existing strategies for analyzing MRSI data. In the following, there is firstly an overview of MRSI data, followed by a description of the SIVIC software package. Two workflows that have been implemented at UCSF in order to streamline the routine use of MRSI in research and clinical studies are presented as examples of the applications of SIVIC. This is followed by a description of an approach for generalizing MRSI data analysis pipelines.

2. Features of MRSI Data

Working with MRSI data has unique requirements compared with anatomical and functional images. In a volumetric sense, MRSI data is at least 4-dimensions, comprising 3 spatial and at least one spectral dimension. Dynamic and multichannel MRSI acquisitions result in data with 5 or more dimensions. Reconstruction, postprocessing, and quantification of such data require specialized algorithms for generating and evaluating spectral data. Once reconstructed, the MRSI data are typically visualized by displaying a frequency spectrum at each spatial location (Figure 1(a)). Dynamic MRSI requires analysis of MRSI data at multiple time points and is conveniently represented as frequency specific plots reflecting the dynamic behavior of individual metabolites (Figure 1(b)). This means that specialized tools are required to represent the data and correlate it with other types of images.

MRSI data are often encoded in vendor specific formats or private DICOM SOP classes. This introduces a major obstacle in managing the data and developing software that will work with data acquired on scanners from multiple vendors. In contrast, anatomical images are typically encoded as standard DICOM MR Image Storage SOP instances. This enables existing DICOM infrastructures to be used for data transmission between devices, storage of images in PACS, and visualization with standardized image viewing applications. MRSI data, on the other hand, require special workflow protocols that are separate from the standard workflows. Raw MRSI data is typically manually copied from the scanner's hard drive following an exam, processed offline, and rendered by an analyst, and the resulting screen captures are transmitted to PACS as DICOM Secondary Capture Image Storage SOP instances for radiologists to view in the reading room. Since the MRSI data are delivered to PACS separately from the rest of the exam, it may be necessary to notify the radiologist by e-mail, complicating their ability to read exams efficiently. Not only does this require extra workstations, storage, and personnel, but it results in inefficient delivery of results that are required for patient care.

From a research perspective, the use of vendor-specific MRSI data formats hinders the development and validation of spectroscopic and metabolic imaging methods as there are limited software packages capable of reading, reconstructing, processing, displaying, and exporting data that are encoded in all of the most common data formats. This poses an obstacle to comparing data from multiple scanners and complicates the comparison of reconstruction, processing, and quantification algorithms using data from different scanner vendors. Though not widely implemented, the DICOM standard does define an information object definition (IOD) for encoding MRSI data [13], which could greatly simplify the use of MRSI if more widely adopted. Several freely available software projects address different aspects of these problems. jMRUI [16] is a closed-source package that supports reading, analysis, and visualization of MRSI data from multiple vendors as well as DICOM MRI and

MRS data. The MIDAS package [17] is an open-source project that supports GE, Philips, and Siemens data and is distributed with an MRSI acquisition sequence implemented for each of these vendor platforms that MIDAS is capable of reconstructing and processing. TARQUIN [18] is an open-source package for spectral quantification that understands multiple vendor formats as well as the DICOM MR spectroscopy standard. Though these software packages provide needed functionality for the analysis of MRSI data, none of them provide a complete scanner-to-PACS workflow. The following sections describe the open-source software framework and application suite that were developed at UCSF to implement the DICOM MR spectroscopy (MRS) standard and to address MRSI analysis and workflow needs.

3. The SIVIC Software Suite

SIVIC is an extensible, open-source, freely available, and cross-platform software suite designed to support all aspects of MRSI data analysis and visualization. It comprises a set of C++ libraries that support the various stages of analysis including data IO (input-output), algorithm pipelines, and visualization (Figure 2). This set of libraries is called the svk, for SIVIC Kit. Many of the svk C++ classes extend base classes from the visualization toolkit (VTK) for 3D visualization [19] or DCMTK [20], which provides low-level DICOM support. VTK is widely used in other medical imaging software enabling svk classes to be compatible with those packages. This compatibility is important for the development of SIVIC plug-ins to applications such as 3D Slicer [21]. The svk IO layer is a key component of SIVIC, enabling it to work with data from multiple formats and export data to the DICOM standard. Figure 3 lists the data formats currently supported by SIVIC. The svk IO layer will be discussed in more detail below.

The classes in the svk libraries can be used to construct flexible MRSI applications that work with data from multiple vendor sources. In addition to providing these building blocks, the project provides a suite of applications that are built from the libraries. The most important application is the standalone SIVIC graphical user interface (GUI). This supports reading MRI and MRSI data, MRSI reconstruction, processing algorithms such as apodization, zero filling, and phasing, visualization of MRSI data and acquisition constructs such as the voxel grid, volume localization, and sat band placement and also supports exporting data to supported formats. The SIVIC GUI is also provided in the form of a plug-in for the OsiriX [15, 22, 23] open-source PACS and medical imaging package. This enables it to be used for visualization of MRSI data together with the storage management functionality provided by OsiriX PACS. A plugin for 3D Slicer [24, 25] is currently under development. SIVIC also provides command line tools [26] for converting between different file formats and for applying reconstruction, postprocessing, and quantification algorithms. Source-code and binary releases for OsX, Windows, and Linux are freely available from sourceforge: http://sourceforge.net/projects/sivic/. The software is released under a BSD license, which enables it to

(a)

(b)

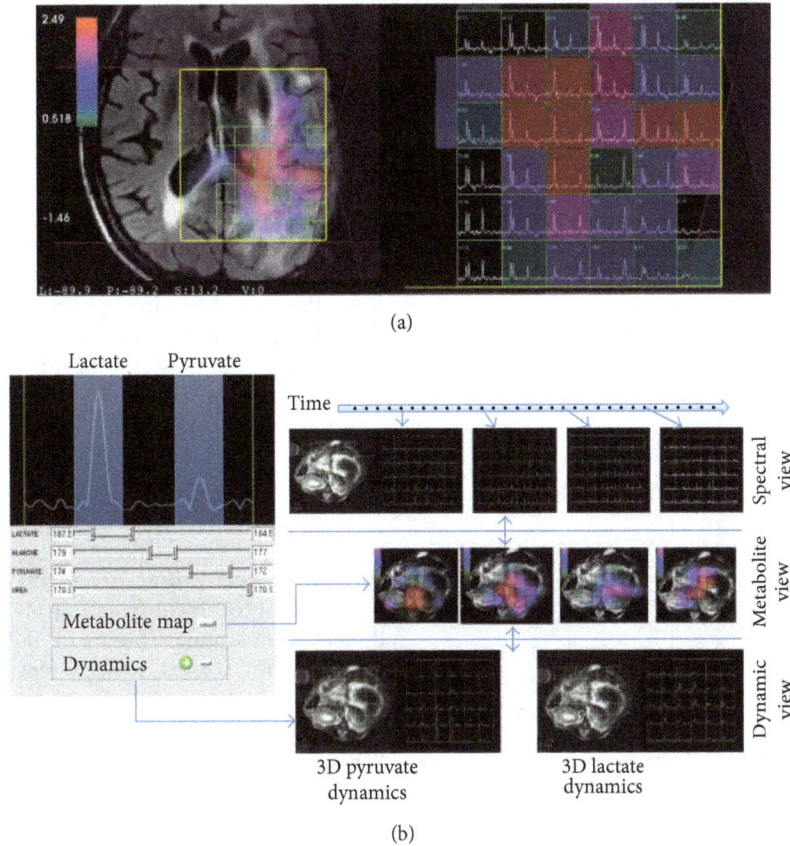

FIGURE 1: Multidimensional MRSI data visualization. (a) 4D brain MRSI data in SIVIC. Spectra from individual voxels are shown on the right. The left panel shows the spatial localization of each MRSI voxel on a reference anatomical image. The color overlay is a 3D metabolite map derived from spectral quantification of individual peaks. (b) 5D dynamic MRSI data. Metabolite peaks are derived from each point in a time series of 4D MRSI volumes. 3D dynamics of individual metabolites are represented by time curves in the bottom row for two different metabolites. The example at the bottom is from hyperpolarized ^{13}C MRSI of a rat.

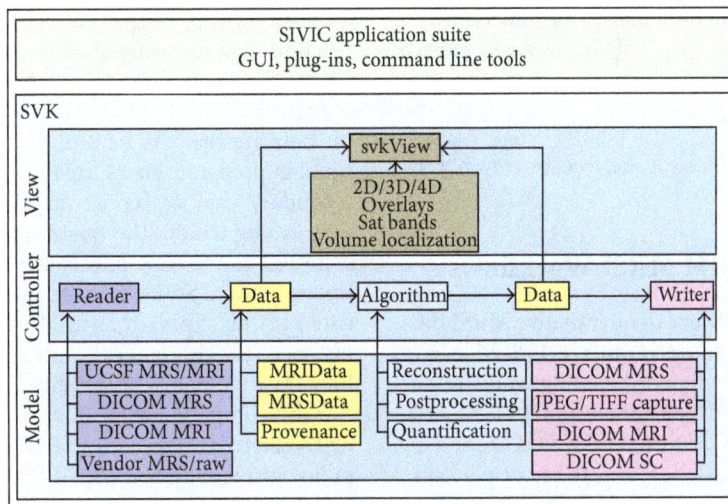

FIGURE 2: SIVIC software suite components. SIVIC applications (top) are built using the SIVIC Kit (svk) bottom. The svk is a C++ library representing a model, view, controller (MVC) design. View classes provide components that graphically display data and acquisition constructs represented by svkImageData objects (yellow). The controller layer utilizes svk IO (readers, writers) and svk algorithm classes to provide analysis functionality. The underlying svk model is represented by specific implementations of IO, algorithm, and data structure classes. Some specific examples of each class hierarchy are shown in the model (bottom box).

Format	Read*	Write
DICOM MR spectroscopy storage	✓	✓
DICOM MR image storage	✓	✓
DICOM enhanced MR image storage	✓	✓
DICOM secondary capture		✓
DICOM raw storage	✓	✓
GE P-files ($9x$–$23x$)**	✓	
GE.shf	✓	
GE postage stamp MRS	✓	
GE signa MRI	✓	
Siemens.rda	✓	
Siemens.IMA****	✓	
Varian.fdf	✓	
Varian FID ***	✓	
Philips MRS	1	
JPEG		✓
TIFF		✓
EPS †		✓
PDF †		✓
SVG †		✓

* Version numbers indicate future target release

** PSD specific, currently supports: probe-p, presscsi, mbrease. UCSF sequences. Others on request.

*** PSD specific, currently supports: UCSF compressed sensing, 2DCSI. Others on request.

**** IMA representing MR Image Storage SOP class

† Requires user to compile functionality from source code.

FIGURE 3: File formats supported by the svk IO layer are shown. SIVIC provides support for parsing raw data formats such as the GE P-file and Varian FID files, though interpreting the data may be sequence specific requiring customization to svk reader software classes. Version numbers indicate target SIVIC release to provide support.

be freely used in open- or closed-source, free, or commercial applications.

4. SIVIC Enabled DICOM MRSI Workflows

Current workflows for the delivery of quantitative MRSI data from the scanner to the reading room are inflexible and inefficient processes. Because standard reading workstations are incapable of rendering the high-dimensional MRSI data, they are typically rendered in the form of DICOM Secondary Capture Image Storage SOP instance reports and displayed as screen capture images. These images are limiting because they are static objects and cannot be further manipulated or analyzed. Even for product sequences that are reconstructed and analyzed on the scanner using vendor provided software, it is often desirable to create custom-tailored reports that focus on study-specific content and to generate reports from novel sequences or from analyses not supported by the vendor's

native software. Providing customized DICOM secondary capture reports typically requires taking the data offline and using custom software algorithms. An added complication of such offline analysis is that non-DICOM MRSI data must be retrieved from the scanner using a separate workflow, for example, via SFTP [27], and must be stored separately from the DICOM exam. This results in a decoupling of the actual MRSI data from the rest of the exam and requires significant effort to maintain a searchable record for future retrieval.

In the following, on-scanner and off-scanner MRSI workflows that have been implemented at UCSF with SIVIC are described. A common enabling feature is the use of SIVIC to convert vendor-specific MRSI data to standard DICOM SOP classes that can be transferred from the scanner to PACS, managed with the rest of the exam data, and retrieved for review or additional analysis (Figure 4) using existing DICOM infrastructure or easily accessible open-source tools.

4.1. On-Scanner MRSI Workflow. This section describes a workflow for reconstructing and analyzing MRSI data directly on a scanner (Figure 5). Raw data are acquired and written to the scanner's file system in a vendor-specific file format. The SIVIC GUI is configured to start from customizable push buttons directly on the console. Once started, SIVIC loads the raw MRSI data and can optionally load 3D DICOM MR image storage reference images (Figure 6). Raw data from a phantom acquisition are shown in the right panel. The left panel shows the voxel grid spatially referenced to the reference image. The yellow box represents the PRESS volume localization, and sat bands are shown in purple. Once loaded into the GUI, the MRSI data may be preprocessed with apodization filters, zero-filled, reconstructed, and phased. The resulting spectra may then be quantified to obtain maps that represent the spatial distribution of various metabolites (Figure 7). For computationally demanding reconstructions, data are securely staged on a computational cluster [28] for batch processing using SIVIC's command line tools, and the results are returned to the scanner in near real time where they can be loaded for review in the SIVIC GUI. At this stage, the data are ready to be sent to PACS. If the data have been suitably prepared for radiological interpretation, a DICOM secondary capture report may be generated for review in the reading room. The quantified metabolite maps may be exported as DICOM MR Image Storage, or Enhanced MR Image Storage SOP instances, and the reconstructed MRSI data may be exported as a DICOM MR Spectroscopy SOP instance. The original raw data are encapsulated in DICOM Raw Data Storage SOP instances.

The complete exam, now in DICOM format, can then be transferred to an offline PACS system. Once in PACS, a radiologist may review the DICOM secondary capture report together with other anatomical or functional images. From a research workstation, the original raw or reconstructed data may be retrieved for additional processing and analysis. Figure 8 shows an entire imaging exam including MRI, SC, MRSI, and raw data in OsiriX and DCM4CHEE [29] PACS. The entire exam including MRSI data and derived 3D metabolite maps is now archived in PACS, which is

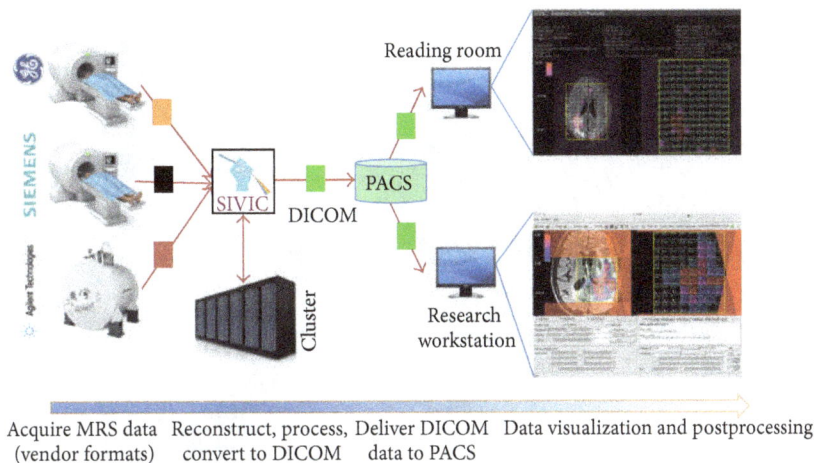

Acquire MRS data   Reconstruct, process,   Deliver DICOM   Data visualization and postprocessing
(vendor formats)   convert to DICOM   data to PACS

FIGURE 4: Generalized DICOM MRSI workflow. MRS data is acquired and encoded in vendor specific formats (red, orange, and pink). SIVIC tools reconstruct data and/or convert to DICOM format (green) to send to PACS. DICOM data can be retrieved for visualization in the reading room or on a research workstation for processing and visualization using the SIVIC GUI or command line tools.

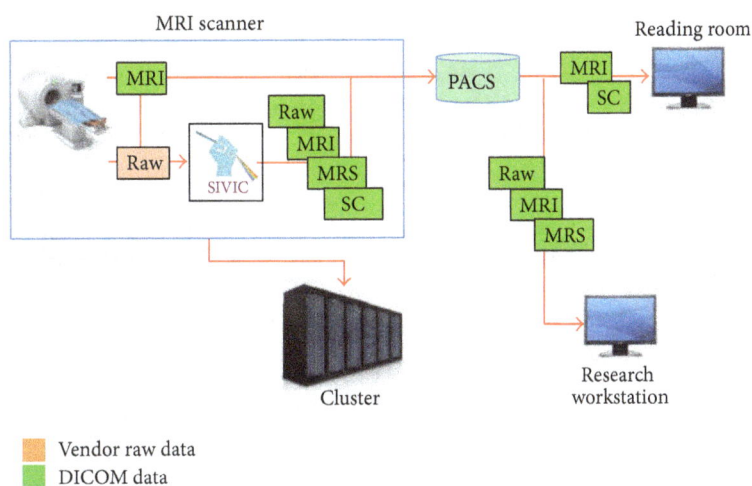

■ Vendor raw data
■ DICOM data

FIGURE 5: On-scanner MRSI workflow. SIVIC running on the scanner reads raw MRSI vendor data and anatomical DICOM MRI images. MRSI data is reconstructed and DICOM MRS, DICOM MRI metabolite maps, and DICOM secondary capture (SC) images are exported and sent to PACS. DICOM SC and DICOM MRI images are viewed in the reading room. DICOM MRI (anatomical and metabolite maps) and DICOM MRS images may be viewed on a research workstation running SIVIC or other DICOM applications. CPU intensive on-scanner reconstruction may require a computational cluster for real-time analysis during an exam.

a major benefit for data management. A key point here is that the derived metabolite maps are 3D DICOM images which can be treated on an equal footing with other 3D imaging data to correlate MRSI with other data in a multimodal analysis (Figure 9). Specialized software such as SIVIC is still required for visualization of DICOM MRSI data, however, in principle any software package that implements the DICOM MR spectroscopy standard will be capable of interpreting it. The SIVIC plug-in for OsiriX permits the MRSI data to be visualized from within OsiriX PACS. Several other freely available software packages such as TARQUIN [18, 30] and jMRUI [16, 31] also support the reading of DICOM MRS data and provide capabilities that are complimentary to SIVIC.

4.2. Off-Scanner MRSI Workflow. A workflow for reconstructing and analyzing MRSI data using an external workstation and transferring the resulting images is shown in Figure 10. In this scenario, raw data are encapsulated in Raw Data Storage SOP instances using the svk_create_dcmraw utility on the scanner and transferred to an offline PACS. The resulting DICOM raw data storage instances, together with the other DICOM data from the exam, are retrieved to a workstation where SIVIC tools process and reconstruct the data as described above. The DICOM SC report is sent back to PACS where it can be retrieved for review in the reading room.

4.3. Workflow Discussion. MRSI data from patients with brain tumors are routinely acquired on GE MRI scanners at UCSF using product as well as novel acquisition methods developed in our research groups [32, 33]. These are converted to DICOM Raw Data Storage SOP instances using svk_create_dcmraw and pushed, together with other DICOM data, to a research DCM4CHEE PACS.

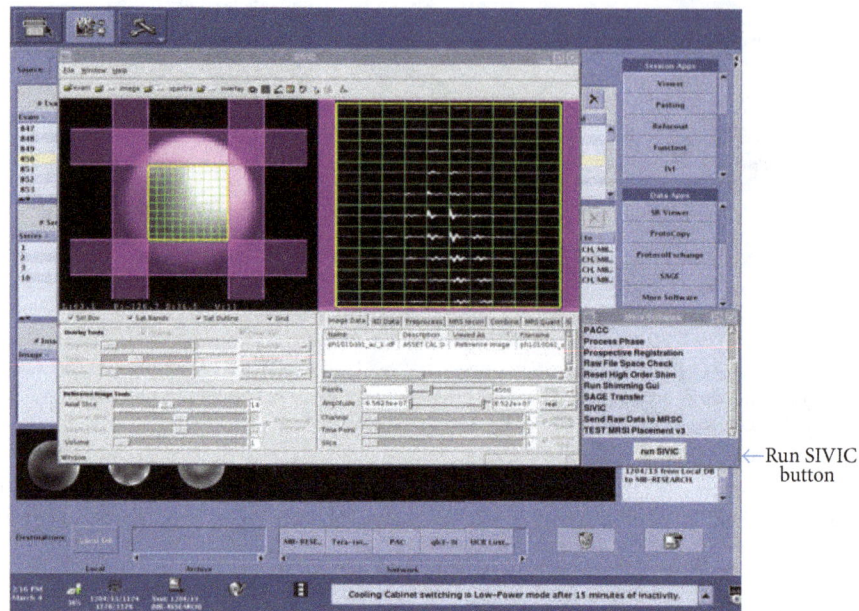

FIGURE 6: SIVIC GUI running on a GE 7T scanner console. Raw data from a phantom acquisition is shown in the right SIVIC panel. The left SIVIC panel shows the MRSI voxel grid spatially referenced to the reference image. The yellow box represents the PRESS volume localization, and purple regions represent sat bands. The SIVIC GUI is configured to run from configurable menu buttons on the scanner's operator console (right side).

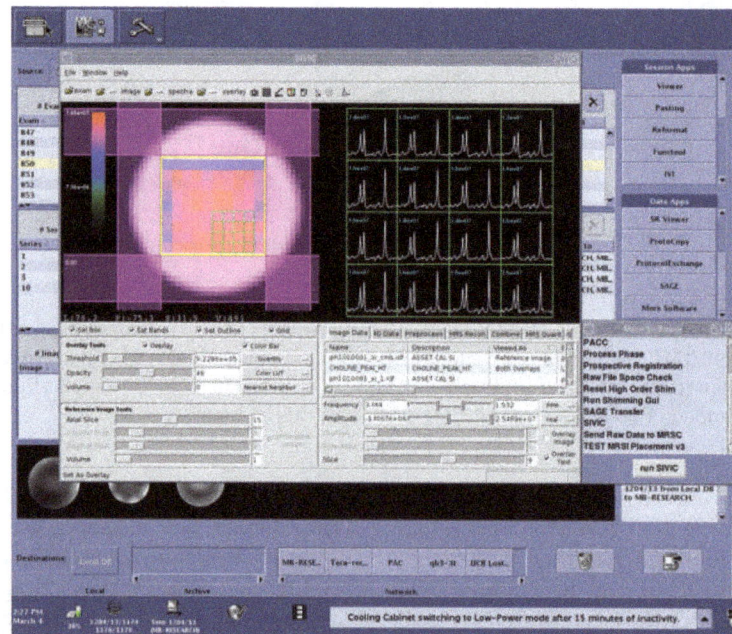

FIGURE 7: Phantom MRS data reconstructed and quantified using the SIVIC GUI on a 7T GE scanner console. The right panel shows spectra from the 16 selected voxels. The voxels are spatially referenced to the image in the left panel. The color overlay on the left is a metabolite map representing the choline peak height. The blue text above the spectra gives the exact value of the current overlay for each voxel.

The DICOM exam is retrieved to a Linux workstation for processing. Details of the spectroscopic data processing pipeline are beyond the scope of this paper and are described here only at a high level. MRSI data is unencapsulated from the DICOM raw data storage object, and the file integrity is confirmed by the SHA1 digest. The unencapsulated raw data are converted to DICOM MR spectroscopy Storage instances with the command line svk_gepfile_reader utility. Apodization and zero filling as well as spatial and spectral Fourier transforms are performed within SIVIC. In addition to these methods, SIVIC supports zero and first-order phase correction, HSVD baseline removal, sum-of-squares coil

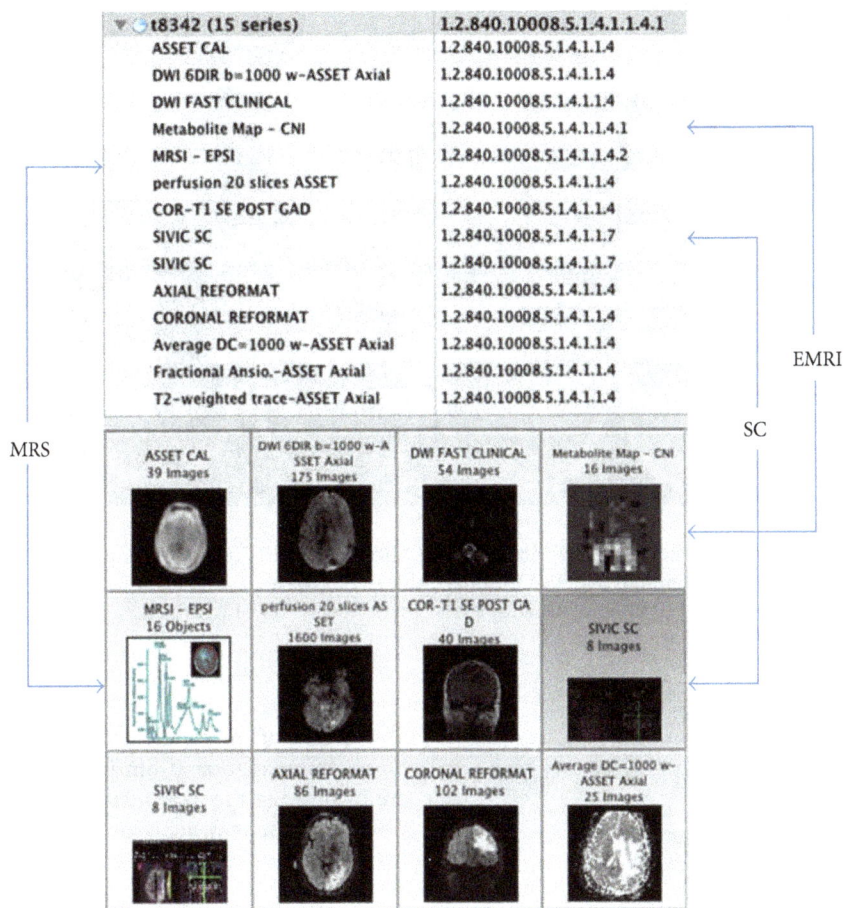

(a)

(b)

Figure 8: DICOM MRSI exam in OsiriX PACS (a) and DCM4CHEE PACS (b): Raw Data Storage SOP class (1.2.840.10008.5.1.4.1.1.66, RAW), reconstructed MRSI, MR Spectroscopy SOP class (1.2.840.10008.5.1.4.1.1.4.2, MRS), Secondary Capture SOP class (1.2.840.10008.5.1.4.1.1.7, SC), metabolite maps (Enhanced MR Image Storage SOP class (1.2.840.10008.5.1.4.1.1.4.1, EMRI).

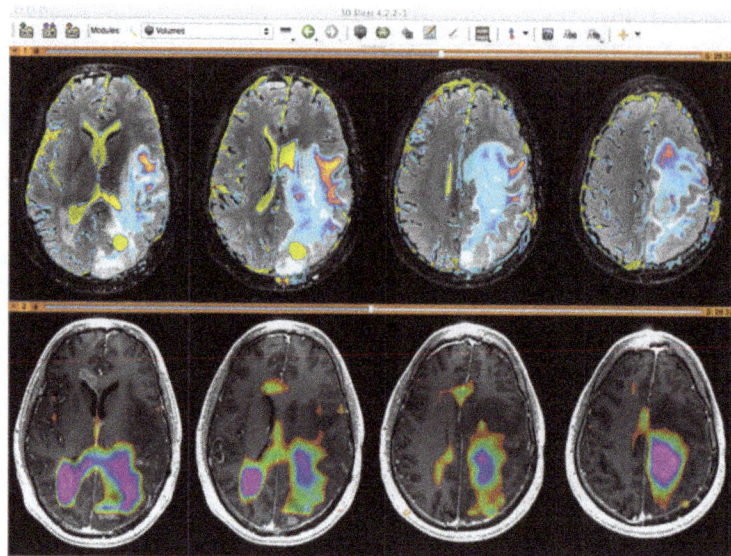

FIGURE 9: CNI metabolite maps (bottom color overlay) derived from MRSI data in SIVIC are exported as standard DICOM MR Image Storage SOP instances, which can be loaded into 3D DICOM image analysis software packages (shown here in 3D Slicer). Derived maps are thus amenable to multimodal analysis. The top panel shows ADC maps (color) on FLAIR images. The bottom panel shows the same anatomical locations on a T1 contrast enhanced image.

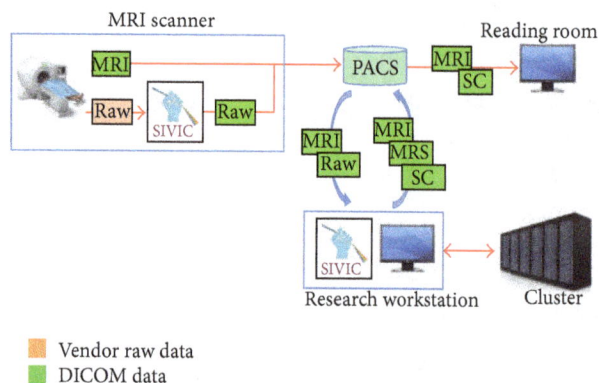

FIGURE 10: Off-scanner MRSI workflow. SIVIC command line tools running on the scanner convert vendor raw MRS data to DICOM Raw Data Storage SOP instances. Anatomical MRI and raw DICOM data is sent to PACS. A research workstation retrieves DICOM images from PACS. MRSI data is reconstructed and DICOM MRS, DICOM MRI metabolite maps and DICOM secondary capture (SC) images are exported and sent to PACS. DICOM SC and DICOM MRI data is viewed in the reading room. DICOM MRI (anatomical and metabolite maps) and DICOM MRS images may be viewed on a research workstation running SIVIC or other DICOM applications.

combination, and peak height and integrated area metabolite quantification. Registration, segmentation, and other standard image processing algorithms are already implemented in other packages and are not reimplemented within SIVIC. Metabolite maps are exported from SIVIC as standard 3D images and can be processed using any number of available tools. The final processed MRSI data and MRI data are loaded into the SIVIC GUI in order to create a DICOM secondary capture report for radiological review as shown in Figure 11.

The format of the report and its contents have been based on recommendations from neuroradiologists at UCSF who are involved in the treatment of patients with brain cancers. Over the past year approximately 400 brain MRSI reports have been sent to the UCSF clinical PACS for review using this method.

A limitation of such workflows is that not all PACS implementations currently support the storage of Raw Data Storage SOP class or the MR Spectroscopy Storage SOP class, however many do, such as DCM4CHEE [34], OsiriX [35], Carestream [36], Philips [37], and Agfa [38]. Furthermore, reading workstations are still not capable of directly rendering MRSI data, which necessitates the use of DICOM secondary capture image reports. However, the ability to couple the raw and processed MRSI data with the DICOM record is a major benefit, making the data accessible to applications that implement the DICOM MRS standard.

5. Modular Vendor Neutral MRSI Analysis Software

Another major goal of SIVIC is to provide a flexible, vendor neutral MRSI analysis package that facilitates the validation of metabolic imaging methods and the dissemination of novel MRSI methods broadly within the community. The approach taken to achieve this is to separate vendor- and acquisition-specific details from generalized downstream reconstruction and analysis algorithms. All pipelines are thus divided into a data-reading component that is vendor and sequence specific, followed by a vendor and sequence neutral component representing the downstream processing pipeline as shown in Figure 12.

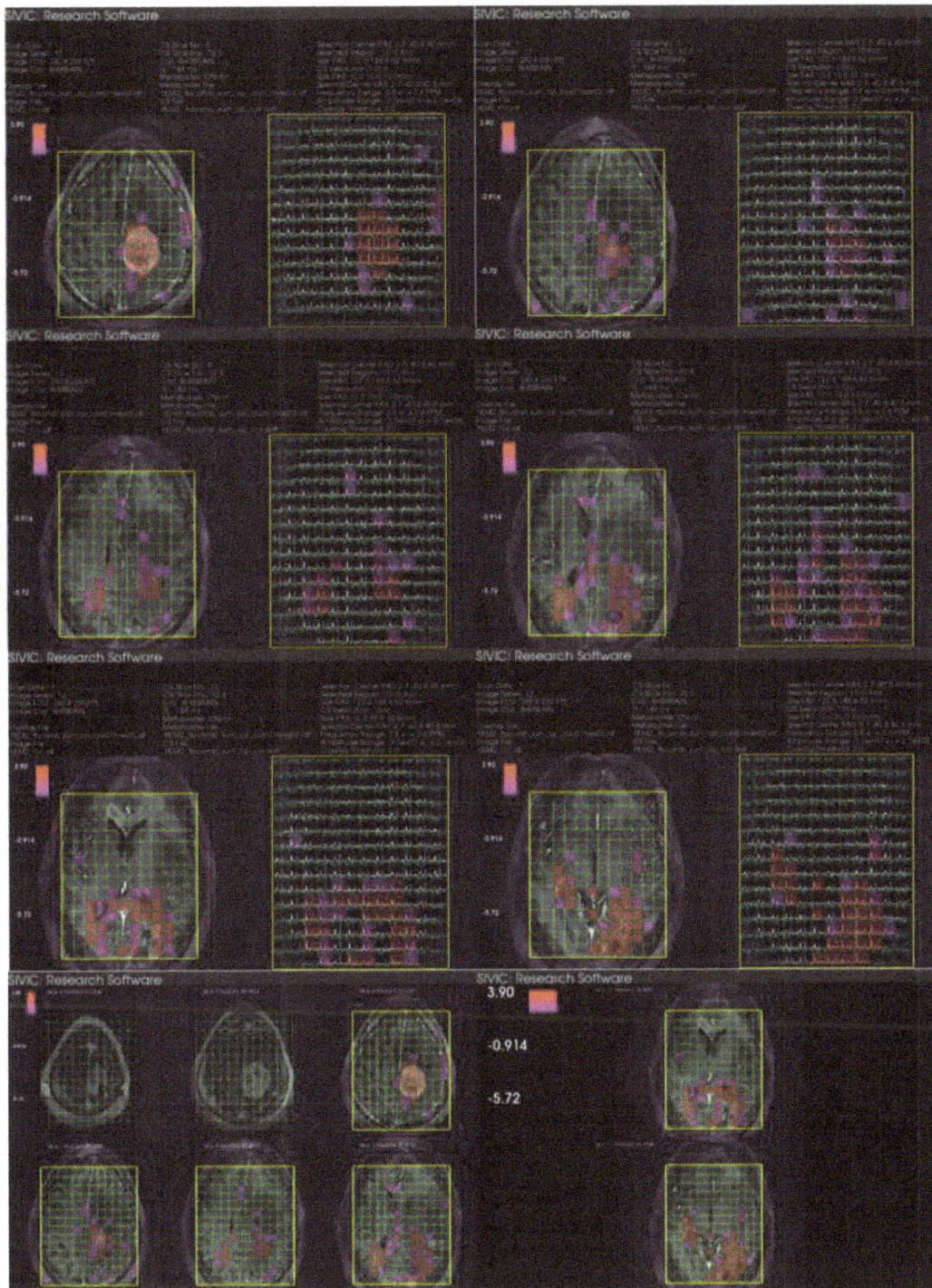

FIGURE 11: SIVIC generated DICOM secondary capture report for UCSF MRS exam. The series consists of 8 images shown here. The color overlay represents the choline to NAA index. Spatial referencing to T1 postcontrast image, volume localization (yellow), and sat bands (purple shading) are shown. The final two images are summary representations of the acquisition referenced to the anatomical images.

Variability in data loading reflects differences in (i) data formats and (ii) acquisition methods. These differences are handled modularly within SIVIC's svkImageReader2 class hierarchy [39] in the following way. The process is split into two parts, reading the raw data file and interpreting its contents using a data mapping class. SIVIC implements readers for multiple vendor formats, and their responsibility is to parse a vendor's file format, but without making any interpretation of the content. Once the raw data has been parsed the data mapper is used to interpret the vendor- and acquisition-specific details such that the output of the svkImageReader2 (e.g., svkMrsImageData) consists of data

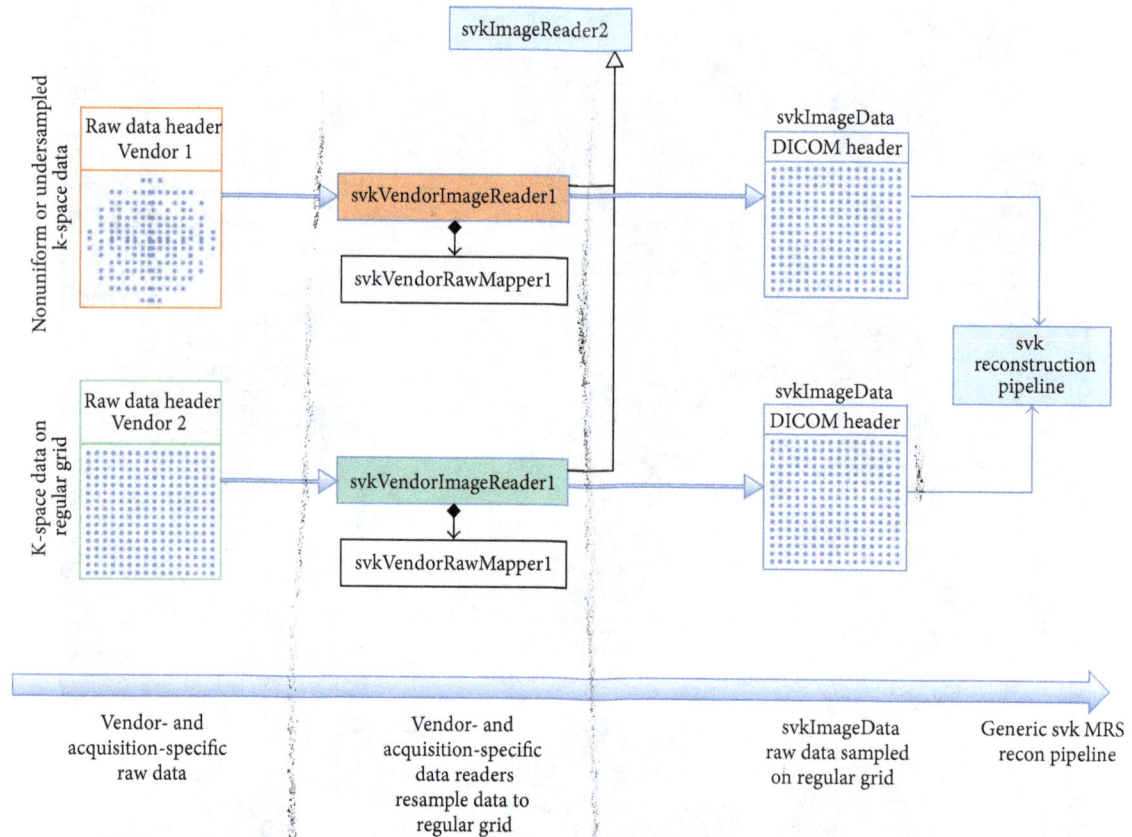

FIGURE 12: svk raw data readers handle acquisition-specific data reorganization. This includes vendor-specific header parsing and acquisition-specific data reordering and resampling. The output of an svkImageReader is always an svkImageData object, represented by a DICOM header and data sampled on a regular grid that is suitable for FFT-based reconstruction. This permits the use of a common set of independent downstream reconstruction and processing algorithms, independent of the acquisition sequence or vendor data format. An svkImageReaderFactory reads the raw data files to create the appropriate type of svkImageReader for the specific input format and acquisition type. Vendor- and acquisition-specific readers load data and associated mappers resample data to a regular grid.

sampled on a regularly spaced grid suitable for the Fourier transform reconstruction and acquisition-neutral processing [40]. Because the output of the readers has been standardized in this way, the SIVIC algorithms can be tested using data from multiple sources.

The svk reader classes are modular at multiple levels. The vendor-specific readers only need to be implemented once per vendor data format. Mappers are more complex, yet the underlying algorithms utilized by the mappers to accomplish data reordering or resampling exist as separate svk algorithm classes that may be reused to accomplish the same task in similar data acquired on different vendor's scanners. For example, linear phase correction algorithms, required to correct for time delays in EPSI frequency sampling [32], may be used to make this correction on EPSI data from any vendor. This modularity is of great value and enables svk readers to be adapted for use with data from different vendors. At UCSF, this has enabled SIVIC software initially developed to read EPSI data acquired on a Varian animal scanner to be adapted easily for use on data acquired from a clinical GE scanner as studies transitioned from animal validation to human trials.

6. Conclusions

The SIVIC software framework and application suite presented here comprise a widely accessible software package designed to facilitate the routine incorporation of MRSI data into imaging studies. This is accomplished by providing tools for converting MRSI data from nonstandard vendor-specific formats to the standard DICOM MR Spectroscopy SOP class. The use of this standard enables existing DICOM infrastructures to manage MRSI data together with other components of the exam, rather than requiring separate storage, transmission, and searching infrastructures. Two MRSI workflows that have been implemented at UCSF to analyze and deliver quantitative MRSI data from scanner to the clinical PACS and reading room in over 400 brain tumor exams were described. These workflows store GE raw data as DICOM Raw Data Storage SOP instances, reconstructed MRSI data as DICOM MR Spectroscopy Storage SOP instances, metabolic image maps as DICOM Enhanced MR Image Storage SOP instances and reports as DICOM Secondary Capture Image Storage SOP instances. DICOM MRSI data are maintained in a research PACS. This simplifies ongoing and retrospective analysis of imaging studies containing MRSI data. The encoding of derived 3D metabolite maps as DICOM MR Image Storage SOP instances enables them to be used by standard DICOM image analysis software, thus providing a straightforward mechanism to integrate metabolic data with other anatomical and functional imaging data as part of a multimodal analysis.

The use of the DICOM MR Spectroscopy SOP class to encode MRSI data increases data accessibility to any application that implements the DICOM MRS standard. As has been demonstrated here, this allows MRSI data to be managed by conventional PACS solutions and enables MRSI analysis software to be used for evaluation of data from multiple sources. SIVIC extends the interoperability to data originally encoded in vendor-specific formats and thus enables a common set of software algorithms and visualization tools to be used with data from multiple sources. Tools developed on one scanner platform can thus be relatively easily ported to other scanner platforms. This facilitates the transition of methods from animal models to human models and streamlines the use of MRSI analysis in multicenter trials. Other dynamic imaging modalities can also benefit from the type of high dimensional visualization tools used here for display of MRSI data. For example, MR perfusion studies track the time evolution of contrast in a 3D volume, and SIVIC has been adapted to display such data sets both as 3D arrays of time curves as well as 3D maps representing derived perfusion parameters.

The distribution of SIVIC as a free open-source software package that runs on all major operating system has been shown to foster interinstitutional MRSI research studies as research MRSI acquisition sequences can be distributed together with the software required for reconstruction and visualization of data acquired with novel MRSI methods. These collaborations provide important feedback for the project that acts to stabilize the distributions and improve functionality. The project encourages community participation and welcomes collaborative input.

Acknowledgments

This work was supported by the NIH P41EB013598, NIH P01 CA11816, and NIH R01 CA127612.

References

[1] D. T. Okuda, R. Srinivasan, J. R. Oksenberg et al., "Genotype-phenotype correlations in multiple sclerosis: HLA genes influence disease severity inferred by 1HMR spectroscopy and MRI measures," *Brain*, vol. 132, no. 1, pp. 250–259, 2009.

[2] A. Laprie, I. Catalaa, E. Cassol et al., "Proton magnetic resonance spectroscopic imaging in newly diagnosed glioblastoma: predictive value for the site of postradiotherapy relapse in a prospective longitudinal study," *International Journal of Radiation Oncology Biology Physics*, vol. 70, no. 3, pp. 773–781, 2008.

[3] J. Chang, S. Thakur, G. Perera et al., "Image-fusion of MR spectroscopic images for treatment planning of gliomas," *Medical Physics*, vol. 33, no. 1, pp. 32–40, 2006.

[4] E. Westman, L.-O. Wahlund, C. Foy et al., "Magnetic resonance imaging and magnetic resonance spectroscopy for detection of early Alzheimers Disease," *Journal of Alzheimer's Disease*, vol. 26, no. 3, pp. 307–319, 2011.

[5] S. Josan, D. Spielman, Y.-F. Yen, R. Hurd, A. Pfefferbaum, and D. Mayer, "Fast volumetric imaging of ethanol metabolism in rat liver with hyperpolarized [1-^{13}C]pyruvate," *NMR in Biomedicine*, vol. 25, no. 8, pp. 993–999, 2012.

[6] I. Park, G. Tamai, M. C. Lee et al., "Patterns of recurrence analysis in newly diagnosed glioblastoma multiforme after three-dimensional conformal radiation therapy with respect to pre-radiation therapy magnetic resonance spectroscopic findings," *International Journal of Radiation Oncology Biology Physics*, vol. 69, no. 2, pp. 381–389, 2007.

[7] T. Sankar, Z. Caramanos, R. Assina et al., "Prospective serial proton MR spectroscopic assessment of response to tamoxifen for recurrent malignant glioma," *Journal of Neuro-Oncology*, vol. 90, no. 1, pp. 63–76, 2008.

[8] A. Stadlbauer, E. Moser, S. Gruber, C. Nimsky, R. Fahlbusch, and O. Ganslandt, "Integration of biochemical images of a tumor into frameless stereotaxy achieved using a magnetic resonance imaging/magnetic resonance spectroscopy hybrid data set," *Journal of Neurosurgery*, vol. 101, no. 2, pp. 287–294, 2004.

[9] A. A. Tzika, "Proton magnetic resonance spectroscopic imaging as a cancer biomarker for pediatric brain tumors," *International Journal of Oncology*, vol. 32, no. 3, pp. 517–526, 2008.

[10] F. W. Crawford, I. S. Khayal, C. McGue et al., "Relationship of pre-surgery metabolic and physiological MR imaging parameters to survival for patients with untreated GBM," *Journal of Neuro-Oncology*, vol. 91, no. 3, pp. 337–351, 2009.

[11] K. Pinker, A. Stadlbauer, W. Bogner, S. Gruber, and T. H. Helbich, "Molecular imaging of cancer: MR spectroscopy and beyond," *European Journal of Radiology*, vol. 81, no. 3, pp. 566–577, 2012.

[12] DICOM, http://medical.nema.org/.

[13] DICOM Standard Part 3PS 3.3-2011, section A.36.3.3, http://medical.nema.org/standard.html.

[14] SIVIC, http://sourceforge.net/projects/sivic/.

[15] J. C. Crane, M. P. Olson, and S. J. Nelson, "Open source DICOM MR spectroscopy software framework and plug-in for osiriX," in *RSNA Annual Meeting*, 2009.

[16] jMRUI, http://www.mrui.uab.es/mrui/mrui_Overview.shtml.

[17] MIDAS, http://mrir.med.miami.edu:8000/midas/.

[18] TARQUIN, http://tarquin.sourceforge.net/.

[19] VTK, http://www.vtk.org/.

[20] DCMTK, http://dicom.offis.de/dcmtk.php.en.

[21] 3D Slicer, http://www.slicer.org/.

[22] OsiriX, http://www.osirix-viewer.com/.

[23] SIVIC plug-in for OsiriX, http://sourceforge.net/projects/sivic/files/osirix_plugin/.

[24] Slicer project week, 2010, http://www.na-mic.org/Wiki/index.php/2010_Summer_Project_Week_MRSI_module_and_SIVIC_interface.

[25] Slicer project week, 2011, http://www.na-mic.org/Wiki/index.php/2011_Winter_Project_Week:MRSI_module_and_SIVIC_interface.

[26] SIVIC command line tools, http://sivic.sourceforge.net/libsvk/html/index.html.

[27] SFTP, http://en.wikipedia.org/wiki/SSH_File_Transfer_Protocol.

[28] J. C. Crane, F. W. Crawford, and S. J. Nelson, "Grid enabled magnetic resonance scanners for near real-time medical image processing," *Journal of Parallel and Distributed Computing*, vol. 66, no. 12, pp. 1524–1533, 2006.

[29] DCM4CHEE, http://www.dcm4che.org/confluence/display/ee2/Home.

[30] M. Wilson, G. Reynolds, R. A. Kauppinen, T. N. Arvanitis, and A. C. Peet, "A constrained least-squares approach to the automated quantitation of in vivo ^{1}H magnetic resonance spectroscopy data," *Magnetic Resonance in Medicine*, vol. 65, no. 1, pp. 1–12, 2011.

[31] D. Stefan, F. D. Cesare, A. Andrasescu et al., "Quantitation of magnetic resonance spectroscopy signals: the jMRUI software package," *Measurement Science and Technology*, vol. 20, no. 10, Article ID 104035, 2009.

[32] C. H. Cunningham, D. B. Vigneron, A. P. Chen et al., "Design of flyback echo-planar readout gradients for magnetic resonance spectroscopic imaging," *Magnetic Resonance in Medicine*, vol. 54, no. 5, pp. 1286–1289, 2005.

[33] S. J. Nelson, E. Ozhinsky, Y. Li, I. W. Park, and J. Crane, "Strategies for rapid in vivo ^{1}H and hyperpolarized ^{13}C MR spectroscopic imaging," *Journal of Magnetic Resonance*, vol. 229, pp. 187–197, 2013.

[34] DCM4CHEE conformance, http://www.dcm4che.org/docs/conformance/dcm4chee-cs.pdf.

[35] OsiriX conformance, http://www.osirix-viewer.com/DICOM-ConformanceStatements.pdf.

[36] http://www.carestream.com/pacsvl1_dicom_8g8913.pdf.

[37] Philips conformance, http://incenter.medical.philips.com/doclib/getdoc.aspx?func=ll&objid=9332344&objaction=open.

[38] Agfa impax 6.5 conformance, http://www.agfahealthcare.com/global/en/he/library/libraryopen?ID=28653428.

[39] svkImageReader2 classes, http://sivic.sourceforge.net/libsvk/html/hierarchy.html.

[40] D. Sundararajan, *Digital Signal Processing: Theory and Practice*, World Scientific, 2003.

5

Computer Aided Diagnostic Support System for Skin Cancer: A Review of Techniques and Algorithms

Ammara Masood and Adel Ali Al-Jumaily

School of Electrical, Mechanical and Mechatronic Engineering, University of Technology, Broadway Ultimo, Sydney, NSW 2007, Australia

Correspondence should be addressed to Ammara Masood; ammara.masood@student.uts.edu.au

Academic Editor: Michael W. Vannier

Image-based computer aided diagnosis systems have significant potential for screening and early detection of malignant melanoma. We review the state of the art in these systems and examine current practices, problems, and prospects of image acquisition, preprocessing, segmentation, feature extraction and selection, and classification of dermoscopic images. This paper reports statistics and results from the most important implementations reported to date. We compared the performance of several classifiers specifically developed for skin lesion diagnosis and discussed the corresponding findings. Whenever available, indication of various conditions that affect the technique's performance is reported. We suggest a framework for comparative assessment of skin cancer diagnostic models and review the results based on these models. The deficiencies in some of the existing studies are highlighted and suggestions for future research are provided.

1. Introduction

The incidence of melanoma skin cancer has been increasing over the past few decades [1–3]. Estimated 76,250 new cases of invasive melanoma were diagnosed in USA in 2012, with an estimated number of 9,180 that result in death [4]. Australia has one of the highest rates of skin cancer in the world. Over 1,890 Australians die from skin cancer each year [5]. Melanoma is capable of deep invasion. The most dangerous characteristic of melanoma is that it can spread widely over the body via the lymphatic vessels and blood vessels. Thus, early diagnosis of melanoma is a key factor for the prognosis of the disease.

The usual clinical practice of melanoma diagnosis is a visual inspection by the dermatologist. Clinical diagnostic accuracy is a bit disappointing [6, 7]. However, dermoscopy [8] is a noninvasive diagnostic technique that links clinical dermatology and dermatopathology by enabling the visualization of morphological features which are not discernible by examination with the naked eye. There are different techniques, like solar scan [9], epiluminescence microscopy (ELM) [10, 11], cross-polarization epiluminescence (XLM),

and side transillumination (TLM) [12, 13], that can greatly increase the morphological details that are visualized. Thus, they provide additional diagnostic criteria to the dermatologist.

Dermoscopy enables better diagnosis as compared to unaided eye [14–16] with an improvement in diagnostic sensitivity of 10–30% [17]. However, it has also been demonstrated that dermoscopy may actually lower the diagnostic accuracy in the hands of inexperienced dermatologists [10, 18–20], since this method requires great deal of experience to differentiate skin lesions [21]. As described in [9, 22] only experts have arrived at 90% sensitivity and 59% specificity in skin lesion diagnosis, while for less trained doctors these figures show significant drop till around 62%-63% for general practitioners.

The main problem is that the diagnosis is highly dependent on subjective judgement and is scarcely reproducible [23, 24]. Several scoring systems and algorithms such as the ABCD-E rule [25–27], the seven-point checklist [28–30], three-point checklist [31], and the Menzies method [32, 33] have been proposed to improve the diagnostic performance of less experienced clinicians. Although this simplification has enabled the development of these diagnostic algorithms with good accuracy, still they showed problems that have not yet been solved. The most important shortcoming is that the purpose for which they were designed was not achieved, because the within- and between-observer concordance is very low, even for expert observers [10, 25, 34, 35]. Despite extensive research in investigating the varied presentations and physical characteristics of melanoma, the clinical diagnostic accuracy remains suboptimal. Thus, a growing interest has developed in the last two decades in the automated analysis of digitized images obtained by ELM techniques to assist clinicians in differentiating early melanoma from benign skin lesions.

Application of computational intelligence methods helps physicians as well as dermatologists in faster data process to give better and more reliable diagnoses. Studies related to the automated classification of pigmented skin lesion images have appeared in the literature as early as 1987 [36]. After some successful experiments on automatic diagnostic systems for melanoma diagnosis [36–42], utility of machine vision and computerized analysis is getting more important every year. The importance of the topic is patent if we analyse the enormous quantity of research works related with the melanoma diagnosis. Numerous computerized diagnostic systems have been reported in the literature where different border detection, feature extraction, selection, and classification algorithms are used. Some researchers [37, 43–48] reviewed and tried to critically examine image analysis techniques for diagnosis of skin cancer and compared diagnostic accuracy of experts dermoscopists with artificial intelligence and computer aided diagnosis. More research, however, is needed to identify and reduce uncertainties in the automatic decision support systems to improve diagnosis accuracy. A comprehensive up-to-date review of automatic diagnostic model for skin lesions is not available. Continuous emergence of new classification algorithms and techniques for dermoscopic image analysis in recent years necessitates such a review.

This paper describes a standard automatic decision support system which is based on semantic analysis of melanoma images and further classification of characteristic objects commonly found in pigmented skin lesions. The aim of this review is to summarize and compare advanced dermoscopic algorithms used for the classification of skin lesions and discuss important issues affecting the success of classification. A brief and comprehensive review of feature extraction and selection algorithms that are so far being used for extracting various features of malignant melanoma is also provided. Analysis of various papers is performed with respect to several criteria, such as lesion segmentation, feature extraction, size of data sets, classification techniques, and performance measures used in reporting the diagnosis results. This paper will provide a framework that represents a comprehensive guideline for selecting suitable algorithms needed for different steps of automatic diagnostic procedure for ensuring timely diagnosis of skin cancer.

The paper is organized as follows. the scheme of a general computer aided diagnosis system is provided. A comprehensive review of the available literature regarding each stage is presented. The different classification algorithms are explained. Performance evaluation measures and model validation details are presented for analysing various algorithms/models and finally concluding comments are provided.

2. Computer-Aided Diagnosis System

Computer aided decision support tools are important in medical imaging for diagnosis and evaluation. Predictive models are used in a variety of medical domains for diagnostic and prognostic tasks. These models are built based on experience which constitutes data acquired from actual cases. The data can be preprocessed and expressed in a set of rules, such as that it is often the case in knowledge-based expert systems, and consequently can serve as training data for statistical and machine learning models.

The general approach of developing a CAD system for the diagnosis of skin cancer is to find the location of a lesion and also to determine an estimate of the probability of a disease. The first step in this paper was to establish a standard general scheme of a CAD system for skin lesions. The proposed scheme is shown in Figure 1. The inputs to the computer aided system are digital images obtained by ELM, with the possibility to add other acquisition system such as ultrasound or confocal microscopy. In the first phase preprocessing of image is done that allows reducing the ill effects and various artifacts like hair that may be present in the dermoscopic images. It is followed by the detection of the lesion by image segmentation technique. Once the lesion is localized, different chromatic and morphological features can be quantified and used for classification.

Differentiation of malignant melanoma images demands very fast image processing and feature extraction and classification algorithms. A detailed research is necessary to make the best choice and to set the benchmarks for diagnostic system development and validation. The following section focuses on the description of the major steps that may be involved in skin cancer diagnosis.

2.1. Image Acquisition/Methods for Screening Skin Lesions. Unaided visual inspection of the skin is often suboptimal for diagnosing melanoma. Numerous imaging modalities are under investigation to determine their usefulness in imaging and ascertaining a correct in vivo diagnosis of melanoma. These include total cutaneous photography, dermoscopy, confocal scanning laser microscopy (CSLM), ultrasound, magnetic resonance imaging (MRI), optical coherence tomography (OCT), and multispectral imaging. Each technique has certain pros and cons. These are now being harnessed to improve early detection. We have provided here a bird eye view of the currently available cutaneous imaging devices and new frontiers in noninvasive automated diagnosis of melanoma in Table 1. Readers may refer to [33, 49–52] for analysing performance comparison of some of the existing screening techniques.

Relative to other specialties, dermatologists have been slow to adopt advanced technologic diagnostic aids. Thus, so far dermoscopy is the fastest growing method to image

TABLE 1: In vivo imaging techniques for the diagnosis of skin cancer.

Method	Advantages	Limitations
Photography [203–205] Total body photograph (2-D TBP 3-D TBP) Baseline photographs of individual lesions	Affordable and easy data management. Monitoring patients with many dysplastic nevi. Useful in the follow-up management and easy comparison for detecting change in size, shape, or color that may be suggestive of malignancy. 3D representation of the patient's entire cutaneous surface may reduce work time and clarify documentation.	Limited morphologic information.
Dermoscopy [8, 10, 19, 123, 206–208] ELM (oil/slide mode and polarizing mode)	Facilitating 20–70% magnification of the skin. Melanoma dermoscopic characteristics are well correlated to histopathologic features. Identifying foci of melanoma for helping pathologist as to where to section the specimen so as to minimize false-negative results as a result of sampling error. Liquid immersion provides increased illumination and resolution and sharper and less distorted colours. Polarizing mode avoids a potential source of nosocomial infections.	Qualitative and potentially subjective. Low magnification in routinely used instruments and the limited scope of observable structures restrict the usefulness and diagnostic applicability of the method.
Multispectral imaging [209–211] Melafind Solar scan Spectrophotometric intracutaneous analysis	Spectral imaging is quantitative and more objective. Less interphysician variability. Melafind can create multispectral sequence of images in less than 3 seconds. SIA scope can help in the diagnosis of lesions as small as 2 mm. Analysing the location, quantity, and distribution of skin chromophores within epidermis and papillary dermis.	Difficult interpretation because of the complexity of the optical processes of scattering and absorption.
Laser-based enhanced diagnosis [212–214] Confocal scanning laser microscopy Reflectance confocal microscopy Spectrally encoded confocal microscopy	In vivo imaging of skin lesions at variable depths in horizontal planes and examination at a quasi-histological resolution without biopsy. High resolution allows imaging of nuclear, cellular, and tissue architecture of the epidermis and underlying dermal structures without a biopsy and allows recognition of abnormal intraepidermal melanocytic proliferation. No tissue damage because of low-power laser.	Processes in the reticular dermis and tumor invasion depth cannot be evaluated reliably. Technically sensitive and expensive to use in routine clinical application. Formal training and experience are required to become proficient in this new technique.
Optical coherence tomography [215–217]	Depth of invasion can be better measured with OCT than CSLM. Noninvasive assessment and monitor of inflammatory skin diseases.	Limited resolution does not allow a differential diagnosis between benign and malignant lesions. Limited to thin tumors because of the strong scattering of epidermic tissue.
Ultrasound imaging [218, 219]	Can provide information about perfusion patterns of lymph nodes and other soft tissues that can be used to stage the tumor.	May overestimate or underestimate tumor thickness; accuracy of results depends heavily on the skill of examiner and anatomic site of lesion.
Magnetic resonance imaging [220–222]	Obtaining information on the depth and extent of the underlying tissue involvement and can be used to measure melanoma thickness or volume.	The need for sufficient resolution and adequate number of images per sequence for discriminating skin lesions.

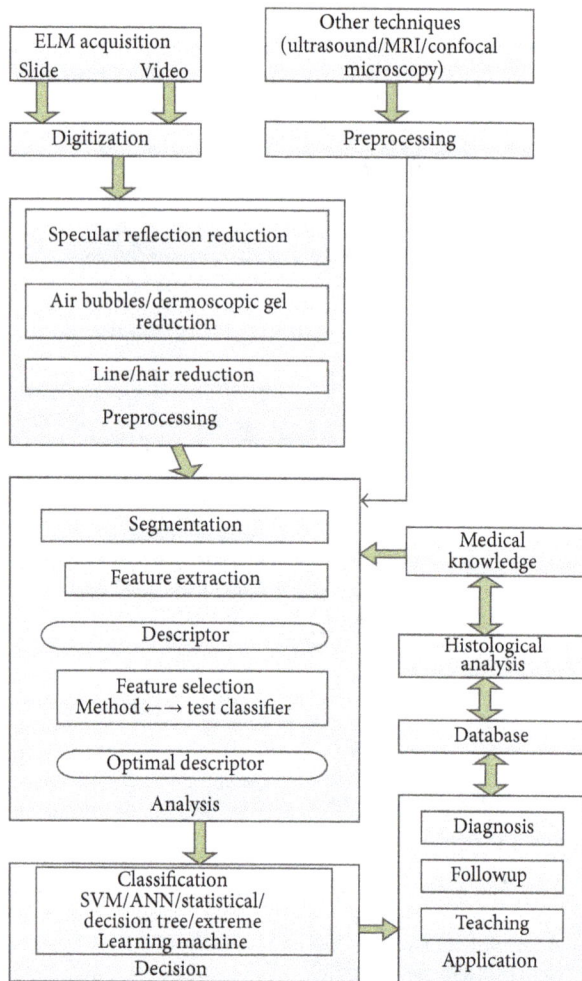

FIGURE 1: Computer aided diagnostic support system for skin cancer diagnosis.

skin. Sometimes simple ELM does not sufficiently increase the diagnostic accuracy in distinguishing pigmented Spitz nevus (PSNs) from melanoma. For obviating the problems of qualitative interpretation, methods based on the mathematical analysis of pigmented skin lesions (PSLs), such as digital dermoscopy analysis (DDA) and D-ELM, have been developed [53, 54]. The visual evaluation of the content of DDA is very complex. Efficient image processing techniques must therefore be developed to help physicians in making a diagnosis. The introduction of digital ELM and sophisticated image processing software has opened up a new horizon in the evaluation of cutaneous benign and malignant pigmented skin lesions (PSLs) as it enables the observation, storage, and objective evaluation of many parameters.

In this paper we have focussed on automatic diagnostic system based on digital dermoscopy images normally collected from different dermoscopy atlases [55, 56] or from dermatologists since it is the most widely used. However, we anticipate that multimodal systems that combine different imaging technologies will further improve the ability to detect melanoma at an earlier stage and reduce the trauma of dermatologic diagnosis.

2.2. Preprocessing. The main processing step towards a complete analysis of pigmented skin lesion is to differentiate the lesion from the healthy skin. Detection of the lesion is a difficult problem in dermatoscopic images as the transition between the lesion and the surrounding skin is smooth and even for trained dermatologist; it is a challenge to distinguish accurately. It has been observed that dermoscopy images often contain artifacts such as uneven illumination, dermoscopic gel, black frames, ink markings, rulers, air bubbles, and intrinsic cutaneous features that can affect border detection such as blood vessels, hairs, and skin lines and texture. These artifacts and extraneous elements complicate the border detection procedure, which results in a loss of accuracy as well as an increase in computational time. Thus, it requires some preprocessing steps to facilitate the segmentation process by the removal of unwanted objects or artifacts and colour space transformation.

Everything that might corrupt the image and consequently affect the results of image processing must be localized and then removed, masked, or replaced. Many approaches can be used that include image resizing, masking, cropping, hair removal (or attenuation), and conversion from RGB color to intensity grey image. It is done to reduce noise and the effect of reflection artifacts. It is meant to facilitate image segmentation by filtering the image and enhancing its important features.

The most straightforward way to remove these artifacts is to smooth the image using a general purpose filter such peer group filter (PGF) [57], mean filters, median filter [58–60], Gaussian filters [61, 62], or anisotropic diffusion filters (ADF). A major issue with these aforementioned filters is that these filters are originally formulated for scalar images. For vector images one can apply a scalar filter to each channel independently and then combine the results, a strategy referred to as marginal filtering. Despite being fast, this scheme introduces color artifacts in the output. An alternative solution is to use filters that treat the pixels as vectors [63]. Another noteworthy thing is setting mask size proportional to the image size to manage a tradeoff between smoothing of image and blurring of edges. Inspite of taking care of all the forementioned things, it is still not guaranteed to get an image free of all artifacts.

An alternative strategy for artifact removal is to use specialized methods for each artifact type. Many methods have been suggested; very few [64–66] discussed different aspects of artifacts together, but none of them have discussed all cases of artifacts. For this rationale, we have presented an overview of effective preprocessing methods, namely, color space transformation, color quantization, contrast enhancement, and artifact removal, which are being used for reducing all the possible ill effects present in the dermoscopic images.

Dermoscopy images are commonly acquired using a digital camera with a dermatoscope attachment. Due to the computational simplicity and convenience of scalar (single channel) processing, the resulting RGB (red-green-blue) color image is often converted to a scalar image using different methods like retaining only the blue channel as lesions are often more prominent in this channel or applying the luminance transformation or Karhunen-Loéve (KL) transformation and retaining the channel with the highest variance. Skin lesions come in a variety of colors but absolute colors are not very useful in segmenting images. Normally the analysis is based on changes in color within the lesion or with the surrounding skin particularly color changes belonging to the lesion boundary. Therefore, it is quite common to transform the images that are in RGB color coordinates into other color spaces like CIEL$^*a^*b^*$, CIEL$^*u^*v^*$, KL, and HSI (Hue-Saturation-Intensity).

Typical 24-bit color images have thousands of colors, which are difficult to handle directly. For this reason color quantization is commonly used as a preprocessing step for color image segmentation [67]. The process of color quantization consists of two-phases palette design (i.e., selection of a small set of colors that represents the original image colors) and pixel mapping (i.e., assignment of one of the palette colors to each input pixel). Celebi et al. [57] showed that, for skin lesion, the color quantization method should reduce the number of colors in image to 20 for getting precise quantization.

One of the factors that complicate the detection of borders in dermoscopy images is insufficient contrast. The contrast of image is enhanced to ensure that edges of the lesion are eminence. Gómez et al. [68] proposed a contrast enhancement method based on independent histogram pursuit (IHP). An easy, yet powerful way to enhance the image contrast is histogram stretching, a mapping of the pixel values onto [0, 255]. Another very popular technique is histogram equalization, which alters pixel values to achieve a uniform distribution. Homomorphic filtering [69], FFT, and high pass filter can be used to compensate for uneven illumination or specular reflection variations in order to obtain the high contrast lesion images.

For the removal of black frames produced in the digitization process, Celebi et al. [59, 70] proposed an iterative algorithm based on the lightness component of the HSL (Hue-Saturation-Lightness) color space. In order to remove air bubbles and dermoscopic gels, adaptive and recursive weighted median filter developed by Dehghani Tafti and Mirsadeghi [71] can be utilized. This type of median filters has an edge persevering capability. A method that can remove bubbles with bright edges was introduced in [72] where the authors utilized a morphological top-hat operator followed by a radial search procedure. Line detection procedure based on the 2D derivatives of Gaussian (DOG) [73] and exemplar-based object removal algorithm [74] can be used for removing dark lines like ruler marking. In most cases, image smoothing effectively removes the skin lines and blood vessels.

One of the most undesirable elements that are most commonly present in dermatoscopic images is hair. Lee et al. [75] and Schmid [76] used mathematical morphology. Fleming et al. [72] applied curvilinear structure detection with various constraints followed by gap filling. Erosion/dilation with straight line segments can efficiently eliminate (or at least weaken the effect of) hairs [77, 78]. Schmid et al. [79, 80] suggested a scheme based on a morphological closing operator, while in [81] they applied to the three components of the $L^*u^*v^*$ uniform color space [82]. Zhou et al. [83] and Wighton et al. [84]. proposed more sophisticated approaches

based on inpainting. However, it is being observed that most of these techniques often leave behind undesirable blurring; disturb the texture of the tumor; and result in color bleeding. Due to these problems, it is very difficult to use the color diffuse image for further skin tumor differentiation. In contrast, a new artifact removal algorithm that focuses on accurate detection of curvilinear artifacts and pays special attention to lesion structure during the removal stage has been introduced by Zhou et al. [85]. This approach effectively removes artifacts such as ruler markings and hair, but it has high computational requirements.

To address all these issues Abbas et al. [64] developed a novel method that automatically detects these visible artifacts and removes them. Abbas et al. [86] presented a comparative study about hair removal methods which indicate that hair-repairing algorithm based on the fast marching method achieves an accurate result.

All the above mentioned strategies are meant to facilitate the segmentation and feature extraction stages which consequently lead to better diagnostic results.

2.3. Segmentation. Segmentation refers to the partitioning of an image into disjoint regions that are homogeneous with respect to a chosen property such as luminance, color, and texture. The goal of segmentation is to simplify and/or change the representation of an image into something that is more meaningful and easier to analyse. Some researchers [87] argued that manual border detection is better than computer-detected borders in order to separate the problems of feature extraction from the problems of automated lesion border detection. However, for the development of automated diagnostic system for skin lesion detection, it is very important to develop automatic segmentation algorithms. As segmentation is a crucial early step in the analysis of lesion images, it has become one of the important areas of research and many algorithms and segmentation techniques are available in the literature. We have briefly provided an overview of various segmentation algorithms being used for dermoscopic image analysis as tabulated in Table 2.

Several comparative studies [59, 61, 66, 88, 89] are also present in the literature which provides performance analysis of several segmentation algorithms. There are several issues that should be kept in mind for selecting a suitable algorithm, for example, scalar versus vector processing, automatic versus semiautomatic, and the number of parameters whose values need to be determined a priori [65]. Interested readers may check relevant references to identify a suitable approach for a specific study.

2.4. Feature Extraction. Melanoma is visually difficult to differentiate from Clark nevus lesions which are benign. It is important to identify the most effective features to extract from melanoma, melanoma in situ and Clark nevus lesions, and to find the most effective pattern-classification criteria and algorithms for differentiating those lesions. Thus, the next stage of the image analysis process is to extract the important features of the image.

The purpose of feature extraction is to reduce the original data set by measuring certain properties, or features, that

TABLE 2: Methods for segmentation of dermoscopic images.

Method	Description	Related references
Thresholding	Determining threshold and then the pixels are divided into groups based on that criterion. It include bilevel and multithresholding	Histogram thresholding ([90, 91, 109, 110, 223, 224]) Adaptive thresholding ([61, 88, 111, 112, 124, 126, 200, 225])
Color-based segmentation algorithms	Segmentation based on color discrimination. Include principle component transform/spherical coordinate transform	[134, 226–230]
Discontinuity-based segmentation	Detection of lesion edges using active contours/radial search techniques/zero crossing of Laplacian of Gaussian (LoG)	Active contours ([58, 62, 64, 88, 231–233]) Radial search ([115, 234, 235]) LoG ([117, 163, 236, 237])
Region-based segmentation	Splitting the image into smaller components then merging subimages which are adjacent and similar in some sense. It includes Statistical region merging, multiscale region growing, and morphological flooding	Split and merge ([238, 239]) SRM ([59, 70, 92, 112]) Multi-scale ([118, 196]) Morphological flooding ([79])
Soft computing	Methods involve the classification of pixels using soft computing techniques including neural networks, fuzzy logic, and evolutionary computation	Fuzzy logic ([60, 76, 80, 85, 140, 157, 200, 240]) Neural Network ([177, 241]) Optimization algorithms ([241–243])

differentiate one input pattern from another. The feature extraction is performed by measurements on the pixels that represent a segmented object allowing various features to be computed. Unfortunately, the feature extraction step is often subject to error. In most of the publications dealing with this topic, many features are extracted to feed a sophisticated classifier, but there is very little discussion about the real meaning of those features and about objective ways to measure them. Thus, we investigate this topic in detail to come up with a guideline for future research.

Different feature extraction methods found in the literature include statistical and model-based and filtering-based methods, among which multichannel filtering is the most efficient and accurate one. Various researchers used principal component analysis (PCA) of a binary mask of the lesion, wavelet packet transform (WPT) [90–94], grey level cooccurrence matrix (GLCM) [61, 95], Fourier power spectrum [96], Gaussian derivative kernels [97], and decision boundary feature extraction [98–100] in order to reduce data redundancy. Some of the typically used filter banks are Laws masks, the dyadic Gabor filter bank, and wavelet transform [101]. A particular problem in the related literature is that a significant number of studies do not report the details of their feature extraction procedure; see Table 6.

The ABCD-E system [25, 26, 102], 7-point checklist [29, 103], 3-point checklist [104], pattern analysis [23], and Menzies method [105] offer alternative approaches in deciding the differentiating features that need to be extracted.

According to the conclusion made by Johr [28], the automatic extraction of characteristics that take into account the rule ABCD [25, 102, 106] is computationally less expensive than the ones that take into account 7-point checklist [29, 103] or the Menzies method [32, 107]. Furthermore, the reliability in the clinical diagnosis is very high for ABCD-E rule. So, most of the automated decision support systems

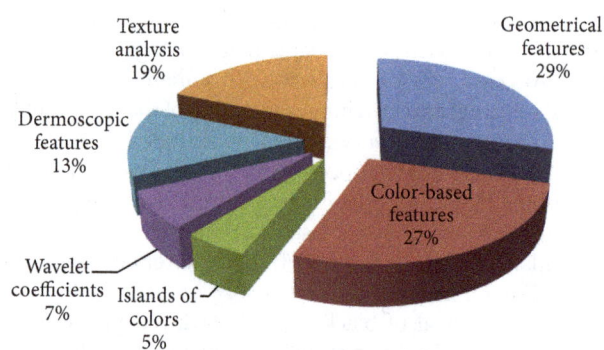

FIGURE 2: Illustration of feature distribution used in dermoscopic studies in the literature.

also use ABCD rule as the base of their feature extraction step. However, ABCD is more prone to over classification of atypical melanocytic nevi as melanomas. Dolianitis et al. [108] showed, in a comparative study, that Menzies method achieved the highest sensitivity, 84.6%, for the diagnosis of melanoma, followed by the 7-point checklist (81.4%), the ABCD rule (77.5%), pattern analysis (68.4%), and assessment of a macroscopic image (60.9%). Pattern analysis and assessment of the macroscopic image showed the highest specificity, 85.3% and 85.4%, respectively. So many researchers [109–114] are trying to develop efficient automatic diagnostic systems based on 7-point criteria and pattern analysis.

Numerous methods for extracting features from clinical skin lesion images have been proposed in the literature as Figure 2 illustrated the distribution of features used in dermoscopic studies. Several studies have also proven the efficiency of border shape descriptors for the detection of malignant melanoma on both clinical- and computer-based evaluation methods [115, 116]. Very simple parameters, such as area and perimeter, are extracted in [117–119]. Measurements of shape features are also used like fragmentation index [120–122], thinness ratio/circularity factor [61, 123–125] asymmetry index [77, 116, 122], aspect ratio [118, 126], compactness [118, 126], symmetry axis [127], bulkiness score [128], irregularity index [129, 130], fractality of borders [117], convex hull ratio [124], and skin line pattern [131]. Some groups use the sharpness of the transition from the lesion interior to the skin [61, 123, 125] as descriptors of the structure and irregularity of the border. Hall et al. [37] calculate fractal dimensions to represent border irregularity. Lacunarity [132] is another measure that can be used to characterize a property of fractals and quantifies aspects of patterns that exhibit changes in structure.

Color features are mainly statistical parameters calculated from different colour channels, like average value and standard deviation of the RGB [120–124] or HSV colour channels [125]. Other color features used in different studies include colour asymmetry [118], centroidal distance [118], and LUV histogram distance [118]. Cotton and Claridge [133] found that all normal skin colours lie on a two-dimensional surface patch within a three- dimensional (3D) colour space (CIE-LMS). Atypical skin structures result in colour coordinates that deviate from the normal surface patch. Some researchers [61, 117, 118, 134, 135] used GLCM-based texture features [136–138] like dissimilarity, contrast, energy, maximum probability, correlation, entropy, and so forth.

Parameters for the description of dermatoscopic structures and ELM criteria are difficult to find in the literature. Major issues are concerned with the difficulty in relating such information as lesion shape and color to medical structures (tissues, vessels, etc.) which experts are more familiar with. Some of the dermoscopic feature extraction studies include atypical pigment networks [72, 110, 139], globules/dots/blotches [72, 140–143], streaks [144], granularity [145], and blue-white veil [87, 146]. It is noteworthy that diagnostic systems based on extraction of critical high level features show an increase in the diagnostic accuracy of computerized dermoscopy image analysis systems. Thus, in addition to general features like area, border, shape, and color, these high level features should also be integrated in the automated diagnostic system to gain greater clinical acceptance.

Some researchers used some unique features for classification, but we know from skin cancer research that a unique feature is not sufficient to diagnose precisely skin cancer and that the combination of different criteria is the key to the early detection of malignant melanoma and other types of skin cancer. The evolution of competing dermoscopic algorithms with variable definitions of specific attributes complicates dermoscopic diagnosis. It is necessary to identify features that are the most reproducible and diagnostically significant and formulate them into a single algorithm.

2.5. Feature Selection. For clinical purposes, it is arguable that parsimony is a desirable feature of a good predictive model [147]. Similarly, features selection is a critical step for successfully distinguishing between malignant melanoma, benign, and dysplastic nevi. Many potential features may be used, but it is important to select a reasonable reduced number

of useful features while eliminating redundant, irrelevant, or noisy features. However, it is important to make sure that there may not be loss of significant information.

From the classification perspective, there are numerous potential benefits associated with feature selection: (i) reduced feature extraction time and storage requirements, (ii) reduced classifier complexity for better generalization behaviour, (iii) increased prediction accuracy, (iv) reduced training and testing times, and (v) enhanced data understanding and visualization.

There are many methods available for feature selection [148] which include principle component analysis [81] and search strategies like sequential forward selection (SFS) [149], sequential backward selection (SBS) [150], plus-l-take-away-r (PTA (l, r)), floating search methods [54, 151], sequential forward floating selection (SFFS), sequential backward floating selection (SBFS)) and Fisher score ranking [135]. All these algorithms use stepwise inclusions and exclusions of features into/from the subset of consideration, but they differ in their strategy of applying them. Although the floating methods are considered to be more intelligent, they are still suboptimal and even more there is no warranty that they yield better results.

In addition to these, some of the filter-based methods include Relief F [152], mutual information-based feature selection (MIFS) [153], and correlation-based feature selection (CFS) [154]. Filter methods are usually very fast and allow one to compare several alternative methods within an optimization framework. It is possible, and also desirable, to use clinical criteria or statistical methods to reduce the number of candidate variables, thus reducing the risk of an overoptimistic model [155].

A particular problem in the related literature is that there is very little number of studies that report the details of their feature selection procedure. Normally we do not find details of feature selection procedures that are used for choosing the appropriate features for skin cancer diagnosis. Handels et al. [156] described feature selection as an optimization problem and compared several approaches including heuristic strategies, greedy and genetic algorithms. Zagrouba and Barhoumi [157] proposed an accelerated system for melanoma diagnosis based on subset feature selection.

The number of features retained by the feature selection algorithm (*k*) is an important parameter. Sometimes a small number of features are not likely to discriminate between the classes well. On the other hand, a large number of features might lead to overfitting. Green et al. [121] showed by calculating correlation coefficients that the size of the lesion is the most important feature in their system. Roß et al. [158] perform a feature selection by the application of the sequential forward selection algorithm. They achieve a tremendous reduction to five features starting with 87 features calculated from surface profiles of skin lesions. Ganster et al. [159] used SBFS and SFFS and showed that the best selection performances were with subset size of between 10 to 15 and performance degrades with subsets size of more than 20 features. On the other hand by inspecting individual sensitivities on the malignant class of several subset sizes, it turns out that an acceptable performance is only achieved with subsets of more than 20 features. While Celebi et al. [118] showed by using CFS feature selection algorithm that AUC peaks can be obtained with the use of 18 features and inclusion of features beyond this value does not add much to the classifier performance.

Rohrer et al. [160] presented a study particularly based on feature selection for melanoma recognition and showed a strong increase in performance for small subsets followed by a slight increase up to medium sized subsets. Larger subsets cause a drop in the recognition rate. Ruiz et al. [126] also confirmed this thing in the evaluation done using SBFS and SFFS and showed that minimum error rate was observed using subset of 6 features and a significant increase in classification error rate is observed by using a subset of more than 20 features.

By inspecting the overall achieved performances one even could imagine that using 5 to 20 features is enough to get acceptable classification results. The aim of feature selection is to find the optimum number of features to obtain the best achievable performance (i.e., recognition rate) in classification. Therefore, the feature selection algorithms should be evaluated to get performance estimation on some standard classifier by applying tenfold cross-validation (XVAL), that is, repeating feature selection ten times with slightly different data for all algorithms.

2.6. Classification. Classification phase of the diagnostic system is the one in charge of making the inferences about the extracted information in the previous phases in order to be able to produce a diagnostic about the input image. There are two different approaches for the classification of dermoscopic images: the first considers only a dichotomous distinction between the two classes (melanoma and benign) and assigns class labels 0 or 1 to data item. The second attempts to model $P(y \mid x)$; this yields not only a class label for a data item, but also a probability of class membership. The most prominent representatives of the first approach are support vector machines. Logistic regression, artificial neural networks, k-nearest neighbours, and decision trees are all members of the second approach, although they vary considerably in building an approximation to $P(y \mid x)$ from data.

We do not intend in this paper to delve deeply into the technical aspects of all the classification algorithms. However, to make the reader analyse the performance of algorithms that are mostly used for dermoscopic image analysis, we believe that it is helpful to air them briefly. Readers who wish to have a detailed description of a specific classification approach should refer to cited references.

2.6.1. K-Nearest Neighbour Algorithm. The K-nearest neighbour classifier [161, 162] is a nonparametric method of pattern recognition. For a lesion belonging to the test set (query vector), it is found that the K vectors are the closest to the query vector in the training set. The unclassified sample is then assigned to the class represented by the majority of the K closest neighbours.

The most critical requirement of the K-nearest neighbour classifier is to have a training set including enough examples of each class of pigmented lesions to adequately represent the full range of measurements that can be expected from each class. Optimizing the procedures of feature selection and weight definition could additionally improve the performance of the K-nearest neighbour classifier [163].

In medicine, most applications use nearest-neighbour algorithms as benchmarks for other machine learning techniques [156, 164]. Classification based on the k-nearest neighbour algorithm differs from the other methods considered here, as this algorithm uses the data directly for classification, without building a model first [162, 165]. The only adjustable parameter in the model is k, the number of nearest neighbours to include in the estimate of class membership, and the value of $P(y \mid x)$ is calculated simply as the ratio of members of class y among the k-nearest neighbours of x. By varying k, the model can be made more or less flexible (small or large values of k, resp.). Generally, the choice of k can only be determined empirically.

K-NN algorithm permits retrieval and visualization of the "most similar" cases to those at hand. This aspect partly resembles the medical reasoning and allows a dermatologist to directly compare unknown lesions with other known skin lesions. This case-based explanation can provide an advantage in areas where black-box models are inadequate. It is well known that k-NN fails in case of irrelevant features. K-NN can also be used for the evaluation of feature subset selection process because it allows incorporating/eliminating characteristics easily and it has low computational cost.

The major drawback of k-nearest neighbour lies in the calculation of the case neighbourhood. Thus, it needs to define a metric that measures the distance between data items. In most application areas, it is not clear how to, other than by trial and error, define a metric in such a way that the relative (but unknown!) importance of data components is reflected in the metric [166].

2.6.2. Decision Trees. The decision tree approach belongs to the supervised machine learning techniques. It is popular for its simplicity in constructing, efficient use in decision making, and simple representation, which is easily understood by humans.

This algorithm repeatedly splits the data set according to a criterion that maximizes the separation of the data, resulting in a tree-like structure [167–171]. It does this by identifying a variable and a threshold in the domain of this variable that can be used to divide the data set into two groups. The best choice of variable and threshold is the one that minimizes the disparity measures in the resulting groups. The most common criterion employed is information gain; this means that at each split, the decrease in entropy due to this split is maximized. The estimate of $P(y \mid x)$ is the ratio of y class elements over all elements of the leaf node that contains data item x. Various modifications of decision trees like ADWAT and LMT are also used for dermoscopic image classification.

Advantages and disadvantages of decision trees in medicine have been widely investigated [172, 173]. The advantage of decision trees over many of the other methods is that they are not black-box models but can easily be expressed as rules. This makes them especially well-suited for medical applications. In many classification tasks decision

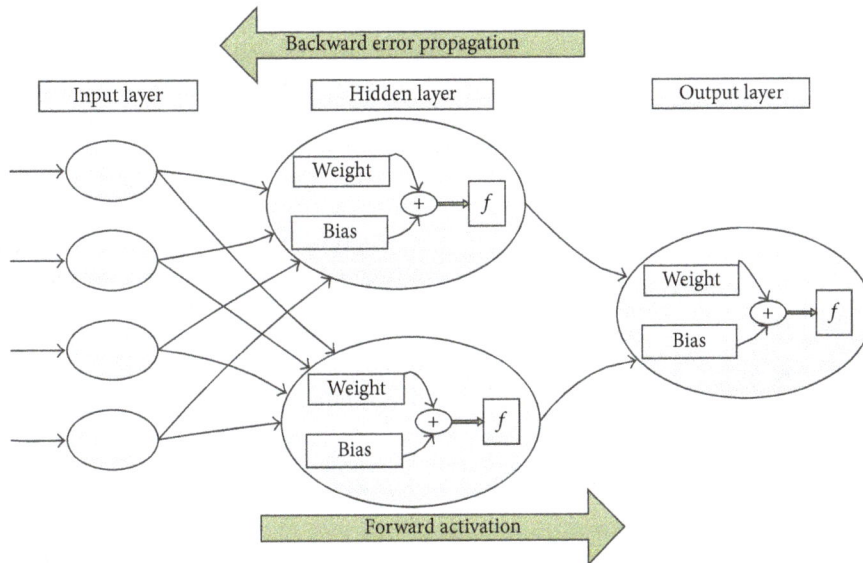

FIGURE 3: Working mechanism of artificial neural network.

tree classifiers have been preferred to other solutions (also including ANN and SVM) because they are often fast to train and apply and generate easy-to-understand rules.

A major disadvantage of decision trees is given by the greedy construction process. In this process at each step, the combination of single best variable and optimal split-point is selected. However, on the other hand if we use multistep look ahead, it considers combinations of variables which may obtain different (and better) results. Given a large training set, decision tree classifiers, in general, generate complex decision rules that perform well on the training data but do not generalize well to unseen data [174]. In such cases, the classifier model is said to have overfit the training data. A further drawback lies in the fact that continuous variables are implicitly discretised by the splitting process, losing information along the way.

2.6.3. Logistic Regression. Logistic regression is an algorithm that constructs a separating hyperplane between two data sets, using the logistic function to express distance from the hyperplane as a probability of class membership.

Although the model is linear in parameters and can thus only calculate linear decision boundaries, it is nevertheless a widely used predictive model in medical applications [155, 175, 176]. The main advantage that this method has over other algorithms is its ease of use (it is implemented in numerous software packages), allowing the interpretation of results as probabilities and variable-selection capability. Dreiseitl et al. [166] showed in a comparative study that logistic regression performs on about the same level as artificial neural networks and support vector machines, which are both capable of implementing nonlinear separating surfaces.

2.6.4. ANN. Artificial neural network [165, 177–180] is one of the great vital parts of soft computing. The ANN consists of several small processing units (the artificial neurons) that

are highly interconnected. Information flow in an ANN is modelled after the human brain. The supervise ANN is an iterative process which requires many presentations of the training set; the system is said to learn from examples. It has conspicuous capacity to obtain idea from complex data and is used to take out patterns and determine trends that are too difficult to be noticed by humans or any other computer skills. A lot of research is being carried out nowadays on dermoscopic image analysis using ANNs.

The general working mechanism for artificial neural network is presented in Figure 3. Many of the early implementations required a significant amount of parameter tuning to achieve satisfactory results, a process that needed too much time and expertise for a nonexpert. Over the past few years, statistically motivated Bayesian methods [181] and implementations of faster learning algorithms [182] have allowed nonexperts use to sophisticated methods that require little to no parameter tuning. Various neural networks-based clustering techniques and algorithms are being used in this regard [183] which include back propagation network (BPN), radial basis function network (RBF) and extreme learning machine (ELM).

2.6.5. Support Vector Machines. Support vector machines (SVMs) are a machine learning paradigm based on statistical learning theory [184, 185]. Performances on par with or exceeding that of other machine learning algorithms have been reported in the medical literature. Algorithmically, support vector machines build optimal separating boundaries between data sets by solving a constrained quadratic optimization problem [186]. While the basic training algorithm can only construct linear separators, different kernel functions (i.e., linear, polynomial, radial basis function, and sigmoid) can be used to include varying degrees of nonlinearity and flexibility in the model. The principle of support vector machine is shown in Figure 4.

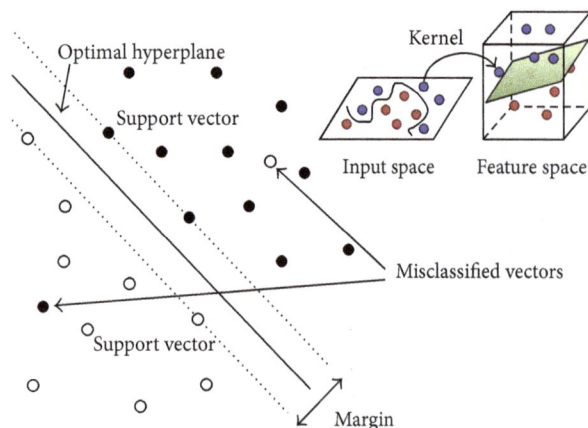

FIGURE 4: Principle of support vector machine.

SVMs have several advantages over the more classical classifiers such as decision trees and neural networks. The support vector training mainly involves optimization of a convex cost function. Therefore, there is no risk of getting stuck at local minima as in the case of back propagation neural networks. SVMs are based on the structural risk minimization (SRM) principle which minimizes the upper bound on the generalization error. Therefore, SVMs are less prone to overfitting when compared to algorithms such as back propagation neural networks that implement the ERM empirical risk minimization principle. Another advantage of SVMs is that they provide a unified framework in which different learning machine architectures (e.g., RBF networks and feed forward neural networks) can be generated through an appropriate choice of kernel [118]. The disadvantage of support vector machines is that the classification result is purely dichotomous, and no probability of class membership is given.

2.6.6. Extreme Learning Machine. Extreme learning machine is the feed forward network [187–189]. It consists of three layers which are similar to the other networks. The only difference is that the hidden elements can be independent from the training data and target functions. Because of this independence of hidden elements, this feed forward network provides better generalization performance and it can learn much faster as compared to the other conventional algorithms.

The important features of extreme learning machine are that even simple math is enough for it. It is a simple tuning-free three-step algorithm. The learning speed is extremely fast. Unlike the traditional classic gradient-based learning algorithms which often face several issues like local minima, improper learning rate, and overfitting. The extreme learning machine tends to reach the solutions straightforward without such trivial issues [190]. This learning algorithm looks much simpler than many other learning algorithms like neural networks and support vector machines.

There is very less work being done on the classification of dermoscopic images using extreme learning machine. Research work done on extreme learning machine shows

that extreme learning machine needs much less training time as compared to popular BP and SVM. The prediction accuracy of ELM is usually slightly better than BP [177] and close to SVM in many applications. Compared with BP and SVM, extreme learning machine can be implemented easily since there is no parameter to be tuned except an insensitive parameter L. It should be noted that many nonlinear activation functions can be used in extreme learning machine. Extreme learning machine needs more hidden nodes than BP but much less nodes than SVM. This implies that extreme learning machine and BP have much shorter response time to unknown data than SVM. So, this can be a good area to dig in for future research.

2.7. Evaluation of Classification Performance. Evaluation of classification results is an important process in the classification procedure. The papers propose that, for skin lesion classification, three different classification tasks should be used as benchmarks: the dichotomous problem for distinguishing common nevi from dysplastic nevi and melanoma, the dichotomous problem for distinguishing melanoma from common nevi and dysplastic nevi, and the trichotomous problem for correctly distinguishing all the three classes.

The two criteria to assess the quality of a classification model are discrimination and calibration. Discrimination is a measure of how well the two classes in the data set are separated and calibration is a measure of how close the predictions of a given model are to the real underlying probability based on expert knowledge. Some of the common measures of analysing discriminatory power of different methods are reported in this paper as can be noticed in Table 3.

Sensitivity and specificity are the most commonly used performance evaluation parameters in the literature. Accuracy can be used as a single parameter, but if there is imbalance between the classes (melanoma, benign), then accuracy is not a suitable approach of evaluation. A better performance measure in unbalanced domains is the receiver operating characteristic (ROC) curve. AUC is a statistically consistent and a more discriminatory measure than accuracy [191, 192]. The log diagnostic odds ratio is also sometimes used in meta-analyses of diagnostic test accuracy studies due to its simplicity (being approximately normally distributed). d_{class} is a measure to compare different classifiers presented by Sboner et al. [193] that enable giving a simple estimation of how useful one classifier is with respect to another. By using this parameter instead of accuracy, out the comparison between classifiers can be carried in an accurate but intuitive way, avoiding the unbalanced class problem.

To provide an unbiased estimate of a model's discrimination and calibration there are some important considerations like the effect of class imbalance, train/test ratio, and cross-validation. Several studies have demonstrated that the accuracy degradation on unbalanced data sets is more severe when the classes overlap significantly [190, 194, 195] which is the case in skin lesion classification. Most classifiers focus on learning the large classes which leads to poor classification accuracy for the small classes such as classifying the minority

TABLE 3: Measures for evaluating performance of a classifier.

Evaluation parameters

$$\text{Accuracy} = \frac{TP + TN}{TP + TN + FP + FN} \times 100\%$$

$$\text{Diagnostic accuracy} = \frac{TP}{TP + FP + FN}$$

$$\text{Sensitivity} = \frac{TP}{TP + FN} \times 100\%$$

$$\text{Specificity} = \frac{TN}{TN + FP} \times 100\%$$

ROC curve – a plot of the true positive TP-rate versus false positive FP-rate

$$\text{Positive predictive value} = \frac{TP}{TP + FP} \times 100\%$$

$$\text{Negative predictive value} = \frac{TN}{TN + FN} \times 100\%$$

$$\text{Error probability} = \frac{FP + FN}{TP + TN + FP + FN} \times 100\%$$

$$\text{Index of suspicion} = \frac{TP + FP}{TP + FN} \times 100\%$$

$$LR_+ = \frac{\text{Sensitivity}}{1 - \text{Specificity}}$$

$$LR_- = \frac{1 - \text{Sensitivity}}{\text{Specificity}}$$

Diagnostic odds ratio [191], $DOR = \dfrac{TP/FN}{FP/TN}$

Distance of a real classifier from the ideal one

$$d_{\text{class}} = \sqrt{(1 - Se)^2 + (1 - Sp)^2}$$

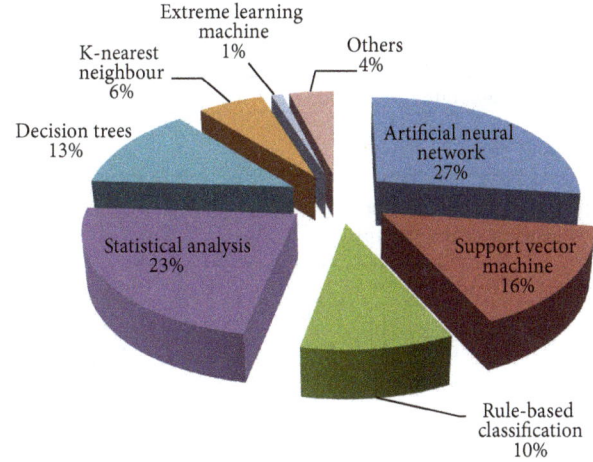

FIGURE 5: Illustration of classification methods as used by existing diagnostic systems.

for skin lesion case, but it has shown to be superior to cross-validation on many other data sets [199].

2.8. Selection of Suitable Classification Method. The increasing number of electronic data bases containing dermoscopic images has led to an increasing interest in their utilization for building classification models that can "learn" from examples. The need to use data and learning techniques in order to make correct diagnosis requires proper choice of the learning algorithms and of their statistical validation. The problem is difficult given the relative paucity of lesion data and consequently the low quality of training data available and the imbalance between the classes.

A variety of statistical and machine learning approaches are used for the classification of dermoscopic images. As illustrated in Table 4, while Figure 5 presents the percentage of classification methods as used by existing diagnostic systems in literature.

Different classification methods have their own merits. The question of which classification approach is suitable for a specific study is not easy to answer. Different classification results may be obtained depending on the classifier(s) chosen, differences in sample sizes, proportion of melanomas in the sample, and the number of features used for discrimination as can be notice in Table 5. Many factors, such as different sources of obtaining dermoscopic images, availability of classification software, time consumption, computational resources, and the number of melanoma and benign images available for training must be taken into account when selecting a classification method for use.

Very few researchers provided comparisons of different classification algorithms using the same set of images [46, 94, 126, 166, 196]. The review of all these comparative studies reveals that MLP gives better performance than Bayesian and kNN classifiers, while SVM with RBF kernel normally outperforms MLP, decision trees, and other statistical methods. The results of an experimental assessment of the different

(melanoma) samples as majority (benign) which implies serious consequences.

Train to test ratio is another important factor effecting the classification result. It has been observed [134] that as the training-set size increases, the results improve. The effect of train/test ratios on classification accuracy is studied in [196] and the best classification results were reached with 70/30 train to test ratio. We observed that over training may also lead to less accuracy.

There are two approaches for selecting training and test data: either to separate test and training feature vectors or pick training feature vectors as a subset of the test vectors. A classification result may be overly optimistic if performance cannot be measured on a data set not used for model building. In the ideal case, testing on a separate data set will provide an unbiased estimate of generalization error. If the original data set is too small for this approach, the recommended strategy is to use cross-validation [197] or bootstrapping [198] to make the best possible use of the limited amount of data. One way is to divide the whole data into n pieces, $n - 1$ pieces used for training, and the last piece as the test set. This process of n-fold cross-validation builds n models; the numbers reported are the averages over all n test sets. The extreme case of using only one data item for testing is known as leave-one-out cross-validation. Bootstrapping is rarely used in the literature

TABLE 4: Classification methods used in the literature for skin cancer diagnosis.

Classification method	Related references
K-nearest neighbour	[124, 126, 163, 166, 200]
Decision trees	[87, 110, 146, 166] ADWAT [93, 244], Logistic Model tree (LMT) [111, 112, 225], CART [46, 245]
Statistical (discriminant analysis/logistic regression/multifactorial analysis)	[80, 96, 120, 134, 141, 231, 246] DA [117, 121, 247, 248] mathematical classifier [249], logistic regression [38, 166, 236, 237, 239, 250] linear classifier [163]
Rule-based classification	[125, 223, 223, 251, 251–254]
Artificial neural network	[41, 90–92, 94, 126, 135, 140, 141, 157, 166, 177, 196, 209, 230, 246, 248, 254–258]
Support vector machine (SVM)	[40, 46, 61, 77, 91, 94, 118, 166, 196, 200, 259, 260]
Extreme learning machine	[177]
Others (Gaussian maximum likelihood, Bayesian classifier)	[46, 126, 200]

designs can be the basis for choosing one of the classifiers as a final solution to the problem.

It had been observed in such design studies that although one of the designs would yield the best performance, the sets of patterns misclassified by the different classifiers would not necessarily overlap. These observations motivated the relatively recent interest in combining classifiers. The idea is not to rely on a single decision making scheme. Instead, all the designs, or their subset, are used for decision making by combining their individual opinions to derive a consensus decision. Some classifier combination schemes have been devised [126, 193, 200] for dermoscopic images and it has been experimentally demonstrated that some of them consistently outperform a single best classifier. However, there is presently inadequate understanding why some combination schemes are better than others and in what circumstances.

3. Model Validation

A vast number of diagnostic algorithms/models are published each year. Such models do not always work well in practice, so it is widely recommended that they need to be validated [201, 202]. To be useful, a prognostic index should be clinically credible and accurate and have generality (i.e., be validated elsewhere), and the study should be described in adequate detail. To gauge the current state of reporting results in the literature, we sampled many papers on dermoscopic images data sets analysis.

We reviewed 31 publications which claimed fully automatic diagnostic models. We found frequent shortcomings both reporting and methodology used. The paper is proposing some criteria as quality assessment criteria which can be noticed in Table 6. It includes lack of calibration in image acquisition, unspecified method for extracting and selecting variables in the model, and risk of overfitting through too few events per variable. Many researchers did not specify the test/train or used uneven number of melanoma and benign images for training which may lead to biased classification. Some articles do not report comparisons and cross-validation; instead they just reported the performance of a single method. It is imperative that these details should be presented in papers as otherwise the validity of the claims in the papers cannot be assessed by the reader.

When assessing the quality of the results obtained using any diagnostic models, the work should consider the quality of the data set employed in model building, the care with which adjustable model parameters were chosen, and the evaluation criteria used to report the results of the modelling process. This is important in distinguishing between overly optimistic claims (such as when performance is reported on the training set) and needlessly pessimistic ones (when model parameters are chosen in a suboptimal manner). The latter is especially common in studies that promote "new" algorithms.

Apart from all this, in order to judge the performance of an automatic diagnostic model it is important to mention who is going to use that model. If automated diagnostic systems will be used by general practitioners or in pharmacies and shopping centres, these systems should be used with very high sensitivity and reasonably good specificity. That is, it should recognize the greatest number of melanomas in early stage, without misclassifying too many nevi so that unnecessary excision of benign lesions could be avoided.

If the target is the expert user, studies should be designed with the aim to help clinicians in distinguishing between benign lesions, dysplastic nevi, and malignant tumors of the skin. An increase in specificity might be the goal for an automated system directed to expert users together with sensitivity at least equal to that achieved by the expert.

Overall, our objective is to get a classifier with the sensibility and the specificity balanced. It should be noted that the ability to diagnose correctly melanoma is by far the most important property that an automated system must have. The consequence of failure to diagnose correctly a malignant tumor may lead to the eventual death of the patient. On the other hand, if we get a classifier with a high sensibility but a low specificity, it is not going to be useful as a screening method to avoid biopsies (an invasive technique). And, off course, we want a classifier with a high sensibility to avoid false negatives.

TABLE 5: Summary of classification performance of some skin cancer detection methods.

Source	year	No. of features selected	Classifier	Total images	Melanoma %	Dysplastic nevi %	Benign	Sens %	Spec %	Accuracy
[249]	1993		CART	353	62		38	94	88	
[49]	1994		CART	404	59		41	90	88	80
[121]	1994	22	D.A.	164	11		89	88	89	
[255]	1994		ANN	200	40	30	30	95	88	
[129]	1994	14	ANN	240 216	50 50	16.7	33.3 50	79.5 86	86.3 85.5	82.9 85.7
[261]	1997		Logistic regression	170	44		56	93	67	
[262]	1998	22	Discriminant analysis	917	7		93	93	95	
[257]	1998	16	ANN	120	32.5	48.4	27.5	90	74	
[263]	1999	26	Discriminant analysis	383	4.7		95.3	100	92	
[258]	1999	26	ANN	44	43.2		56.8	97.7	100	
[117]	1999	13	Discriminant analysis	147	38.8		61.2	88	81	85
[45]	2000	38	ANN	315	13.3		86.7	92.9	97.8	
[159]	2001	21	kNN	5363	1.8	18.8	79.4	87	92	
[211]	2001	13	Linear classification	246	25.6	45.1	29.2	100	85	
[41]	2002	13	ANN	588	36.9		63.1			94
[246]	2002	10	ANN	147	38.8		61.2	93	92.8	
[80]	2003	1	Linear classifier	100	50		50	78	90	
[193]	2003	38	LDA + kNN + decision tree	152	27.6		72.4	81	74	
[163]	2004	10	Linear classifier KNN	840	46.5		53.5	95 98	78 79	
[77]	2004		SVM (third degree polynomial)	977	5.12		94.88	96.4	87.16	
[40]	2005	NR	SVM	477	8.8		91.2	84	72	
[248]	2005	20	ANN Discriminant analysis	34	41	59		86 79	100 90	
[259]	2006	200	SVM	22	45		65			70
[87]	2006	28	Decision tree	224	51.8		48.2	51	97	
[237]	2006	3	LR+ multivariate model + ROC	132	17.4		82.6	60.9	95.4	89.4
[118]	2007	18	SVM	564	15.6		84.4	93.3	92.3	
[239]	2007	2	Logistic regression (LR)	260	17.7	18.1	64.2	91.3	81–91	
[200]	2008	10	Multiple classifiers (SVM, GML, kNN)	358	37.4	32.96	29.6			75.69
[124]	2011	33	kNN	83	55.4		44.6	60.7	80.5	66.7
[126]	2011	6	K-NN Bayesian Multilayered perceptron Combination of three	98	52		48	76.4 76.4 78.4 78.4	70.21 85.11 95.74 97.87	73.47 80.61 86.73 87.76
[135]	2012	12	Multilayer percentron	102	50		50	70.5	87.5	76

Concluding Comments

Our study gives an important contribution to this research area for several reasons. First, it is a study that combines the research being done related to all the steps needed for developing an automatic diagnostic system for skin cancer detection and classification. Second, it presents knowledge that help the researchers judge the importance of high level feature extraction and proper feature selection methods which needs more effort for making correct diagnosis of melanoma. Third, it proposed a frame work that highlights the importance of developing benchmarks and standard approaches for model validation which is generally overlooked in the previously published studies.

TABLE 6: Assessment of diagnostic models based on quality assessment criteria.

Criteria	Details Provided (% of models)	Details not Provided (% of models)
Image calibration	51	49
Preprocessing	45	55
Segmentation	78	22
Feature extraction	71	29
Feature selection	54	46
Test/train ratio	42	58
Taking care of balance in lesion classes for training	32	68
Comparative results	55	45
Cross-validation	29	71

Well-designed studies are needed to ascertain which design features and analysis procedures are likely to lead to a good model. At this time, there are no computers that can replace an experienced clinician's intuition. Nonetheless, logic dictates that with proficient training and programming, automated systems will eventually match, if not exceed, clinical diagnostic accuracy. The refinement of current approaches and development of new techniques will help in improving the ability to diagnose skin cancer and achieving our goal of significant reduction in melanoma mortality rate.

Conflict of Interests

The authors declare that there is no conflict of interests regarding the publication of this paper.

References

[1] R. Siegel, D. Naishadham, and A. Jemal, "Cancer statistics, 2012," *CA: Cancer Journal for Clinicians*, vol. 62, no. 1, pp. 10–29, 2012.

[2] R. Siegel, E. Ward, O. Brawley, and A. Jemal, "Cancer statistics, 2011: the impact of eliminating socioeconomic and racial disparities on premature cancer deaths," *CA: Cancer Journal for Clinicians*, vol. 61, no. 4, pp. 212–236, 2011.

[3] E. Linos, S. M. Swetter, M. G. Cockburn, G. A. Colditz, and C. A. Clarke, "Increasing burden of melanoma in the United States," *Journal of Investigative Dermatology*, vol. 129, no. 7, pp. 1666–1674, 2009.

[4] Society, A.C., "Cancer Facts & Figures 2012," 2012, http://www.cancer.org/acs/groups/content/epidemiologysurveilance/documents/document/acspc-031941.pdf.

[5] C.W.o. Australia, Ed., *Causes of Death 2010*, Australian Bureau of Statistics, Canberra, Australia.

[6] B. Lindelöf and M.-A. Hedblad, "Accuracy in the clinical diagnosis and pattern of malignant melanoma at a dermatological clinic," *The Journal of Dermatology*, vol. 21, no. 7, pp. 461–464, 1994.

[7] C. A. Morton and R. M. Mackie, "Clinical accuracy of the diagnosis of cutaneous malignant melanoma," *British Journal of Dermatology*, vol. 138, no. 2, pp. 283–287, 1998.

[8] G. Argenziano and H. P. Soyer, "Dermoscopy of pigmented skin lesions—a valuable tool for early diagnosis of melanoma," *The Lancet Oncology*, vol. 2, no. 7, pp. 443–449, 2001.

[9] S. W. Menzies, L. Bischof, H. Talbot et al., "The performance of SolarScan: an automated dermoscopy image analysis instrument for the diagnosis of primary melanoma," *Archives of Dermatology*, vol. 141, no. 11, pp. 1388–1396, 2005.

[10] M. Binder, M. Schwarz, A. Winkler et al., "Epiluminescence microscopy: a useful tool for the diagnosis of pigmented skin lesions for formally trained dermatologists," *Archives of Dermatology*, vol. 131, no. 3, pp. 286–291, 1995.

[11] H. Pehamberger, M. Binder, A. Steiner, and K. Wolff, "In vivo epiluminescence microscopy: improvement of early diagnosis of melanoma," *Journal of Investigative Dermatology*, vol. 100, no. 3, 1993.

[12] A. P. Dhawan, R. Gordon, and R. M. Rangayyan, "Nevoscopy: three-dimensional computed tomography of nevi and melanomas in situ by transillumination," *IEEE Transactions on Medical Imaging*, vol. 3, no. 2, pp. 54–61, 1984.

[13] G. Zouridakis, M. D. M. Duvic, and N. A. Mullani, "Transillumination imaging for early skin cancer detection," Tech. Rep. 2005, Biomedical Imaging Lab, Department of Computer Science, University of Houston, Houston, Tex, USA.

[14] M. E. Vestergaard, P. Macaskill, P. E. Holt, and S. W. Menzies, "Dermoscopy compared with naked eye examination for the diagnosis of primary melanoma: a meta-analysis of studies performed in a clinical setting," *British Journal of Dermatology*, vol. 159, no. 3, pp. 669–676, 2008.

[15] P. Carli, V. De Giorgi, E. Crocetti et al., "Improvement of malignant/benign ratio in excised melanocytic lesions in the "dermoscopy era": a retrospective study 1997–2001," *British Journal of Dermatology*, vol. 150, no. 4, pp. 687–692, 2004.

[16] P. Carli, V. De Giorgi, A. Chiarugi et al., "Addition of dermoscopy to conventional naked-eye examination in melanoma screening: a randomized study," *Journal of the American Academy of Dermatology*, vol. 50, no. 5, pp. 683–689, 2004.

[17] J. Mayer, "Systematic review of the diagnostic accuracy of dermatoscopy in detecting malignant melanoma," *Medical Journal of Australia*, vol. 167, no. 4, pp. 206–210, 1997.

[18] D. Piccolo, A. Ferrari, K. Peris, R. Daidone, B. Ruggeri, and S. Chimenti, "Dermoscopic diagnosis by a trained clinician vs. a clinician with minimal dermoscopy training vs. computer-aided diagnosis of 341 pigmented skin lesions: a comparative study," *British Journal of Dermatology*, vol. 147, no. 3, pp. 481–486, 2002.

[19] R. P. Braun, H. S. Rabinovitz, M. Oliviero, A. W. Kopf, and J.-H. Saurat, "Dermoscopy of pigmented skin lesions," *Journal of the American Academy of Dermatology*, vol. 52, no. 1, pp. 109–121, 2005.

[20] H. Kittler, H. Pehamberger, K. Wolff, and M. Binder, "Diagnostic accuracy of dermoscopy," *The Lancet Oncology*, vol. 3, no. 3, pp. 159–165, 2002.

[21] J. D. Whited and J. M. Grichnik, "Does this patient have a mole or a melanoma?" *The Journal of the American Medical Association*, vol. 279, no. 9, pp. 696–701, 1998.

[22] M. Burroni, R. Corona, G. Dell'Eva et al., "Melanoma computer-aided diagnosis: reliability and feasibility study," *Clinical Cancer Research*, vol. 10, no. 6, pp. 1881–1886, 2004.

[23] H. Pehamberger, A. Steiner, and K. Wolff, "In vivo epiluminescence microscopy of pigmented skin lesions. I. Pattern analysis of pigmented skin lesions," *Journal of the American Academy of Dermatology*, vol. 17, no. 4, pp. 571–583, 1987.

[24] A. Steiner, H. Pehamberger, and K. Wolff, "Improvement of the diagnostic accuracy in pigmented skin lesions by epilumines-cent light microscopy," *Anticancer Research*, vol. 7, no. 3B, pp. 433–434, 1987.

[25] F. Nachbar, W. Stolz, T. Merkle et al., "The ABCD rule of dermatoscopy," *Journal of the American Academy of Dermatology*, vol. 30, no. 4, pp. 551–559, 1994.

[26] N. R. Abbasi, H. M. Shaw, D. S. Rigel et al., "Early diagnosis of cutaneous melanoma: revisiting the ABCD criteria," *The Journal of the American Medical Association*, vol. 292, no. 22, pp. 2771–2776, 2004.

[27] J. K. Robinson and R. Turrisi, "Skills training to learn discrimination of ABCDE criteria by those at risk of developing melanoma," *Archives of Dermatology*, vol. 142, no. 4, pp. 447–452, 2006.

[28] R. H. Johr, "Dermoscopy: alternative melanocytic algorithms—the ABCD rule of dermatoscopy, menzies scoring method, and 7-point checklist," *Clinics in Dermatology*, vol. 20, no. 3, pp. 240–247, 2002.

[29] M. F. Healsmith, J. F. Bourke, J. E. Osborne, and R. A. C. Graham-Brown, "An evaluation of the revised seven-point checklist for the early diagnosis of cutaneous malignant melanoma," *British Journal of Dermatology*, vol. 130, no. 1, pp. 48–50, 1994.

[30] V. Dal Pozzo, C. Benelli, and E. Roscetti, "The seven features for melanoma: a new dermoscopic algorithm for the diagnosis of malignant melanoma," *European Journal of Dermatology*, vol. 9, no. 4, pp. 303–308, 1999.

[31] I. Zalaudek, G. Argenziano, H. P. Soyer et al., "Three-point checklist of dermoscopy: an open internet study," *British Journal of Dermatology*, vol. 154, no. 3, pp. 431–437, 2006.

[32] S. W. Menzies, C. Ingvar, K. A. Crotty, and W. H. McCarthy, "Frequency and morphologic characteristics of invasive melanomas lacking specific surface microscopic features," *Archives of Dermatology*, vol. 132, no. 10, pp. 1178–1182, 1996.

[33] M. E. Vestergaard and S. W. Menzies, "Automated diagnostic instruments for cutaneous melanoma," *Seminars in Cutaneous Medicine and Surgery*, vol. 27, no. 1, pp. 32–36, 2008.

[34] P. Carli, V. De Giorgi, L. Naldi et al., "Reliability and inter-observer agreement of dermoscopic diagnosis of melanoma and melanocytic naevi," *European Journal of Cancer Prevention*, vol. 7, no. 5, pp. 397–402, 1998.

[35] I. Stanganelli, M. Burroni, S. Rafanelli, and L. Bucchi, "Intraob-server agreement in interpretation of digital epiluminescence microscopy," *Journal of the American Academy of Dermatology*, vol. 33, no. 4, pp. 584–589, 1995.

[36] N. Cascinelli, M. Ferrario, T. Tonelli, and E. Leo, "A possible new tool for clinical diagnosis of melanoma: the computer," *Journal of the American Academy of Dermatology*, vol. 16, no. 2, pp. 361–367, 1987.

[37] P. N. Hall, E. Claridge, and J. D. M. Smith, "Computer screening for early detection of melanoma—is there a future?" *British Journal of Dermatology*, vol. 132, no. 3, pp. 325–338, 1995.

[38] M. Cristofolini, P. Bauer, S. Boi, P. Cristofolini, R. Micciolo, and M. C. Sicher, "Diagnosis of cutaneous melanoma: accuracy of a computerized image analysis system (Skin View)," *Skin Research and Technology*, vol. 3, no. 1, pp. 23–27, 1997.

[39] S. E. Umbaugh, *Computer Vision in Medicine: Color Metrics and Image Segmentation Methods for Skin Cancer Diagnosis*, Electrical Engineering Department, University of Missouri, Rolla, Mo, USA, 1990.

[40] I. Stanganelli, A. Brucale, L. Calori et al., "Computer-aided diagnosis of melanocytic lesions," *Anticancer Research*, vol. 25, no. 6, pp. 4577–4582, 2005.

[41] P. Rubegni, G. Cevenini, M. Burroni et al., "Automated diagno-sis of pigmented skin lesions," *International Journal of Cancer*, vol. 101, no. 6, pp. 576–580, 2002.

[42] A. J. Sober and J. M. Burstein, "Computerized digital image analysis: an aid for melanoma diagnosis—preliminary investi-gations and brief review," *The Journal of Dermatology*, vol. 21, no. 11, pp. 885–890, 1994.

[43] S. M. Rajpara, A. P. Botello, J. Townend, and A. D. Ormerod, "Systematic review of dermoscopy and digital dermoscopy/ artificial intelligence for the diagnosis of melanoma," *British Journal of Dermatology*, vol. 161, no. 3, pp. 591–604, 2009.

[44] B. Rosado, S. Menzies, A. Harbauer et al., "Accuracy of computer diagnosis of melanoma: a quantitative meta-analysis," *Archives of Dermatology*, vol. 139, no. 3, pp. 361–367, 2003.

[45] P. Bauer, P. Cristofolini, S. Boi et al., "Digital epiluminescence microscopy: usefulness in the differential diagnosis of cuta-neous pigmentary lesions. A statistical comparison between visual and computer inspection," *Melanoma Research*, vol. 10, no. 4, pp. 345–349, 2000.

[46] I. Maglogiannis and C. N. Doukas, "Overview of advanced computer vision systems for skin lesions characterization," *IEEE Transactions on Information Technology in Biomedicine*, vol. 13, no. 5, pp. 721–733, 2009.

[47] R. J. Friedman, D. Gutkowicz-Krusin, M. J. Farber et al., "The diagnostic performance of expert dermoscopists vs a computer-vision system on small-diameter melanomas," *Archives of Der-matology*, vol. 144, no. 4, pp. 476–482, 2008.

[48] A. Blum, I. Zalaudek, and G. Argenziano, "Digital image analysis for diagnosis of skin tumors," *Seminars in Cutaneous Medicine and Surgery*, vol. 27, no. 1, pp. 11–15, 2008.

[49] T. Schindewolf, R. Schiffner, W. Stolz, R. Albert, W. Abmayr, and H. Harms, "Evaluation of different image acquisition techniques for a computer vision system in the diagnosis of malignant melanoma," *Journal of the American Academy of Dermatology*, vol. 31, no. 1, pp. 33–41, 1994.

[50] A. A. Marghoob, L. D. Swindle, C. Z. M. Moricz et al., "Instru-ments and new technologies for the in vivo diagnosis of melanoma," *Journal of the American Academy of Dermatology*, vol. 49, no. 5, pp. 777–797, 2003.

[51] D. S. Rigel, J. Russak, and R. Friedman, "The evolution of melanoma diagnosis: 25 years beyond the ABCDs," *CA: Cancer Journal for Clinicians*, vol. 60, no. 5, pp. 301–316, 2010.

[52] E. L. Psaty and A. C. Halpern, "Current and emerging tech-nologies in melanoma diagnosis: the state of the art," *Clinics in Dermatology*, vol. 27, no. 1, pp. 35–45, 2009.

[53] M. Sasikala and N. Kumaravel, "Comparison of feature selection techniques for detection of malignant tumor in brain images," in *International Conference of IEEE India Council (INDICON '05)*, pp. 212–215, December 2005.

[54] S. Nakariyakul and D. P. Casasent, "Improved forward floating selection algorithm for feature subset selection," in *Interna-tional Conference on Wavelet Analysis and Pattern Recognition (ICWAPR '08)*, pp. 793–798, August 2008.

[55] G. Argenziano, G. S. H, and V. D. Giorgy, *Interactive Atlas of Dermoscopy. Dermoscopy Tutorial: Vascular Structures*, EDRA Medical Publishing & New Media, 2002.

[56] D. J. Eedy, "An atlas of surface microscopy of pigmented skin lesions: dermoscopy," *British Journal of Dermatology*, vol. 149, no. 5, pp. 1093–1093, 2003.

[57] M. E. Celebi, Y. A. Aslandogan, and P. R. Bergstresser, "Unsupervised border detection of skin lesion images," in *International Conference on Information Technology: Coding and Computing (ITCC '05)*, pp. 123–128, April 2005.

[58] M. Silveira and J. S. Marques, "Level set segmentation of dermoscopy images," in *Proceedings of the 5th IEEE International Symposium on Biomedical Imaging: From Nano to Macro (ISBI '08)*, pp. 173–176, May 2008.

[59] M. E. Celebi, H. A. Kingravi, J. Lee et al., "Fast and accurate border detection in dermoscopy images using statistical region merging," in *Medical Imaging 2007: Image Processing*, vol. 6512 of *Proceedings of SPIE*, February 2007.

[60] S. Sookpotharom, "Border detection of skin lesion images based on fuzzy C-means thresholding," in *Proceedings of the 3rd International Conference on Genetic and Evolutionary Computing (WGEC '09)*, pp. 777–780, October 2009.

[61] I. Maglogiannis, E. Zafiropoulos, and C. Kyranoudis, "Intelligent segmentation and classification of pigmented skin lesions in dermatological images," in *Advances in Artificial Intelligence*, G. Antoniou, G. A. Potamias, C. Spyropoulos, and D. Plexousakis, Eds., vol. 3955 of *Lecture Notes in Computer Science*, pp. 214–223, Springer, Berlin, Germany, 2006.

[62] B. Erkol, R. H. Moss, R. J. Stanley, W. V. Stoecker, and E. Hvatum, "Automatic lesion boundary detection in dermoscopy images using gradient vector flow snakes," *Skin Research and Technology*, vol. 11, no. 1, pp. 17–26, 2005.

[63] M. E. Celebi, H. A. Kingravi, and Y. A. Aslandogan, "Nonlinear vector filtering for impulsive noise removal from color images," *Journal of Electronic Imaging*, vol. 16, no. 3, Article ID 033008, 2007.

[64] Q. Abbas, I. Fondón, and M. Rashid, "Unsupervised skin lesions border detection via two-dimensional image analysis," *Computer Methods and Programs in Biomedicine*, vol. 104, no. 3, p. -e15, 2011.

[65] M. E. Celebi, H. Iyatomi, G. Schaefer, and W. V. Stoecker, "Lesion border detection in dermoscopy images," *Computerized Medical Imaging and Graphics*, vol. 33, no. 2, pp. 148–153, 2009.

[66] Q. Abbas, M. E. Celebi, I. Fondón García, and M. Rashid, "Lesion border detection in dermoscopy images using dynamic programming," *Skin Research and Technology*, vol. 17, no. 1, pp. 91–100, 2011.

[67] M. Celenk, "A color clustering technique for image segmentation," *Computer Vision, Graphics and Image Processing*, vol. 52, no. 2, pp. 145–170, 1990.

[68] D. D. Gómez, C. Butakoff, B. K. Ersbøll, and W. Stoecker, "Independent histogram pursuit for segmentation of skin lesions," *IEEE Transactions on Biomedical Engineering*, vol. 55, no. 1, pp. 157–161, 2008.

[69] H. G. Adelmann, "Butterworth equations for homomorphic filtering of images," *Computers in Biology and Medicine*, vol. 28, no. 2, pp. 169–181, 1998.

[70] M. E. Celebi, H. A. Kingravi, H. Iyatomi et al., "Border detection in dermoscopy images using statistical region merging," *Skin Research and Technology*, vol. 14, no. 3, pp. 347–353, 2008.

[71] A. Dehghani Tafti and E. Mirsadeghi, "A novel adaptive recursive median filter in image noise reduction based on using the entropy," in *Proceedings of the IEEE International Conference on Control System, Computing and Engineering (ICCSCE '12)*, pp. 520–523, November 2012.

[72] M. G. Fleming, C. Steger, J. Zhang et al., "Techniques for a structural analysis of dermatoscopic imagery," *Computerized Medical Imaging and Graphics*, vol. 22, no. 5, pp. 375–389, 1998.

[73] Q. Li, L. Zhang, J. You, D. Zhang, and P. Bhattacharya, "Dark line detection with line width extraction," in *Proceedings of the 15th IEEE International Conference on Image Processing (ICIP '08)*, pp. 621–624, October 2008.

[74] A. Criminisi, P. Pérez, and K. Toyama, "Region filling and object removal by exemplar-based image inpainting," *IEEE Transactions on Image Processing*, vol. 13, no. 9, pp. 1200–1212, 2004.

[75] T. Lee, V. Ng, R. Gallagher, A. Coldman, and D. McLean, "DullRazor: a software approach to hair removal from images," *Computers in Biology and Medicine*, vol. 27, no. 6, pp. 533–543, 1997.

[76] P. Schmid, "Segmentation of digitized dermatoscopic images by two-dimensional color clustering," *IEEE Transactions on Medical Imaging*, vol. 18, no. 2, pp. 164–171, 1999.

[77] M. D'Amico, M. Ferri, and I. Stanganelli, "Qualitative asymmetry measure for melanoma detection," in *Proceedings of the 2nd IEEE International Symposium on Biomedical Imaging: Macro to Nano*, pp. 1155–1158, April 2004.

[78] D. H. Chung and G. Sapiro, "Segmenting skin lesions with partial-differential-equations-based image processing algorithms," *IEEE Transactions on Medical Imaging*, vol. 19, no. 7, pp. 763–767, 2000.

[79] P. Schmid, "Lesion detection in dermatoscopic images using anisotropic diffusion and morphological flooding," in *Proceedings of the International Conference on Image Processing (ICIP '99)*, pp. 449–453, October 1999.

[80] P. Schmid-Saugeon, J. Guillod, and J.-P. Thiran, "Towards a computer-aided diagnosis system for pigmented skin lesions," *Computerized Medical Imaging and Graphics*, vol. 27, no. 1, pp. 65–78, 2003.

[81] R. C. Gonzalez and R. E. Woods, *Digital Image Processing*, Prentice Hall, Upper Saddle River, NJ, USA, 2nd edition, 2002.

[82] G. Wyszecki and G. S. W, *Color Science: Concepts and Methods, Quantitative Data and Formulae*, Wiley, New York, NY, USA, 1983.

[83] H. Zhou, M. Chen, R. Gass et al., "Feature-preserving artifact removal from dermoscopy images," in *Medical Imaging 2008: Image Processing*, vol. 6914 of *Proceedings of SPIE*, February 2008.

[84] P. Wighton, T. K. Lee, and M. S. Atkins, "Dermascopic hair disocclusion using inpainting," in *Medical Imaging 2008: Image Processing*, vol. 6914 of *Proceedings of SPIE*, February 2008.

[85] H. Zhou, G. Schaefer, A. H. Sadka, and M. E. Celebi, "Anisotropic mean shift based fuzzy C-means segmentation of dermoscopy images," *IEEE Journal on Selected Topics in Signal Processing*, vol. 3, no. 1, pp. 26–34, 2009.

[86] Q. Abbas, M. E. Celebi, and I. F. García, "Hair removal methods: a comparative study for dermoscopy images," *Biomedical Signal Processing and Control*, vol. 6, no. 4, pp. 395–404, 2011.

[87] M. E. Celebi, H. A. Kingravi, Y. A. Aslandogan, and W. V. Stoecker, "Detection of blue-white veil areas in dermoscopy images using machine learning techniques," in *Medical Imaging 2006: Image Processing*, vol. 6144 of *Proceedings of SPIE*, February 2006.

[88] T. Mendonca, A. R. S. Marcal, A. Vieira et al., "Comparison of segmentation methods for automatic diagnosis of dermoscopy images," in *Proceedings of the 29th Annual International Conference of the IEEE Engineering in Medicine and Biology Society (EMBS '07)*, pp. 6573–6576, 2007.

[89] M. Silveira, J. C. Nascimento, J. S. Marques et al., "Comparison of segmentation methods for melanoma diagnosis in

dermoscopy images," *IEEE Journal on Selected Topics in Signal Processing*, vol. 3, no. 1, pp. 35–45, 2009.

[90] J. Sikorski, "Identification of malignant melanoma by wavelet analysis," in *Proceedings of Student/Faculty Research Day*, Pace University, 2004.

[91] A. Chiem, A. Al-Jumaily, and R. N. Khushaba, "A novel hybrid system for skin lesion detection," in *Proceedings of the 3rd International Conference on Intelligent Sensors, Sensor Networks and Information Processing (ISSNIP '07)*, pp. 567–572, December 2007.

[92] M. K. A. Mahmoud, A. Al-Jumaily, and M. Takruri, "The automatic identification of melanoma by wavelet and curvelet analysis: study based on neural network classification," in *Proceedings of the 11th International Conference on Hybrid Intelligent Systems (HIS '11)*, pp. 680–685, December 2011.

[93] S. V. Patwardhan, A. P. Dhawan, and P. A. Relue, "Classification of melanoma using tree structured wavelet transforms," *Computer Methods and Programs in Biomedicine*, vol. 72, no. 3, pp. 223–239, 2003.

[94] G. Surowka and K. Grzesiak-Kopec, "Different learning paradigms for the classification of melanoid skin lesions using wavelets. in," in *Proceedings of the 29th Annual International Conference of the IEEE Engineering in Medicine and Biology Society (EMBS '07)*, pp. 3136–3139, 2007.

[95] "The GLCM Tutorial," http://www.fp.ucalgary.ca/mhallbey/tutorial.htm.

[96] T. Tanaka, S. Torii, I. Kabuta, K. Shimizu, M. Tanaka, and H. Oka, "Pattern classification of nevus with texture analysis," in *Proceedings of the 26th Annual International Conference of the IEEE Engineering in Medicine and Biology Society (EMBC '04)*, pp. 1459–1462, September 2004.

[97] H. Zhou, M. Chen, and J. M. Rehg, "Dermoscopic interest point detector and descriptor," in *Proceedings of the 6th IEEE International Symposium on Biomedical Imaging: From Nano to Macro (ISBI '09)*, pp. 1318–1321, July 2009.

[98] C. Lee and D. A. Landgrebe, "Decision boundary feature extraction for neural networks," *IEEE Transactions on Neural Networks*, vol. 8, no. 1, pp. 75–83, 1997.

[99] C. Lee and D. A. Landgrebe, "Decision boundary feature extraction for nonparametric classification," *IEEE Transactions on Systems, Man and Cybernetics*, vol. 23, no. 2, pp. 433–444, 1993.

[100] C. Lee and D. A. Landgrebe, "Feature extraction based on decision boundaries," *IEEE Transactions on Pattern Analysis and Machine Intelligence*, vol. 15, no. 4, pp. 388–400, 1993.

[101] X. Yuan, J. Zhang, X. Yuan, and B. P. Buckles, "Multi-scale feature identification using evolution strategies," *Image and Vision Computing*, vol. 23, no. 6, pp. 555–563, 2005.

[102] H. Kittler, M. Seltenheim, M. Dawid, H. Pehamberger, K. Wolff, and M. Binder, "Morphologic changes of pigmented skin lesions: a useful extension of the ABCD rule for dermatoscopy," *Journal of the American Academy of Dermatology*, vol. 40, no. 4, pp. 558–562, 1999.

[103] M. Keefe, D. C. Dick, and R. A. Wakeel, "A study of the value of the seven-point checklist in distinguishing benign pigmented lesions from melanoma," *Clinical and Experimental Dermatology*, vol. 15, no. 3, pp. 167–171, 1990.

[104] H. P. Soyer, G. Argenziano, I. Zalaudek et al., "Three-point checklist of dermoscopy: a new screening method for early detection of melanoma," *Dermatology*, vol. 208, no. 1, pp. 27–31, 2004.

[105] S. W. Menzies, K. Crotty, C. Ingvar, and W. McCarthy, *An Atlas of Surface Microscopy of Pigmented Skin Lesions*, McGraw Hill, New York, NY, USA, 1995.

[106] R. J. Friedman and D. S. Rigel, "The clinical features of malignant melanoma," *Dermatologic Clinics*, vol. 3, no. 2, pp. 271–283, 1985.

[107] S. W. Menzies, K. A. Crotty, and W. H. McCarthy, "The morphologic criteria of the pseudopod in surface microscopy," *Archives of Dermatology*, vol. 131, no. 4, pp. 436–440, 1995.

[108] C. Dolianitis, J. Kelly, R. Wolfe, and P. Simpson, "Comparative performance of 4 dermoscopic algorithms by nonexperts for the diagnosis of melanocytic lesions," *Archives of Dermatology*, vol. 141, no. 8, pp. 1008–1014, 2005.

[109] G. Betta, G. Di Leo, G. Fabbrocini, A. Paolillo, and M. Scalvenzi, "Automated application of the "7-point checklist" diagnosis method for skin lesions: estimation of chromatic and shape parameters," in *Proceedings of the IEEE Instrumentation and Measurement Technology Conference (IMTC '05)*, pp. 1818–1822, May 2005.

[110] G. Di Leo, C. Liguori, A. Paolillo, and P. Sommella, "An improved procedure for the automatic detection of dermoscopic structures in digital ELM images of skin lesions," in *Proceedings of the IEEE International Conference on Virtual Environments, Human-Computer Interfaces, and Measurement Systems (VECIMS '08)*, pp. 190–195, July 2008.

[111] G. Di Leo, A. Paolillo, P. Sommella, and G. Fabbrocini, "Automatic diagnosis of melanoma: a software system based on the 7-point check-list," in *Proceedings of the 43rd Annual Hawaii International Conference on System Sciences (HICSS '10)*, January 2010.

[112] V. De Vita, G. L. Di Leo, G. Fabbrocini, C. Liguori, A. Paolillo, and P. Sommella, "Statistical techniques applied to the automatic diagnosis of dermoscopic images," *ACTA IMEKO*, vol. 1, no. 1, pp. 7–18, 2012.

[113] G. Betta, G. Di Leo, G. Fabbrocini, A. Paolillo, and P. Sommella, "Dermoscopic image-analysis system: estimation of atypical pigment network and atypical vascular pattern," in *Proceedings IEEE International Workshop on Medical Measurement and Applications (MeMeA '06)*, pp. 63–67, April 2006.

[114] G. Fabbrocini, G. Betta, G. Di Leo et al., "Epiluminescence image processing for melanocytic skin lesion diagnosis based on 7-point check-list: a preliminary discussion on three parameters," *The Open Dermatology Journal*, vol. 4, pp. 110–115, 2010.

[115] J. E. Golston, W. V. Stoecker, R. H. Moss, and I. P. S. Dhillon, "Automatic detection of irregular borders in melanoma and other skin tumors," *Computerized Medical Imaging and Graphics*, vol. 16, no. 3, pp. 199–203, 1992.

[116] W. V. Stoecker, W. W. Li, and R. H. Moss, "Automatic detection of asymmetry in skin tumors," *Computerized Medical Imaging and Graphics*, vol. 16, no. 3, pp. 191–197, 1992.

[117] L. Andreassi, R. Perotti, P. Rubegni et al., "Digital dermoscopy analysis for the differentiation of atypical nevi and early melanoma: a new quantitative semiology," *Archives of Dermatology*, vol. 135, no. 12, pp. 1459–1465, 1999.

[118] M. E. Celebi, H. A. Kingravi, B. Uddin et al., "A methodological approach to the classification of dermoscopy images," *Computerized Medical Imaging and Graphics*, vol. 31, no. 6, pp. 362–373, 2007.

[119] H. Ganster, M. Gelautz, A. Pinz et al., "Initial results of automated melanoma recognition," in *Proceedings of the 9th Scandinavian Conference on Image Analysis*, Swedish Society for Automated Image Analysis, Uppsala, Sweden, 1995.

[120] J. F. Aitken, J. Pfitzner, D. Battistutta, O. 'Rourke PK, A. C. Green, and N. G. Martin, "Reliability of computer image analysis of pigmented skin lesions of Australian adolescents," *Journal of Cancer*, vol. 78, no. 2, pp. 252–257, 1996.

[121] A. Green, N. Martin, J. Pfitzner, M. O'Rourke, and N. Knight, "Computer image analysis in the diagnosis of melanoma," *Journal of the American Academy of Dermatology*, vol. 31, no. 6, pp. 958–964, 1994.

[122] H. C. Lee, *Skin Cancer Diagnosis Using Hierarchical Neural Networks and Fuzzy Logic*, Department of Computer Science, University of Missouri, Rolla, Mo, USA, 1994.

[123] S. Seidenari, M. Burroni, G. Dell'Eva, P. Pepe, and B. Belletti, "Computerized evaluation of pigmented skin lesion images recorded by a videomicroscope: comparison between polarizing mode observation and oil/slide mode observation," *Skin Research and Technology*, vol. 1, no. 4, pp. 187–191, 1995.

[124] K. Ramlakhan and Y. Shang, "A mobile automated skin lesion classification system," in *Proceedings of the 23rd IEEE International Conference on Tools with Artificial Intelligence (ICTAI '11)*, pp. 138–141, November 2011.

[125] N. Cascinelli, M. Ferrario, R. Bufalino et al., "Results obtained by using a computerized image analysis system designed as an aid to diagnosis of cutaneous melanoma," *Melanoma Research*, vol. 2, no. 3, pp. 163–170, 1992.

[126] D. Ruiz, V. Berenguer, A. Soriano, and B. Sánchez, "A decision support system for the diagnosis of melanoma: a comparative approach," *Expert Systems with Applications*, vol. 38, no. 12, pp. 15217–15223, 2011.

[127] P. Schmid-Saugeon, "Symmetry axis computation for almost-symmetrical and asymmetrical objects: application to pigmented skin lesions," *Medical Image Analysis*, vol. 4, no. 3, pp. 269–282, 2000.

[128] E. Claridge, P. N. Hall, M. Keefe, and J. P. Allen, "Shape analysis for classification of malignant melanoma," *Journal of Biomedical Engineering*, vol. 14, no. 3, pp. 229–234, 1992.

[129] F. Ercal, A. Chawla, W. V. Stoecker, H.-C. Lee, and R. H. Moss, "Neural network diagnosis of malignant melanoma from color images," *IEEE Transactions on Biomedical Engineering*, vol. 41, no. 9, pp. 837–845, 1994.

[130] T. K. Lee, D. I. McLean, and M. S. Atkins, "Irregularity index: a new border irregularity measure for cutaneous melanocytic lesions," *Medical Image Analysis*, vol. 7, no. 1, pp. 47–64, 2003.

[131] Z. She and P. Fish, "Analysis of skin line pattern for lesion classification," *Skin Research and Technology*, vol. 9, no. 1, pp. 73–80, 2003.

[132] S. Gilmore, R. Hofmann-Wellenhof, J. Muir, and H. P. Soyer, "Lacunarity analysis: a promising method for the automated assessment of melanocytic naevi and melanoma," *PloS ONE*, vol. 4, no. 10, Article ID e7449, 2009.

[133] S. D. Cotton and E. Claridge, "Developing a predictive model of human skin coloring," in *Medical Imaging 1996: Physics of Medical Imaging*, vol. 2708 of *Proceedings of SPIE*, pp. 814–825, February 1996.

[134] N. Dawei, "Classification of melanoma and clark nevus skin lesions based on Medical Image Processing Techniques," in *Proceedings of the 3rd International Conference on Computer Research and Development (ICCRD '11)*, pp. 31–34, March 2011.

[135] M. S. Mabrouk, M. A. Sheha, and A. Sharawy, "Automatic detection of melanoma skin cancer using texture analysis," *International Journal of Computer Applications*, vol. 42, no. 20, pp. 22–26, 2012.

[136] J. R. J. Kontinen and R. M. MacKie, "Texture features in the classification of melanocytic lesions," in *Proceedings of the 9th International Conference on Image Analysis and Processing (ICIAP '97)*, Springer, Florence, Italy, 1997.

[137] R. M. Haralick, K. Shanmugam, and I. Dinstein, "Textural features for image classification," *IEEE Transactions on Systems, Man and Cybernetics*, vol. 3, no. 6, pp. 610–621, 1973.

[138] D. A. Clausi, "An analysis of co-occurrence texture statistics as a function of grey level quantization," *Canadian Journal of Remote Sensing*, vol. 28, no. 1, pp. 45–62, 2002.

[139] B. Shrestha, J. Bishop, K. Kam et al., "Detection of atypical texture features in early malignant melanoma," *Skin Research and Technology*, vol. 16, no. 1, pp. 60–65, 2010.

[140] A. Khan, K. Gupta, R. J. Stanley et al., "Fuzzy logic techniques for blotch feature evaluation in dermoscopy images," *Computerized Medical Imaging and Graphics*, vol. 33, no. 1, pp. 50–57, 2009.

[141] W. V. Stoecker, K. Gupta, R. J. Stanley, R. H. Moss, and B. Shrestha, "Detection of asymmetric blotches (asymmetric structureless areas) in dermoscopy images of malignant melanoma using relative color," *Skin Research and Technology*, vol. 11, no. 3, pp. 179–184, 2005.

[142] G. Pellacani, C. Grana, R. Cucchiara, and S. Seidenari, "Automated extraction and description of dark areas in surface microscopy melanocytic lesion images," *Dermatology*, vol. 208, no. 1, pp. 21–26, 2004.

[143] S. O. Skrøvseth, T. R. Schopf, K. Thon et al., "A computer aided diagnostic system for malignant melanomas," in *Proceedings of the 3rd International Symposium on Applied Sciences in Biomedical and Communication Technologies (ISABEL '10)*, November 2010.

[144] H. Mirzaalian, T. K. Lee, and G. Hamarneh, "Learning features for streak detection in dermoscopic color images using localized radial flux of principal intensity curvature," in *Proceedings of the IEEE Workshop on Mathematical Methods in Biomedical Image Analysis (MMBIA '12)*, pp. 97–101, January 2012.

[145] W. V. Stoecker, M. Wronkiewiecz, R. Chowdhury et al., "Detection of granularity in dermoscopy images of malignant melanoma using color and texture features," *Computerized Medical Imaging and Graphics*, vol. 35, no. 2, pp. 144–147, 2011.

[146] M. E. Celebi, H. Iyatomi, W. V. Stoecker et al., "Automatic detection of blue-white veil and related structures in dermoscopy images," *Computerized Medical Imaging and Graphics*, vol. 32, no. 8, pp. 670–677, 2008.

[147] W. Sauerbrei, "The use of resampling methods to simplify regression models in medical statistics," *Journal of the Royal Statistical Society. Series C*, vol. 48, no. 3, pp. 313–329, 1999.

[148] I. Guyon, S. Gunn, M. Nikravesh, and L. A. Zadeh, Eds., *Feature Extraction: Foundations and Applications*, Springer, Dordrecht, The Netherlands, 2006.

[149] A. W. Whitney, "A direct method of nonparametric measurement selection," *IEEE Transactions on Computers*, vol. 20, no. 9, pp. 1100–1103, 1971.

[150] T. G. D. Marill, "On the effectiveness of receptors in recognition systems," *IEEE Transactions on Information Theory*, vol. 9, no. 1, pp. 11–17, 1963.

[151] P. Pudil, J. Novovičová, and J. Kittler, "Floating search methods in feature selection," *Pattern Recognition Letters*, vol. 15, no. 11, pp. 1119–1125, 1994.

[152] I. Kononenko, E. Simec, and I. K. Edvard, "Induction of decision trees using RELIEFF," in *CISM Courses and Lectures No. 363,*

G. Della Riccia, R. Kruse, and R. Viertl, Eds., Heidelberg, Germany, 1994.

[153] R. Battiti, "Using mutual information for selecting features in supervised neural net learning," *IEEE Transactions on Neural Networks*, vol. 5, no. 4, pp. 537–550, 1994.

[154] M. A. Hall, *Correlation-Based Feature Selection for Machine Learning*, University of Waikato, 1999.

[155] F. E. Harrell Jr. and K. L. Lee, "Regression modelling strategies for improved prognostic prediction," *Statistics in Medicine*, vol. 3, no. 2, pp. 143–152, 1984.

[156] H. Handels, T. Roß, J. Kreusch, H. H. Wolff, and S. J. Pöppl, "Feature selection for optimized skin tumor recognition using genetic algorithms," *Artificial Intelligence in Medicine*, vol. 16, no. 3, pp. 283–297, 1999.

[157] E. Zagrouba and W. Barhoumi, "An accelerated system for melanoma diagnosis based on subset feature selection," *Journal of Computing and Information Technology*, vol. 13, no. 1, pp. 69–82, 2005.

[158] Th. Roß, H. Handels, J. Kreusch, H. Busche, H. H. Wolf, and S. J. Pöppl, "Automatic classification of skin tumours with high resolution surface profiles," in *Proceeding of the 6th International Conference on Computer Analysis of Images and Patterns*, vol. 970 of *Lecture Notes in Computer Science*, pp. 368–375, Springer, Berlin, Germany, 1995.

[159] H. Ganster, A. Pinz, R. Röhrer, E. Wildling, M. Binder, and H. Kittler, "Automated melanoma recognition," *IEEE Transactions on Medical Imaging*, vol. 20, no. 3, pp. 233–239, 2001.

[160] R. Rohrer, H. Ganster, A. Pinz, and M. Binder, "Feature selection in melanoma recognition," in *Proceedings of the 14th International Conference on Pattern Recognition*, vol. 2, pp. 1668–1670, 1998.

[161] T. Cover and P. Hart, "Nearest neighbor pattern classification," *IEEE Transactions on Information Theory*, vol. 13, no. 1, pp. 21–27, 1967.

[162] B. V. Dasarathy, *Nearest Neighbor (NN) Norms: NN Pattern Classification Techniques*, 1991.

[163] M. Burroni, R. Corona, G. Dell'Eva et al., "Melanoma computeraided diagnosis: reliability and feasibility study," *Clinical Cancer Research*, vol. 10, no. 6, pp. 1881–1886, 2004.

[164] E. A. El-Kwae, J. E. Fishman, M. J. Bianchi, P. M. Pattany, and M. R. Kabuka, "Detection of suspected malignant patterns in three-dimensional magnetic resonance breast images," *Journal of Digital Imaging*, vol. 11, no. 2, pp. 83–93, 1998.

[165] B. D. Ripley, *Pattern Recognition and Neural Networks*, Cambridge University Press, Cambridge, UK, 1996.

[166] S. Dreiseitl, L. Ohno-Machado, H. Kittler, S. Vinterbo, H. Billhardt, and M. Binder, "A comparison of machine learning methods for the diagnosis of pigmented skin lesions," *Journal of Biomedical Informatics*, vol. 34, no. 1, pp. 28–36, 2001.

[167] J. R. Quinlan, *C4.5: Programs for Machine Learning*, Morgan Kaufmann, Los Altos, Calif, USA, 1993.

[168] J. Gehrke, "Classification and regression trees," in *Encyclopedia of Data Warehousing and Mining*, pp. 192–195, IGI Global, 2nd edition, 2009.

[169] W.-Y. Loh, "Classification and regression trees." *Wiley Interdisciplinary Reviews: Data Mining and Knowledge Discovery*, vol. 1, no. 1, pp. 14–23, 2011.

[170] N. Speybroeck, "Classification and regression trees," *International Journal of Public Health*, vol. 57, no. 1, pp. 243–246, 2012.

[171] X. Wu and V. Kumar, "CART: classification and regression trees," in *The Top Ten Algorithms in Data Mining*, pp. 179–203, CRC Press, Boca Raton, Fla, USA, 2009.

[172] M. Zorman, M. M. Štiglic, P. Kokol, and I. Malčić, "The limitations of decision trees and automatic learning in real world medical decision making," *Journal of Medical Systems*, vol. 21, no. 6, pp. 403–415, 1997.

[173] D. E. Clark, "Computational methods for probabilistic decision trees," *Computers and Biomedical Research*, vol. 30, no. 1, pp. 19–33, 1997.

[174] T. Oates and D. Jensen, "Large datasets lead to overly complex models: an explanation and a solution," in *Proceedings of the of the 4th International Conference on Knowledge Discovery and Data Mining*, AAAI Press, New York, NY, USA, 1998.

[175] D. J. Spiegelhalter, "Probabilistic prediction in patient management and clinical trials," *Statistics in Medicine*, vol. 5, no. 5, pp. 421–433, 1986.

[176] D. Altman, *Practical Statistics for Medical Research*, Chapman & Hall, London, UK, 1991.

[177] G. S. Vennila, L. P. Suresh, and K. L. Shunmuganathan, "Dermoscopic image segmentation and classification using machine learning algorithms," in *Proceedings of the International Conference on Computing, Electronics and Electrical Technologies (ICCEET '12)*, 2012.

[178] S. S. Cross, R. F. Harrison, and R. L. Kennedy, "Introduction to neural networks," *The Lancet*, vol. 346, no. 8982, pp. 1075–1079, 1995.

[179] C. M. Bishop, *Neural Networks for Pattern Recognition*, Clarendon, Oxford, UK, 1995.

[180] J. A. Freeman and D. M. Skapura, *Neural Networks, Algorithms, Applications and Programming Techniques*, Computation and Neural Systems Series, Addison-Wesley, 2002.

[181] R. M. Neal, *Bayesian Learning for Neural Networks*, Springer, New York, NY, USA, 1996.

[182] C. M. Bishop, *Neural Networks for Pattern Recognition*, Oxford University Press, London, UK, 1995.

[183] L. Fausett, *Fundamentals of Neural Network: Architectures, Algorithms and Applications*, Prentice Hall, Englewood Cliffs, NJ, USA, 1994.

[184] V. N. Vapnik, *Statistical Learning Theory*, Wiley, New York, NY, USA, 1998.

[185] V. N. Vapnik, *The Nature of Statistical Learning Theory*, Springer, New York, NY, USA, 2nd edition, 2000.

[186] N. S.-T. J. Cristianini, *An Introduction to Support Vector Machines and Other Kernel-Based Learning Methods*, Cambridge University Press, Cambridge, UK, 2000.

[187] G.-B. Huang, Q.-Y. Zhu, and C.-K. Siew, "Extreme learning machine: a new learning scheme of feedforward neural networks," in *Proceedings of the IEEE International Joint Conference on Neural Networks*, pp. 985–990, July 2004.

[188] Q.-Y. Zhu, A. K. Qin, P. N. Suganthan, and G.-B. Huang, "Evolutionary extreme learning machine," *Pattern Recognition*, vol. 38, no. 10, pp. 1759–1763, 2005.

[189] G.-B. Huang, Q.-Y. Zhu, and C.-K. Siew, "Extreme learning machine: theory and applications," *Neurocomputing*, vol. 70, no. 1–3, pp. 489–501, 2006.

[190] A. Bharathi and A. M. Natarajan, "Cancer classification using modified extreme learning machine based on anova features," *European Journal of Scientific Research*, vol. 58, no. 2, pp. 156–165, 2011.

[191] J. Huang and C. X. Ling, "Using AUC and accuracy in evaluating learning algorithms," *IEEE Transactions on Knowledge and Data Engineering*, vol. 17, no. 3, pp. 299–310, 2005.

[192] C. X. Ling, J. Huang, and H. Zhang, "AUC: a better measure than accuracy in comparing learning algorithms," in *Proceedings of the 16th Conference of the Canadian Society for Computational Studies of Intelligence*, Y. Xiang and C.-D. Brahim, Eds., pp. 329–341, Springer, June 2003.

[193] A. Sboner, C. Eccher, E. Blanzieri et al., "A multiple classifier system for early melanoma diagnosis," *Artificial Intelligence in Medicine*, vol. 27, no. 1, pp. 29–44, 2003.

[194] N. Japkowicz, "Learning from imbalanced data sets: a comparison of various strategies," in *Proceedings of the AAAI Workshop on Learning from Imbalanced Data Sets*, AAAI Press, 2000.

[195] R. C. Prati, G. E. A. P. A. Batista, and M. C. Monard, "Class imbalances versus class overlapping: an analysis of a learning system behavior," in *Proceedings of the 3rd Mexican International Conferenceon Artificial Intelligence*, R. Monroy, G. Arroyo-Figueroa, L. E. Sucar, and J. H. S. Azuela, Eds., pp. 312–321, Springer, April 2004.

[196] M. O. Karol Przystalski, L. Nowak, and G. Surowka, "Decision support system for skin cancer diagnosis," in *Proceedings of the 9th Internaltional Symposium on Operations Research and It's Applications (ISORA '10)*, Chengdu-Jiuzhaigou, China, 2010.

[197] M. Schumacher, N. Holländer, and W. Sauerbrei, "Resampling and cross-validation techniques: a tool to reduce bias caused by model building?" *Statistics in Medicine*, vol. 16, no. 24, pp. 2813–2827, 1997.

[198] R. W. Johnson, "An introduction to the bootstrap," *Teaching Statistics*, vol. 23, no. 2, pp. 49–54, 2001.

[199] B. Efron, "The estimation of prediction error: covariance penalties and cross-validation," *Journal of the American Statistical Association*, vol. 99, no. 467, pp. 619–632, 2004.

[200] M. M. Rahman, P. Bhattacharya, and B. C. Desai, "A multiple expert-based melanoma recognition system for dermoscopic images of pigmented skin lesions," in *Proceedings of the 8th IEEE International Conference on BioInformatics and BioEngineering (BIBE '08)*, 2008.

[201] Y. Vergouwe, E. W. Steyerberg, M. J. C. Eijkemans, and J. D. Habbema, "Validity of prognostic models: when is a model clinically useful?" *Seminars in Urologic Oncology*, vol. 20, no. 2, pp. 96–107, 2002.

[202] D. G. Altman and P. Royston, "What do we mean by validating a prognostic model?" *Statistics in Medicine*, vol. 19, no. 4, pp. 453–473, 2000.

[203] K. S. Nehal, S. A. Oliveria, A. A. Marghoob et al., "Use of and beliefs about baseline photography in the management of patients with pigmented lesions: a survey of dermatology residency programmes in the United States," *Melanoma Research*, vol. 12, no. 2, pp. 161–167, 2002.

[204] N. E. Feit, S. W. Dusza, and A. A. Marghoob, "Melanomas detected with the aid of total cutaneous photography," *British Journal of Dermatology*, vol. 150, no. 4, pp. 706–714, 2004.

[205] W. Slue, A. W. Kopf, and J. K. Rivers, "Total-body photographs of dysplastic nevi," *Archives of Dermatology*, vol. 124, no. 8, pp. 1239–1243, 1988.

[206] M. Stante, V. De Giorgi, P. Cappugi, B. Giannotti, and P. Carli, "Non-invasive analysis of melanoma thickness by means of dermoscopy: a retrospective study," *Melanoma Research*, vol. 11, no. 2, pp. 147–152, 2001.

[207] D. Massi, V. De Giorgi, and H. P. Soyer, "Histopathologic correlates of dermoscopic criteria," *Dermatologic Clinics*, vol. 19, no. 2, pp. 259–268, 2001.

[208] F. Stauffer, H. Kittler, C. Forstinger, and M. Binder, "The dermatoscope: a potential source of nosocomial infection?" *Melanoma Research*, vol. 11, no. 2, pp. 153–156, 2001.

[209] M. Carrara, A. Bono, C. Bartoli et al., "Multispectral imaging and artificial neural network: mimicking the management decision of the clinician facing pigmented skin lesions," *Physics in Medicine and Biology*, vol. 52, no. 9, article 018, pp. 2599–2613, 2007.

[210] M. Carrara, S. Tomatis, A. Bono et al., "Automated segmentation of pigmented skin lesions in multispectral imaging," *Physics in Medicine and Biology*, vol. 50, no. 22, pp. N345–N357, 2005.

[211] M. Elbaum, A. W. Kopf, H. S. Rabinovitz et al., "Automatic differentiation of melanoma from melanocytic nevi with multispectral digital dermoscopy: a feasibility study," *Journal of the American Academy of Dermatology*, vol. 44, no. 2, pp. 207–218, 2001.

[212] A. Lorber, M. Wiltgen, R. Hofmann-Wellenhof et al., "Correlation of image analysis features and visual morphology in melanocytic skin tumours using in vivo confocal laser scanning microscopy," *Skin Research and Technology*, vol. 15, no. 2, pp. 237–241, 2009.

[213] A. Gerger, R. Hofmann-Wellenhof, H. Samonigg, and J. Smolle, "In vivo confocal laser scanning microscopy in the diagnosis of melanocytic skin tumours," *British Journal of Dermatology*, vol. 160, no. 3, pp. 475–481, 2009.

[214] R. Hofmann-Wellenhof, E. M. T. Wurm, V. Ahlgrimm-Siess et al., "Reflectance confocal microscopy—state-of-art and research overview," *Seminars in Cutaneous Medicine and Surgery*, vol. 28, no. 3, pp. 172–179, 2009.

[215] J. Welzel, "Optical coherence tomography in dermatology: a review," *Skin Research and Technology*, vol. 7, no. 1, pp. 1–9, 2001.

[216] M. C. Pierce, J. Strasswimmer, B. H. Park, B. Cense, and J. F. De Boer, "Advances in optical coherence tomography imaging for dermatology," *Journal of Investigative Dermatology*, vol. 123, no. 3, pp. 458–463, 2004.

[217] M. Mogensen, L. Thrane, T. M. Jørgensen, P. E. Andersen, and G. B. E. Jemec, "OCT imaging of skin cancer and other dermatological diseases," *Journal of Biophotonics*, vol. 2, no. 6-7, pp. 442–451, 2009.

[218] L. Serrone, F. M. Solivetti, M. F. Thorel, L. Eibenschutz, P. Donati, and C. Catricalà, "High frequency ultrasound in the preoperative staging of primary melanoma: a statistical analysis," *Melanoma Research*, vol. 12, no. 3, pp. 287–290, 2002.

[219] A. Blum, M.-H. Schmid-Wendtner, V. Mauss-Kiefer, J. Y. Eberle, C. Kuchelmeister, and D. Dill-Müller, "Ultrasound mapping of lymph node and subcutaneous metastases in patients with cutaneous melanoma: results of a prospective multicenter study," *Dermatology*, vol. 212, no. 1, pp. 47–52, 2005.

[220] J. Mäurer, F. D. Knollmann, D. Schlums et al., "Role of high-resolution magnetic resonance imaging for differentiating melanin-containing skin tumors," *Investigative Radiology*, vol. 30, no. 11, pp. 638–643, 1995.

[221] I. Ono and F. Kaneko, "Magnetic resonance imaging for diagnosing skin tumors," *Clinics in Dermatology*, vol. 13, no. 4, pp. 393–399, 1995.

[222] S. El Gammal, R. Hartwig, S. Aygen, T. Bauermann, C. El Gammal, and P. Altmeyer, "Improved resolution of magnetic resonance microscopy in examination of skin tumors," *Journal of Investigative Dermatology*, vol. 106, no. 6, pp. 1287–1292, 1996.

[223] H. Motoyama, T. Tanaka, M. Tanaka, and H. Oka, "Feature of malignant melanoma based on color information," in *SICE Annual Conference*, pp. 399–402, August 2004.

[224] L. Xu, M. Jackowski, A. Goshtasby et al., "Segmentation of skin cancer images," *Image and Vision Computing*, vol. 17, no. 1, pp. 65–74, 1999.

[225] G. Di Leo, G. Fabbrocini, A. Paolillo, O. Rescigno, and P. Sommella, "Towards an automatic diagnosis system for skin lesions: estimation of blue-whitish veil and regression structures," in *Proceedings of the 6th International Multi-Conference on Systems, Signals and Devices (SSD '09)*, March 2009.

[226] S. E. Umbaugh, R. H. Moss, and W. V. Stoecker, "An automatic color segmentation algorithm with application to identification of skin tumor borders," *Computerized Medical Imaging and Graphics*, vol. 16, no. 3, pp. 227–235, 1992.

[227] G. A. Hance, S. E. Umbaugh, R. H. Moss, and W. V. Stoecker, "Unsupervised color image segmentation," *IEEE Engineering in Medicine and Biology Magazine*, vol. 15, no. 1, pp. 104–110, 1996.

[228] S. E. Umbaugh, R. H. Moss, W. V. Stoecker, and G. A. Hance, "Automatic color segmentation algorithms: with application to skin tumor feature identification," *IEEE Engineering in Medicine and Biology Magazine*, vol. 12, no. 3, pp. 75–82, 1993.

[229] M. M. Rahman, B. C. Desai, and P. Bhattacharya, "Image retrieval-based decision support system for dermatoscopic images," in *Proceedings of the 19th IEEE International Symposium on Computer-Based Medical Systems (CBMS 2006)*, pp. 285–290, June 2006.

[230] M. Ogorzałek, L. Nowak, G. Surowka, and A. Alekseenko, "Melanoma in the clinic—diagnosis, management and complications of malignancy," in *Modern Techniques for Computer-Aided Melanoma Diagnosis*, InTech, 2011.

[231] C. Grana, G. Pellacani, R. Cucchiara, and S. Seidenari, "A new algorithm for border description of polarized light surface microscopic images of pigmented skin lesions," *IEEE Transactions on Medical Imaging*, vol. 22, no. 8, pp. 959–964, 2003.

[232] B. Erkol, R. H. Moss, R. J. Stanley, W. V. Stoecker, and E. Hvatum, "Automatic lesion boundary detection in dermoscopy images using gradient vector flow snakes," *Skin Research and Technology*, vol. 11, no. 1, pp. 17–26, 2005.

[233] M. K. A. Mahmoud and A. Al-Jumaily, "Segmentation of skin cancer images based on gradient vector flow (GVF) snake," in *Proceedings of the IEEE International Conference on Mechatronics and Automation (ICMA '11)*, pp. 216–220, August 2011.

[234] J. E. Golston, R. H. Moss, and W. V. Stoecker, "Boundary detection in skin tumor images: an overall approach and a radial search algorithm," *Pattern Recognition*, vol. 23, no. 11, pp. 1235–1247, 1990.

[235] Z. Zhang, W. V. Stoecker, and R. H. Moss, "Border detection on digitized skin tumor images," *IEEE Transactions on Medical Imaging*, vol. 19, no. 11, pp. 1128–1143, 2000.

[236] M. Burroni, P. Sbano, G. Cevenini et al., "Dysplastic naevus vs. in situ melanoma: digital dermoscopy analysis," *British Journal of Dermatology*, vol. 152, no. 4, pp. 679–684, 2005.

[237] A. G. Manousaki, A. G. Manios, E. I. Tsompanaki et al., "A simple digital image processing system to aid in melanoma diagnosis in an everyday melanocytic skin lesion unit. A preliminary report," *International Journal of Dermatology*, vol. 45, no. 4, pp. 402–410, 2006.

[238] A. J. Round, A. W. G. Duller, and P. J. Fish, "Colour segmentation for lesion classification," in *Proceedings of the 19th Annual International Conference of the IEEE Engineering in Medicine and Biology Society*, pp. 582–585, November 1997.

[239] T. Fikrle and K. Pizinger, "Digital computer analysis of dermatoscopical images of 260 melanocytic skin lesions; perimeter/area ratio for the differentiation between malignant melanomas and melanocytic nevi," *Journal of the European Academy of Dermatology and Venereology*, vol. 21, no. 1, pp. 48–55, 2007.

[240] A. Masood and A. A. Al-Jumaily, "Fuzzy C mean thresholding based level set for automated segmentation of skin lesions," *Journal of Signal and Information Processing*, vol. 4, pp. 66–71, 2013.

[241] J. Liu and B. Zuo, "The segmentation of skin cancer image based on genetic neural network," in *Proceedings of the WRI World Congress on Computer Science and Information Engineering (CSIE '09)*, pp. 594–599, April 2009.

[242] N. Situ, X. Yuan, G. Zouridakis, and N. Mullani, "Automatic segmentation of skin lesion images using evolutionary strategy," in *Proceedings of the 14th IEEE International Conference on Image Processing (ICIP '07)*, pp. 277–280, September 2007.

[243] I. Cruz-Aceves, J. G. Aviña-Cervantes, J. M. López-Hernández, and S. E. González-Reyna, "Multiple active contours driven by particle swarm optimization for cardiac medical image segmentation," *Computational and Mathematical Methods in Medicine*, vol. 2013, Article ID 132953, 13 pages, 2013.

[244] S. V. Patwardhan, S. Dai, and A. P. Dhawan, "Multi-spectral image analysis and classification of melanoma using fuzzy membership based partitions," *Computerized Medical Imaging and Graphics*, vol. 29, no. 4, pp. 287–296, 2005.

[245] C. Garbe, P. Büttner, J. Bertz et al., "Primary cutaneous melanoma. Identification of prognostic groups and estimation of individual prognosis for 5093 patients," *Cancer*, vol. 75, no. 10, pp. 2484–2491, 1995.

[246] P. Rubegni, M. Burroni, G. Cevenini et al., "Digital dermoscopy analysis and artificial neural network for the differentiation of clinically atypical pigmented skin lesions: a retrospective study," *Journal of Investigative Dermatology*, vol. 119, no. 2, pp. 471–474, 2002.

[247] R. Marchesini, N. Cascinelli, M. Brambilla et al., "In vivo spectrophotometric evaluation of neoplastic and non-neoplastic skin pigmented lesions. II: discriminant analysis between nevus and melanoma," *Photochemistry and Photobiology*, vol. 55, no. 4, pp. 515–522, 1992.

[248] I. Maglogiannis, S. Pavlopoulos, and D. Koutsouris, "An integrated computer supported acquisition, handling, and characterization system for pigmented skin lesions in dermatological images," *IEEE Transactions on Information Technology in Biomedicine*, vol. 9, no. 1, pp. 86–98, 2005.

[249] T. Schindewolf, W. Stolz, R. Albert, W. Abmayr, and H. Harms, "Classification of melanocytic lesions with color and texture analysis using digital image processing," *Analytical and Quantitative Cytology and Histology*, vol. 15, no. 1, pp. 1–11, 1993.

[250] W. H. Clark Jr., D. E. Elder, D. Guerry IV et al., "Model predicting survival in stage I melanoma based on tumor progression," *Journal of the National Cancer Institute*, vol. 81, no. 24, pp. 1893–1904, 1989.

[251] R. J. Stanley, R. H. Moss, W. Van Stoecker, and C. Aggawal, "A fuzzy-based histogram analysis technique for skin lesion discrimination in dermatology clinical images," *Computerized Medical Imaging and Graphics*, vol. 27, no. 5, pp. 387–396, 2003.

[252] J. Chen, R. J. Stanley, R. H. Moss, and W. Van Stoecker, "Colour analysis of skin lesion regions for melanoma discrimination in clinical images," *Skin Research and Technology*, vol. 9, no. 2, pp. 94–104, 2003.

[253] R. J. Stanley, W. V. Stoecker, and R. H. Moss, "A relative color approach to color discrimination for malignant melanoma

detection in dermoscopy images," *Skin Research and Technology*, vol. 13, no. 1, pp. 62–72, 2007.

[254] R. Joe Stanley, W. V. Stoecker, R. H. Moss et al., "A basis function feature-based approach for skin lesion discrimination in dermatology dermoscopy images," *Skin Research and Technology*, vol. 14, no. 4, pp. 425–435, 2008.

[255] M. Binder, A. Steiner, M. Schwarz, S. Knollmayer, K. Wolff, and H. Pehamberger, "Application of an artificial neural network in epiluminescence microscopy pattern analysis of pigmented skin lesions: a pilot study," *British Journal of Dermatology*, vol. 130, no. 4, pp. 460–465, 1994.

[256] R. Husemann, S. Tolg, K. Hoffmann et al., "Computerized diagnosis of skin cancer using neural networks," *Melanoma Research*, vol. 6, p. S30, 1996.

[257] M. Binder, H. Kittler, A. Seeber, A. Steiner, H. Pehamberger, and K. Wolff, "Epiluminescence microscopy-based classification of pigmented skin lesions using computerized image analysis and an artificial neural network," *Melanoma Research*, vol. 8, no. 3, pp. 261–266, 1998.

[258] H. Handels, T. Roß, J. Kreusch, H. H. Wolff, and S. J. Pöppl, "Computer-supported diagnosis of melanoma in profilometry," *Methods of Information in Medicine*, vol. 38, no. 1, pp. 43–49, 1999.

[259] X. Yuan, Z. Yang, G. Zouridakis, and N. Mullani, "SVM-based texture classification and application to early melanoma detection," in *Proceedings of the 28th Annual International Conference of the IEEE Engineering in Medicine and Biology Society (EMBS '06)*, pp. 4775–4778, New York, NY, USA, September 2006.

[260] S. Gilmore, R. Hofmann-Wellenhof, and H. P. Soyer, "A support vector machine for decision support in melanoma recognition," *Experimental Dermatology*, vol. 19, no. 9, pp. 830–835, 2010.

[261] S. W. Menzies, L. M. Bischof, G. Peden et al., "Automated instrumentation for the diagnosis of invasive melanoma: image analysis of oil epiluminescence microscopy," in *Skin Cancer and UV-Radiation*, pp. 1064–1070, Springer, Berlin, Germany, 1997.

[262] S. Seidenari, G. Pellacani, and P. Pepe, "Digital videomicroscopy improves diagnostic accuracy for melanoma," *Journal of the American Academy of Dermatology*, vol. 39, no. 2, pp. 175–181, 1998.

[263] S. Seidenari, G. Pellacani, and A. Giannetti, "Digital videomicroscopy and image analysis with automatic classification for detection of thin melanomas," *Melanoma Research*, vol. 9, no. 2, pp. 163–171, 1999.

6

Robust Diffeomorphic Mapping via Geodesically Controlled Active Shapes

Daniel J. Tward,[1] **Jun Ma,**[1,2] **Michael I. Miller,**[3] **and Laurent Younes**[3]

[1] *Department of Biomedical Engineering, Johns Hopkins University, Baltimore, MD 21218, USA*
[2] *Siemens Healthcare, Hoffman Estates, Chicago, IL 60192, USA*
[3] *Center for Imaging Science, Johns Hopkins University, Baltimore, MD 21218, USA*

Correspondence should be addressed to Daniel J. Tward; dtward@cis.jhu.edu

Academic Editor: Kenji Suzuki

This paper presents recent advances in the use of diffeomorphic active shapes which incorporate the conservation laws of large deformation diffeomorphic metric mapping. The equations of evolution satisfying the conservation law are geodesics under the diffeomorphism metric and therefore termed geodesically controlled diffeomorphic active shapes (GDAS). Our principal application in this paper is on robust diffeomorphic mapping methods based on parameterized surface representations of subcortical template structures. Our parametrization of the GDAS evolution is via the initial momentum representation in the tangent space of the template surface. The dimension of this representation is constrained using principal component analysis generated from training samples. In this work, we seek to use template surfaces to generate segmentations of the hippocampus with three data attachment terms: surface matching, landmark matching, and inside-outside modeling from grayscale T1 MR imaging data. This is formulated as an energy minimization problem, where energy describes shape variability and data attachment accuracy, and we derive a variational solution. A gradient descent strategy is employed in the numerical optimization. For the landmark matching case, we demonstrate the robustness of this algorithm as applied to the workflow of a large neuroanatomical study by comparing to an existing diffeomorphic landmark matching algorithm.

1. Introduction

There have been many approaches to segmentation in medical imaging, including both the active shape methods pioneered by Kass et al. [1] and template based approaches pioneered by Dann et al. [2]. For studying images made up of simple homogeneous structures such as anatomical structures, local active evolution methods [1, 3–5] which are encoded through their boundary representations are natural. In such methods, the complexity of the representation is reduced from an encoding based on the dimension of the extrinsic background space containing the object, to the dimension of the boundary.

Given the line of work in template based computational anatomy which has emphasized the important role of diffeomorphisms for defining bijective correspondence between coordinate systems, it is natural to constrain the iterative methods of active shapes so that shape evolution preserves the original topology of the template. This is the intention of the diffeomorphic active contour (DAC) approaches taken by Younes et al. [6–8], including in the local evolution equations the diffeomorphism constraint. DAC methods, in a form similar to the original methods of Christensen et al. and Trouvé [9, 10], only optimize for the final position of the deformable template and not for the evolution process that leads to it. The approach adopted herein results in an entire trajectory through shape space, allowing basic prior knowledge, that is, proximity to a template, to be incorporated in the estimate of a shape.

The trajectories considered are geodesic flows, which are deduced from the Riemannian structure associated to large deformation diffeomorphic metric mapping (LDDMM) [10–12]. Geodesics are characterized by a conservation law [7, 13–16] on the "momentum" associated to the evolution, where we describe in Section 2 what is meant by momentum in this context. This allows a further reduction in complexity from a time varying flow to a single initial condition: an initial momentum vector. In other words, a target shape is represented as the endpoint of a geodesic flow from a template and can be encoded by one such vector. In this setting, knowledge of shape variability is straightforwardly incorporated via prior distributions on initial momentum. We call these connections geodesically controlled diffeomorphic active shapes (GDAS).

In this paper, we examine robust LDDMM via geodesically controlled diffeomorphic active shape models. The GDAS method allows us to introduce prior distributions so as to support the diffeomorphic large deformations of unconstrained LDDMM (taking advantage of the reduction in complexity from a time varying flow to an initial condition), while at the same time constraining the mapping, so it is indexed to neuroanatomical shapes such as the subcortical structures (taking advantage of the reduction in complexity from background space to structure boundaries). We demonstrate that these mappings are robust to small variations associated with the MRI measures of the structures. This is accomplished by constraining the initial momentum of the GDAS solutions to be in the span of a finite-dimensional basis constructed from PCA associated with large-scale surface-based [17] anatomical studies and by penalizing our initial momentum estimates in basis directions of low variability as recently also derived in Qiu et al.'s work [18].

As with the classical active shape methods (described for example in [19–25]), we pose the GDAS problem in the variational setting with the data term used for matching derived from various representations of a partition of the "scenes" including (i) collection of structures defined via triangulated meshes, (ii) a collection of structures defined through feature points, and (iii) a collection of homogeneous structures defined via inside-outside appearance model [26–30]. In case (iii), the process is iteratively driven by a voxel's likelihood of being interior or exterior of the region of interest (ROI), with the shape controlled by the conservation law geodesic dynamics. In our model, the appearance likelihood at each voxel only depends on whether the voxel is inside or outside the surface. It is estimated from the MRI training samples and modelled as Gaussian mixtures [31, 32] learned with the expectation maximization algorithm.

Vailliant et al. [33] first proposed this framework in a discussion of statistics on diffeomorphisms, and more recently Qiu et al. [18] addressed this problem and derived an algorithm for the case of surface-to-surface matching. Here, we consider a general data attachment term and provide a variational solution. We develop and implement a gradient descent algorithm for the case of surface matching, landmark matching, and grayscale image segmentation. A lack of robustness is an important challenge to high dimensional registration and a barrier to its automation and use in high throughput studies. We show that GDAS provides an efficient method for constraining LDDMM to incorporate the finite-dimensionality of typical shape variation and emphasize the robust performance of our methods on challenging biological datasets

2. Geodesic Diffeomorphic Evolution for Active Surfaces

In our region-of-interest (ROI) approaches to subcortical structure analysis in the human brain, our goal is to robustly segment anatomical structures (in particular neuroanatomical structures such as the hippocampus, caudate nucleus, etc.) from the surrounding environment using a given set of data (such as manually placed landmarks within an ROI, coarse segmentations, or MR images). Typically, anatomical structures have their own characteristic shapes and appearance which must be learned from training data to successfully perform segmentation.

2.1. Conservation Law Controlled Diffeomorphic Evolution. The methodology of tangent space representation has been a powerful tool in computational anatomy, since it was proposed in [16]. In this context, evolution of visual structures, like points, curves, surfaces, and images is governed by geodesic equations. By the law of momentum conservation, the initial state of the equations determines the entire trajectory of evolution and can be used as a representation of the trajectory endpoint. We refer to [16, 34] for more details and context in shape spaces modeled as homogeneous spaces under diffeomorphic action and describe here a special form of the associated equations that will be adapted to our needs.

For a triangulated surface S_0 in $\mathbb{R}^3$ with vertices $x_1, \ldots, x_L$, the initial momentum $\rho(0) : S_0 \to \mathbb{R}^3$ can be represented by a vector a_l at each vertex through $\rho(0) = \sum_{l=1}^{L} a_l \delta(x_l)$. One can derive the geodesic equation for the evolution of S_0, which is equivalent to the geodesic equation for point sets [16]. We define a radially symmetric smoothing kernel K on $\mathbb{R}^3 \times \mathbb{R}^3$. A typical choice, used here, is

$$K(x, y) = \exp\left(-\frac{\|x - y\|^2}{2\tau^2}\right). \tag{1}$$

With $K(x, y) = \gamma(\|x - y\|^2)$, we denote $\gamma_{kl} = \gamma(\|x_k - x_l\|^2)$, and $\gamma'_{kl} = \gamma'(\|x_k - x_l\|^2)$. The geodesic evolution satisfies

$$\frac{dx_k}{dt} = \sum_{l=1}^{L} \gamma_{kl} a_l,$$

$$\frac{da_k}{dt} = -2\sum_{l=1}^{L} \gamma'_{kl} (a_l \cdot a_k)(x_k - x_l), \tag{2}$$

where the notation $a \cdot b$ refers to the usual dot product between vectors in $\mathbb{R}^3$. Once the initial position of the vertices, $x(0) = (x_1(0), \ldots, x_L(0))$, and the *initial momentum vector*, $\alpha(0) = (a_1(0), \ldots, a_L(0))$, are provided, the evolution of the point set is uniquely determined. The endpoints of the evolution $x(1) = (x_1(1), x_2(1), \ldots, x_L(1))$ correspond to the deformed surface $S(1)$. It can be shown that (2) has solutions over arbitrary time intervals [34]. Equation (2) induces a diffeomorphism, ϕ, that interpolates the evolution of the vertices via the equation

$$\frac{d\phi}{dt}(t,x) = \sum_{l=1}^{L} K\left(\phi\left(t,x\right),x_l\right) a_l. \tag{3}$$

The conservation law associated to (2) then takes the form $a_l(t) = D\phi(t,x_l)^{-T} a_l(0)$.

Hence, we are able to represent a shape by an initial momentum vector (as opposed to a function or distribution) and a template. Furthermore, the variability of shapes can be described from probabilistic properties of initial momentum. This is the basic representation for the tangent space PCA of shapes.

2.2. Finite Dimensional Representation via PCA in the Tangent Space. Clearly, as the discretization of the surface gets fine, the dimension of the control point representation of the momentum goes to infinity. We want to characterize the main modes of statistical variations in our data, of which there is a small number up to some acceptable error. This enables us to write the momentum vector in a finite dimensional span regardless of the discretization.

It is natural to do this empirically based on training samples. PCA depends on the definition of an inner product in the considered space. In our context, the inner product derives from the Riemannian metric that led to the geodesic equation. Details of corresponding PCA have been described previously [33].

We calculate a population template T using the approach in [35], but several other algorithms are available [36–38]. We denote the inner product between two initial momentum vectors α and $\tilde{\alpha}$, as $\langle \alpha, \tilde{\alpha} \rangle_T$. Assume we have recovered mean initial momentum vector $\bar{\alpha}$, D orthonormal prinicipal components u_i (with $\langle u_i, u_j \rangle_T = \delta_{ij}$), and an estimate of variance along each component λ_i. We note that any initial momentum vector α can be projected onto the principal space as

$$\text{proj}(\alpha) = \bar{\alpha} + \sum_{i=1}^{D} k_i u_i, \quad \text{where } k_i = \langle \alpha - \bar{\alpha}, u_i \rangle_T. \tag{4}$$

By parameterizing our deformations with respect to the k_i, the variability of the surface shape is constrained by the principal space generated from the training set.

3. Segmentation Algorithms

3.1. Variational Formulation of Volumetric Segmentation. We formulate segmentation problems within an energy minimizing scheme. The energy includes two terms: one term is to constrain the shape in the principal space, with appropriate weights derived from PCA, and the other term regulates the error of mismatch, which we will define in a general sense here and show specific examples in Sections 3.2 to 3.4.

We introduce some notation. Let $\Omega \subset \mathbb{R}^3$ be the background space. Let T denote the template, which will be assumed to be a closed surface. After learning, the selected principal space of initial momentum is spanned by D orthonormal vectors $u_1, u_2, \ldots, u_D$ corresponding to decreasing eigenvalues $\lambda_1, \lambda_2, \ldots, \lambda_D$.

Our goal is to segment the region-of-interest (ROI) from Ω using a deformable model; that is, we want to deform the template T, so that it overlaps with the boundary of the ROI. We assume that T is a triangulated surface, with vertex set $x^0 = (x_1^0, \ldots, x_L^0)$. For an initial momentum α, we let x^α denote the solution at time $t = 1$ of (2) initialized with $x_k(0) = x_k^0$ and $a_k(0) = \alpha$. We let S^α denote the triangulated surface that inherits the topology of T with displaced vertices x^α.

We now describe the two terms in our energy that balance the prior knowledge we have of the diffeomorphic deformation with the accuracy of the segmentation. The initial momentum α is constrained to the principal space and takes the form $\alpha(0) = \bar{\alpha} + \sum_{n=1}^{D} k_n u_n$. This prior knowledge is regulated by the coefficients of principal components, scaled by eigenvalues, resulting in the first term of our cost function:

$$E_1 = \sum_{n=1}^{D} \frac{k_n^2}{\lambda_n}. \tag{5}$$

We define the accuracy of segmentation based on some function E_2 of only available data (e.g., an image, a set of landmarks, or a surface) and the configuration of our deformed template S^α. For the time being, we assume that the derivative of this function with respect to each of the x_i^α is known, and we denote the vector of this derivative by $\partial E_2 / \partial x^\alpha$.

Our goal is to find the optimal coefficients $k_1, k_2, \ldots, k_D$ that minimize the energy:

$$E = E_1 + \frac{1}{\sigma^2} E_2. \tag{6}$$

The variational problem is solved by calculating the derivative of E with respect to each coefficient k_n. The derivative of E_1 is trivial:

$$\frac{\partial E_1}{\partial k_n} = \frac{2k_n}{\lambda_n}. \tag{7}$$

The derivative of E_2 can be calculated by the chain rule

$$\frac{\partial E_2}{\partial k_n} = \left(\frac{\partial E_2}{\partial x^\alpha}\right)^T \left(\frac{\partial x^\alpha}{\partial \alpha}\right) u_n$$
$$= \left(\frac{\partial E_2}{\partial \alpha}\right)^T u_n. \tag{8}$$

While the term $\partial x^\alpha / \partial \alpha$ is unknown, its product with $\partial E_2 / \partial x^\alpha$ (which we denote as $\partial E_2 / \partial \alpha$) can be calculated numerically by solving a system of linear ordinary differential equations. This adjoint method has become common in this context and is derived, for example, in [35]. It is described for completeness in Appendix B. The derivative of E is given by

$$\frac{\partial E}{\partial k_n} = \frac{2k_n}{\lambda_n} + \frac{1}{\sigma^2} \left(\frac{\partial E_2}{\partial \alpha}\right)^T u_n. \tag{9}$$

We now discuss three applications and explain examples of E_2 and their gradients.

3.2. Robust Surface Matching.

3.2. Robust Surface Matching. In challenging surface mapping applications, it can be necessary to regularize the mappings to avoid undesirable results, and GDAS provides a powerful method for doing so.

In particular, volumetric segmentations of neuroanatomy are often readily available. Converting them to an isosurface for analysis and display is standard, and GDAS provides a method to convert such an isosurface to one reflecting the typicality and variability of a population, rather than features of the volumetric data with an unnatural voxelized structure. Our goal here is to provide a tool to correct for such erroneous segmentations.

This application is essentially equivalent to that presented in [18]. We retain it here as it is the most natural application of GDAS (priors learned from surface matching are used to regularize surface matching), to develop a notation consistent with that for our other applications and to demonstrate robust performance on poorly behaved datasets.

3.2.1. Notation. The deformed template surface S^α is triangulated with vertices $x_1^\alpha, \ldots, x_L^\alpha$. Suppose the template surface has M faces denoted as $F = (f_1, \ldots, f_M)$. Each face is represented by an ordered triple of vertices: $f = (x_{f,1}^\alpha, x_{f,2}^\alpha, x_{f,3}^\alpha)$. We define oriented edges on face f by

$$
\begin{aligned}
e_{f,1}^\alpha &= x_{f,2}^\alpha - x_{f,3}^\alpha, \\
e_{f,2}^\alpha &= x_{f,3}^\alpha - x_{f,1}^\alpha, \\
e_{f,3}^\alpha &= x_{f,1}^\alpha - x_{f,2}^\alpha,
\end{aligned}
\tag{10}
$$

the area-weighted normal to face f by

$$
N_f^\alpha = \frac{1}{2} e_{f,3}^\alpha \times e_{f,2}^\alpha,
\tag{11}
$$

and the face center by

$$
c_f^\alpha = \frac{1}{3} \left(x_{f,1}^\alpha + x_{f,2}^\alpha + x_{f,3}^\alpha \right).
\tag{12}
$$

Similarly, suppose the target surface has L' vertices $y_1, \ldots, y_L$ and M' faces denoted as $F' = (f_1', \ldots, f_{M'}')$, with oriented edges $e_{f',1}', e_{f',2}', e_{f',3}'$, area-weighted normals given by $N_{f'}'$, and face center $c_{f'}'$.

Similarly to the case for velocity fields, we define a smoothing kernel K_S (S for "surface") of the form in (1) to be used for comparing two surfaces.

3.2.2. Energy. Following [17], we embed surface matching in a more general "current matching" problem. This results in an energy to be minimized taking into account closeness between two surfaces, as well as orientation of normals:

$$
\begin{aligned}
E_2 = &\sum_{i=1}^{M} \sum_{j=1}^{M} N_i^{\alpha T} K_S \left(c_i^\alpha, c_j^\alpha \right) N_j^\alpha \\
&- 2 \sum_{i=1}^{M} \sum_{j=1}^{M'} N_i^{\alpha T} K_S \left(c_i^\alpha, c_j' \right) N_j' \\
&+ \sum_{i=1}^{M'} \sum_{j=1}^{M'} N_i'^{T} K_S \left(c_i', c_j' \right) N_j'.
\end{aligned}
\tag{13}
$$

The constant σ^2 in (6) is determined heuristically.

3.2.3. Energy Gradient. We refer the reader to [17] for the derivation of this energy gradient and present the result only here:

$$
\begin{aligned}
&\left. \frac{\partial E_2}{\partial x^\alpha} \right|_k \\
&= \sum_{f: x_k^\alpha = x_{f,i}^\alpha} \left[\sum_{j=1}^{M} e_{f,i}^\alpha \times K_S \left(c_j^\alpha, c_f^\alpha \right) N_j^\alpha \right. \\
&\qquad + \frac{2}{3} \left(N_f^{\alpha T} \frac{\partial}{\partial c_f^\alpha} K_S \left(c_j^\alpha, c_f^\alpha \right) \right) N_j^\alpha \\
&\qquad - \sum_{j=1}^{M'} e_{f,i}^\alpha \times K_S \left(c_j', c_f^\alpha \right) N_j' \\
&\qquad \left. - \frac{2}{3} \left(N_f^{\alpha T} \frac{\partial}{\partial c_f^\alpha} K_S \left(c_j', c_f^\alpha \right) \right) N_j' \right],
\end{aligned}
\tag{14}
$$

where the first sum is over faces f for which x_k^α is a vertex, and the symbol i is reserved for the index of that vertex on each such face ($i \in \{1, 2, 3\}$).

3.3. Robust Landmark Matching.

3.3. Robust Landmark Matching. A further application of our framework involves ROI analysis methods based on diffeomorphic landmark matching. Given a template surface containing K landmarks located on vertices, a trained technician places corresponding landmarks in T1 MR images. Diffeomorphic landmark matching provides a segmentation of the structure of interest in each T1 image by applying the landmark-based transformation to the entire template surface. This procedure is advantageous, because it provides a compromise between the speed of automatic segmentation and the accuracy of hand segmentation.

However, variability in landmark placement and sparsity of landmarks can occasionally lead to unsatisfactory segmentation results and to a time-consuming quality control stage where such segmentations are fixed manually. We propose to regularize the problem, taking into account landmark placement variability based on voxel size, as well as shape variability learned from PCA.

3.3.1. Notation. For simplicity, we assume that landmarks on the template are chosen among the vertices of its representation as a triangulated surface. We denote by $X_i(t) = x_{l(i)}(t)$ the ith landmark, which is placed on a template vertex $l(i)$ and flowed according to (2) up to time t. Therefore, $X_i(1) = x_{l(i)}^\alpha$. We define the corresponding landmark placed on the target image as Y_i.

3.3.2. Energy. We assume that the only available information on the targets is landmarks at positions homologous to those on the template. The accuracy of segmentation is then based on the squared distance between deformed template and target landmarks, leading to the term

$$E_2 = \sum_{i=1}^{K} \left\| X_i(1) - Y_i \right\|^2. \tag{15}$$

The weighting parameter is chosen on the order of voxel size $\sigma^2 = ((\Delta x/2)^2 + (\Delta y/2)^2 + (\Delta z/2)^2)/3$ (equal to 0.4475 for our application) where Δx, Δy, and Δz are the target image's voxel dimension.

3.3.3. Energy Gradient. The variation of E_2 with respect to the kth deformed template vertex is 0 if this vertex does not correspond to a landmark, and $2(X_k - Y_k) = 2(x_{l(k)}^\alpha - Y_k)$ if it does. That is,

$$\frac{\partial E_2}{\partial x_\alpha}\bigg|_k = \begin{cases} 0 & k \text{ is not a landmark,} \\ 2\left(x_k^\alpha - Y_j\right) & k \text{ is the } j\text{th landmark.} \end{cases} \tag{16}$$

3.4. Robust Image Segmentation. We seek to automatically segment subcortical structures from MR images. For simplicity, we assume that such structures are relatively homogenous throughout and therefore chose an appearance model for voxel intensities that depend on location only through whether they are inside the structure or not. To perform image segmentation, we seek to partition the space into high integrated voxel-likelihood under such an inside-outside model. The approach can be generalized to more complex appearance models (involving higher order image features, e.g.) in a straightforward way.

3.4.1. Appearance Model. Gaussian mixtures are widely employed to model voxel intensity of medical imaging. That is, a p.d.f of intensity I at a certain location in the tissue is in the form of

$$p(I; x) = \sum_{q=1}^{Q} \pi_q(x) \frac{1}{\sqrt{2\pi\sigma_q^2(x)}} \exp\left(-\frac{\left(I - \mu_q(x)\right)^2}{2\sigma_q^2(x)}\right), \tag{17}$$

where π_q, μ_q, and σ_q^2 denote the weight, mean and variance of qth (out of Q) Gaussian component, respectively.

In our work, we assume that the intensities at all points of the interior region (resp., exterior region) of the surfaces share the same mixed Gaussian distribution and the p.d.f's are denoted as p_{int} and p_{ext}, respectively.

Given the number of mixture components, the maximum likelihood estimator for the parameters can be computed using the EM algorithm [39]. Our estimation of p_{int} and p_{ext} (using mixtures of Gaussians) is performed on the basis of training images with manual segmentation, in which the collection of all intensity values of voxels inside (resp., outside) the ROI are used for p_{int} (resp., p_{ext}).

3.4.2. Energy. We define the accuracy of segmentation using integrals of likelihood of being misclassified, and we define the mismatch:

$$E_2 = \int_{x \in \text{int}(S)} \log\left(p_{\text{ext}}\left(I(x)\right)\right) dx \\ + \int_{x \in \text{ext}(S)} \log\left(p_{\text{int}}\left(I(x)\right)\right) dx, \tag{18}$$

where we denote the interior and exterior of a closed surface S by $\text{int}(S)$ and $\text{ext}(S)$, respectively.

The constant σ^2 in (6) is determined heuristically.

3.4.3. Energy Gradient. The energy gradient is derived in Theorem A.1 in Appendix A. With $g(y) = \log[p_{\text{ext}}(y)/p_{\text{int}}(I(y))]$ and $m_{f,i}^\alpha$ the midpoint of the ith edge of face f, we have

$$\frac{\partial E_2}{\partial x^\alpha}\bigg|_k = \sum_{f: x_k^\alpha = x_{f,i}^\alpha} \frac{1}{2|N_f|} \int_f g(y) \left(m_{f,i}^\alpha - y\right) \times e_{f,i}^\alpha \, d\sigma_f. \tag{19}$$

3.5. Numerical Implementation. We use gradient descent to optimize the PCA coefficients and iteratively update k_n with $k_n - \epsilon(\partial E/\partial k_n)$ until convergence. The discretization of the surface integrals in (19) is simply performed by replacing $g(y)(m_{f,i}^\alpha - y) \times e_{f,i}^\alpha$ by its value at $y = c_f^\alpha$, the center of face f, with

$$\frac{1}{2}\left(m_{k,f}^\alpha - c_f^\alpha\right) \times e_{k,f}^\alpha = \frac{1}{3}N_f^\alpha. \tag{20}$$

This yields the approximation

$$\frac{\partial E_2}{\partial x^\alpha}\bigg|_k = \frac{1}{3} \sum_{f: x_k \in f} g\left(c_f^\alpha\right) N_f^\alpha, \tag{21}$$

that has been used in our implementation.

We summarize these steps in Algorithm 1. The complete procedure, including training, is summarized in Algorithm 2.

4. Experimental Methods

To demonstrate the proposed algorithm, for each of the three data attachment terms, we use data being processed as part of many of our region-of-interest (ROI) biological studies in schizophrenia, depression, Alzheimer's disease, ADHD, and autism [40–45] (for landmark matching and image segmentation) and Alzheimer's Disease Neuroimaging Initiative (ADNI) study (for surface matching and PCA

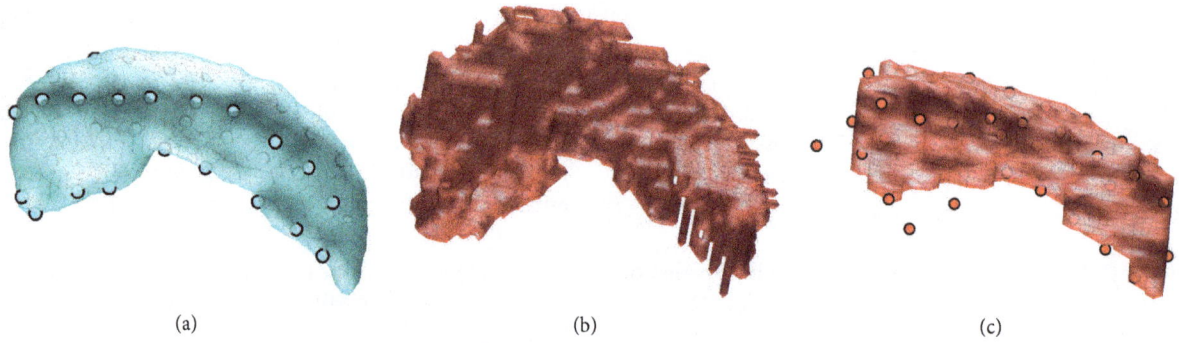

(a)   (b)   (c)

FIGURE 1: (a) Template hippocampus for ADNI dataset. (b) Hippocampus isosurface from example volumetric parcellation. (c) Isosurface of example hippocampus manual segmentation for our landmark datasets.

In order to find an initial momentum α minimizing (6)
    (1) Initialize with $x(0)$ being vertices of template T and $\alpha = \overline{\alpha}$.
    (2) For the current system, update matrices $J(t)$ and $J(t)^*$ according to (B.1) and (19).
    (3) Compute the gradient $\partial E_2/\partial x^\alpha$, for example using (14), (16), or (21).
    (4) Solve system (B.3) backward in time with initial condition $\eta_x(1) = \partial E_2/\partial x^\alpha$ and $\eta_\alpha(1) = 0$.
    (5) Replace k_n by $k_n - \epsilon((2k_n/\lambda_n) + (1/\sigma^2)\, u_n \cdot \eta_\alpha(0))$, ϵ being optimized with a line search.
    (6) Update the initial momentum $\alpha = \overline{\alpha} + \sum_{n=1}^{D} k_n u_n$, and solve (2) initialized at
        α, to obtain the updated surface S^α.
Iterate steps 2 to 6 until numerical convergence or reaching the maximum iteration limit.

ALGORITHM 1: Geodesically controlled diffeomorphic segmentation algorithm.

training). Shown in the accompanying figures are 5 examples demonstrating the robustness constraints imposed by performing large deformation mapping in the span of the first few PCA dimensions learned from our empirical mappings. For the case of landmark matching, we have integrated it into the workflow of several large neuroanatomical studies (e.g., [46]). We therefore include this application as a case study, quantifying performance in detail and demonstrating improvement we expect to gain. Our hypothesis when beginning this work was that the GDAS algorithm would exhibit increased robustness compared to more standard methods, without significantly sacrificing accuracy.

Data used in the preparation of this paper were obtained from the ADNI database (http://adni.loni.ucla.edu/). The ADNI was launched in 2003 by the National Institute on Aging (NIA), the National Institute of Biomedical Imaging and Bioengineering (NIBIB), the Food and Drug Administration (FDA), private pharmaceutical companies, and nonprofit organizations, as a \$60-million, 5-year public-private partnership. The primary goal of ADNI has been to test whether serial magnetic resonance imaging (MRI), positron emission tomography (PET), other biological markers, and clinical and neuropsychological assessment can be combined to measure the progression of mild cognitive impairment (MCI) and early Alzheimer's disease (AD). Determination of sensitive and specific markers of very early AD progression is intended to aid researchers and clinicians to develop new treatments and monitor their effectiveness, as well as lessen the time and cost of clinical trials.

The Principal Investigator of this initiative is Michael W. Weiner, MD, VA Medical Center and University of California San Francisco, CA, USA. ADNI is the result of efforts of many coinvestigators from a broad range of academic institutions and private corporations, and subjects have been recruited from over 50 sites across the US and Canada. The initial goal of ADNI was to recruit 800 adults, ages 55 to 90, to participate in the research, approximately 200 cognitively normal older individuals to be followed for 3 years, 400 people with MCI to be followed for 3 years, and 200 people with early AD to be followed for 2 years. For up-to-date information, see http://www.adni-info.org/.

4.1. Principal Component Analysis. Given a template and a set of target surfaces (650 for the ADNI study), we perform principal component analysis on initial momentum data as described in Section 2.2. The same ADNI template and PCA model will be used in each of our applications, even for data taken from other datasets. We plot the variance as a function of number of dimensions and identify the number of dimensions required to account for 95% of the variance.

4.2. Surface Matching Study. As part of the ADNI study, volumetric parcellations (performed using Freesurfer, described, e.g., in [47]) of whole brains are available at a series of time points. The $t = 0$ data has been studied and a template (see Figure 1(a)) as well as a population of initial momenta data has been calculated [48]. To study their changing shapes over time, we wish to convert such binary

(A) Training.
    (1) Generate a template surface T from N surfaces $S_1, \ldots, S_N$ using the method in [35].
    (2) Map T to the N surfaces and obtain the initial momenta α_n, $n = 1, \ldots, N$. Compute the.
       mean momentum $\bar{\alpha}$ and perform PCA in the tangent space as described in Section 2.2.
    (3) Estimate the constant σ^2, and other terms required for E_2 (e.g., estimate the density
       function p_{int} and p_{ext} for interior and exterior of ROI from training images as described in Section 3.4.1).
(B) Segmentation.
    (1) Initialize the template surface T, and register the target data to it (e.g., through a
       similitude matching, rigid motion × scale).
    (2) Run Algorithm 1 to optimize the initial momentum α.
    (3) The result of segmentation is the deformed surface S^α. Apply the inverse of the
       transformation in step 1 if necessary.

ALGORITHM 2: Geodesically controlled diffeomorphic active shapes.

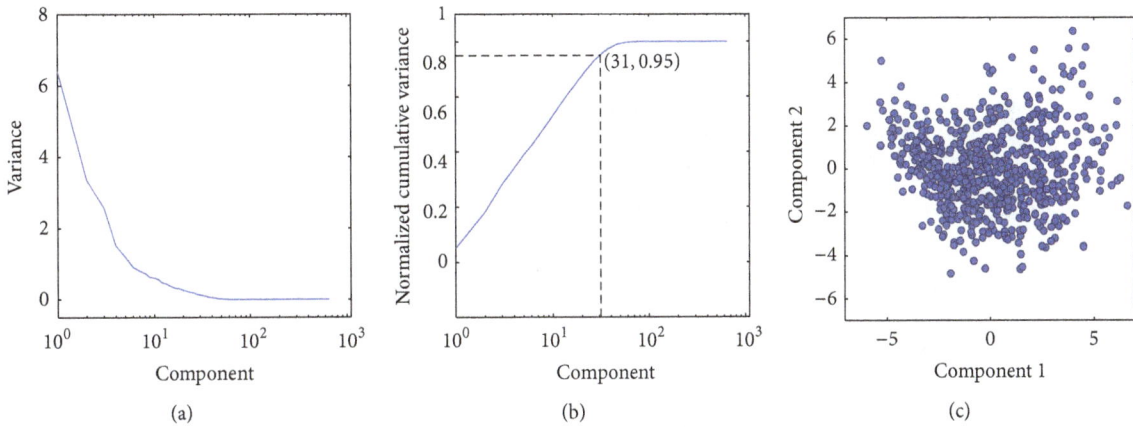

(a)   (b)   (c)

FIGURE 2: (a) The variance of each PCA coefficient in the left hippocampus ADNI population. (b) The normalized cumulative variance indicating the number of dimensions accounting for 95% of the variability. Note the semilog scale in (a) and (b). (c) A scatter plot of the first two PCA coefficients for this population.

segmentations to surfaces. However, the voxelized nature of the segmentations makes simple isosurfaces unacceptable (as shown in Figure 1(b)).

We therefore employ the technique of matching our template to such an isosurface, using the constraints of a smooth deformation regularized by PCA to avoid the unnatural appearance of the isosurface. We show example results from our GDAS surface matching algorithm, and compare them to typical results from the traditional surface matching LDDMM algorithm.

4.3. Landmark Matching Study. Our segmentation pipeline for our ROI methods is described in [40–44, 46]. The relevant portion (the landmark matching phase) for one such study is summarized here. Thirty-eight landmarks are placed along the left and right hippocampi in 441 0.93 × 0.93 × 2.0 mm T1 images of the brain. The first was placed at the tip of the head of the hippocampus (the center of the most anterior slice containing the hippocampus in a T1 image), and the second was placed at the tip of the tail of the hippocampus (the center of the most posterior slice containing the hippocampus). The distance between these two was then divided into 9 slices from anterior to posterior,

and on each slice 4 landmarks were placed at the superior, inferior, medial, and lateral margins of the hippocampus. This manual procedure takes approximately 10 minutes for a trained technician to complete, as compared to over 2 hours for a full hand segmentation of images of this size.

In the existing segmentation and analysis pipeline, a template surface was chosen as the left hippocampus for a single subject, and a manual segmentation and resulting isosurface were generated for this case. After a similitude alignment (including reflecting right hippocampi to match left) landmark LDDMM [49] was used to map this template to each target, defining a segmentation surface and binary image for each patient.

However, this procedure was found to suffer from lack of robustness, and roughly 30 out of 441 cases were unacceptable. A laborious phase of quality control was necessary involving identifying problematic or distorted segmentations, manually editing their binary images, and regenerating isosurfaces.

To measure whether our prior model provides enough robustness to avoid such issues, we chose 5 challenging cases of left hippocampi (as identified during quality control inspection), where manual intervention was required

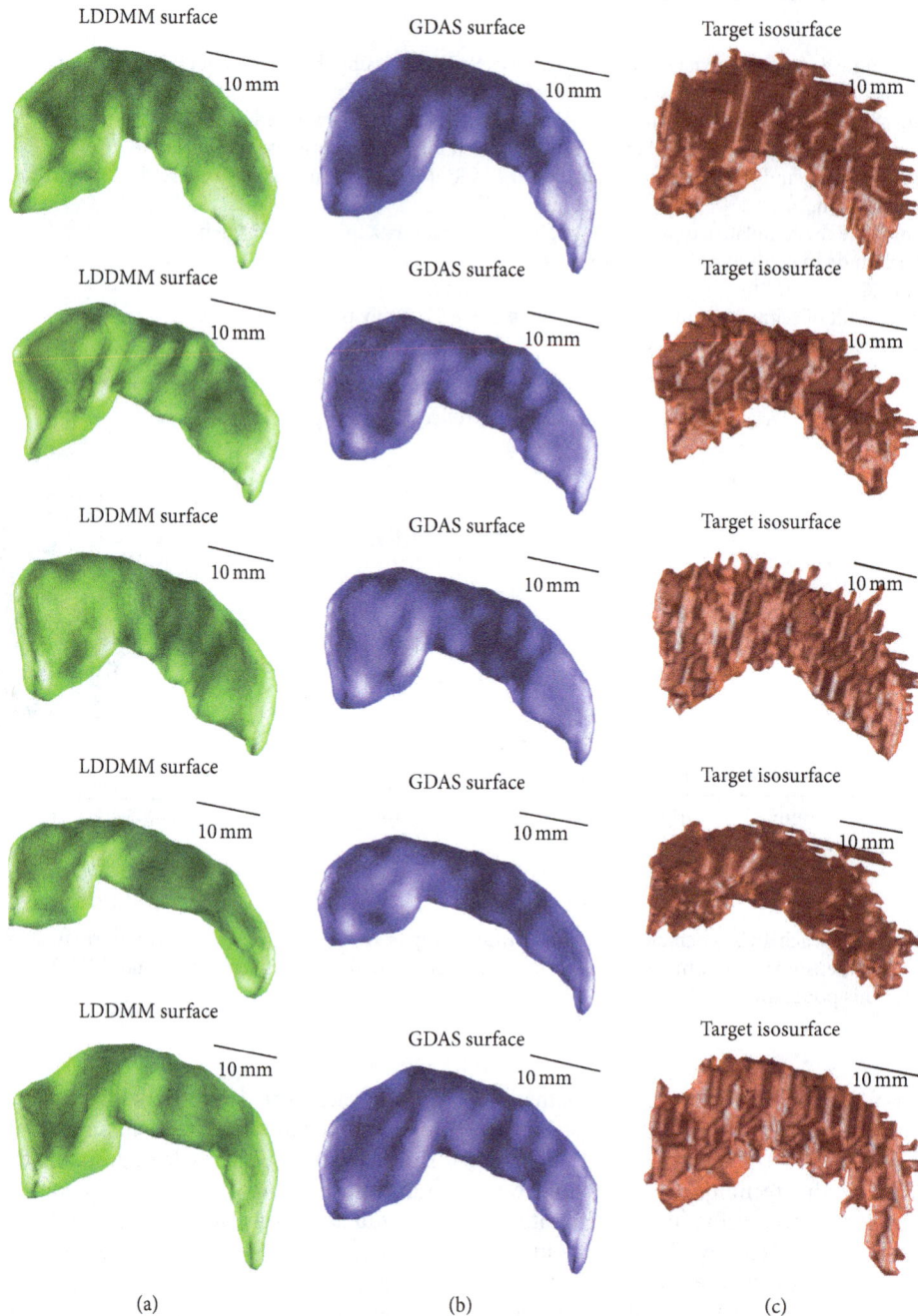

FIGURE 3: Examples of hippocampus surfaces resulting from using (left/green) surface LDDMM and (center/blue) GDAS surface matching. The target isosurface is shown at the right (red).

and 11 typical cases, and we examined the performance improvement using the proposed algorithm rather than that outlined above. These cases were manually segmented by a trained technician to provide a gold standard, and associated isosurfaces were generated for further evaluation. Furthermore, for 3 cases requiring intervention and 2 typical cases (those illustrated in Figure 4), a second manual segmentation was obtained to give a sense of interrater variability.

Note that the segmentations that are shown here do not constitute the final output of the ROI pipeline described in [40], in which they would be further processed. That

is, the results of standard landmark mapping shown here are not reflective of the final segmentations. However, we expect improvement at this stage to contribute to overall improvement.

The template with its associated landmarks is shown in Figure 1(a). In Figure 1(c), an example isosurface generated from a manual segmentation is shown together with its associated landmarks. Note that landmarks were placed on template surface vertices, but the target landmarks were placed independently (by a different technician) from the gold standard manual segmentation. Figure 1 shows

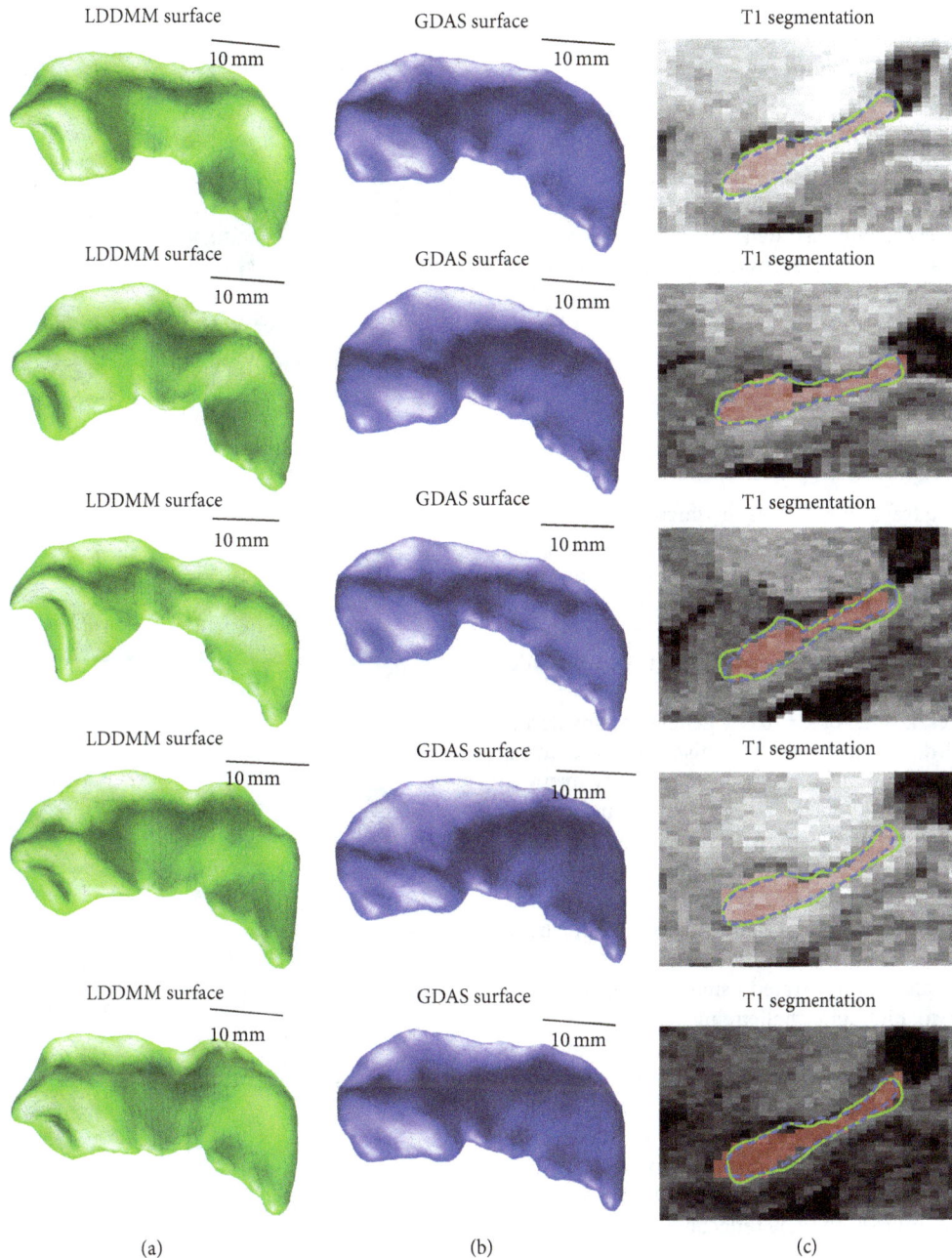

FIGURE 4: Segmentation results for standard landmark matching (left/green/solid) and GDAS landmark matching (center/blue/broken) for 5 examples (first 3 were identified for quality control; final 2 were not). Segmentations overlaid with corresponding T1 image and "ground truth" (red highlight) are shown in the right column.

the uncertainty of landmark placement, particularly in the region of the hippocampus' head and demonstrates the need to include landmark placement variability in the segmentation algorithm. In these figures and throughout this paper, the color cyan will be used for the template, red for the target, blue for our new results, and green for results using existing algorithms.

4.4. Image Segmentation Study. To demonstrate the capabilities of the GDAS image segmentation algorithm, 5 examples for the same dataset as the landmark matching study are

shown. We anticipate that good initial alignment will be important for high quality segmentations, and so the same landmark based similitude registration as above will be used to initialize the target data in this study.

We use 4 outside and 3 inside components for our Gaussian mixture model. The mixture model is trained based on gold standard segmentations from the remaining cases in a "leave-one-out" fashion. A histogram equalization intensity transformation is applied to each T1 image to match the first training sample, based on data from a neighborhood (±5 voxels) around the landmarks, before estimating mixture model coefficients. A similar histogram equalization is applied to the target image (to match the first training sample) before beginning the segmentation process.

4.5. Analysis Methods. In analyzing results, we seek to demonstrate two main ideas. First, the accuracy of GDAS is comparable to existing methods, and second its robustness is improved. Accuracy is demonstrated using three techniques. First, we use visual inspection. Second, κ scores [50] are used to compare our results to gold standard segmentations. This score is defined by

$$\kappa = \frac{p_{\text{agree}} - p_{\text{random}}}{1 - p_{\text{random}}}, \qquad (22)$$

where p_{agree} is the fraction of voxels in which the given segmentation agrees with the manual segmentation, and p_{random} is the fraction you would expect by random chance (based only on the volumes of foreground and background). We calculate κ scores using a Monte-Carlo method, generating uniformly distributed points and checking if they are inside one or both segmentations. For applications involving subcortical structures, a value of $\kappa = 0.8$ is generally considered quite good. Third, surface-to-surface distance cumulative distribution functions (c.d.f.s) are used to quantify average proximity of surfaces. At each vertex on each surface, we calculate the distance to the nearest vertex on the other surface and analyze the distribution of these distances. We examine entire c.d.f.s and also examine thresholds: distance at which 50% of vertices are closer than and distance at which 80% of vertices are closer than.

Robustness is also demonstrated using visual inspection, with care taken to highlight challenging regions. Surface-to-surface distance histograms are also restricted to such regions, highlighting challenging areas rather than averaging over the entire surface. Additionally, we quantify surface smoothness by measuring integrated sum of squares of principal curvatures over the deformed template surface (this quantity is scale invariant); the assumption being that smoother surfaces more accurately reflect natural anatomy in these applications.

Further, to overcome limitations surrounding the accuracy of manual segmentation and to emphasize the robustness of our algorithm, we evaluate its performance on simulated data. Five hippocampal shapes are generated according to the PCA model in Section 4.1, and landmarks are placed on the vertices shown in Figure 1(a) with additive Gaussian noise of variance 0.01, 0.1, 1, 10, and 100 times that of the weighting parameter discussed in Section 3.3.2. Traditional LDDMM landmark matching as well as GDAS is run on this dataset using the same parameters as for our real data, emulating a scenario where errors in landmark placement are unknown beforehand. We demonstrate robustness by reporting κ scores as a function of landmark noise for both algorithms. Lastly, we show the accuracy at which PCA coefficients are recovered using Mahalanobis distance, and P values corresponding to such distances are shown for real and simulated data.

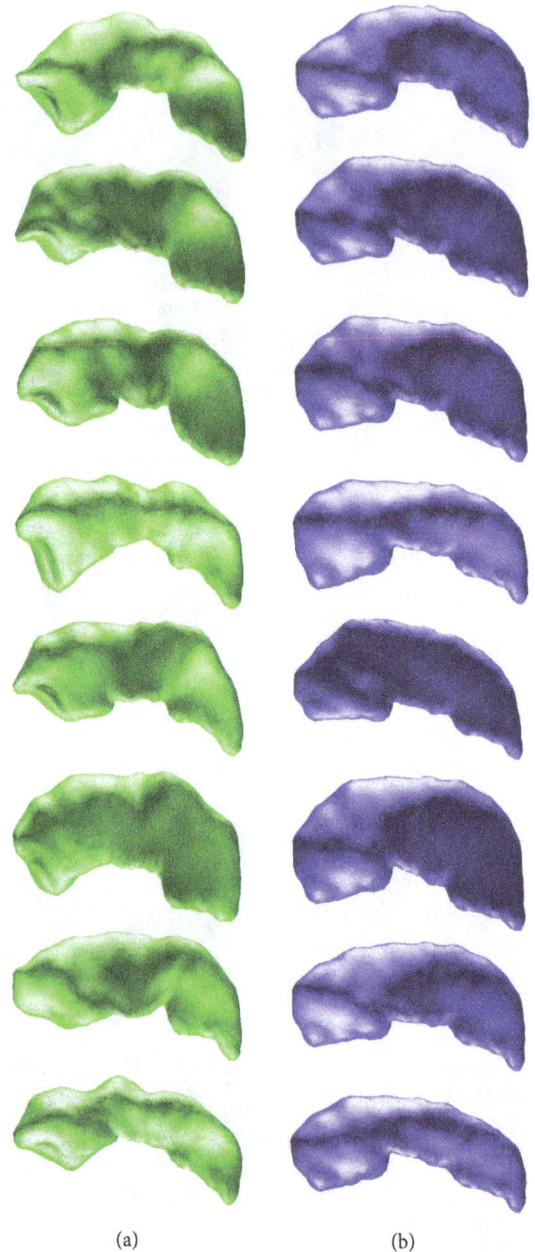

(a)   (b)

FIGURE 5: Segmentation results for standard landmark matching (left/green) and GDAS landmark matching (right/blue), for an additional 8 examples demonstrating GDAS overcoming common pitfalls.

5. Results

5.1. Principal Component Analysis. After performing tangent space PCA with the left hippocampus for the ADNI dataset, we found 31 dimensions characterized 95% of the variability for this population (to be contrasted with 1184×3 dimensions associated with a momentum vector at each vertex of the discretized surface). This is illustrated in Figure 2.

5.2. Examples: Surface Matching. For 5 examples, the outcomes of traditional LDDMM surface matching [17] and

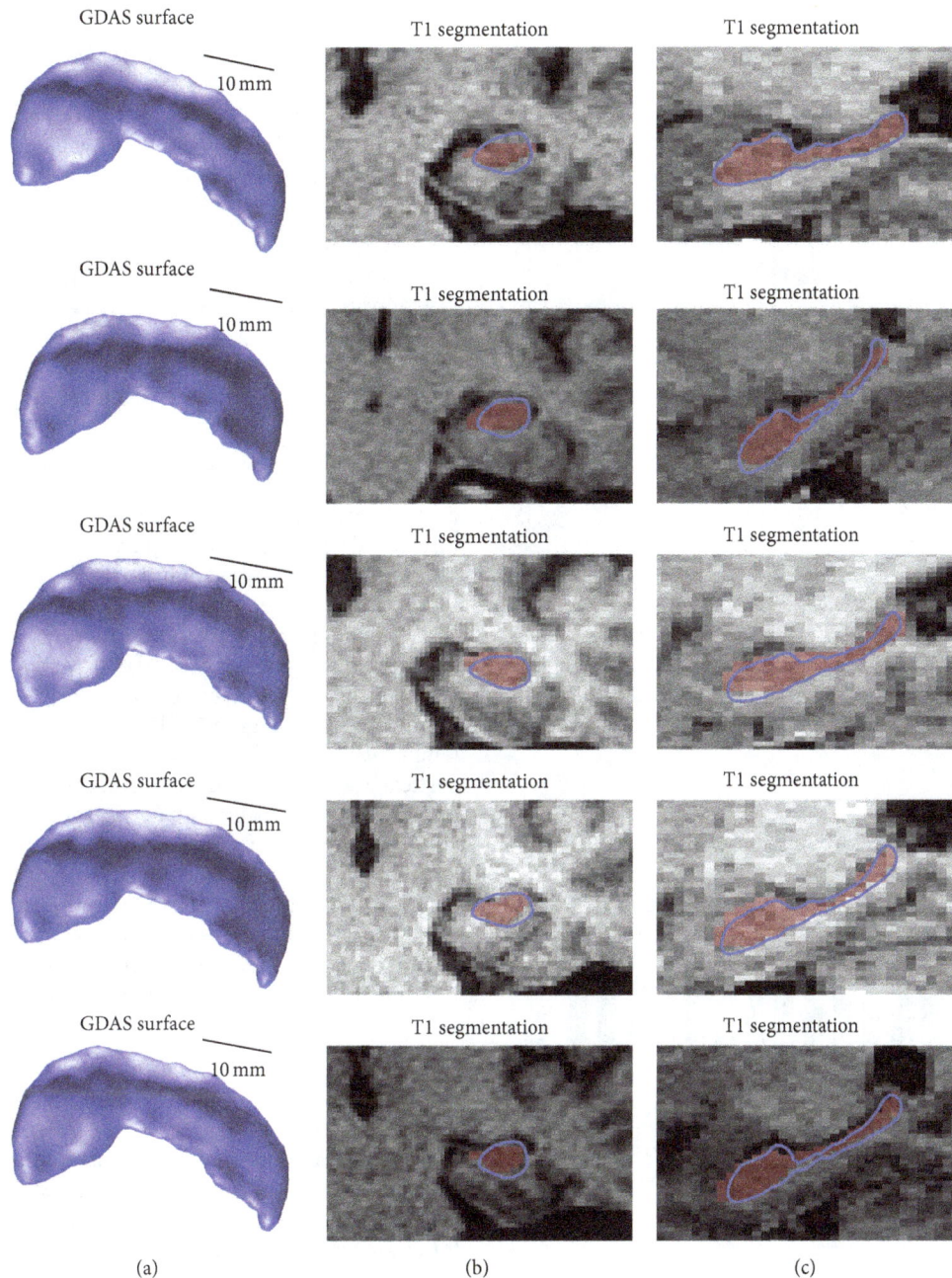

FIGURE 6: Example segmentations of T1 images using GDAS image segmentation based on inside-outside modelling. The resulting surfaces are shown on the left-hand side, and T1 images with gold standard (red highlight) and segmentation (blue curve) are shown in coronal (center) and sagittal (right) views.

GDAS surface matching are shown in Figure 3, with target isosurfaces shown on the right-hand side. Qualitatively speaking, the traditional LDDMM result tends to produce squared off hippocampal heads (left side in figure) due to outlier voxels, as well as an overestimation of the medial margin (bottom of figure) due to overfitting an outlier "ribbon" of voxels.

The constraints imposed in GDAS surface matching result in a useful and accurate segmentation reflective of the population being analyzed. The "fingerlike" and "ribbonlike" projections reflecting the voxelized structure of the target isosurface, as well as the set of constraints used in Freesurfer that are designed for an unrelated application, do not significantly influence the resulting surface.

5.3. *Examples: Robust Landmark Matching.* For 3 cases requiring quality control and 2 typical cases, the outcome of landmark matching is shown in Figure 4. Traditional landmark matching is shown on the left side (green), while GDAS landmark matching is shown in the center column

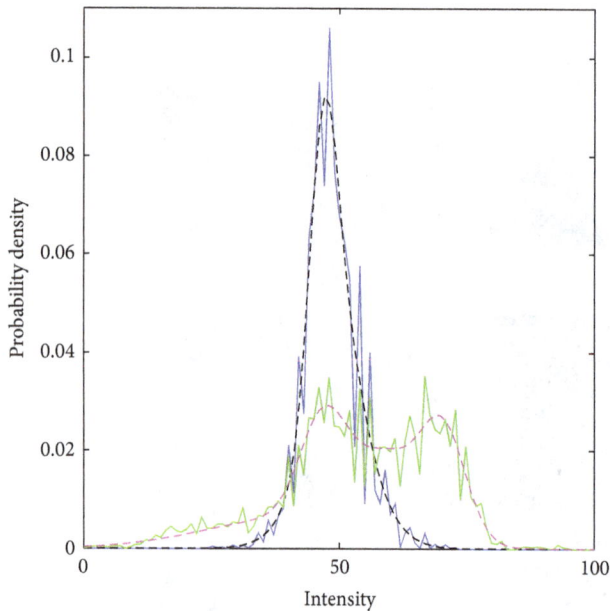

FIGURE 7: Mixture modeling is shown for inside (narrow curve, red/blue) and outside (broad curve, magenta/green) T1 voxel intensities (after histogram equalization). The T1 data is shown with broken lines and the mixture model with solid lines.

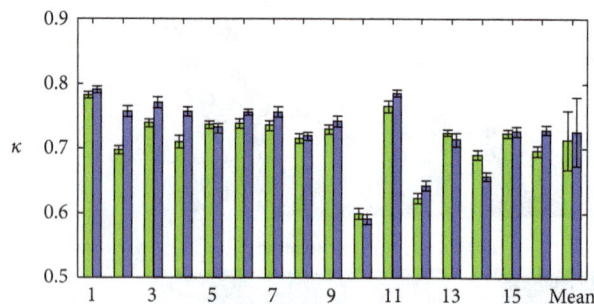

FIGURE 8: Kappa scores are shown for each of the 16 patients examined, with mean and standard deviation shown on the right. Green/left of pair: typical landmark matching; blue/right of pair: GDAS landmark matching.

(blue). In the right-hand column, the surfaces are shown overlaid on a T1 image, with the gold standard segmentation shown in red.

Qualitatively, the improvement of the GDAS algorithm over traditional landmark matching is evident. Large distortions at the head of the hippocampus are common where landmark placement can be quite variable. Along the length of the hippocampus, deformations with scale characteristic of the distance between landmarking planes are easily seen. These issues are still common in those surfaces not requiring quality control. The GDAS algorithm avoids each of these pitfalls, avoiding overfitting landmarks while maintaining shape variability characteristic of the population.

Because poor performance of traditional landmark LDDMM motivated this analysis, we also display (in less detail) results for an additional 8 patients selected randomly

from among those identified as performing poorly. These are shown in Figure 5 with traditional LDDMM results shown in the left column and GDAS results shown in the right column. It is evident that the distortions seen in the top three rows of Figure 4 are typical for this dataset, and that the GDAS results avoid these distortions in a similar manner.

5.4. Examples: Image Segmentation. An example of the results of Gaussian mixture modeling is shown as probability density functions in Figure 7. Measured data (after histogram equalization) is shown as a solid curve, and the results of mixture modeling as dashed curve. The Gaussian mixture parameters are quite similar in all cases examined. The "inside" region (narrow curve, blue and red) is a unimodal distribution describing subcortical gray matter. The challenge of this application can be seen from the "outside" region (broad curve, green and magenta), which is a more heterogenous mixture. It describes cerebrospinal fluid and white matter, as well as cortical gray matter and partial-volume voxels whose intensities are quite similar to the "inside".

Five example segmentation results are shown in Figure 6. The performance appears satisfactory, an achievement considering the large overlap between inside and outside histograms seen in Figure 7. The PCA prior can prevent the template surface from deforming to erroneously include cortical gray matter in many cases, even though it is similar or identical in intensity to subcortical gray matter. This simple inside/outside model could likely be improved, for example, by including a heterogenous appearance model, or combining landmarks and intensity information in cost functions. However, this will be the subject of future research. The purpose of this section was to demonstrate the extensibility of the GDAS framework to a varied range of applications.

5.5. Evaluation: ROI Method Case Study. For the landmark matching application, we describe in detail the performance of the GDAS algorithm as compared to our existing method.

The overlap on a large scale is quantified by κ scores, as shown in Figure 8 for each of the 16 test cases. The GDAS results tend to be similar, but better on average than those for landmark LDDMM. For typical landmark matching, the mean and standard deviation of κ is 0.7131 ± 0.0457, and for GDAS landmark matching, it is 0.7268 ± 0.0531. The difference is statistically significant ($P < 0.05$ in Student's paired t-test).

For those cases with two raters, we examine the second κ score, which differed from the first by 2.66% on average, to understand interrater variability. We present κ scores, averaged over the two raters in Table 1. In each case, the GDAS method performs superiorly for both raters, and this is reflected in the increased average κ scores from 0.732 to 0.751. Despite this improvement, it is interesting to note that the κ overlap between the two manual segmentations is comparable to that between the results of the two segmentation methods.

Examining overlap voxel by voxel, as in Figure 8, shows our algorithm making a small improvement in accuracy. However, the relatively larger improvement in robustness

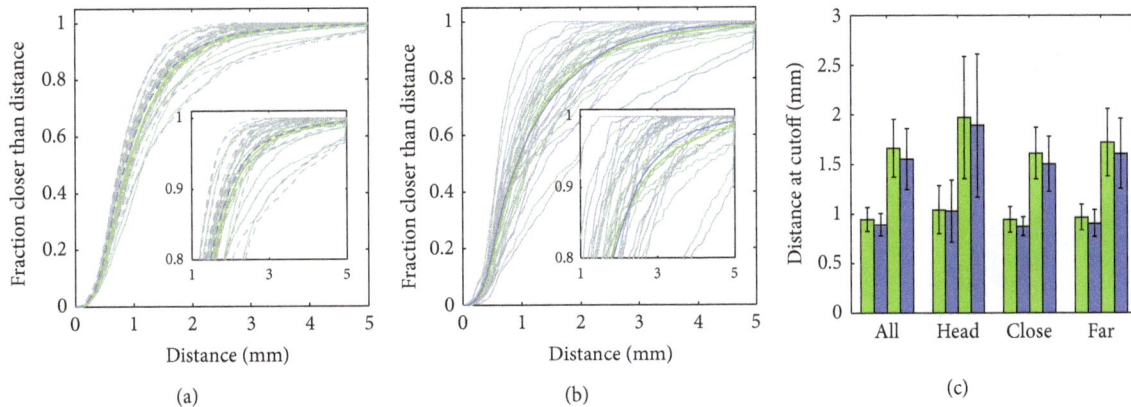

FIGURE 9: Surface-to-surface distance c.d.f.s including (a) all vertices and (b) only vertices within 10 mm of head landmark. Inset shows same data zoomed to ≥80%. Plot (c) shows the 50% (left pair in a set of four) and 80% (right pair in a set) crossing for the vertices shown in (a) ("All") and (b) ("Head"), as well as within 2.5 mm of any landmark ("Close") or not ("Far"). Green/solid/left of pair: traditional LDDMM; blue/broken/right of pair: GDAS.

TABLE 1: Interrater variability is examined by presenting κ overlap between various pairs of data (indicated in the left column).

Case	1	2	3	4	5	Average
LDDMM versus Manual Segs.	0.780	0.743	0.718	0.719	0.702	0.732
GDAS versus Manual Segs.	0.784	0.768	0.752	0.721	0.731	0.751
Manual Segs.	0.866	0.853	0.813	0.800	0.784	0.823
LDDMM versus GDAS	0.832	0.820	0.830	0.827	0.829	0.828

can be seen when examining surface shapes globally such as in Figures 4 and 5 and contrasting with expectations from knowledge of neuroanatomy. The region around the head was seen to be particularly challenging to segment in the traditional landmark case, and distortions occurring at the scale of landmark spacing give the impression that certain regions are "left behind." To quantify accuracy globally, while acknowledging these specifically challenging areas, we use surface-to-surface-distance histograms and associated c.d.f.s.

These c.d.f.s are shown for all 16 patients (unsaturated colors, green: standard landmark matching, blue: GDAS) in Figure 9(a). Combining all vertices gives a single c.d.f indicative of the whole population (saturated colors). A CDF closer to the top left reflects a better segmentation. In Figure 9(b), we show the same analysis, but restricted to vertices within 10 mm of the head landmark. This analysis was repeated (not shown) with vertices restricted to those within 2.5 mm of any landmark, and those not within 2.5 mm of any landmark.

For each patient, the 50% and 80% crossings were measured and are plotted in Figure 9(c). In each set of four bars, the left two show 50% crossings, and the right two show 80% crossings. A smaller value indicates a better segmentation, but the 50% crossing indicates a "typical" region, while the 80% crossing indicates an "outlier" region. Our hypothesis was that the GDAS algorithm would show improvement in outlier regions, at the cost of poorer performance in typical regions. However, the data shows better performance from GDAS in all regions examined. This is likely due to traditional

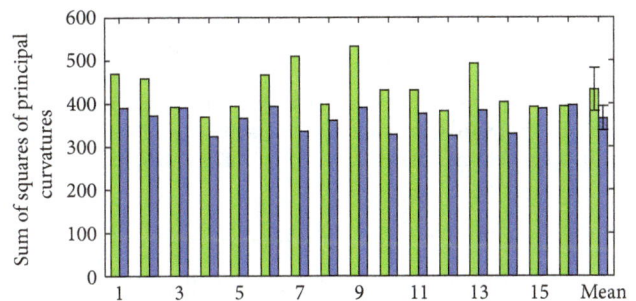

FIGURE 10: Integrated sum of squares of principal curvatures is shown for the 16 patients examined, as well as means and standard deviations. Green/left of pair: typical landmark matching; blue/right of pair: GDAS landmark matching.

LDDMM overfitting landmark placement inaccuracies, while GDAS finds an appropriate balance between landmark matching accuracy and shape variability. Differences show statistical significance ($P < 0.05$ in a Student's paired t-test) with the exception of vertices close to the head (50%: $P = 0.4073$, 80%: $P = 0.0895$).

To further quantify the more natural shapes produced by GDAS, we examine the curvature of the resulting segmentations. For each patient examined, the integrated sum of squares of principal curvatures is shown in Figure 10. In all but one case, the GDAS algorithm results in surfaces with less curvature. The differences are statistically significant ($P < 0.0001$ in a Student's paired t-test).

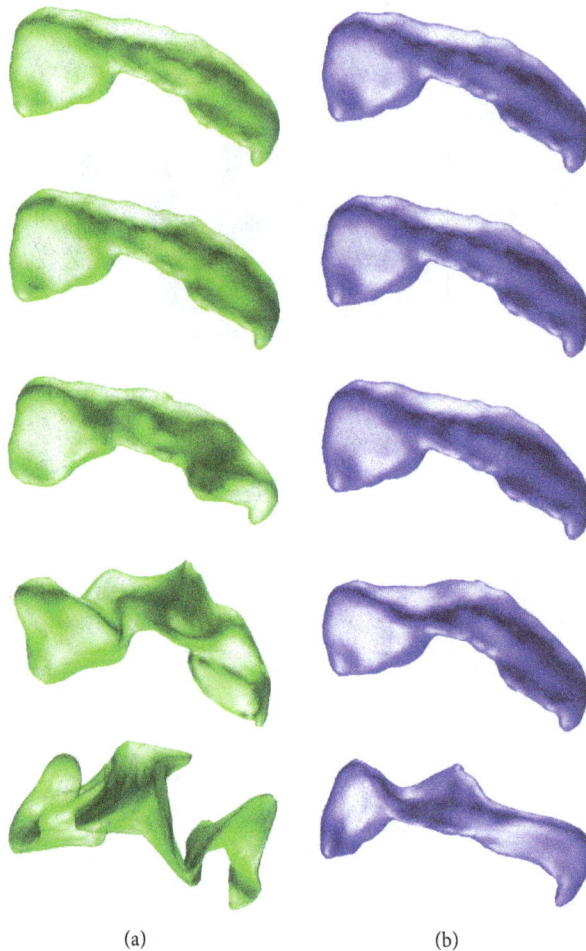

(a)   (b)

FIGURE 11: Example result from simulated data. (a) Standard landmark matching, (b) GDAS landmark matching. Landmark variance from top to bottom: 0.004475, 0.04475, 0.4475, 4.475, and 44.75.

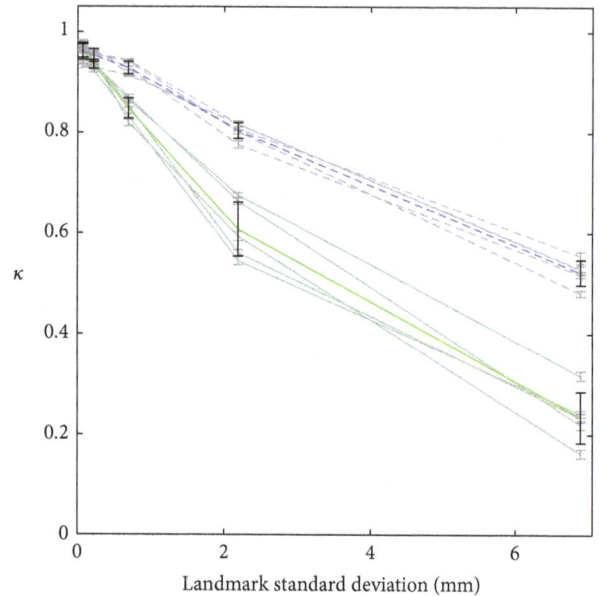

FIGURE 12: Kappa scores are shown for the 5 simulated cases (desaturated) and mean and standard deviation (saturated), as a function of landmark noise. Green/bottom: standard landmark matching; blue/top: GDAS landmark matching.

5.6. Evaluation: Simulated Data. To further quantify the performance and robustness of our landmark matching algorithm, we evaluate it using simulated data such that the gold standard segmentation can be precisely known. Figure 11 shows example results of our landmark matching algorithms as described in Section 4.5, with traditional landmark matching shown on the left side (green) and GDAS landmark matching shown on the right side (blue). From top to bottom, the additive noise in landmark placement increases from 1/10 to 10 times that expected from voxel size in our case study (variance 0.004475, 0.04475, 0.4475, 4.475, and 44.75). At low levels of landmark uncertainty, the two algorithms give very similar results. However, as landmark uncertainty increases, the performance of GDAS exhibits a graceful decline, while that of traditional LDDMM demonstrates a precipitous drop. Note that third row gives a level of landmark uncertainty comparable to that in our case study.

Figure 12 shows κ scores as a function of landmark noise for each of the five simulated cases (desaturated colors), as well as for the average performance (saturated colors). Consistent with our expectations of improved robustness, we see

a much smaller variability in κ scores for GDAS. Furthermore, consistent with our earlier discussion of accuracy, we see poor performance of traditional LDDMM due to overfitting untrustworthy data. Note that the third data point (close to the left-hand side of the figure) corresponds to a level of landmark uncertainty comparable to that in our case study.

For the GDAS results, we can also express accuracy by measuring the error in PCA coefficients recovered by the algorithm. A natural way to do this is through the Mahalanobis distance (treating the inverse of the covariance matrix as a bilinear symmetric operator defining an inner product). Loosely, this distance is the square root of the sum of squares of differences in PCA coefficients; each being first divided by its respective standard deviation. At the five levels of landmark noise examined, the distance between the true coefficients and those recovered by GDAS (summed over the 31 coefficients) is given by 0.8100, 2.0484, 4.0477, 5.5894, and 5.7708 standard deviations. However, the lower order coefficients, which contribute more to overal shape, are recovered with more accuracy than the higher ones. The first coefficient is recovered with an error of 0.0154, 0.0259, 0.1422, 0.4338, and 0.6215 standard deviations, and the first 5 with an error of 0.0813, 0.2791, 0.5213, 1.6052, 2.0663 standard deviations.

This highlights a potential future direction for the GDAS framework. We calculate the Mahalanobis distance from the origin for each of the 650 patients in our ADNI training set and use the empirical distribution to calculate P values. A sample of these patients is shown in Figure 13(a). Surfaces are colored by their P value and binned for P between the values $\{0, 0.01, 0.05, 0.1, 0.5, 1\}$. Each column represents one bin, and five-example cases per bin are shown. It is evident that such

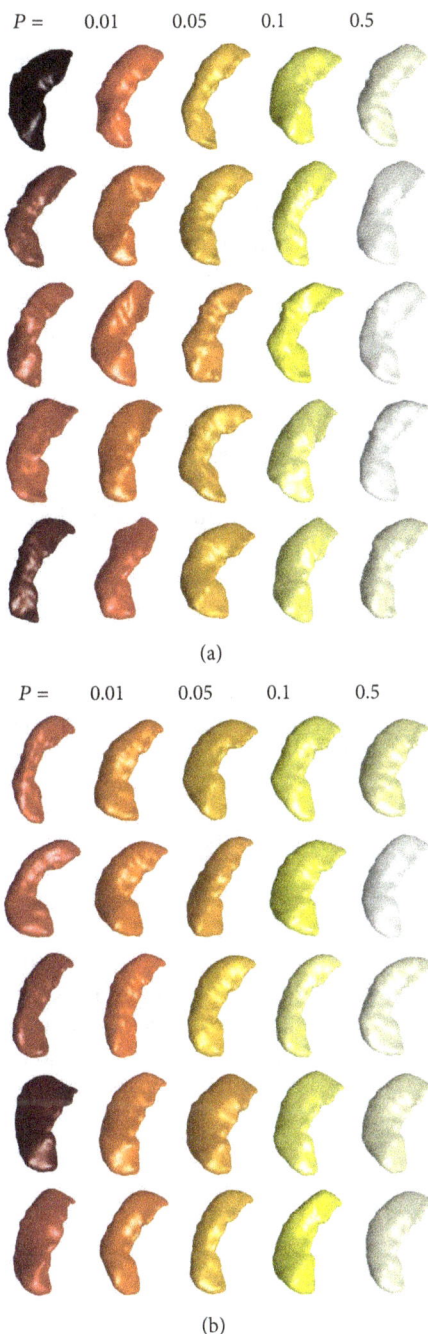

Figure 13: Population of left hippocampus surfaces binned by P value from ADNI dataset. (a) Real patient data. (b) Simulated data.

a distance is descriptive of the naturalness of anatomical shapes, with low P values corresponding to unnatural shapes. Using such a tool to identify outliers for targeted quality control is the subject of future research.

An extension of this idea is the ability to generate random anatomical shapes and quantify their typicality with P values. Some examples are shown in Figure 13(b), with format paralleling what was discussed above. This tool demonstrates the generative nature of the GDAS framework and may prove to be useful for didactic or other purposes.

6. Conclusion

Volumetric segmentation has played an essential role in computer-based interpretation of medical images. There have been many approaches published to address this challenge [1, 51–58]. Most segmentation methods use a combination of shape constraint and data attachment to achieve their goals. Data attachment can be based on geometric data, gray levels, edge detection [59], or unstructured segmentation like K-Means [60] or Gaussian Mixtures [61].

In this paper, we have demonstrated applications of the GDAS framework with data attachment based on landmarks, surfaces, and likelihood ratios from grayscale values. For the case of landmark matching, we demonstrated how it could be used to remove or hasten a laborious quality control phase of large-scale neuroanatomical studies. We quantified its improvement over an existing method based on accuracy, as well as robustness. As is typical of Bayesian analysis, we originally expected to see a tradeoff between accuracy and robustness. However, our results showed improvements in both, likely due to overfitting to noisy data in the standard method, reducing accuracy.

The GDAS algorithm shows improvement over traditional landmark matching in κ scores and surface-to-surface distances, as compared to the gold standard segmentation. Qualitatively, improvements are particularly noticeable in the region around the hippocampus' head (where landmark placement is uncertain). The segmentations resulting from GDAS appear natural, reflecting the typicality and variability of the population from which the PCA basis was determined. This naturalness was quantified in terms of reduced curvature as compared to the traditional method and can be understood in terms of Mahalanobis distance P values.

We have found in large sample studies that robustness is accommodated by our GDAS methods controlled by the PCA dimensions empirically trained from samples of subcortical anatomy. In a study with over 400 hand placements of landmarks in hippocampus and amygdala, we have found that robust GDAS detects our failed landmark based mappings using P-values, supporting the notion that it provides direct method for quality control of large deformation mappings. Exploring this possibility will be the subject of future research.

Our method is based on the geodesically controlled diffeomorphism constraints associated with the momentum conservation law. Encoding structure via prior distributions which are empirically trained has a longstanding tradition in active shape and appearance modeling [4, 62], defined on landmark structures as well as on higher dimensional structures as proposed in [3, 63, 64]. Our principal contribution here has been to encode the diffeomorphism constraint into the standard active shape models. By incorporating the conservation law controls, we not only inherit the power of diffeomorphic transfer of the submanifold surface in the background 3D space, as has been described in [7, 8], but also obtain the metric structure property. Along the geodesic path connecting templates and targets; the metric structure of the large space is maintained.

These properties have been explicitly modelled in our own methods previously using deformable templates acted upon by diffeomorphisms and embedding them into the associated metric space structures [12, 65]. These formulations have tended to explicitly model the transformations on the entire dense background space Ω, working to minimize a cost function accumulated over the entire space. In the setting where the template consists of a collection of homogeneous substructures, we would expect to obtain similar formulations as described herein. In fact, Qiu and Miller [48] have used dense deformations for statistical modeling in such settings via their support on the boundaries of the cortical substructures.

Appendices

A. Image Segmentation Energy Gradient

Theorem A.1. *The gradient of* (18) *with respect to the kth deformed template vertex is given by* (19).

In the proof of the theorem, we will use the following lemma (see [34] for a proof).

Lemma A.2. *Let S be a surface and v a smooth function on S with values in* $\mathbb{R}^3$. *For small* $\epsilon > 0$, *let* S_ϵ *denote the surface* $S + \epsilon v_{|_S}$. *Let h be a smooth vector field on* $\mathbb{R}^3$. *One has*

$$
\partial_\epsilon \left(\int_{S_\epsilon} h^T n_\epsilon d\sigma_\epsilon \right)\Big|_{\epsilon=0}
$$
$$
= \int_{\partial S} \det(\tau, h, v)\, d\ell + \int_S (\nabla \cdot h)\, v^T n\, d\sigma,
$$
(A.1)

where τ *is the positively oriented tangent to the boundary of S,* n_ϵ *and* σ_ϵ, *respectively, denote the unit normal and the area form on* S_ϵ, *and* $\nabla \cdot h$ *is the divergence of h.*

Proof of Theorem 1. First notice that by adding and subtracting $\int_{x \in \text{int}(S)} \log [p_{\text{int}}(I(x))] dx$, we can rewrite the energy as

$$
E_2 = \int_{x \in \text{int}(S)} g(x)\, dx + \text{cst},
$$
(A.2)

where the constant, cst, has gradient zero.

Define surface faces and normals as in Section 3.2.1. Note that the unit normal on a face is $n_f^\alpha = N_f^\alpha / |N_f^\alpha|$, the area of face f being $|N_f^\alpha|$. A generic point in face f takes the form

$$
y = \lambda_1 x_{f,1}^\alpha + \lambda_2 x_{f,2}^\alpha + \lambda_3 x_{f,3}^\alpha,
$$
(A.3)

with $\lambda_1, \lambda_2, \lambda_3 \geq 0$ and $\lambda_1 + \lambda_2 + \lambda_3 = 1$. These coefficients are explicitly given by

$$
\lambda_j N_f = \frac{1}{2} \left(m_{f,j}^\alpha - y \right) \times e_{f,j}^\alpha.
$$
(A.4)

A variation $x_k^\alpha \mapsto x_k^\alpha + \epsilon \eta_k$ for $k = 1, \ldots, L$ implies for such a y the transformation $y + \epsilon v(y)$ with

$$
v(y) = \lambda_1 \eta_{f,1} + \lambda_2 \eta_{f,2} + \lambda_3 \eta_{f,3}.
$$
(A.5)

The mapping v which is defined this way is a continuous vector field on S and smooth (linear) over each face. Introduce a function h such that $\nabla \cdot h = g$ (such an h always exists). By Stokes theorem, we have

$$
E_2 = \int_S \left(h^T n \right) d\sigma + \text{cst}.
$$
(A.6)

We can decompose this integral over all faces and apply (A.1) in Lemma A.2 to each face. Summing the result over the faces and noting that the boundary terms cancel (because the tangents of two neighbor faces are in opposite directions), we find

$$
\left(\frac{dE_2}{dx^\alpha} \right)^T \eta = \sum_{f \in F} \int_f g\, (v \cdot n_f)\, d\sigma_f.
$$
(A.7)

Replacing v by its expression and reordering the sum over the vertices yield

$$
\left(\frac{dE_2}{dx^\alpha} \right)^T \eta
$$
$$
= \sum_{k=1}^L \eta_k^T \left(\sum_{f : x_k^\alpha = x_{f,i}^\alpha} \frac{1}{2 |N_f|} \int_f g(y) \left(m_{f,i}^\alpha - y \right) \times e_{f,i}^\alpha d\sigma_f \right).
$$
(A.8)

Equation (19) follows, completing the proof.

B. Adjoint Method

We need the following definitions, associated to the variation of (2) and its transpose. Applying an infinitesimal variation $\alpha \to \alpha + \delta\alpha$ in the initial condition induces infinitesimal variations $a + \delta a$ and $x + \delta x$, and the pair $(\delta x, \delta a)$ obeys the following differential system, that can be obtained from a formal variation of (2):

$$
\frac{d\delta x_k(t)}{dt} = \sum_{l=1}^L \gamma_{kl} \delta a_l + 2\gamma_{kl}' a_l (x_k - x_l) \cdot (\delta x_k - \delta x_l),
$$

$$
\frac{d\delta a_k(t)}{dt} = \sum_{l=1}^L -2\gamma_{kl}' (a_l \cdot \delta a_k + \delta a_l \cdot a_k)(x_k - x_l)
$$
$$
- 2\sum_{l=1}^L \gamma_{kl}' (a_l \cdot a_k)(\delta x_k - \delta x_l)
$$
$$
- 4\sum_{l=1}^L \gamma_{kl}'' (a_l \cdot a_k)(x_k - x_l)
$$
$$
\times ((x_k - x_l) \cdot (\delta x_k - \delta x_l)),
$$
(B.1)

with $\gamma_{kl}'' = \gamma''(\|x_k - x_l\|^2)$ (recall that $\gamma_{kl}, \gamma_{kl}'$ are short for $\gamma(\|x_k - x_l\|^2)$ and $\gamma'(\|x_k - x_l\|^2)$).

This linear system can be rewritten in matrix form:

$$
\frac{d}{dt} \begin{pmatrix} \delta x \\ \delta \alpha \end{pmatrix} = J(t) \begin{pmatrix} \delta x \\ \delta \alpha \end{pmatrix}.
$$
(B.2)

We let $\zeta(x^0, \alpha, \rho)$ denote the solution at $t = 1$ of (B.1) initialized at $\delta x(0) = 0$ and $\delta\alpha(0) = \rho$, solved along with (2) initialized with (x^0, α). We define the dual variation $\zeta^*(x^0, \alpha, \xi)$ as follows. First, solve (2) with initial conditions $x(0) = x^0$ and $a(0) = \alpha$. Then, solve

$$\frac{d}{dt}\begin{pmatrix} \eta_x \\ \eta_\alpha \end{pmatrix} = -J(t)^* \begin{pmatrix} \eta_x \\ \eta_\alpha \end{pmatrix}, \tag{B.3}$$

from time $t = 1$ to time $t = 0$ with $\eta_x(1) = \xi$ and $\eta_\alpha(1) = 0$, and set

$$\zeta^*\left(x^0, \alpha, \xi\right) = \eta_\alpha(0). \tag{B.4}$$

We state without proof the following lemma, which is a consequence of the theory of linear differential systems (cf. [34, 35] for a proof).

Lemma A.3. *For dynamic system* (2), *let* $dx^\alpha / d\alpha$ *denote the Jacobian matrix of the nonlinear transformation* $\alpha \mapsto x^\alpha$, *represented as a 3L by 3L matrix. One has, for a momentum vector* ρ,

$$\left(\frac{dx^\alpha}{d\alpha}\right)\rho = \zeta\left(x^0, \alpha, \rho\right), \tag{B.5}$$

and, for a vector $\xi \in \mathbb{R}^{3L}$,

$$\left(\frac{dx^\alpha}{d\alpha}\right)^T \xi = \zeta^*\left(x^0, \alpha, \xi\right). \tag{B.6}$$

In our application, setting $\xi = \partial E_2 / \partial x^\alpha$, we retreive

$$\begin{aligned} \left(\frac{\partial E_2}{\partial \alpha}\right) &= \left(\frac{\partial x^\alpha}{\partial \alpha}\right)^T \left(\frac{\partial E_2}{\partial x^\alpha}\right) \\ &= \zeta^*\left(x^0, \alpha, \frac{\partial E_2}{\partial x^\alpha}\right), \end{aligned} \tag{B.7}$$

which is used in calculating the energy gradient.

Acknowledgments

This work is partially supported by R24-HL085343, R01-EB000975, P41-EB015909, R01-EB008171, R01-MH084803, U01-AG033655, U01-NS082085, and the Julie Payette (NSERC) Natural Sciences and Engineering Research Council of Canada Research Scholarship. Some data collection and sharing for this project were funded by the Alzheimer's Disease Neuroimaging Initiative (ADNI) (National Institutes of Health Grant U01 AG024904). ADNI is funded by the National Institute on Aging the National Institute of Biomedical Imaging and Bioengineering and through generous contributions from the following: Abbott; Alzheimer's Association; Alzheimer's Drug Discovery Foundation; Amorfix Life Sciences Ltd.; AstraZeneca; Bayer HealthCare; BioClinica, Inc.; Biogen Idec Inc.; Bristol-Myers Squibb Company; Eisai Inc.; Elan Pharmaceuticals Inc.; Eli Lilly and Company; F. Hoffmann-La Roche Ltd. and its affiliated company Genentech, Inc.; GE Healthcare; Innogenetics N.V.; Janssen Alzheimer Immunotherapy Research & Development, LLC.; Johnson & Johnson Pharmaceutical Research & Development LLC.; Medpace, Inc.; Merck & Co., Inc.; Meso Scale Diagnostics, LLC.; Novartis Pharmaceuticals Corporation; Pfizer Inc.; Servier; Synarc Inc.; and Takeda Pharmaceutical Company. The Canadian Institutes of Health Research are providing funds to support ADNI clinical sites in Canada. Private sector contributions are facilitated by the Foundation for the National Institutes of Health (http://www.fnih.org/). The grantee organization is the Northern California Institute for Research and Education, and the study is coordinated by the Alzheimer's Disease Cooperative Study at the University of California, San Diego, CA, USA. ADNI data are disseminated by the Laboratory for Neuro Imaging at the University of California, Los Angeles, CA, USA. This research was also supported by NIH Grants P30 AG010129 and K01 AG030514. Data used in preparation of this paper were obtained from the Alzheimer's Disease Neuroimaging Initiative (ADNI) database (http://adni.loni.ucla.edu/). As such, the investigators within the ADNI contributed to the design and implementation of ADNI and/or provided data but did not participate in the analysis or writing of this report. A complete listing of ADNI investigators can be found at http://adni.loni.ucla.edu/wp-content/uploads/how_to_apply/ADNI_Acknowledgement_List.pdf.

References

[1] M. Kass, A. Witkin, and D. Terzopoulos, "Snakes: active contour models," *International Journal of Computer Vision*, vol. 1, no. 4, pp. 321–331, 1988.

[2] R. Dann, J. Hoford, S. Kovacic, M. Reivich, and R. Bajcsy, "Evaluation of elastic matching system for anatomic (CT, MR) and functinal (PET) cerebral images," *Journal of Computer Assisted Tomography*, vol. 13, no. 4, pp. 603–611, 1989.

[3] L. H. Staib and J. S. Duncan, "Boundary finding with parametrically deformable models," *IEEE Transactions on Pattern Analysis and Machine Intelligence*, vol. 14, no. 11, pp. 1061–1075, 1992.

[4] T. F. Cootes, C. J. Taylor, D. H. Cooper, and J. Graham, "Active shape models-their training and application," *Computer Vision and Image Understanding*, vol. 61, no. 1, pp. 38–59, 1995.

[5] U. Grenander and M. I. Miller, "Representations of knowledge in complex systems," *Journal of the Royal Statistical Society B*, vol. 56, no. 4, pp. 549–603, 1994.

[6] Z. Sirong, L. Younes, J. Zweck, and J. T. Ratnanather, "Diffeomorphic surface flows: a novel method of surface evolution," *SIAM Journal on Applied Mathematics*, vol. 68, no. 3, pp. 806–824, 2007.

[7] L. Younes, F. Arrate, and M. I. Miller, "Evolutions equations in computational anatomy," *NeuroImage*, vol. 45, no. 1, pp. S40–S50, 2009.

[8] F. Arrate, J. Tilak Ratnanather, and L. Younes, "Diffeomorphic active contours," *SIAM Journal on Imaging Sciences*, vol. 3, no. 2, pp. 176–198, 2010.

[9] G. E. Christensen, R. D. Rabbitt, and M. I. Miller, "Deformable templates using large deformation kinematics," *IEEE Transactions on Image Processing*, vol. 5, no. 10, pp. 1435–1447, 1996.

[10] A. Trouvé, "Diffeomorphisms groups and pattern matching in image analysis," *International Journal of Computer Vision*, vol. 28, no. 3, pp. 213–221, 1998.

[11] P. Dupuis, U. Grenander, and M. I. Miller, "Variational problems on flows of diffeomorphisms for image matching," *Quarterly of Applied Mathematics*, vol. 56, no. 3, pp. 587–600, 1998.

[12] M. I. Miller, A. Trouvé, and L. Younes, "On the metrics and Euler-Lagrange equations of computational anatomy," *Annual Review of Biomedical Engineering*, vol. 4, pp. 375–405, 2002.

[13] V. I. Arnold, "Sur la geomerie differentielle des groupes de lie de dimension infinie et ses applications a l'hydrodynamique des uides parfaits," *Annales De L'Institut Fourier*, vol. 16, no. 1, pp. 319–361, 1966.

[14] D. D. Holm, J. E. Marsden, and T. S. Ratiu, "The euler-poincaré equations and semidirect products with applications to continuum theories," *Advances in Mathematics*, vol. 137, no. 1, pp. 1–81, 1998.

[15] J. E. Marsden and T. S. Ratiu, *Introduction to Mechanics and Symmetry*, Springer, 1999.

[16] M. I. Miller, A. Trouvé, and L. Younes, "Geodesic shooting for computational anatomy," *Journal of Mathematical Imaging and Vision*, vol. 24, no. 2, pp. 209–228, 2006.

[17] M. Vaillant and J. Glaunès, "Surface matching via currents," in *Proceedings of Information Processing in Medical Imaging*, vol. 3565, 2005.

[18] A. Qiu, L. Younes, and M. Miller, "Principal component based diffeomorphic surface mapping," *IEEE Transactions on Medical Imaging*, vol. 31, pp. 302–3311, 2012.

[19] T. Cootes and C. Taylor, "Active shape models smart snakes," in *Proceedings of the British Machine Vision Conference*, pp. 266–275, Citeseer, 1992.

[20] A. M. Baumberg and D. C. Hogg, "An efficient method for contour tracking using active shape models," in *Proceedings of the IEEE Workshop on Motion of Non-Rigid and Articulated Objects*, pp. 194–199, Citeseer, November 1994.

[21] T. Cootes, A. Hill, C. Taylor, and J. Haslam, "Use of active shape models for locating structures in medical images," *Image and Vision Computing*, vol. 12, no. 6, pp. 355–365, 1994.

[22] N. Duta and M. Sonka, "Segmentation and interpretation of MR brain images: an improved active shape model," *IEEE Transactions on Medical Imaging*, vol. 17, no. 6, pp. 1049–1062, 1998.

[23] B. Van Ginneken, A. F. Frangi, J. J. Staal, B. M. Ter Haar Romeny, and M. A. Viergever, "Active shape model segmentation with optimal features," *IEEE Transactions on Medical Imaging*, vol. 21, no. 8, pp. 924–933, 2002.

[24] C. Davatzikos, X. Tao, and D. Shen, "Hierarchical active shape models, using the wavelet transform," *IEEE Transactions on Medical Imaging*, vol. 22, no. 3, pp. 414–423, 2003.

[25] D. Rueckert, A. Frangi, and J. Schnabel, "Automatic construction of 3d statistical deformation models using non-rigid registration," in *Proceedings of the Medical Image Computing and Computer-Assisted Intervention (MICCAI '01)*, pp. 77–84, Springer, 2010.

[26] U. Grenander, Y. Chow, and D. M. Keenan, *Hands: A Pattern Theoretic Study of Biological Shapes*, Springer, 1991.

[27] U. Grenander and M. I. Miller, "Representation of knowledge in complex systems (with discussion section)," *Journal of the Royal Statistical Society*, vol. 56, no. 4, pp. 569–603, 1994.

[28] S. C. Zhu, "Region competition: unifying snakes, region growing, and bayes/mdl for multiband image segmentation," *IEEE Transactions on Pattern Analysis and Machine Intelligence*, vol. 18, no. 9, pp. 884–900, 1996.

[29] T. F. Chan and L. A. Vese, "Active contours without edges," *IEEE Transactions on Image Processing*, vol. 10, no. 2, pp. 266–277, 2001.

[30] G. Sapiro, *Geometric Partial Differential Equations and Image Analysis*, Cambridge University Press, 2001.

[31] R. Guillemaud and M. Brady, "Estimating the bias field of MR images," *IEEE Transactions on Medical Imaging*, vol. 16, no. 3, pp. 238–251, 1997.

[32] W. M. Wells III, W. E. L. Crimson, R. Kikinis, and F. A. Jolesz, "Adaptive segmentation of mri data," *IEEE Transactions on Medical Imaging*, vol. 15, no. 4, pp. 429–442, 1996.

[33] M. Vaillant, M. I. Miller, L. Younes, and A. Trouvé, "Statistics on diffeomorphisms via tangent space representations," *NeuroImage*, vol. 23, no. 1, pp. S161–S169, 2004.

[34] L. Younes, *Shapes and Diffeomorphisms*, Applied Mathematical Sciences, Springer, 2010.

[35] J. Ma, M. I. Miller, and L. Younes, "A bayesian generative model for surface template estimation," *International Journal of Biomedical Imaging*, vol. 2010, Article ID 974957, 14 pages, 2010.

[36] H. Le, "Mean size-and-shapes and mean shapes: a geometric point of view," *Advances in Applied Probability*, vol. 27, pp. 44–55, 1995.

[37] E. Klassen, A. Srivastava, W. Mio, and S. H. Joshi, "Analysis of planar shapes using geodesic paths on shape spaces," *IEEE Transactions on Pattern Analysis and Machine Intelligence*, vol. 26, no. 3, pp. 372–383, 2004.

[38] P. T. Fletcher, S. Venkatasubramanian, and S. Joshi, "Robust statistics on Riemannian manifolds via the geometric median," in *Proceedings of the 26th IEEE Conference on Computer Vision and Pattern Recognition (CVPR '08)*, pp. 1–8, June 2008.

[39] C. Bishop, *Pattern Recognition and Machine Learning*, Springer, New York, NY, USA, 2006.

[40] J. W. Haller, A. Banerjee, G. E. Christensen et al., "Three-dimensional hippocampal MR morphometry with high-dimensional transformation of a neuroanatomic atlas," *Radiology*, vol. 202, no. 2, pp. 504–510, 1997.

[41] J. G. Csernansky, L. Wang, D. Jones et al., "Hippocampal deformities in schizophrenia characterized by high dimensional brain mapping," *American Journal of Psychiatry*, vol. 159, no. 12, pp. 2000–2006, 2002.

[42] J. A. Posener, L. Wang, J. L. Price et al., "High-dimensional mapping of the hippocampus in depression," *American Journal of Psychiatry*, vol. 160, no. 1, pp. 83–89, 2003.

[43] J. G. Csernansky, M. K. Schindler, N. R. Splinter et al., "Abnormalities of thalamic volume and shape in schizophrenia," *American Journal of Psychiatry*, vol. 161, no. 5, pp. 896–902, 2004.

[44] J. G. Csernansky, L. Wang, J. Swank et al., "Preclinical detection of Alzheimer's disease: hippocampal shape and volume predict dementia onset in the elderly," *NeuroImage*, vol. 25, no. 3, pp. 783–792, 2005.

[45] M. A. Munn, J. Alexopoulos, T. Nishino et al., "Amygdala volume analysis in female twins with major depression," *Biological Psychiatry*, vol. 62, no. 5, pp. 415–422, 2007.

[46] M. M. Mielke, N. J. Haughey, V. V. Ratnam Bandaru et al., "Plasma ceramides are altered in mild cognitive impairment and predict cognitive decline and hippocampal volume loss," *Alzheimer's and Dementia*, vol. 6, no. 5, pp. 378–385, 2010.

[47] B. Fischl, "FreeSurfer," *Neuroimage*, vol. 62, no. 2, pp. 774–781, 2012.

[48] A. Qiu and M. I. Miller, "Multi-structure network shape analysis via normal surface momentum maps," *NeuroImage*, vol. 42, no. 4, pp. 1430–1438, 2008.

[49] S. C. Joshi and M. I. Miller, "Landmark matching via large deformation diffeomorphisms," *IEEE Transactions on Image Processing*, vol. 9, no. 8, pp. 1357–1370, 2000.

[50] J. R. Landis and G. G. Koch, "The measurement of observer agreement for categorical data," *Biometrics*, vol. 33, no. 1, pp. 159–174, 1977.

[51] D. L. Pham, C. Xu, and J. L. Prince, "Current methods in medical image segmentation," *Annual Review of Biomedical Engineering*, vol. 2, no. 2000, pp. 315–337, 2000.

[52] S. Osher and J. A. Sethian, "Fronts propagating with curvature-dependent speed: algorithms based on Hamilton-Jacobi formulations," *Journal of Computational Physics*, vol. 79, no. 1, pp. 12–49, 1988.

[53] S. Z. Li, *Markov Random Field Modeling in Computer Vision*, Springer, 1995.

[54] F. L. Bookstein, "Principal warps: Thin-plate splines and the decomposition of deformations," *IEEE Transactions on Pattern Analysis and Machine Intelligence*, vol. 11, pp. 567–585, 1992.

[55] D. Rueckert, "Nonrigid registration using free-form deformations: application to breast mr images," *IEEE Transactions on Medical Imaging*, vol. 18, no. 8, pp. 712–721, 1999.

[56] B. Fischl, D. H. Salat, E. Busa et al., "Whole brain segmentation: automated labeling of neuroanatomical structures in the human brain," *Neuron*, vol. 33, no. 3, pp. 341–355, 2002.

[57] B. Fischl, D. H. Salat, A. J. W. Van Der Kouwe et al., "Sequence-independent segmentation of magnetic resonance images," *NeuroImage*, vol. 23, no. 1, pp. S69–S84, 2004.

[58] X. Han and B. Fischl, "Atlas renormalization for improved brain MR image segmentation across scanner platforms," *IEEE Transactions on Medical Imaging*, vol. 26, no. 4, pp. 479–486, 2007.

[59] M. Unser, "Multigrid adaptive image processing," in *Proceedings of the IEEE International Conference on Image Processing*, vol. 1, pp. 49–52, October 1995.

[60] A. Kumar, A. Yezzi, S. Kichenassamy, P. Olver, and A. Tannenbaum, "Active contours for visual tracking: a geometric gradient based approach," in *Proceedings of the 34th IEEE Conference on Decision and Control*, vol. 1, pp. 4041–4046, December 1995.

[61] C. E. Priebe, M. I. Miller, and J. Tilak Ratnanather, "Segmenting magnetic resonance images via hierarchical mixture modelling," *Computational Statistics and Data Analysis*, vol. 50, no. 2, pp. 551–567, 2006.

[62] T. F. Cootes, G. J. Edwards, and C. Taylor, "Active appearance models," *IEEE Transactions on Pattern Analysis and Machine Intelligence*, vol. 23, pp. 681–685, 2001.

[63] A. Srivastava, A. Jain, S. Joshi, and D. Kaziska, "Statistical shape models using elastic-string representations," in *Proceedings of the 7th Asian conference on Computer Vision (ACCV '06)*, vol. 3851 of *Lecture Notes in Computer Science*, pp. 612–621.

[64] D. Cremers, T. Kohlberger, and C. Schnörr, "Shape statistics in kernel space for variational image segmentation," *Pattern Recognition*, vol. 36, no. 9, pp. 1929–1943, 2003.

[65] U. Grenander and M. I. Miller, "Computational anatomy: an emerging discipline," *Quarterly of Applied Mathematics*, vol. 56, no. 4, pp. 617–694, 1998.

7

Improving Image Quality in Medical Images Using a Combined Method of Undecimated Wavelet Transform and Wavelet Coefficient Mapping

Du-Yih Tsai,[1] **Eri Matsuyama,**[1] **and Hsian-Min Chen**[2]

[1] *Department of Radiological Technology, Graduate School of Health Sciences, Niigata University, 2-746 Asahimachi-dori, Niigata 951-8518, Japan*
[2] *Department of Biomedical Engineering, College of Engineering, Hungkuang University, Taichung 43302, Taiwan*

Correspondence should be addressed to Du-Yih Tsai; tsai@clg.niigata-u.ac.jp

Academic Editor: J. C. Chen

We propose a method for improving image quality in medical images by using a wavelet-based approach. The proposed method integrates two components: image denoising and image enhancement. In the first component, a modified undecimated discrete wavelet transform is used to eliminate the noise. In the second component, a wavelet coefficient mapping function is applied to enhance the contrast of denoised images obtained from the first component. This methodology can be used not only as a means for improving visual quality of medical images but also as a preprocessing module for computer-aided detection/diagnosis systems to improve the performance of screening and detecting regions of interest in images. To confirm its superiority over existing state-of-the-art methods, the proposed method is experimentally evaluated via 30 mammograms and 20 chest radiographs. It is demonstrated that the proposed method can further improve the image quality of mammograms and chest radiographs, as compared to two other methods in the literature. These results reveal the effectiveness and superiority of the proposed method.

1. Introduction

Denoising and contrast enhancement operations are two of the most common and important techniques for medical image quality improvement. Because of their importance, there has been an enormous amount of research dedicated to the subject of noise removal and image enhancement [1–4].

With regard to image denoising, some approaches using discrete wavelet transform (DWT) have been proposed [5–7]. The DWT is very efficient from a computational point of view, but it is shift variant. Therefore, its denoising performance can change drastically if the starting position of the signal is shifted. In order to achieve shift invariance, researchers have proposed the undecimated DWT (UDWT) [8–10]. Mencattini et al. reported a UDWT-based method for the reduction of noise in mammographic images [11]. The reported method was robust and effective. However, the method was not advantageous in terms of computational aspects. Zhao et al. proposed an image denoising method

based on Gaussian and non-Gaussian distribution assumptions for wavelet coefficients [12]. Huang et al. reported on a denoising method which involves directly selecting the thresholds for denoising by evaluating some statistical properties of the noise [13]. Recently, Matsuyama et al. proposed a modified UDWT approach to mammographic denoising [14]. The results demonstrated that the method could further improve image quality and decrease image processing time.

As regard to the improvement of contrast enhancement, various image enhancement techniques have been proposed [15–20]. These techniques can be divided into several categories, including histogram equalization [15, 16], region-based [17], fuzzy [18], genetic algorithm [19], and adaptive methodology [20]. Wavelet-based approaches to enhancement of digital images have been also reported [21–25]. Tsai et al. proposed a method which employs an exponential-type mapping function to the wavelet coefficients of digital chest images and then reconstructs an enhanced image with the mapped wavelet coefficients [22, 23]. Lee et al. used a sigmoid-type mapping function for wavelet coefficient weighting adjustment to improve the contrast of medical images [25]. The method was applied to chest radiographs, mammograms, and chest CT images. The method showed a statistically significant superiority over the exponential-type mapping function.

In this study, we expanded upon the previously suggested modified UDWT method [14] and combined it with the sigmoid-type mapping function [25]. By combining the two methods together in sequence, an effective algorithm for both image denoising and enhancement could be obtained. Original images were first denoised using the modified UDWT, followed by image enhancement using the wavelet coefficient mapping function. Finally, a denoised and contrast enhanced image was reconstructed by the inverse wavelet transform. In this study, we investigated the effectiveness of the proposed method by comparing it with two methods in the literature [14, 25].

2. Methods and Materials

2.1. Combined Method of Undecimated Discrete Wavelet Transform and Wavelet Coefficient Mapping.

Figure 1 shows a flowchart of our proposed method. In the first phase, denoising was applied to original images using our newly adopted UDWT. In the second phase, image enhancement was performed using a sigmoid-type transfer function for wavelet coefficient mapping. Sections 2.1.1 and 2.1.2 describe the two phases of the proposed method, respectively.

2.1.1. Extended Undecimated Discrete Wavelet Transform Method.

The UDWT is a wavelet transform algorithm designed to overcome the lack of translation invariance of the DWT. Unlike the DWT, the UDWT does not incorporate the downsampling operations. Thus, the approximation coefficients (low-frequency coefficients) and detailed coefficients (high-frequency coefficients) at each level are the same length as the original signal. The basic algorithm of the conventional UDWT is that it applies the transform at each point of the image and saves the detailed coefficients and uses the approximation coefficients for the next level. The size of the coefficients array does not diminish from level to level. This decomposition operation is further iterated up to a higher level. There are major differences between the modified UDWT method [14] and the conventional UDWT method. First, the conventional UDWT decomposes the original image (level 0) into one low-frequency band and three high-frequency bands for each resolution level with the same size as the original image. The decompositions are usually conducted up to resolution level 4. In contrast, the modified UDWT method only needs to perform the computation up to resolution level 2 and repeat the computation only one time [14, 26]. Second, the conventional UDWT thresholded the detailed coefficients at all 4 levels with the same thresholding value, while the modified UDWT method utilizes the hierarchical correlation of the coefficients between level 1 and level 2 of the three detailed coefficients for thresholding. In other

words, the thresholding values vary and are dependent on the nature of the noise.

The extended UDWT method adopted in the present study was based on the modified UDWT [14]. The method we used mainly consisted of the following steps (see Figure 1).

(1) Perform two-dimensional UDWT to the original image to obtain wavelet coefficients up to level 2.

(2) Calculate the hierarchical correlations of the detailed coefficients between level 1 and level 2 for the three subbands. The correlations for the three detailed subbands are given as

$$\left| \text{Coef}_{\text{lev\_1}}(p,q) \times \text{Coef}_{\text{lev\_2}}(p,q) \right|, \tag{1}$$

where p and q are the new coordinates after wavelet transform. $\text{Coef}_{\text{lev\_1}}$ and $\text{Coef}_{\text{lev\_2}}$ are wavelet coefficients of level 1 and level 2, respectively.

(3) Determine threshold values for each detailed subband. The determination procedure is as follows

(a) Generate a correlation image $\text{Img}_{\text{Cor}}(p,q)$ for each detailed subband:

$$\text{Img}_{\text{Cor}}(p,q) \\ = \left| \text{Coef}_{\text{lev}_1}(p,q) \times \text{Coef}_{\text{lev}_2}(p,q) \right|. \tag{2}$$

(b) Find the maximum value in each row in the horizontal (x-) direction of the obtained correlation image for each of the three detailed subbands.

(c) Compute the mean of the maximum values obtained from all rows in the x-direction of the correlation image. The mean is denoted by Mean_{max}

(d) Eliminate those correlation values greater than $0.8 \times \text{Mean}_{\text{max}}$. These excluded values are considered signal data. The value of 0.8 was determined empirically through experiments.

(e) Compute the standard deviation σ from the remaining correlation values.

(f) Determine the threshold value by use of the following formula:

$$\text{THR} = 1.6 \times \sigma. \tag{3}$$

The value of 1.6 was determined empirically through experiments.

(4) Apply the determined threshold values to the correlation values:

$$\text{New Coef}_{\text{lev\_1}}(p,q) \\ = \begin{cases} \text{Coef}_{\text{lev\_1}}(p,q), & \text{if } \left| \text{Coef}_{\text{lev\_1}} \times \text{Coef}_{\text{lev\_2}} \right| \geq \text{THR}, \\ 0, & \text{otherwise}, \end{cases}$$

$$\tag{4}$$

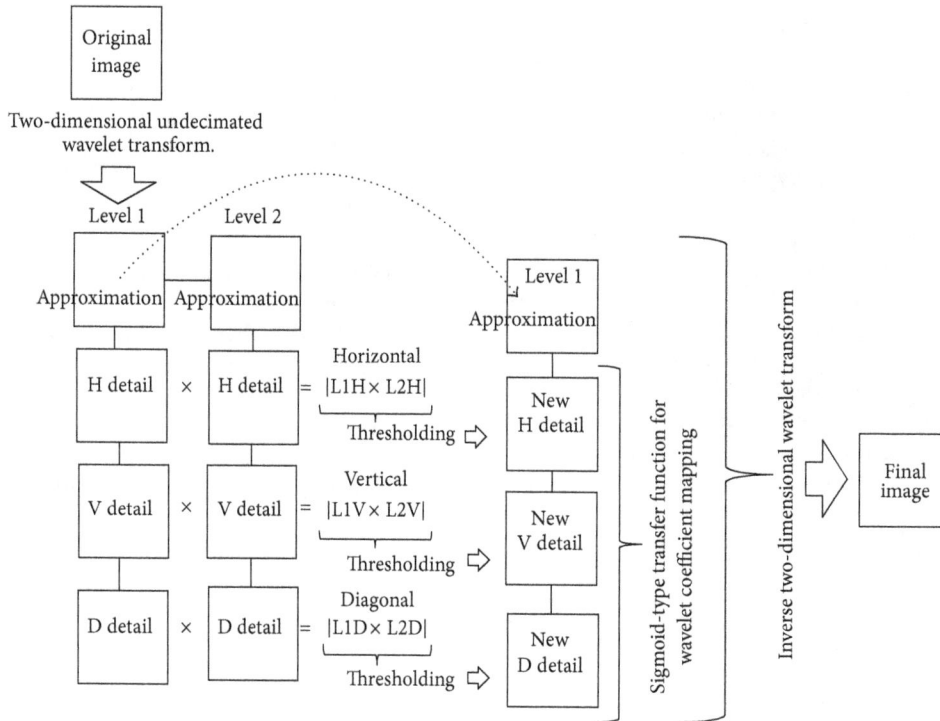

FIGURE 1: A flowchart summarizing the processing procedure for the proposed algorithm.

where New $\text{Coef}_{\text{lev\_1}}(p,q)$ is the newly obtained, modified coefficient for level 1. The modified coefficients of the horizontal, vertical, and diagonal subbands are, respectively, obtained. It should be noted that the threshold operation was only applied to the detailed components. The reason is that the detailed components mainly contain the noise and high-frequency information, whereas the approximation component that mainly contains low-frequency information remains unchanged.

(5) Perform the inverse wavelet transform to reconstruct the denoised image with the approximation coefficient of level 1 and the three newly obtained detailed coefficients of level 1.

In a previous study [14], we evaluated six comparatively popular wavelet basis functions, namely, discrete FIR approximation of Meyer wavelet (dmey), Daubechies order 2 (db2), Symlets order 7 (sym7), Coiflets order 1 (coif1), Coiflets order 5 (coif5), and biorthogonal 6.8 (bior6.8), as candidates for selection as the most suitable basis function for the UDWT. The evaluation results showed that wavelet-processed images with db2 basis function provided the best results among the six basis functions. Thus, we selected db2 basis function for the proposed method [14, 25, 26].

2.1.2. Wavelet Coefficient Mapping. A sigmoid-type transfer curve with a one-to-one mapping function was used for enhancement of image contrast [25]. The mapping function was determined based on the following considerations: (a) wavelet coefficients having high values are heavily weighted

because they carry more useful information; (b) the coefficients at low levels are heavily weighted because they carry detailed information, such as edge information; and (c) the approximation coefficients are not manipulated to prevent image distortion [23, 25].

The input coefficient $w_{\text{input}}^{j}(m,n)$ of level j at position (m,n) was manipulated using the sigmoid-type transfer curves of wavelet coefficients. The mapping function is given by

$$
\begin{aligned}
&w_{\text{output}}^{j}(m,n)\\
&= a \times \frac{1}{1 + \left\{ 1/\exp\left[\left(w_{\text{input}}^{j}(m,n) - c \right)/b \right] \right\}}\\
&\quad \times w_{\text{input}}^{j}(m,n),
\end{aligned}
\tag{5}
$$

where $w_{\text{output}}^{j}(m,n)$ represents output coefficient. a, b, and c are constants and are determined depending on the extent of enhancement to be added. In practice, (6) is used as the mapping function instead of (5). In (6), the values of the coefficients are expressed in terms of percentage for the ease of computation:

$$
\begin{aligned}
w_{\text{output}}^{j} &= a \times \frac{1}{1 + \left[1/\exp\left(\left(w_{\text{input}}^{j} - c \right)/b \right) \right]}\\
&\quad \times w_{\text{input}}^{j}\ [\%].
\end{aligned}
\tag{6}
$$

Here, w_{input}^{j} is the input value expressed in terms of percentage. This value makes the mean of the absolute values of the coefficients at level j equal to 50%. Notation w_{output}^{j} is the corresponding output value expressed in terms of percentage. By utilization of percentage, the constants a, b, and c could be used independent of image characteristics. The value of constant a was obtained using (7):

$$a = 2 - \frac{(j-1)}{N}, \tag{7}$$

where N represents the maximum decomposition level. Consequently, the lower the wavelet decomposition level j, the greater the gradient of the transfer curve becomes. As a result, the wavelet coefficients at low-decomposition levels that contain information about edges of an image are highly weighted. The constant c was determined by use of (8):

$$c = d + b \times \log_e (a - 1.0), \tag{8}$$

where d is a constant used for determining the inflection point of the sigmoid curve, and b represents a constant used for determining the gradient of the sigmoid curve. The values of b and d used in this study were 20 and 25, respectively [23].

2.2. Image Data. To evaluate and validate our proposed method, we used two standard digital databases: a mammogram database and a chest radiograph database. The former was from the Mammographic Image Analysis Society (MIAS) [27] and the latter was from the Japanese Society of Radiological Technology [28]. Patient informed consent was not required. A total of 30 mammograms obtained from the database were used for investigation of the effectiveness of the proposed method. The matrix size of each image was 1024 × 1024 pixels with 8-bit gray-level resolution. The matrix size of each chest radiograph was 2048 × 2048 pixels with 12-bit gray-level resolution. From the radiograph database, 20 chest images were used for the present study.

Other than the described image data, we also prepared another data set by purposely adding a zero-mean Gaussian noise with a standard deviation of 0.01 to the obtained 30 mammograms and 20 chest radiographs. The purpose of using the images with external added noise was to clearly demonstrate the effectiveness of the proposed method by comparing the pixel-value profiles along the horizontal direction of processed images. As for visual perceptual evaluation, in order to keep visual evaluation clinically practical, images without adding external noise were used for visual assessment.

2.3. Visual Perceptual Evaluation. A visual perceptual evaluation was designed for performance analysis. We used Scheffe's method of paired comparison to evaluate the preference of overall image quality [29, 30]. The visual evaluation was made by five experienced radiological technologists (ranging from 20 to 25 years of experience). In the case of mammograms, the obtained 30 mammograms from the data set were processed using the proposed method, the modified UDWT method, and the sigmoid-type wavelet coefficient mapping method. Thus, a total of 90 images were used for image quality evaluation. All images were evaluated on a pair of

widely used medical 3 M monochrome liquid-crystal display monitors. Each observer reviewed the images independently. The reading time was limited to less than 20 seconds for each reading. The observers independently evaluated one pair of images, which were shown on the monitors one at a time, using a 5-point grading scale (−2 points to +2 points). If the image shown on the left was much better than that shown on the right in terms of overall image quality, the left image was given +2 points; the left image was given +1 point when it was slightly better than the right one; the left image was given 0 points, when both images were of the same image quality. Conversely, if the image shown on the left was much poorer than that shown on the right in terms of overall image quality, the left image was given −2 points; the left image was given −1 point when it was slightly poorer than the right one. Comparisons were made by use of three possible combinations, that is, modified UDWT/sigmoid mapping, modified UDWT/proposed method, and sigmoid mapping/proposed method combinations. Each pair of images was determined randomly. In addition, the two paired images (left side versus right side) were arranged on a random basis.

The same procedures were performed for the case of chest radiographs.

2.4. Quantitative Evaluation. In order to compare objectively the performance of the proposed algorithm against two published algorithms [14, 25], in this study we adopted four image quality metrics. The 4 metrics are the mean-to-standard-deviation (MSR), the contrast to noise ratio (CNR), contrast improvement ratio (CIR), and peak signal-to-noise ratio (PSNR). They are briefly described as follows.

The MSR [31, 32] in a desired region of interest (DROI) is defined as

$$\text{MSR} = \frac{\mu_d}{\sigma_d}, \tag{9}$$

where μ_d and σ_d are the mean and standard deviation computed in the DROI. The CNR [31, 32] is defined as

$$\text{CNR} = \frac{|\mu_d - \mu_\mu|}{\sqrt{0.5 \left(\sigma_d^2 + \sigma_\mu^2 \right)}}, \tag{10}$$

where μ_μ and σ_μ are the mean and the standard deviation computed in an undesired region of interest (UROI) such as background. Both the MSR and CNR measurements are proportional to the medical image quality.

The CIR [33] is a quantitative measurement of the contrast improvement and is defined as

$$\text{CIR} = \frac{\sum_i \sum_j |c(i,j) - c'(i,j)^2|}{\sum_i \sum_j c(i,j)^2}, \tag{11}$$

where $c(i,j)$ and $c'(i,j)$ are the local contrast values of original and enhanced images, respectively. The local contrast $c(i,j)$ is defined by the difference of mean values in two

TABLE 1: Results of mammogram scoring for the three combinations by the five observers.

Combination		Observer					
		a	b	c	d	e	Sum
Sigmoid	UDWT	−1.1	−0.87	0	−1.2	−1.2	−4.37
Sigmoid	Proposed	−1.57	−1.4	−1.67	−1.47	−1.6	−7.71
UDWT	Proposed	−1.33	−1.27	−1.47	−1.3	−1.5	−6.87

TABLE 2: Results of chest radiograph scoring for the three combinations by the five observers.

Combination		Observer					
		a	b	c	d	e	Sum
Sigmoid	UDWT	−1	−0.4	−0.1	−0.95	−1.25	−3.7
Sigmoid	Proposed	−1.7	−1.4	−1.35	−1.4	−1.65	−7.5
UDWT	Proposed	−1.5	−1.35	−1.5	−1.4	−1.55	−7.3

rectangular windows centered on a pixel at the coordinate (i, j). In detail the $c(i, j)$ is given by

$$c(i, j) = \frac{|p(i, j) - a(i, j)|}{|p(i, j) + a(i, j)|}, \quad (12)$$

where p and a are the average values of pixels within a 3×3 region and a 7×7 surrounding neighborhood, respectively. The greater the CIR value, the better the enhancement result.

The PSNR [34] in decibels is adopted for measuring the performance of denoising and is given by

$$\text{PSNR} = 10 \log_{10} \frac{M \times N \times T^2}{\sum_i \sum_j [d(i, j) - d'(i, j)]^2}, \quad (13)$$

where $M \times N$ is the size of the image, T^2 is the maximum possible value that can be obtained by the image signal, $d(i, j)$ and $d'(i, j)$ are the pixel-values of original and processed images, respectively. The higher the PSNR value, the better the performance of denoising.

3. Results

In this study, we used 30 mammograms and 20 chest radiographs to evaluate the proposed method by comparing it to two other existing methods: a modified UDWT method [14] and a sigmoid-type wavelet coefficient (STWC) mapping method [25]. The results of a previous study showed that by use of a modified UDWT method the computation time can be reduced to approximately 1/10 that of the conventional UDWT method. In addition, the results of visual assessment indicated that the images processed with the modified UDWT method showed statistically significant superior image quality over those processed with the conventional UDWT method [14]. The STWC mapping method demonstrated that it offers considerably improved enhancement capability as compared to the conventional enhancement methods, such as the fast Fourier transform method, the conventional wavelet-based method, and the conventional exponential-type wavelet coefficient mapping method [25].

Figure 2 shows two sets of example images of mammograms and chest radiographs. Original images are shown in

the upper row of the figure and corresponding images are shown in the lower row with external noise added. Figure 3 illustrates an example of image processing results obtained from the mammogram shown in Figure 2(e). Figures 3(a), 3(b), and 3(c) are resulting images processed by using the proposed method, the modified UDWT method, and the STWC mapping method, respectively.

Figure 4 shows the x-direction profiles of the processed images traced from the lines indicated on the images of Figures 3(a)–3(c). Figures 4(a)–4(c) illustrate the profiles of the images processed by the proposed method, the modified UDWT method, and STWC mapping method, respectively. The x-direction profile of the original image traced from the line indicated on the image of Figure 2(e) is also shown in the figures for comparison. Figures 4(d)–4(f) show the magnified views of the profiles corresponding to the positions indicated by the dotted circles in Figures 4(a)–4(c), respectively. The pixel-value profile of the image obtained with the proposed method and that of the image obtained with the modified UDWT method are shown in Figure 4(g). The pixel-value profile of the image obtained with the proposed method and that of the image obtained with the STWC mapping method are shown in Figure 4(h). It is obvious from Figure 4(g) that the pixel-value profile of the image processed by the proposed method is much more enhanced at the edges than that of the image processed by the modified UDWT method. It is also apparent from Figure 4(h) that the noise has been significantly reduced by employing the proposed method.

Similarly, Figure 5 illustrates an example of image processing obtained from the chest radiograph shown in Figure 2(g). Figures 5(a), 5(b), and 5(c) are resulting images processed by using the proposed method, the modified UDWT method, and the STWC mapping method, respectively.

Figure 6 shows the x-direction profiles of the processed images traced from the lines indicated on the images of Figures 5(a)–5(c). Figures 6(a)–6(c) illustrate the profiles of the images processed by the proposed method, the modified UDWT method, and the STWC mapping method, respectively. The x-direction profile of the original image traced from the line indicated on the image of Figure 2(g) is also shown in the figures for comparison. Figures 6(d)-6(f) show the magnified views of the profiles corresponding to the positions indicated by the dotted circles in Figures 6(a)–6(c). The pixel-value profile of the image obtained with the proposed method and that of the image obtained with the modified UDWT method are shown in Figure 6(g). The pixel-value profile of the image obtained with the proposed method and that of the image obtained with the STWC mapping method are shown in Figure 6(h). It is obvious from Figure 6(g) that the pixel-value profile of the image processed by the proposed method is much more enhanced at the edges than that of the image processed by the modified UDWT method. It is also apparent from Figure 6(h) that the noise has been significantly reduced by employing the proposed method.

The results of scoring for the three combinations by the five observers are listed in Tables 1 and 2 for mammograms and chest radiographs, respectively. As described earlier, if

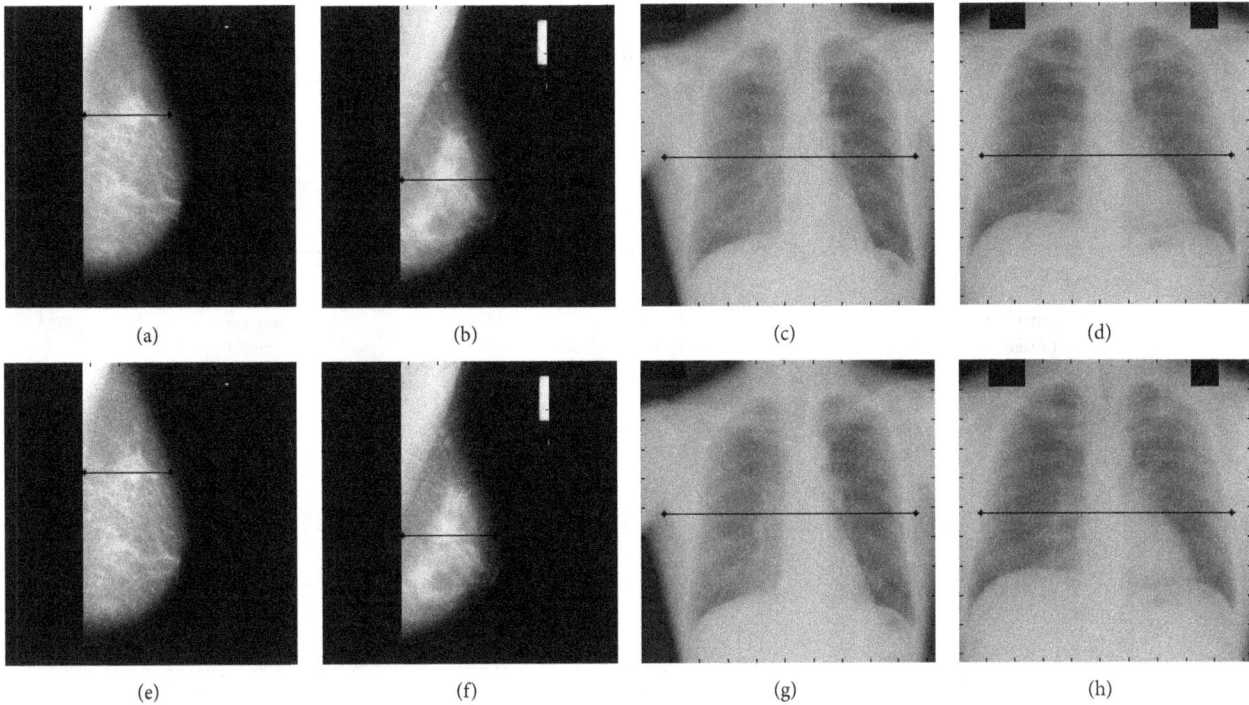

FIGURE 2: Examples of images used for this study. Images shown in the upper row are original images: (a) and (b) are two mammograms and (c) and (d) are two chest radiographs. The corresponding images are in the lower row with external added noise.

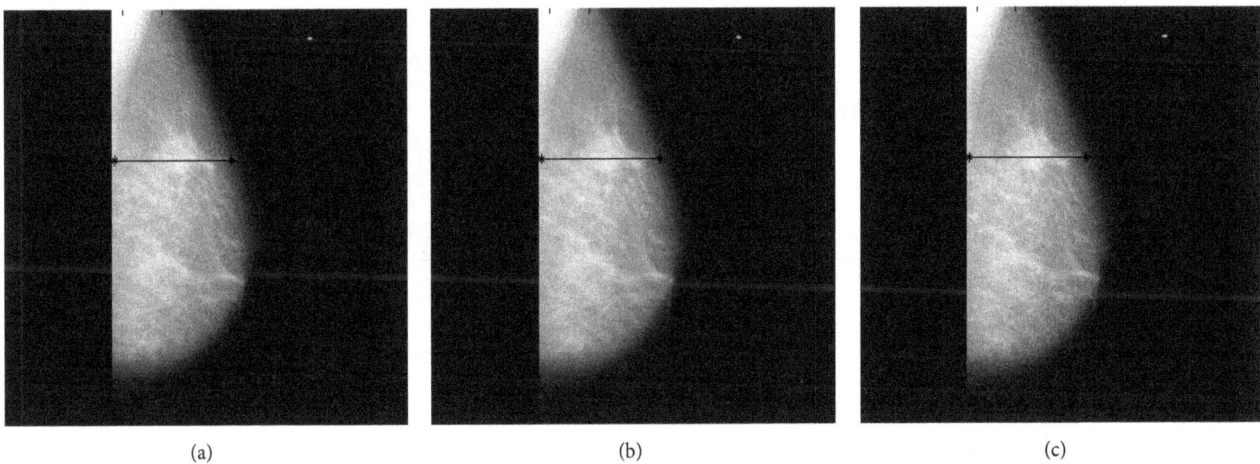

FIGURE 3: Image processing results for mammograms. (a) Image processed by the proposed method, (b) image processed by the modified UDWT method, and (c) image processed by the sigmoid-type wavelet coefficient mapping method.

the left image of the paired images (two-image combination) was poorer than the right image in terms of overall image quality, it received a negative score. Table 1 summarizes the visual results for the case of mammograms. As indicated by the preference scores shown in the rightmost column of the table, the images processed by the proposed method were judged to have the best quality. Figure 7 illustrates visual evaluation results using Scheffe's method of paired comparisons. The results are shown by a preference ranking map for the three image groups, namely, the proposed method, the modified UDWT method, and the STWC mapping method.

The figures shown on the horizontal line of the map are average preference degrees of the three groups. The average preference degrees were obtained from the average main effects by use of the data shown in Table 1. The images processed by the proposed method show the highest ranking, followed by those processed by the modified UDWT method and those processed by the STWC mapping method. A two-tailed F test was used to measure statistical significance. The difference between the processed images of the proposed method and those of the modified UDWT method was statistically significant ($P < 0.05$). The difference between the

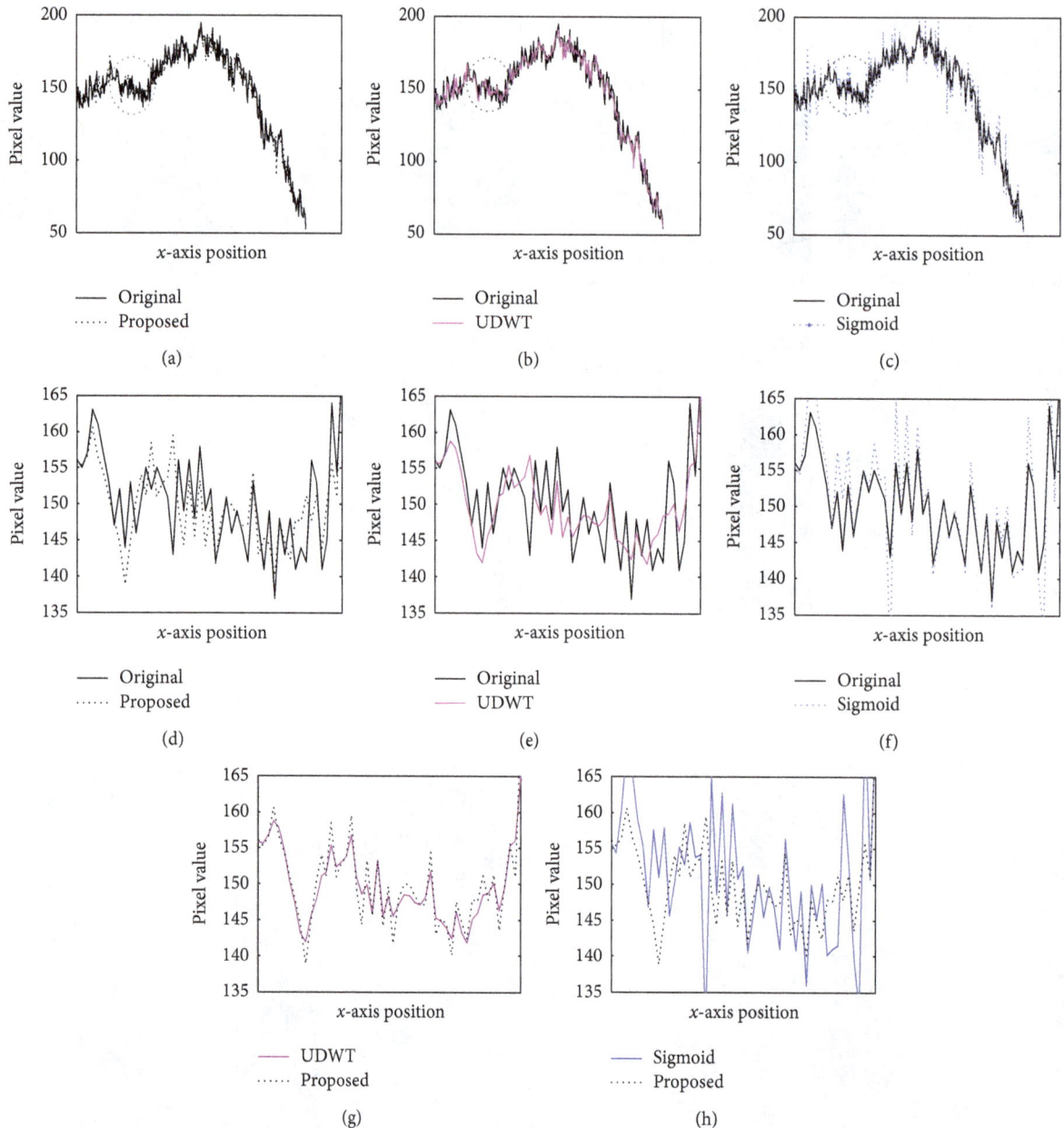

FIGURE 4: An example showing pixel-value profiles from original and processed mammograms. (a)–(c) Original versus processed by the proposed method, the modified UDWT method, and the sigmoid-type wavelet coefficient mapping method, respectively. The profiles were measured along the horizontal lines (black lines) as shown in Figures 3(a)–3(c). (d)–(f) Corresponding magnified profiles indicated by circles as shown in (a)–(c), respectively. (g) Profiles of two processed images; the solid line indicates the profile of an image processed by the modified UDWT method, and the dotted line indicates that by the proposed method. (h) Profiles of two processed images; the solid line indicates the profile of an image processed by the sigmoid-type wavelet coefficient mapping method, and the dotted line indicates that by the proposed method.

processed images of the proposed method and those of the STWC mapping method was also statistically significant ($P <$ 0.01). However, there was no significant difference between the processed images of the modified UDWT method and those of the STWC mapping method.

Table 2 summarizes the visual results for the case of chest radiographs. As shown in the rightmost column of the table, the images processed by the proposed method were judged to

have the best quality. Figure 8 shows visual evaluation results using Scheffe's method of paired comparisons. As shown in the figure, the images processed by the proposed method show the highest ranking, followed by those processed by the modified UDWT method and those processed by the STWC mapping method. The difference between the processed images of the proposed method and those of the modified UDWT method and the difference between the processed

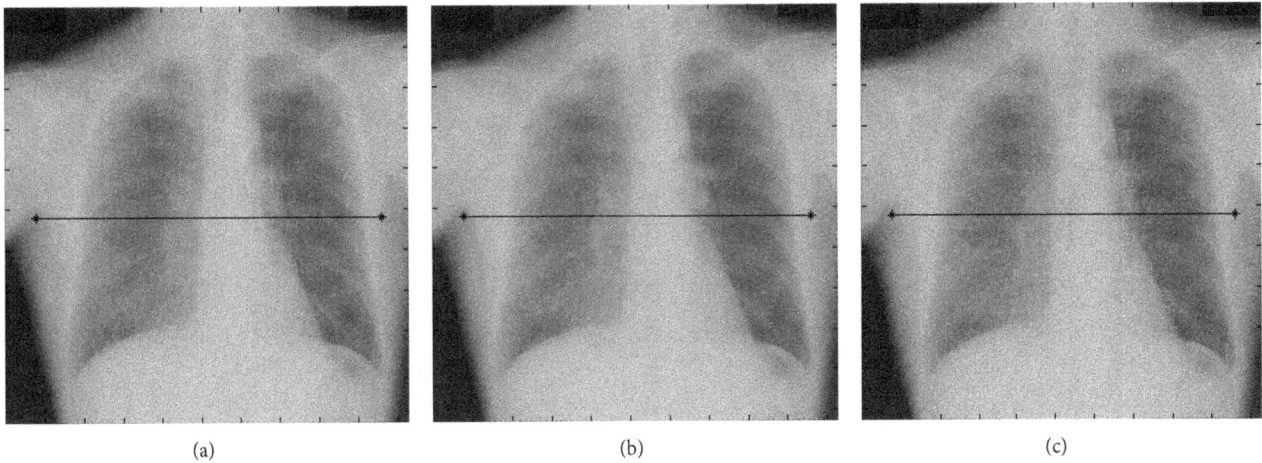

(a)	(b)	(c)

FIGURE 5: Image processing results for chest radiographs. (a) Image processed by the proposed method, (b) image processed by the modified UDWT method, and (c) image processed by the sigmoid-type wavelet coefficient mapping method.

TABLE 3: Comparison of image processing methods in terms of 4 quantitative quality metrics for mammograms.

Method	MSR	CNR	CIR	PSNR
UDWT	5.80	8.18	0.28	38.35
Sigmoid	6.09	7.64	0.29	36.39
Proposed	6.24	8.24	0.67	37.98

TABLE 4: Comparison of image processing methods in terms of 4 quantitative quality metrics for chest radiographs.

Method	MSR	CNR	CIR	PSNR
UDWT	6.36	2.21	0.46	37.61
Sigmoid	6.32	2.17	0.53	36.66
Proposed	6.46	2.29	0.71	36.76

images of the proposed method and those of the STWC mapping method were statistically significant ($P < 0.01$). However, there was no significant difference between the processed images of the modified UDWT method and those of the STWC mapping method.

Tables 3 and 4 summarize the quantitative evaluation results for the proposed method and two published methods in terms of MSR, CNR, CIR, and PSNR metrics. As described in Section 2.4 the MSR and CNR measurements are proportional to the medical image quality. It is obvious from the tables that both MSR and CNR values of the images processed by the proposed method give the best results as compared to those processed by the other two methods. The CIR is a metric used for evaluating the contrast improvement. It is noted from the results shown in Tables 3 and 4 that the proposed method shows the greatest value, followed by the sigmoid mapping and modified UDWT. The reason why the proposed method is superior to the sigmoid mapping method is due to the fact that the images processed by the proposed method have been denoised prior to mapping operation. In the case of PSNR measurement, the results listed in the tables show that the modified UDWT method was slightly

better than both the proposed method and sigmoid mapping method from the point of view of denoising performance. The reason might be because some residual (unremoved) noise has also enhanced at enhancement operation. This results in the decrease of PSNR value. However, the images processed by the proposed method showed the best overall image quality in terms of both denoising and contrast enhancement when looking into the values of the MSR and CNR as shown in Tables 3 and 4.

4. Discussion and Conclusion

In this study, we proposed an algorithm which combines the modified UDWT method and the sigmoid-type wavelet coefficient mapping method. The results of visual evaluation, as illustrated in Figures 7 and 8, suggested that the proposed method was significantly superior to the two previously reported methods. It is apparent from Figures 4(g) and 4(h) and Figures 6(g) and 6(h) that the proposed method combines the advantages of the two methods: denoising and contrast enhancement. The results of the quantitative evaluation also showed that the proposed method outperformed over the two other methods.

By using our proposed method, the computation time can be reduced to 2 seconds (personal computer, DELL, OPTIPLEX 960), approximately 1/10 of the computing time compared to the conventional UDWT method. The reason for enabling reduction of processing time lies in the following fact: in the conventional UDWT method, the decomposition and composition processes are usually conducted up to resolution level 4. That is, the method needs to process a total of 12 images (3 detailed coefficients for each of the 4-resolution levels) for wavelet transforms and inverse transforms and it results in time consumption. In contrast, the proposed method only needs to perform the process up to resolution level 2 and repeat the calculation one time. Therefore, only 6 images (3 detailed components for each of the 2-resolution levels) were required for processing. As a

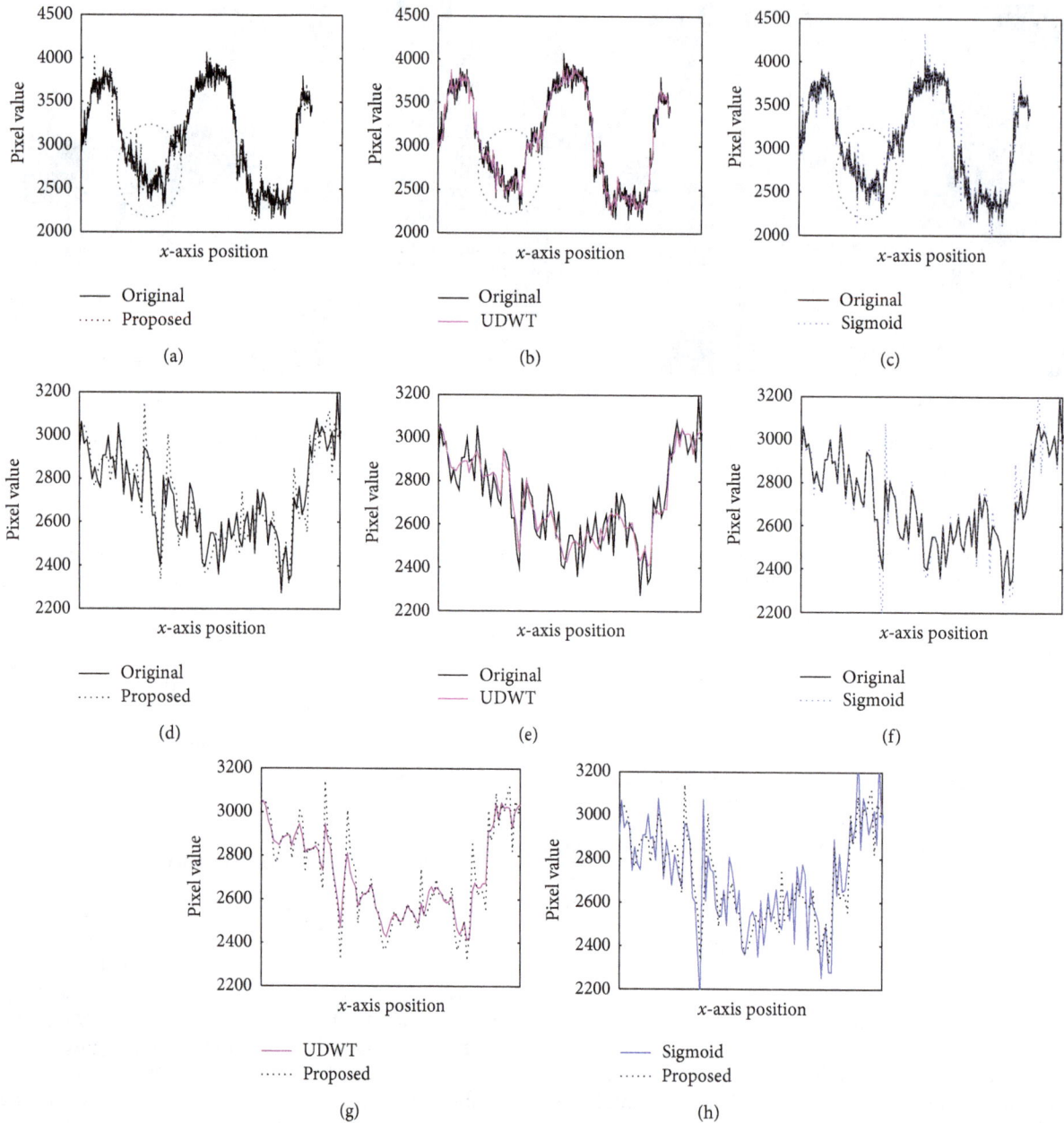

FIGURE 6: An example showing pixel-value profiles from original and processed chest radiographs. (a)–(c) Original versus processed by the proposed method, the modified UDWT method, and the sigmoid-type wavelet coefficient mapping method, respectively. The profiles were measured along the horizontal lines (black lines) as shown in Figures 5(a)–5(c). (d)–(f) Corresponding magnified profiles indicated by circles as shown in (a)–(c), respectively. (g) Profiles of two processed images; the solid line indicates the profile of an image processed by the modified UDWT method, and the dotted line indicates that by the proposed method. (h) Profiles of two processed images; the solid line indicates the profile of an image processed by the sigmoid-type wavelet coefficient mapping method, and the dotted line indicates that by the proposed method.

result, the computing time using the proposed method can be much reduced.

This study has several limitations. First, we only applied the proposed method to mammograms and chest radiographs. In order to validate the versatility of the proposed algorithm, application of the proposed method to other images obtained from different modalities, such as ultrasound, digital radiography, and SPECT is needed. Second, the value shown in (3) used for determining threshold value and

that shown in (8) used for determining the gradient of the sigmoid curve were empirically selected. A method for automated selection is desirable. Finally, our dataset contained only 30 mammograms and 20 chest radiographs. A larger dataset may enable us to better evaluate the performance of the proposed method.

In summary, we proposed a method for improving image quality in medical images by using a wavelet-based approach. The proposed method integrated two components: image

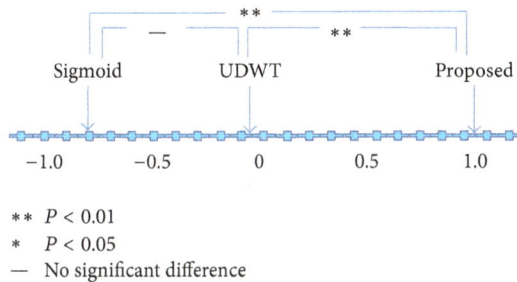

FIGURE 7: Preference ranking map for the three image groups: STWC-mapping-method-processed, modified-UDWT-processed, and proposed-method-processed mammograms.

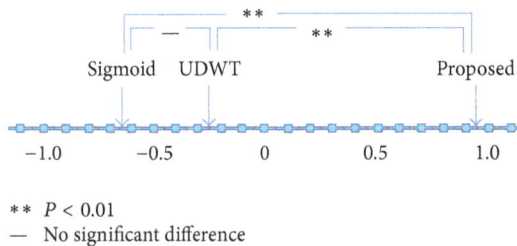

FIGURE 8: Preference ranking map for the three image groups: STWC-mapping-method-processed, modified-UDWT-processed, and proposed-method-processed chest radiographs.

denoising and image enhancement. In the first component, a modified undecimated discrete wavelet transform was used to eliminate the noise. In the second component, a wavelet coefficient mapping function was applied to enhance the contrast of denoised images obtained from the first component. We examined the performance of the proposed method by comparing it with two previously reported methods. The results of visual assessment indicated that the images processed by the proposed UDWT method showed statistically significant superior image quality over the other two methods. The results of quantitative assessment also showed that the proposed UDWT method outperformed over the two other methods. Our research results demonstrated the superiority and effectiveness of the proposed method. This methodology can be used not only as a means for improving visual quality of medical images but also as a preprocessing module for computer-aided detection/diagnosis systems to improve the performance of screening and detecting regions of interest in images.

Conflict of Interests

The authors declare that there is no conflict of interests regarding the publication of this paper.

Acknowledgments

This research was supported in part by a Grant-in-Aid for Scientific Research (23602004) from the Japan Society for the Promotion of Sciences (JSPS). The authors also would like to thank the observers for their participation in visual evaluation.

References

[1] A. Mencattini, M. Salmeri, R. Lojacono, M. Frigerio, and F. Caselli, "Mammographic images enhancement and denoising for breast cancer detection using dyadic wavelet processing," *IEEE Transactions on Instrumentation and Measurement*, vol. 57, no. 7, pp. 1422–1430, 2008.

[2] J. Scharcanski and C. R. Jung, "Denoising and enhancing digital mammographic images for visual screening," *Computerized Medical Imaging and Graphics*, vol. 30, no. 4, pp. 243–254, 2006.

[3] D.-Y. Tsai, Y. Lee, and R. Chiba, "An improved adaptive neighborhood contrast enhancement method for medical images," in *Proceedings of the 3rd IASTED International Conference on Medical Engineering*, pp. 59–63, BioMed, February 2005.

[4] B.-W. Yoon and W.-J. Song, "Image contrast enhancement based on the generalized histogram," *Journal of Electronic Imaging*, vol. 16, no. 3, Article ID 033005, 2007.

[5] I. K. Fodor and C. Kamath, "Denoising through wavelet shrinkage: an empirical study," *Journal of Electronic Imaging*, vol. 12, no. 1, pp. 151–160, 2003.

[6] C. B. R. Ferreira and D. L. Borges, "Analysis of mammogram classification using a wavelet transform decomposition," *Pattern Recognition Letters*, vol. 24, no. 7, pp. 973–982, 2003.

[7] D. Cho, T. D. Bui, and G. Chen, "Image denoising based on wavelet shrinkage using neighbor and level dependency," *International Journal of Wavelets, Multiresolution and Information Processing*, vol. 7, no. 3, pp. 299–311, 2009.

[8] J. E. Fowler, "The redundant discrete wavelet transform and additive noise," *IEEE Signal Processing Letters*, vol. 12, no. 9, pp. 629–632, 2005.

[9] J.-L. Starck, J. Fadili, and F. Murtagh, "The undecimated wavelet decomposition and its reconstruction," *IEEE Transactions on Image Processing*, vol. 16, no. 2, pp. 297–309, 2007.

[10] X.-Y. Wang, H.-Y. Yang, and Z.-K. Fu, "A new wavelet-based image denoising using undecimated discrete wavelet transform and least squares support vector machine," *Expert Systems with Applications*, vol. 37, no. 10, pp. 7040–7049, 2010.

[11] A. Mencattini, G. Rabottino, M. Salmeri, R. Lojacono, and B. Sciunzi, "Denoising and enhancement of mammographic images under the assumption of heteroscedastic additive noise by an optimal subband thresholding," *International Journal of Wavelets, Multiresolution and Information Processing*, vol. 8, no. 5, pp. 713–741, 2010.

[12] P. Zhao, Z. Shang, and C. Zhao, "Image denoising based on Gaussian and non-Gaussian assumption," *International Journal of Wavelets, Multiresolution and Information Processing*, vol. 10, no. 2, Article ID 1250014, 2012.

[13] Z. Huang, B. Fang, X. He, and L. Xia, "Image denoising based on the dyadic wavelet transform and improved threshold," *International Journal of Wavelets, Multiresolution and Information Processing*, vol. 7, no. 3, pp. 269–280, 2009.

[14] E. Matsuyama, D.-Y. Tsai, Y. Lee et al., "A modified undecimated discrete wavelet transform based approach to mammographic image denoising," *Journal of Digital Imaging*, vol. 26, pp. 748–758, 2013.

[15] W. Kim, J. You, and J. Jeong, "Contrast enhancement using histogram equalization based on logarithmic mapping," *Optical Engineering*, vol. 51, no. 6, Article ID 067002, 2012.

[16] A. Papadopoulos, D. I. Fotiadis, and L. Costaridou, "Improvement of microcalcification cluster detection in mammography utilizing image enhancement techniques," *Computers in Biology and Medicine*, vol. 38, no. 10, pp. 1045–1055, 2008.

[17] R. M. Rangayyan, L. Shen, Y. Shen et al., "Improvement of sensitivity of breast cancer diagnosis with adaptive neighborhood contrast enhancement of mammograms," *IEEE Transactions on Information Technology in Biomedicine*, vol. 1, no. 3, pp. 161–170, 1997.

[18] J. Jiang, B. Yao, and A. M. Wason, "Integration of fuzzy logic and structure tensor towards mammogram contrast enhancement," *Computerized Medical Imaging and Graphics*, vol. 29, no. 1, pp. 83–90, 2005.

[19] S. Hashemi, S. Kiani, N. Noroozi, and M. E. Moghaddam, "An image contrast enhancement method based on genetic algorithm," *Pattern Recognition Letters*, vol. 31, no. 13, pp. 1816–1824, 2010.

[20] D.-Y. Tsai, Y. Lee, and R. Chiba, "An improved adaptive neighborhood contrast enhancement method for medical images," in *Proceedings of the 3rd IASTED International Conference on Medical Engineering*, pp. 59–63, February 2005.

[21] R. N. Strickland and H. Hahn, "Wavelet transforms for detecting microcalcifications in mammograms," *IEEE Transactions on Medical Imaging*, vol. 15, no. 2, pp. 218–229, 1996.

[22] D.-Y. Tsai, Y. Lee, and S. Sakaguchi, "A preliminary study of wavelet-coefficient transfer curves for the edge enhancement of medical images," *Transactions of the Japanese Society for Medical and Biological Engineering*, vol. 40, no. 2, pp. 86–90, 2002.

[23] D.-Y. Tsai and Y. Lee, "A method of medical image enhancement using wavelet-coefficient mapping functions," in *Proceedings of the International Conference on Neural Networks and Signal Processing (ICNNSP '03)*, pp. 1091–1094, December 2003.

[24] P. Heinlein, J. Drexl, and W. Schneider, "Integrated wavelets for enhancement of microcalcifications in digital mammography," *IEEE Transactions on Medical Imaging*, vol. 22, no. 3, pp. 402–413, 2003.

[25] Y. Lee, D. -Y. Tsai, and T. Suzuki, "Contrast enhancement of medical images using sigmoid-type transfer curves for wavelet coefficient weighting adjustment," *Medical Imaging and Information Science*, vol. 25, no. 3, pp. 48–53, 2008.

[26] E. Matsuyama, D. Y. Tsai, Y. Lee, and N. Takahashi, "Comparison of a discrete wavelet transform method and a modified undecimated discrete wavelet transform method for denoising of mammograms," in *Proceedings of 34th Annual International Conference of the IEEE EMBS*, pp. 3403–3406, 2013.

[27] Mammographic Image Analysis Society, http://peipa.essex.ac.uk/info/mias.html.

[28] Japanese Society of Radiological Technology, 2012, http://www.jsrt.or.jp/jsrt-db/eng.php.

[29] H. Scheffe, *The Analysis of Variance*, John Wiley & Sons, New York, NY, USA, 1959.

[30] G. C. Canavos and J. A. Koutrouvelis, *An Introduction to the Design & Analysis of Experiments*, Pearson Prentice Hall, 2008.

[31] P. Bao and L. Zhang, "Noise reduction for magnetic resonance images via adaptive multiscale products thresholding," *IEEE Transactions on Medical Imaging*, vol. 22, no. 9, pp. 1089–1099, 2003.

[32] G. Cincotti, G. Loi, and M. Pappalardo, "Frequency decomposition and compounding of ultrasound medical images with wavelet packets," *IEEE Transactions on Medical Imaging*, vol. 20, no. 8, pp. 764–771, 2001.

[33] Y.-P. Wang, Q. Wu, K. R. Castleman, and Z. Xiong, "Chromosome image enhancement using multiscale differential operators," *IEEE Transactions on Medical Imaging*, vol. 22, no. 5, pp. 685–693, 2003.

[34] F. Luisier, T. Blu, and M. Unser, "A new SURE approach to image denoising: interscale orthonormal wavelet thresholding," *IEEE Transactions on Image Processing*, vol. 16, no. 3, pp. 593–606, 2007.

8

A Comparative Study of Theoretical Graph Models for Characterizing Structural Networks of Human Brain

Xiaojin Li,[1] **Xintao Hu,**[1] **Changfeng Jin,**[2] **Junwei Han,**[1] **Tianming Liu,**[3] **Lei Guo,**[1] **Wei Hao,**[2] **and Lingjiang Li**[2]

[1] *School of Automation, Northwestern Polytechnical University, Xi'an 710071, China*
[2] *Department of Psychiatry, The Mental Health Institute, The Second Xiangya Hospital, Central South University, Changsha, China*
[3] *Department of Computer Science and Bioimaging Research Center, University of Georgia, Athens, GA 30602, USA*

Correspondence should be addressed to Lingjiang Li; llj2920@163.com

Academic Editor: Jie Tian

Previous studies have investigated both structural and functional brain networks via graph-theoretical methods. However, there is an important issue that has not been adequately discussed before: what is the optimal theoretical graph model for describing the structural networks of human brain? In this paper, we perform a comparative study to address this problem. Firstly, large-scale cortical regions of interest (ROIs) are localized by recently developed and validated brain reference system named Dense Individualized Common Connectivity-based Cortical Landmarks (DICCCOL) to address the limitations in the identification of the brain network ROIs in previous studies. Then, we construct structural brain networks based on diffusion tensor imaging (DTI) data. Afterwards, the global and local graph properties of the constructed structural brain networks are measured using the state-of-the-art graph analysis algorithms and tools and are further compared with seven popular theoretical graph models. In addition, we compare the topological properties between two graph models, namely, stickiness-index-based model (STICKY) and scale-free gene duplication model (SF-GD), that have higher similarity with the real structural brain networks in terms of global and local graph properties. Our experimental results suggest that among the seven theoretical graph models compared in this study, STICKY and SF-GD models have better performances in characterizing the structural human brain network.

1. Introduction

The human brain is intrinsically organized into distinct large-scale functional networks, and cognitive functions arise from the dynamic interactions of distributed brain areas operating in these networks [1]. New advances in neuroimaging techniques have shown the possibility of systematic exploring the human brain formal complex network perspective. Graph theory provides a theoretical framework in which the topological properties of the brain networks can be examined such as centrality, clustering, efficiency, hierarchy, modularity, robustness, small-worldness, and synchronizability [2], and it can reveal important information about both the global and local organizations of the human brain networks. The improved characterization of brain networks achieved via graph-theoretical methods provides not only parsimonious accounts of normal cognitive processes [3], but also novel insights into psychiatric and neurological disorders such as Alzheimer's disease [4, 5], multiple sclerosis [6], and attention-deficit disorder [7].

Many complex systems show remarkably similar macroscopic behaviors despite profound differences in the microscopic details of the elements of each system or their mechanisms of interaction [2]. In this paper, we focus on an important issue that has not been adequately addressed before: what graph models can best possibly describe the structures of brain networks. In this way, the model provides a possible explanation for a key challenge for systems neuroscience: how to understand the complex network organization of the brain on the basis of neuroimaging data [8]. For instance, previous studies have demonstrated the small-worldness [9] and scale free properties of human brain networks [10].

In brain network studies, the methods for identifying regions of interest (ROIs), that is, the network nodes, can be generally classified into four categories. The first group is manual labeling by experts based on experience and domain knowledge. This method is widely used; however, it may not be reproducible due to both intersubject and intrasubject variations [11]. The second group is data-driven methods, which clusters ROIs from the brain image itself [12, 13]. However, it might be sensitive to the clustering parameters used in many data-driven approaches. The third group of methods identifies activated brain regions as ROIs by task-based functional magnetic resonance imaging (task-based fMRI), and it is regarded as the benchmark approach for ROI identification. However, task-based fMRI itself has limitations such as being time-consuming and expensive. Additionally, different patterns may be shown in group-based activation maps from an individual's activation map [14]. In short, it remains quite challenging to accurately localize ROIs for each individual by using standard analysis of task-based fMRI data [15]. The last group methods are cortical parcellation based on image/surface registration, whose limitations have been comprehensively discussed in [16, 17].

In this paper, we apply our recently developed brain reference system, named Dense Individualized and Common Connectivity-based Cortical Landmarks (DICCCOL) [18] which discovers 358 consistent and corresponding ROIs across subjects based on diffusion tensor imaging (DTI) data, to localize the ROIs for each participated subject. DICCCOL possess intrinsically established structural and functional correspondences (universal), while their locations and sizes are determined in each individual's space (individualized). With the identified brain ROIs, the structural brain network is constructed for each subject based on the corresponding DTI data. Then, through the large network analysis tool GraphCrunch2 [19], we evaluate the fitness of seven popular theoretical graph models for describing the real brain network by measuring both the global and local graph properties of the constructed brain networks and compare them with those graph models. The graph models are as follows: (1) Erdős-Rényi random graph (ER) [20]; (2) Erdős-Rényi random graph with the same degree distribution as the input data (ER-DD) [19, 21]; (3) geometric random graph (GEO) [22, 23]; (4) geometric gene duplication model (GEO-GD) [24]; (5) scale-free Barabási-Albert preferential attachment model (SF) [25]; (6) scale-free gene duplication model (SF-GD) [26]; (7) stickiness-index-based model (STICKY) [27]. Those graph models will be explained in detail in Section 2.

Our experimental results suggest that the SF-GD model fits the real brain network the best in terms of global and local graph properties. We also demonstrate that the real brain network also has the STICKY property. In summary, the SF-GD model, combined with its STICKY property, can best describe graph properties of the real brain network and also can indirectly describe the mechanism of structural network from biological properties. Importantly, the results are consistent across populations.

2. Materials and Methods

2.1. Data Acquisition and Preprocessing. DTI datasets for 104 healthy subjects including three age groups of adolescents

(28), young adults (53), and elderly normal brains (23) were acquired on a 3T GE Signal magnetic resonance imaging (MRI) scanner. Acquisition parameters for the scans were as follows: 256×256 matrix, 3 mm slice thickness, $240\,mm^2$ field of view (FOV), 50 slices, 15 diffusion weighted imaging (DWI) volumes, and B value = 1000. The preprocessing of DTI data included brain skull removal, motion correction, and eddy current correction [28]. After pre-processing, fiber tracking was reconstructed via MEDINRIA [29]. Then, The grey matter (GM)/white matter (WM) cortical surface was reconstructed according to the brain tissue segmentation map based on the DTI data [30].

2.2. Structural Brain Network Construction. The structural brain network of each subject is represented as an unweighted undirected graph $G = (V, E)$ in which $V = \{v_i, i = 1, 2, 3, \dots, N\}$ is the set of nodes and $E = \{e_{ij}, i, j = 1, 2, 3, \dots, N\}$ is the set of edges, where N is the number of nodes in the network. The nodes in V are identified via DICCCOL system [18], and the elements in E are measured for each ROI pair independently. Specifically, DICCCOL employs a novel data-driven strategy to discover, from DTI datasets, dense and common cortical landmarks [18]. The basic idea is that we optimize the localizations of each DICCCOL landmark in individual subjects by maximizing the groupwise consistency of their white matter fiber connectivity patterns. We obtain 358 DICCCOL ROIs for each subject and regard them as network nodes. White matter fibers obtained via the deterministic DTI tractography are projected onto the reconstructed cortical surface and the number of fibers connecting the ROI pair is used to measure the structural connectivity between the ROI pairs. Thus, a structural connectivity matrix is obtained for each subject. A predefined threshold T is applied on the connectivity matrix to remove the noise and errors in fiber tracking. Note that T is the same for all the subjects. After thresholding the structural connectivity matrix, we obtained the adjacency matrix $A_{N \times N}$ for each subject. In the adjacency matrix, two nodes v_i and v_j are connected if $a_{ij} = 1$; otherwise, $a_{ij} = 0$. The self-loops are currently ignored in the constructed structural brain networks.

Following the procedure described above, we constructed structural brain networks for 28 adolescents, 53 adults and 23 elders. Figure 1 shows exemplar brain networks in different groups.

2.3. Graph Models. In this study, we compared the topological properties of the constructed structural brain networks with those of 7 typical graph models via GraphCrunch2 [19], a tool for complex network analysis. GraphCrunch2 implements the following network models: (1) Erdős-Rényi random graph model (ER): ER graph is generated by using the Library of Efficient Data Types and Algorithms- (LEDA-) based random graph generator [19]. ER graph can provide a rigorous definition of what it means for a property to hold for almost all graphs, or be used in the probabilistic method to prove the existence of graphs satisfying various properties [20]. (2) Erdős-Rényi random graph with the same degree distribution as the input data (ER-DD): ER-DD graph is generated by using the "stubs method" [19]. In

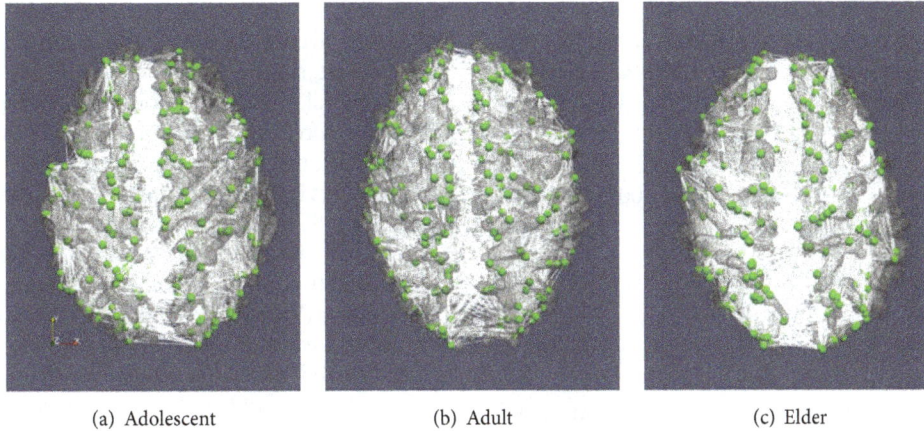

(a) Adolescent (b) Adult (c) Elder

FIGURE 1: Examples of structural brain networks in different groups. (a) Adolescent group. (b) Adult group. (c) Elder group. The nodes are represented by green spheres and the edges are represented by white lines. The constructed structural brain networks are overlaid on the corresponding cortical surfaces reconstructed from DTI data.

brief, according to the degree distribution of the real-world network being modeled, the number of "stubs" (to be filled by edges) is assigned to each node in the model network. After that, edges are created between randomly picked pairs of nodes. At last, the number of "stubs" left available at the corresponding "end-nodes" of the edge is decreased by one [19, 21]. (3) Geometric random graph model (GEO): in GEO graph, nodes correspond to uniformly randomly distributed points in a metric space and if the corresponding points are close enough in the metric space, according to some distance norm, the edges are created between pairs of nodes [22, 23]. (4) Geometric gene duplication model (GEO-GD): GEO-GD graph is the extension of geometric random graph, in which the principles of gene duplications and mutations are incorporated [19]. Every model determines the principle by which the network is grown from a small seed network and adds new nodes intended to model gene duplications and mutations [24]. (5) Scale-free Barabási-Albert preferential attachment model (SF) [25]: the most important characteristic in a scale-free network is the relative commonness of vertices with a degree that greatly exceeds the average. The highest-degree nodes are named "hubs." The scale-free property strongly correlates with the robustness of network. The hierarchy allows for a fault-tolerant behavior [26]. (6) Scale-free gene duplication model (SF-GD): SF-GD model is an evolution of SF model. The tolerance of SF-GD to damage is determined by the scale-free nature of its multifractal distribution. However, they present novel properties: multifractal features are inherited in a model of growing networks [26]. (7) Stickiness-index-based model (STICKY): STICKY graph is based on stickiness indices that summarize node connectivities and the complexities of normalized degree of nodes in networks. The stickiness framework produces a convenient, parameter-free random network [27].

According to the input structural brain network, GraphCrunch2 repeatedly generates a number of instances of the defined graph models and measures the global and local graph properties that infer the similarity/dissimilarity between the input graph and each of the generated model graph instances. In our experiments, the number of repeatedly generated instances is 10. The global and local graph properties implemented in GraphCrunch2 will be introduced in the next section.

2.4. *Topological Properties of Graphs.* We calculated both global and local topological graph properties for the constructed structural brain networks and the 7 graph models. Statistical analysis was conducted to explore which graph model can best describe the constructed brain networks. In this paper, the following global properties are examined: (1) Pearson correlation coefficients between the degree distributions [31]; (2) average shortest path length difference ratio; (3) average clustering coefficient difference ratio. The local graph properties include the relative graphlet frequency (RGF) distance [23] and the graphlet degree distribution (GDD) agreement [32]. We briefly provide the definitions of these measurements below.

2.4.1. *Global Graph Properties.* Define the degree k_i of a node i as the number of neighbors it has in the network. The topological property of a graph can be obtained in terms of the degree distribution $P(k)$ [2]. The degree distribution is one of indirect measures that reflect the network robustness to insult [8]. We compute Pearson correlation coefficients between the degree distributions of the graph model and the real brain network as the similarities between them in the aspect of degree distributions. Shortest path length plays an important role in characterizing the internal structure of a graph. Shortest path length of a node pair is defined as the path between two nodes in a graph that the number of its constituent edges is minimized. The average of the shortest path length, also known as characteristic path length, is the mean of the shortest paths over all node pairs [2] and is the most widely used measure to functional integration [8]. The clustering coefficient of node i is defined as $C_i = 2E_{\text{neighbor},i}/(k_i(k_i-1))$, where $E_{\text{neighbor},i}$ is the number of edges between neighbors of i. The average clustering coefficient C

is the mean of C_i over all nodes [2]. In this paper, we use average shortest path length difference ratio (PathDiff) and average clustering coefficient difference ratio (ClustDiff) to measure the difference between graph models and the real brain networks:

$$\text{PathDiff} = \frac{\left|\text{Path}_{\text{model}} - \text{Path}_{\text{real}}\right|}{\text{Path}_{\text{real}}} \times 100\% \qquad (1)$$

$$\text{ClustDiff} = \frac{\left|C_{\text{model}} - C_{\text{real}}\right|}{C_{\text{real}}} \times 100\%, \qquad (2)$$

where $\text{Path}_{\text{model}}$ and $\text{Path}_{\text{real}}$ are the average of shortest path of models and real brain networks, respectively and C_{model} and C_{real} are the average of clustering coefficient of models and real brain networks, respectively. Smaller difference indicates higher similarity between two networks.

2.4.2. Local Graph Properties. In addition to above global properties, we also measured the local graph properties to evaluate the fitness of the graph models to the real brain networks. In this paper, the local graph properties include RGF distance and GDD agreement.

Graphlet degree distribution agreement (GDD agreement) [32] is a similarity measure between topologies of two networks based on graphlet degree vector distributions. GraphCrunch2 computes 2–5 nodes graphlets [19]. By calculating the fitness of each of the 73 GDDs of the networks under comparison, GDD agreement contains 73 similarity constraints. High GDD agreement between two networks indicates that they are similar [19]. In general, GDD agreement is a local heuristic metric for measuring network structure. It imposes 73 highly structured constraints, and thus it increases the chances that two networks are truly similar if they are similar with respect to this measure [32].

Relative graphlet frequency distance (RGF distance) [23] is a measure that compares the frequencies of appearance of all 2 to 5 node graphlets in two networks [19]. Since there are 30 possible graphlets on up to 5 nodes, RGF distance includes 30 similarity constraints by examining the fit of 30 graphlets frequencies between two networks. The similarity between two graphs only depends on the differences between relative frequencies of graphlets. Smaller RGF distance indicates higher similarity between networks [19].

3. Results and Discussion

3.1. Topological Graph Properties

3.1.1. Global Graph Properties. Figure 2(a) shows the Pearson correlation coefficients between the degree distributions of the constructed brain networks and the 7 graph models for 28 subjects in the adolescent group. Note that the ER-DD model needs to be excluded because it has the same degree distribution as the input graph. It is seen that the Pearson correlation of degree distribution is approaching to 1. Figure 2(a) indicates that the STICKY model and SF-GD model have a high correlation with the real structural brain networks. The difference ratio of average shortest path length and average clustering coefficient are shown in Figures 2(b) and 2(c),

respectively. It is seen that the SF-GD and STICKY models have lower average shortest path length difference ratio and average clustering coefficient difference ratio.

In general, the comparison of global topological properties between real structural brain networks and the 7 graph models demonstrates the superiority of SF-GD and STICKY graph models in characterizing the structural brain networks. SF-GD and STICKY graph models share common features, namely, "inheritance" and "variance": when the new nodes are created, the son nodes inherit the connectivities of their parent nodes ("duplication" and "stickiness"). Meanwhile, the son nodes have new connectivities with other nodes which are not linked with their parent nodes "divergence." These characteristics could indirectly describe the biologically important properties of the mechanism of structural brain network. In the process of brain development, the new neurons are created and contain both functional and structural features. In this way, the specific regions of the brain which have specific function are formed, and the functions of these regions are improved and enhanced, such as the visual association area, motor speech area, and olfactory area. Meanwhile, the new neurons brought additional connectivities with other neurons in different regions; therefore, they enhanced the cooperation and coordination ability of different regions in human brain. The "stickiness" indicates that the important neurons which have large degree in structural brain network will maintain the original functional and structural features during brain development. On the other hand, the SF-GD network shares common features with other scale-free networks, and its tolerance to damage is determined by the scale-free nature of its multifractal distribution. Therefore, it also means that, during development, the brain not only maintains the functional integrity, but also is with increased stability. The SF-GD model has the lowest average shortest path length difference ratio indicates that "divergence" feature enhanced the interactions among different regions during brain development.

3.1.2. Local Graph Properties. The RGF distance and GDD agreement of the 7 graph models, in comparison with the real structural brain networks for the adolescent group with 28 subjects, are shown in Figures 3(a) and 3(b), respectively. It is seen that the GEO-GD model has the lowest GDD agreements when compared with the real brain networks, and there is no significant difference among the rest of the graph models. It is also shown that STICKY, SF, and SF-GD graph models have lower RGF distance, indicating their superior performance in characterizing the real structural brain networks. It is notable that GraphCrunch2 only calculates 2–5 nodes graphlets of the networks, as mentioned previously. In real brain networks, the connectivity patterns are complex and there exist graphlets with size over 5 nodes. Nevertheless, the local graph properties of RGF distance and GDD agreement demonstrate that STICKY, SF, and SF-GD graph models have higher similarity to the real structural brain networks, especially for the STICKY model. This result reflects that the "stickiness" feature plays an important role in brain development, and it might be the main reason that brain maintains regional and group integrity.

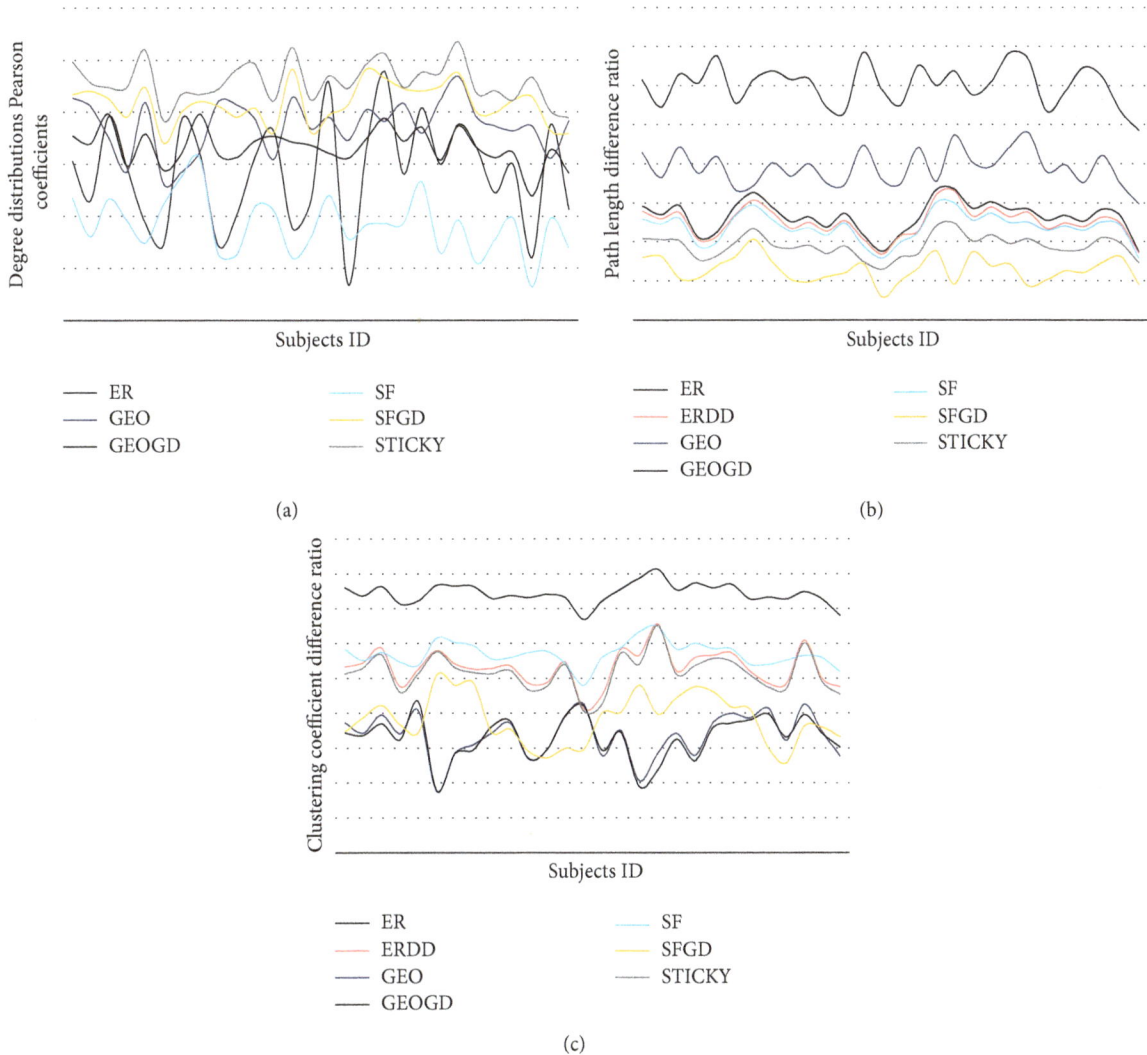

FIGURE 2: The global graph properties of 7 network models compared with real brain networks (28 subjects). (a) The Pearson correlation coefficients between the degree distributions. Higher value means the graph model can describe the real brain network better. (b) Average shortest path length difference ratio. (c) Average clustering coefficient difference ratio. Lower value means the graph model can describe the real brain network better. The x-axis is subject index.

In summary, the results of global and local topological properties indicate that the SF-GD and STICKY graph model fit the brain network data better; that is, the SF-GD and STICKY models have better performance in the description of structural brain networks. Since SF-GD and STICKY are not in conflict [27], we can also regard the stickiness as a property of the real brain network.

3.2. SF-GD versus Sticky. The global and local topological properties presented in the previous section indicate that SF-GD and STICKY graph models have comparable performance in describing the real structural brain networks. In this section, we present a further comparison study between SF-GD and STICKY by evaluating two topological properties of complex graph which were not implemented in GraphCrunch2, namely, (1) small-worldness [9]; (2) global efficiency [2]. Small-worldness has been reported as one of the most important properties of both the functional

and structural human brain networks in previous studies. Small-worldness networks are defined as networks that are significantly more clustered than random networks, yet have approximately the same characteristic path length as random networks. More generally, small-world networks should be simultaneously highly integrated and segregated [33]. This property is often analyzed by considering the fraction of nodes in the network that have a particular number of connections going into them. The average inverse shortest path length is a related measure known as the global efficiency. Some authors have claimed that the global efficiency may be a superior measure of integration [34]. Unlike the characteristic path length, the global efficiency can be more meaningfully computed on disconnected networks. Zero efficiency corresponds to infinite length of paths between disconnected nodes [8]. Figure 4 shows the mean of small-worldness and global efficiency in the adolescent group. It indicates that the SF-GD model has lower discrepancy

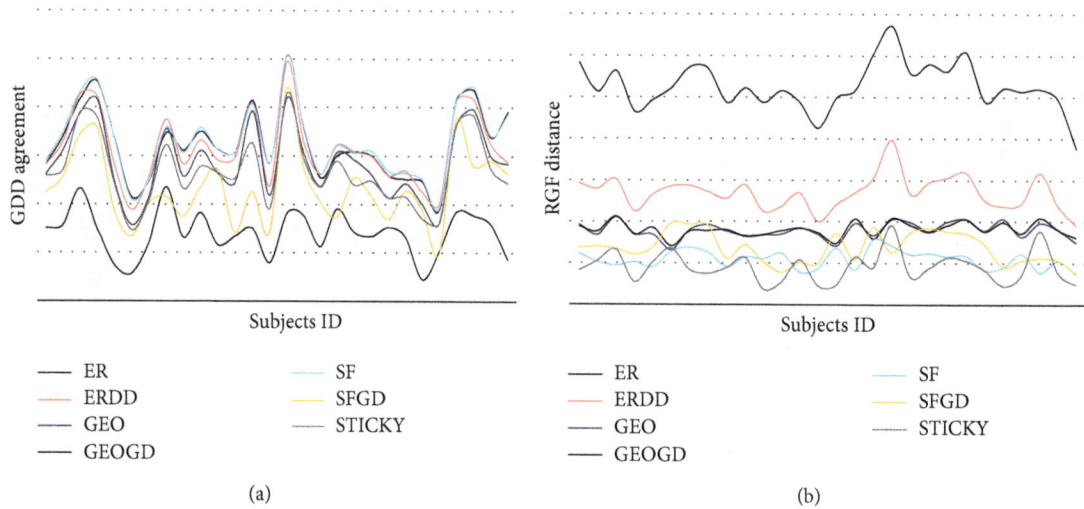

(a)

(b)

FIGURE 3: The local graph properties of 7 network models for 28 adolescents. The x-axis is subject index. (a) GDD-agreement. Higher value indicates higher similarity. (b) RGF-distance. Higher value indicates lower similarity.

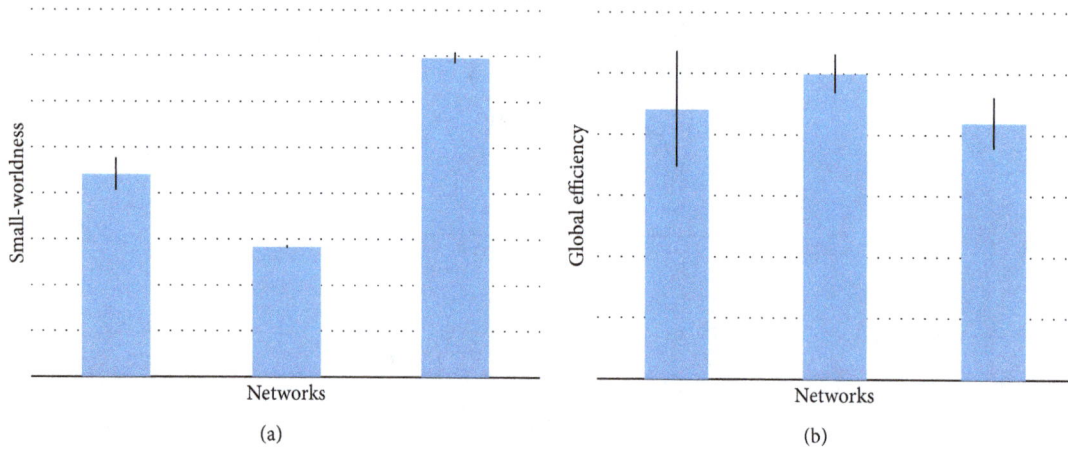

(a)

(b)

FIGURE 4: The comparison of small-worldness and global efficiency between SF-GD, STICKY and the real brain networks. (a) Small-worldness. (b) Global efficiency.

TABLE 1: Average RGF distance in different groups.

Nodes	ER	ERDD	GEO	GEOGD	SF	SFGD	STICKY
Adolescent	3.13 ± 0.29	1.85 ± 0.21	1.39 ± 0.10	1.40 ± 0.09	1.05 ± 0.10	1.18 ± 0.18	0.95 ± 0.19
Adult	3.03 ± 0.29	1.80 ± 0.21	1.43 ± 0.10	1.45 ± 0.10	0.98 ± 0.11	1.07 ± 0.19	0.95 ± 0.18
Elderly	2.93 ± 0.22	1.79 ± 0.19	1.43 ± 0.09	1.47 ± 0.11	0.91 ± 0.10	0.98 ± 0.16	0.98 ± 0.17

TABLE 2: Average GDD agreement in different groups.

Nodes	ER	ERDD	GEO	GEOGD	SF	SFGD	STICKY
Adolescent	0.71 ± 0.04	0.71 ± 0.04	0.69 ± 0.04	0.62 ± 0.02	0.71 ± 0.04	0.67 ± 0.04	0.68 ± 0.04
Adult	0.71 ± 0.04	0.71 ± 0.04	0.69 ± 0.04	0.62 ± 0.03	0.71 ± 0.04	0.67 ± 0.04	0.68 ± 0.04
Elderly	0.72 ± 0.06	0.71 ± 0.05	0.70 ± 0.05	0.61 ± 0.03	0.72 ± 0.06	0.66 ± 0.05	0.68 ± 0.05

TABLE 3: Average Pearson correlation coefficients of degree distributions in different groups.

Nodes	ER	ERDD	GEO	GEOGD	SF	SFGD	STICKY
Adolescent	0.17 ± 0.20	0.97 ± 0.05	0.35 ± 0.10	0.27 ± 0.07	-0.04 ± 0.11	0.43 ± 0.08	0.52 ± 0.08
Adult	0.18 ± 0.17	0.98 ± 0.03	0.35 ± 0.10	0.25 ± 0.07	-0.08 ± 0.09	0.43 ± 0.09	0.51 ± 0.09
Elderly	0.16 ± 0.15	0.98 ± 0.05	0.35 ± 0.08	0.22 ± 0.04	-0.10 ± 0.09	0.43 ± 0.08	0.49 ± 0.08

TABLE 4: Average shortest path length difference ratio in different groups.

Nodes	ER	ERDD	GEO	GEOGD	SF	SFGD	STICKY
Adolescent	0.13 ± 0.02	0.13 ± 0.02	0.19 ± 0.02	0.30 ± 0.02	0.12 ± 0.02	0.06 ± 0.02	0.09 ± 0.01
Adult	0.13 ± 0.02	0.12 ± 0.02	0.19 ± 0.03	0.30 ± 0.03	0.12 ± 0.02	0.06 ± 0.02	0.09 ± 0.02
Elderly	0.12 ± 0.01	0.12 ± 0.01	0.20 ± 0.02	0.31 ± 0.03	0.10 ± 0.01	0.05 ± 0.02	0.08 ± 0.01

TABLE 5: Average clustering coefficient difference ratio in different groups.

Nodes	ER	ERDD	GEO	GEOGD	SF	SFGD	STICKY
Adolescent	0.74 ± 0.03	0.53 ± 0.05	0.33 ± 0.06	0.33 ± 0.06	0.57 ± 0.04	0.38 ± 0.07	0.52 ± 0.05
Adult	0.73 ± 0.03	0.52 ± 0.05	0.38 ± 0.05	0.37 ± 0.05	0.55 ± 0.03	0.34 ± 0.07	0.51 ± 0.05
Elderly	0.72 ± 0.02	0.53 ± 0.04	0.40 ± 0.05	0.39 ± 0.05	0.54 ± 0.03	0.32 ± 0.03	0.52 ± 0.04

compared with the real brain networks in both small-worldness and global efficiency. This result to some extent demonstrates that SF-GD graph model is relatively more suitable in characterizing the human brain networks than STICKY graph model.

3.3. Topological Graph Properties across Groups. As a reproducibility study, we compared the topological properties of the brain networks across three different groups (adolescents, adults, and elders). The results are shown in Tables 1, 2, 3, 4, and 5. The trend is almost the same and the difference across the three groups is relatively small. It is also seen that the SF-GD model has higher correlation coefficients of degree distributions, lower average shortest path length difference ratio, and average clustering coefficient difference ratio in all the three groups. It indicates that SF-GD model is the most similar network to the real structural brain networks. The STICKY model also has higher similarity to real brain networks in terms of GDD agreement and RGF distance.

4. Conclusion

In this paper, we compared the global and local graph properties, as well as the topological properties of structural human brain networks to 7 representative graph models. The objective is to explore which graph model can best describe structural human brain networks.

Our experimental results demonstrated that SF-GD graph model in general has the best performance in characterizing the structural networks of the human brain, followed by STICKY graph model. SF-GD graph model is based on the hypothesis of evolution by duplications and divergence of the genes which produce proteins [26]. It reproduces the topological properties of the protein-protein interaction networks (PIN) with noticeable accuracy. Our experimental results also showed that the STICKY model has high GDD agreement, high Pearson correlation coefficients of the degree distributions, and low RGF distance and average shortest path length difference ratio when compared with SF-GD graph model. The STICKY model was also widely used in the investigation of protein-protein interaction networks, and the stickiness index can essentially capture the abundance and popularity of binding domains on a protein.

Since SF-GD and STICKY are not in conflict [27], we can also regard the stickiness as a property of the real brain network. In SF-GD model, networks revolute by duplication of nodes, and as a node is duplicated, it inherits most of the neighbors (interactions) of its parent nodes but gains some new neighbors as well [26]. Combined with stickiness index, a duplicated node would inherit its parents' stickiness index along with many of the parents' neighbors, and it would gain new neighbors in proportion to its inherited stickiness index and stickiness indices of the nodes already in the network [27]. The characteristics of "duplication," "divergence," and "stickiness" may explain the mechanism of structural brain network from biologically important properties shaped by natural selection. The "duplication" and "stickiness" make sure that the new neurons are created and contain both the functional and structural features. On the other hand, the "divergence" ensures that the new neurons have new connectivities with other neurons in different regions in order to enhance the cooperation and coordination ability of different regions in the human brain. This provides explanation why both STICKY and SF-GD models are suitable for describing the human brain networks; that is, the human brain networks are similar to SF-GD model and have STICKY property at the same time.

References

[1] M. D. Fox, A. Z. Snyder, J. L. Vincent, M. Corbetta, D. C. van Essen, and M. E. Raichle, "The human brain is intrinsically organized into dynamic, anticorrelated functional networks," *Proceedings of the National Academy of Sciences of the United States of America*, vol. 102, no. 27, pp. 9673–9678, 2005.

[2] E. Bullmore and O. Sporns, "Complex brain networks: graph theoretical analysis of structural and functional systems," *Nature Reviews Neuroscience*, vol. 10, no. 3, pp. 186–198, 2009.

[3] S. L. Bressler and V. Menon, "Large-scale brain networks in cognition: emerging methods and principles," *Trends in Cognitive Sciences*, vol. 14, no. 6, pp. 277–290, 2010.

[4] Y. He, Z. Chen, and A. Evans, "Structural insights into aberrant topological patterns of large-scale cortical networks in Alzheimer's disease," *Journal of Neuroscience*, vol. 28, no. 18, pp. 4756–4766, 2008.

[5] C. J. Stam, B. F. Jones, G. Nolte, M. Breakspear, and P. Scheltens, "Small-world networks and functional connectivity in

Alzheimer's disease," *Cerebral Cortex*, vol. 17, no. 1, pp. 92–99, 2007.

[6] Y. He, A. Dagher, Z. Chen et al., "Impaired small-world efficiency in structural cortical networks in multiple sclerosis associated with white matter lesion load," *Brain*, vol. 132, no. 12, pp. 3366–3379, 2009.

[7] L. Wang, C. Zhu, Y. He et al., "Altered small-world brain functional networks in children with attention-deficit/hyperactivity disorder," *Human Brain Mapping*, vol. 30, no. 2, pp. 638–649, 2009.

[8] E. Bullmore, A. Barnes, D. S. Bassett et al., "Generic aspects of complexity in brain imaging data and other biological systems," *NeuroImage*, vol. 47, no. 3, pp. 1125–1134, 2009.

[9] D. J. Watts and S. H. Strogatz, "Collective dynamics of 'small-world' networks," *Nature*, vol. 393, no. 6684, pp. 440–442, 1998.

[10] R. Cohen and S. Havlin, "Scale-free networks are ultra-small," *Physical Review Letters*, vol. 90, no. 5, Article ID 058701, 2003.

[11] K. Amunts, A. Malikovic, H. Mohlberg, T. Schormann, and K. Zilles, "Brodmann's areas 17 and 18 brought into stereotaxic space: where and how variable?" *NeuroImage*, vol. 11, no. 1, pp. 66–84, 2000.

[12] C. F. Beckmann, M. DeLuca, J. T. Devlin, and S. M. Smith, "Investigations into resting-state connectivity using independent component analysis," *Philosophical Transactions of the Royal Society B*, vol. 360, no. 1457, pp. 1001–1013, 2005.

[13] Y. Zang, T. Jiang, Y. Lu, Y. He, and L. Tian, "Regional homogeneity approach to fMRI data analysis," *NeuroImage*, vol. 22, no. 1, pp. 394–400, 2004.

[14] K. Li, L. Guo, D. Zhu, X. Hu, J. Han, and T. Liu, "Individual functional ROI optimization via maximization of group-wise consistency of structural and functional profiles," *Neuroinformatics*, vol. 10, no. 3, pp. 225–242, 2012.

[15] K. Li, L. Guo, C. Faraco et al., "Visual analytics of brain networks," *NeuroImage*, vol. 61, no. 1, pp. 82–97, 2012.

[16] X. Hu, D. Zhu, P. Lv, K. Li et al., "Fine-granularity functional interaction signatures for characterization of brain conditions," *Neuroinformatics*, vol. 11, no. 3, pp. 301–317, 2013.

[17] T. Liu, "A few thoughts on brain ROIs," *Brain Imaging and Behavior*, vol. 5, no. 3, pp. 189–202, 2011.

[18] D. Zhu, K. Li, L. Guo et al., "DICCCOL: dense individualized and common connectivity-based cortical landmarks," *Cerebral Cortex*, vol. 23, no. 4, pp. 786–800, 2013.

[19] O. Kuchaiev, A. Stevanović, W. Hayes, and N. Pržulj, "Graph-Crunch 2: software tool for network modeling, alignment and clustering," *BMC Bioinformatics*, vol. 12, article 24, 2011.

[20] P. Erdos and A. Renyi, "On the evolution of random graphs," *Publicationes Mathematicae*, vol. 6, pp. 290–297, 1959.

[21] M. Molloy and B. Reed, "A critical point of random graphs with a given degree sequence," *Random Structures and Algorithms*, vol. 6, no. 2-3, pp. 161–180, 1995.

[22] M. Penrose, *Random Geometric Graphs*, Oxford University Press, New York, NY, USA, 2003.

[23] N. Przulj, D. G. Corneil, and I. Jurisica, "Modeling interactome: scale-free or geometric?" *Bioinformatics*, vol. 20, no. 18, pp. 3508–3515, 2004.

[24] N. Przulj, O. Kuchaiev, A. Stevanovic, and W. Hayes, "Geometric evolutionary dynamics of protein interaction networks," in *Proceedings of the Pacific Symposium on Biocomputing*, pp. 178–189, Stanford, Calif, USA, 2010.

[25] A.-L. Barabasi and R. Albert, "Emergence of scaling in random networks," *Science*, vol. 286, no. 5439, pp. 509–512, 1999.

[26] A. Vazqueza, A. Flamminia, A. Maritana, and A. Vespignani, "Modeling of protein interaction networks," *Complexus*, vol. 1, no. 1, pp. 38–44, 2003.

[27] N. Przulj and D. J. Higham, "Modelling protein-protein interaction networks via a stickiness index," *Journal of the Royal Society Interface*, vol. 3, no. 10, pp. 711–716, 2006.

[28] D. Zhang, L. Guo, G. Li et al., "Automatic cortical surface parcellation based on fiber density information," in *Proceedings of the 7th IEEE International Symposium on Biomedical Imaging (ISBI '10)*, pp. 1133–1136, Xi'an, China, April 2010.

[29] http://www-sop.inria.fr/asclepios/software/MedINRIA/.

[30] T. Liu, H. Li, K. Wong, A. Tarokh, L. Guo, and S. T. C. Wong, "Brain tissue segmentation based on DTI data," *NeuroImage*, vol. 38, no. 1, pp. 114–123, 2007.

[31] C. Bishop, *Pattern Recognition and Machine Learning*, Springer, Cambridge, Mass, USA, 2006.

[32] N. Przulj, "Biological network comparison using graphlet degree distribution," *Bioinformatics*, vol. 23, no. 2, pp. e177–e183, 2007.

[33] M. D. Humphries and K. Gurney, "Network "small-world-ness": a quantitative method for determining canonical network equivalence," *Plos ONE*, vol. 3, no. 4, Article ID e2051, 2008.

[34] S. Achard and E. Bullmore, "Efficiency and cost of economical brain functional networks," *Plos Computational Biology*, vol. 3, no. 2, article e17, 2007.

9

Comparison of User-Directed and Automatic Mapping of the Planned Isocenter to Treatment Space for Prostate IGRT

Zijie Xu,[1] Ronald Chen,[1] Andrew Wang,[1] Andrea Kress,[1] Mark Foskey,[1,2] An Qin,[3] Timothy Cullip,[1] Gregg Tracton,[1] Sha Chang,[1] Joel Tepper,[3] Di Yan,[3] and Edward Chaney[1,2]

[1] Department of Radiation Oncology, CB 7512, University of North Carolina, Chapel Hill, NC 27599 7512, USA
[2] Morphormics, Inc., 240 Leigh Farm Road, Durham, NC 27707, USA
[3] Department of Radiation Oncology, William Beaumont Hospital, Royal Oak, MI, USA

Correspondence should be addressed to Edward Chaney; chaney@med.unc.edu

Academic Editor: Xishi Huang

Image-guided radiotherapy (IGRT), adaptive radiotherapy (ART), and online reoptimization rely on accurate mapping of the radiation beam isocenter(s) from planning to treatment space. This mapping involves rigid and/or nonrigid registration of planning (pCT) and intratreatment (tCT) CT images. The purpose of this study was to retrospectively compare a fully automatic approach, including a non-rigid step, against a user-directed rigid method implemented in a clinical IGRT protocol for prostate cancer. Isocenters resulting from automatic and clinical mappings were compared to reference isocenters carefully determined in each tCT. Comparison was based on displacements from the reference isocenters and prostate dose-volume histograms (DVHs). Ten patients with a total of 243 tCTs were investigated. Fully automatic registration was found to be as accurate as the clinical protocol but more precise for all patients. The average of the unsigned x, y, and z offsets and the standard deviations (σ) of the signed offsets computed over all images were (avg. $\pm$ σ (mm)): 1.1 ± 1.4, 1.8 ± 2.3, 2.5 ± 3.5 for the clinical protocol and 0.6 ± 0.8, 1.1 ± 1.5 and 1.1 ± 1.4 for the automatic method. No failures or outliers from automatic mapping were observed, while 8 outliers occurred for the clinical protocol.

1. Introduction

Image-guided radiotherapy (IGRT) [1], off-line adaptive radiotherapy (ART) [2], and online reoptimization [3] involve pretreatment imaging, taken here to be CT imaging. A procedure held in common by all three methods is registration of the planning (pCT) and treatment (tCT) images to map the planned isocenter to treatment space. Accuracy and precision of this step are important for delivering an accumulated dose distribution that closely matches the treatment plan. Mapping methods involve at least rigid registration. Ideally a nonrigid step would be included to account for differences in organ shape between planning and treatment times (Figure 1). The composite of the rigid, and possibly nonrigid, matrices is then used to map the planned isocenter to the tCT.

Quantitative evaluation of isocenter mapping methods is muddled by the lack of gold standards [4]. In the absence of standards, this work retrospectively compared a fully automatic method against a user-assisted procedure used in a clinical protocol for IGRT for prostate cancer. The study focused on tCTs from a conventional diagnostic scanner due to the availability of clinical data. However, the approach applies to kilovoltage cone-beam CT (CBCT) images as illustrated later.

2. Methods

2.1. Clinical Protocol. The clinical protocol (Table 1) was practiced over the period 2005–2008 at the University of North Carolina (UNC) as part of the routine workflow during evaluation of a CT-on-rails system [5] (Primatom, Siemens Medical Solutions, Concord, CA). The Primatom system consists of a conventional CT scanner, a set of rails between the

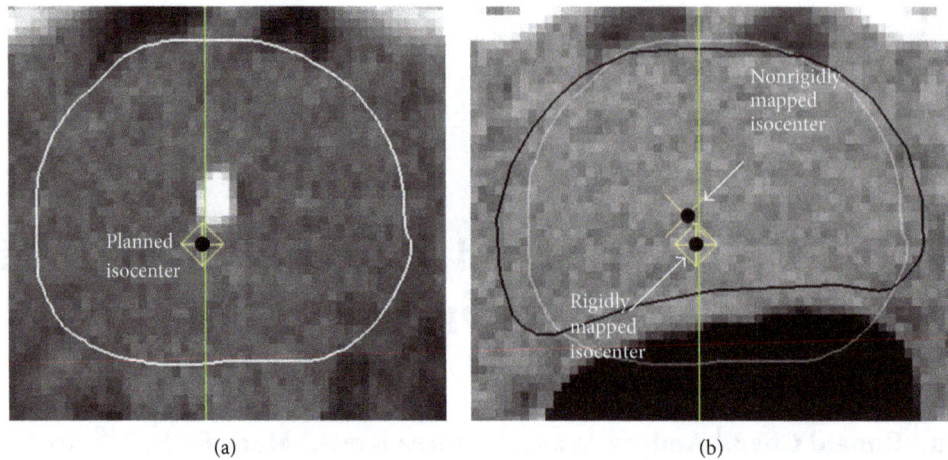

(a)   (b)

FIGURE 1: (a) Axial slice from the pCT showing planning prostate (white) and isocenter (black). (b) Corresponding slice from the tCT showing the prostate (black) segmented by automatic nonrigid model deformation. The rigidly mapped isocenter comes from translating the planning prostate (dim white) to the tCT. The nonrigidly mapped isocenter comes from applying the deformation matrix resulting from autosegmentation to the planned isocenter.

TABLE 1: Isocenter Mapping Methods.

	Clinical mapping	Automatic mapping
1	CT simulate. Align patient with laser beams intersecting at simulated isocenter. Tattoo skin at centers of lateral and anterior laser beams.	Import pCT, structure sets, and isocenter to MxAnatomy. Fit models to planning contours.
2	Plan. Place crosshairs at planned isocenter in axial slice. Mark skin contour at lateral and anterior intersections with crosshairs.	Acquire tCT using standard procedures.
3	Prepare patient for treatment imaging. Tape BBs to anterior and lateral skin tattoos. Acquire tCT with laser beams centered on BBs.	Import tCT. Rigidly register pCT with pCT using automatic multiscale procedure.
4	Import tCT to PLanUNC. Autoregister imaged BBs in tCT with skin marks in pCT from Step 2.	Autosegment prostate in tCT.
5	Inspect registration by comparing prostate contours in pCT with intensity patterns in the tCT. Manually edit registration to get best match between contours and tCT intensities.	Determine correspondences between pCT and tCT prostate models.
6	Convert manual x, y, z edits from Step 5 to table shifts relative to laser beams. Apply shifts >3 mm and treat.	Map isocenter label from pCT to tCT via correspondence from Step 5 (2).

scanner and the linac, and a dual-purpose imaging/treatment couch that moves along the rails. Patients under the IGRT protocol were imaged before treatment, and the couch was rolled from the CT scanner into the image-guided treatment position. The fixed geometry between the scanner and linac allows cross calibration of the patient laser alignment systems, and the rails facilitate moving the couch from the scanner into treatment position with minimal time delay or mechanical disturbance of patient geometry.

All patients underwent simulation using a Philips AcQSim CT system [6] (Philips Healthcare, Andover, MA). The planning isocenter was localized during simulation, and the anterior and lateral laser crosshairs were tattooed according to standard practice. Treatment planning and calculation of hypothetically delivered dose were accomplished with PlanUNC [7, 8]. (PLanUNC is a set of modular software tools for external beam treatment planning and dose calculation

development at UNC.) During planning the dosimetrist placed the computer crosshairs at the planned isocenter and then marked reference points in the pCT at the intersections of the computer crosshairs with the skin (Figure 2). These reference points defined the geometrically correct positions of the anterior and lateral laser crosshairs based on patient geometry at planning time. Before acquisition of each tCT, the patient was positioned by aligning the tattoos on the patient's skin with the CT laser crosshairs. After alignment, steel BBs were taped to the skin at the center of each laser's crosshairs (AP, R&L lat). Assuming accurate laser calibration, this placement allows the treatment isocenter for the initial patient position to be inferred from the imaged BBs. Immediately after imaging, the tCT was imported to the planning system and the physicist defined the BB centers via point and click on a computer display screen. The planning system then automatically registered the tCT and pCT by

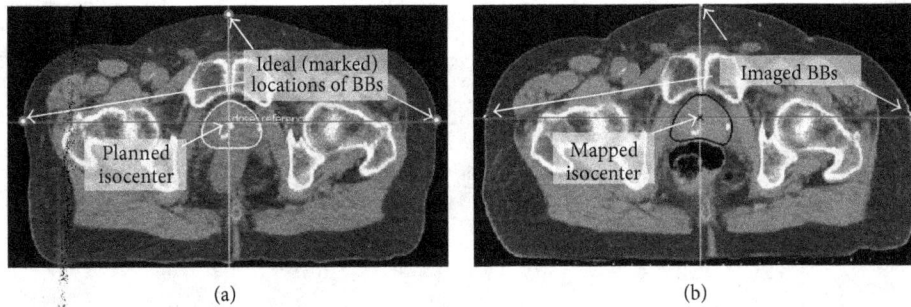

FIGURE 2: (a) Axial slice from the pCT showing planned isocenter inside the prostate (white contour) and the marked locations of BBs. (b) Corresponding slice from the tCT showing the autosegmented prostate (black), nonrigidly mapped isocenter, and imaged BBs.

matching the BBs in the tCT with the ideal locations marked in the pCT. The algorithm minimized $\sum$(distance between corresponding points)^2. The final step was interactive rigid registration of the prostate ROIs using the planning contours for reference. Table tilt around the lateral axis and rotation around the craniocaudal axis were not allowed in the final two steps because rotational errors were not handled during patient setup. Since the prostate was not contoured in the tCT, the final step relied on human judgment to match the pCT intensities and contours with the tCT intensity patterns in the prostate ROI. Table displacements were computed by comparing the coordinates of the mapped isocenter after BB registration with the coordinates after interactive prostate-based registration. The displacements were used to reposition the treatment table. Assuming accurate registration and repositioning, and no changes in patient anatomy between tCT imaging and treatment times, this procedure registered the mapped planned isocenter with the treatment isocenter. In typical practice of IGRT, displacements are implemented only when they exceed a predefined threshold. In the UNC protocol, the threshold was 3 mm along a given axis. However, for comparison purposes this study assumed that the displacements were applied without error regardless of magnitude.

2.2. Automatic Mapping Method.

Automapping (Table 1) was performed using a beta version of ARTSuite (Morphormics, Inc. Chapel Hill, NC) installed at UNC. (Effective July 16, 2012, Morphormics, Inc. became a wholly owned subsidiary of Accuray, Inc., Sunnyvale, CA.) ARTSuite is a DICOM-RT compliant software system developed to support IGRT, ART, and online reoptimization with tools for autosegmentation of pCTs and tCTs, nonrigid mapping between treatment and planning spaces, and dose accumulation and analysis.

Automapping (Figure 3) involved three major steps: (1) multiscale rigid registration of the previously segmented pCT to the tCT, (2) model-based autosegmentation of the prostate in the tCT [9, 10], and (3) nonrigid mapping of the planning isocenter to the tCT using a transformation that included the rigid registration matrix and a nonstatistical, nonrigid diffeomorphism determined from correspondences between the pCT and tCT prostate models.

2.3. Patient Data.

Ten patients with a total of 243 tCTs were investigated. All pCTs were acquired with contrast in the bladder, and one patient had contrast in the bladder and rectum. The pixel dimensions in the axial plane were 1 mm × 1 mm, and the slice thickness was 3 mm for pCTs and tCTs.

All patients were treated with step-and-shoot IMRT using an anterior and six oblique fields to ~75 Gy prescribed to a point or isodose curve. Treatment typically included a boost starting ~50 Gy to reach the final dose. Margins of 5 mm and 3 mm were applied to the planning target volume for the initial and boost plans, respectively.

2.3.1. Model Fitting to Prostate Contours.

This study assumed that the manually drawn prostate contours in the pCT were true at treatment time. To facilitate model-based segmentation of the tCTs as described below, a prostate model was fit to each set of planning contours, using an approach based on prostate shape statistics described by Merck et al. [11]. This process yielded a custom prostate atlas for each patient that was used during registration and segmentation of tCTs. Contours were represented as many short line segments joined together. This representation caused small differences between a contour and a model at sharp vertices where two line segments joined. These differences were less than 0.2 mm per contour on average and were caused by smoothness constraints that forced the model to have continuous curvature.

2.3.2. Multiscale Rigid Registration.

The overall rigid registration approach has similarities with that of Court and Dong [12] and Smitsmans et al. [13], discussed later in Section 3. To minimize compute time, registration progresses from coarse to fine scale in three steps. The output of each step serves as a prior for the following step. Step (1) aligns the skin bounding boxes and registers the images by sliding the image data in the bounding box in the pCT along the box for the tCT. The registration algorithm computes the voxel count per slice in a predefined intensity window and aligns the images by finding the best match between graphs of voxel count versus slice position for each image pair. A bone window performs best but can fail when a "bright" contrast medium is used for the pCT. In such cases, Step (1) is ignored and the algorithm starts

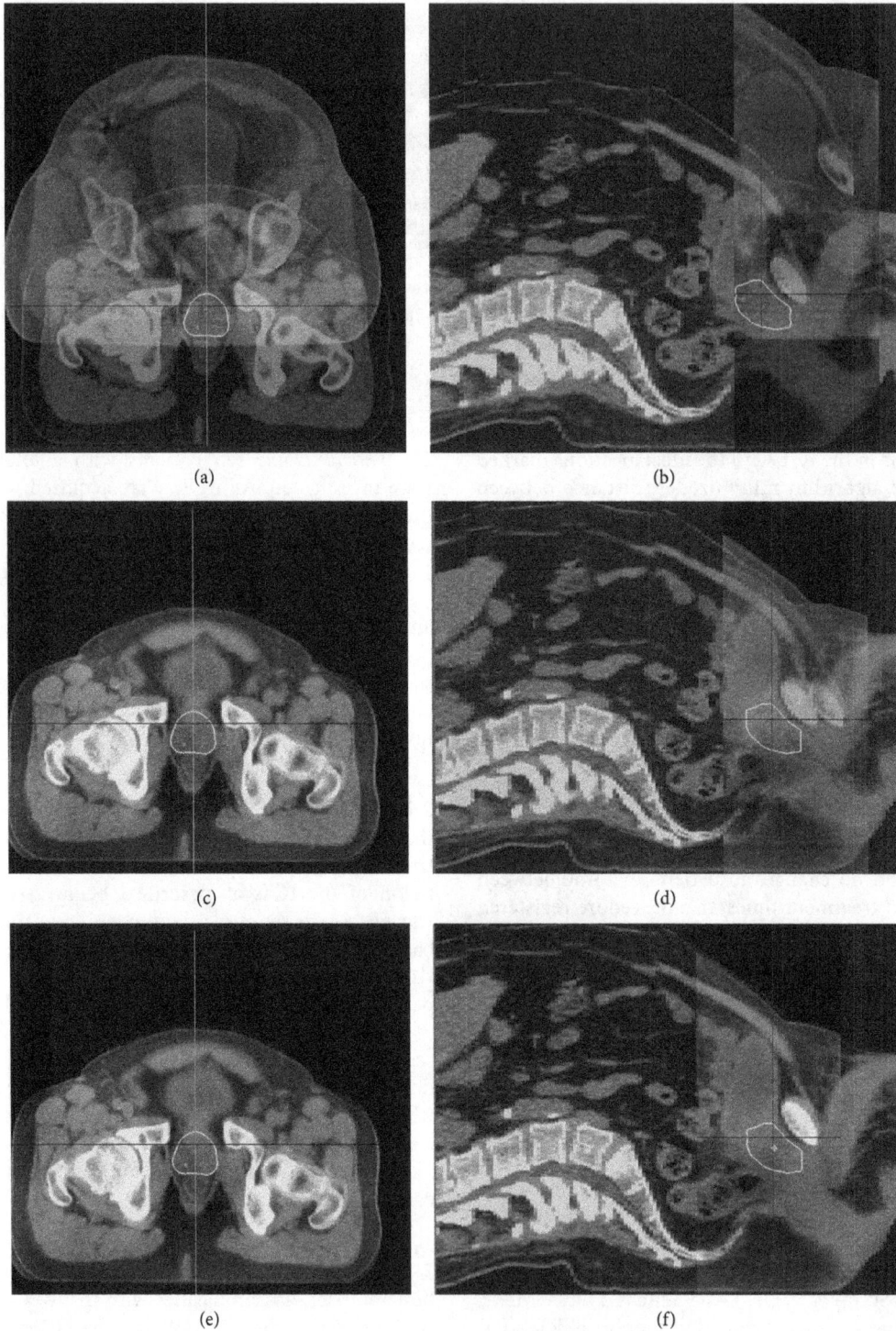

FIGURE 3: Multiscale registration of a pCT with a CBCT. The planning prostate segmentation is white. ((a), (b)) Blended axial and sagittal slices of unregistered images. ((c), (d)) Axial and sagittal slices of images registered via Step (1). ((e), (f)) Axial and sagittal slices of images registered via mutual information in the prostate ROI (Step (3)). In this example, there is little difference between the second and third steps.

over at Step (2), which optimizes global mutual information (MI) using a gradient descent approach [14]. To avoid convergence to a distant optimum, the algorithm is run multiple times with different starting points. The result with the best score over all runs is selected as the output. Step (3) is similar to Step (2) but with MI computed over an ROI defined by the atlas prostate model. As in the clinical procedure, rotations during automatic registration were not allowed explicitly. However, the segmentation step treated rotation as a nonrigid deformation in images with adequate intensity information.

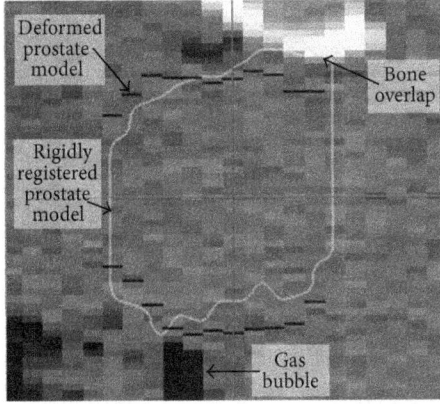

FIGURE 4: Midsagittal slice from a tCT illustrating how prostate rotation is treated as a deformation. The white outline is the atlas prostate after automatic registration to the tCT. The black dashes are the deformed atlas in the tCT.

In Figure 4, for example, the rigidly registered prostate model overlaps pubic bone anteriorly, causing the model to deform in a manner that avoids overlap with both the bone and the gas bubble in the rectum.

2.3.3. Model-Based Autosegmentation. The model used to represent the prostate consists of a chain of so-called medial atoms (Figure 5). A full collection of atoms for an organ is called a medial-representation (m-rep) [9]. The chain configuration is well suited for objects that are more or less tube-like, including objects with closed ends. Each prostate atom has a hub and 16 spokes radiating to the organ surface. Additional hubs and spokes can be interpolated as needed. The skeletal framework serves as an organ-relative coordinate system with a formalism for converting back and forth between model and image coordinates [9, 15]. After deformation of the starting model in a target image, corresponding positions are defined by pairing points in the starting and deformed models that have the same model-relative coordinates (Figure 5). The nonrigid transformation matrix can be specified in image coordinates in terms of a standard displacement vector field [16], where each vector originates on a voxel in the reference image and terminates on its postdeformation position in the target image. In contrast to voxel-scale deformations, the model approach is statistical at the scale of an organ but nonstatistical at voxel scale, eliminating small-scale artifacts [16].

Segmentation of the prostate in the tCT is necessary to determine corresponding points in the pCT and tCT. The algorithm transfers the atlas model to the tCT using the rigid registration matrix, and autosegmentation proceeds in a statistical framework based on Bayes' theorem [9]. A conjugate gradient algorithm seeks to find the optimal model $\underline{M}_{\mathrm{opt}}$ such that

$$\underline{M}_{\mathrm{opt}} = \underset{\underline{M} \in s}{\operatorname{argmax}} \left[\log p\left(\underline{M}\right) + \log p\left(\underline{I} \mid \underline{M}\right) \right], \qquad (1)$$

where $\underline{M}$ is the currently deformed model in the trained shape space s [11], $\underline{I}$ is the target image intensity pattern relative to $\underline{M}$, $p(\underline{M})$ is the probability of $\underline{M}$ (geometric typicality), and $p(\underline{I} \mid \underline{M})$ is the probability of $\underline{I}$ given $\underline{M}$ (image match [17]).

2.3.4. Mapping the Isocenter. The rationale for using a model to map the isocenter stems from several considerations: (1) during planning the isocenter is positioned relative to the prostate; (2) a point in an image can be more accurately found by relying on regional image features that are correlated spatially with the point rather than using local information near the point itself [18]; and (3) the trainable models used in this study provide a means for determining both the rigid and nonrigid components of the mapping transformation. The mapping step is straightforward and involves labeling the point in the tCT that has the same prostate-relative coordinates as the planned isocenter using (2):

$$\mathrm{VAL}'_{\mathrm{Mapped}} \left(M'\left(i', j', k'\right) \right) = \mathrm{VAL}\left(M\left(i, j, k\right)\right), \qquad (2)$$

where $M, M' = $ prostate models in pCT and tCT, respectively, i, j, k and i', j', k' are corresponding positions in M- and M'-relative coordinates, VAL = value of scalar, for example, label, dose, or intensity, in the pCT at M-relative position i, j, k, and $\mathrm{VAL}'_{\mathrm{Mapped}} = $ value of scalar mapped to M'-relative position i', j', k'.

2.4. Reference tCT Isocenters. The clinical and automapping protocols yielded two independent sets of tCT isocenters. To compare these sets, a reference isocenter was determined for each tCT by repeating the automapping procedure with human supervision. The main task was to reposition and/or edit the autosegmented prostate as necessary to achieve the best match with the tCT image data while generally preserving the global shape and volume defined by the planning contours. Every rigid registration and prostate segmentation were evaluated and edited based on human judgment, after which the tCT isocenter from (2) was accepted without modification. This procedure was performed without the pressure of clinical time constraints over ~8 months by two physicists and a dosimetrist working as a team. In general, the dosimetrist and one of the physicists made the initial pass, and the results from that pass were reviewed at a later time by the second physicist. The team met about once a week to discuss and review ongoing progress. Results from the dosimetrist/physicists team were periodically evaluated by one or two radiation oncologists based on the criterion of clinical reasonableness; that is, given the planning contours as truth, would the radiation oncologist judge the location and shape of the prostate in the tCT to be clinically reasonable? This criterion eliminated a potential source of interobserver bias and variability and effectively served the need for clinical standards. Only a few tCTs per patient were reviewed because of the large number of cases and the fact that the position and shape of the prostate in a given tCT are expected to be strongly correlated with other tCTs for the same patient.

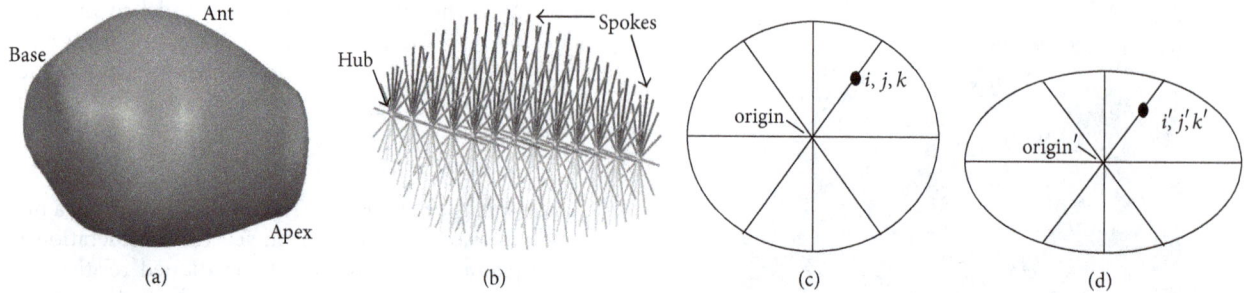

FIGURE 5: (a) Lateral oblique view of the surface of a prostate model. (b) Internal tubular skeleton showing a chain of 13 atoms, each comprising a hub and 16 spokes that touch the prostate surface. (c) and (d) Illustration of corresponding points in reference and deformed models. (c) Reference model with point at i, j, k. (d) Deformed model with corresponding point at i', j', k'. The points are on the same spoke and they have the same fractional distance from the origin (atom hub).

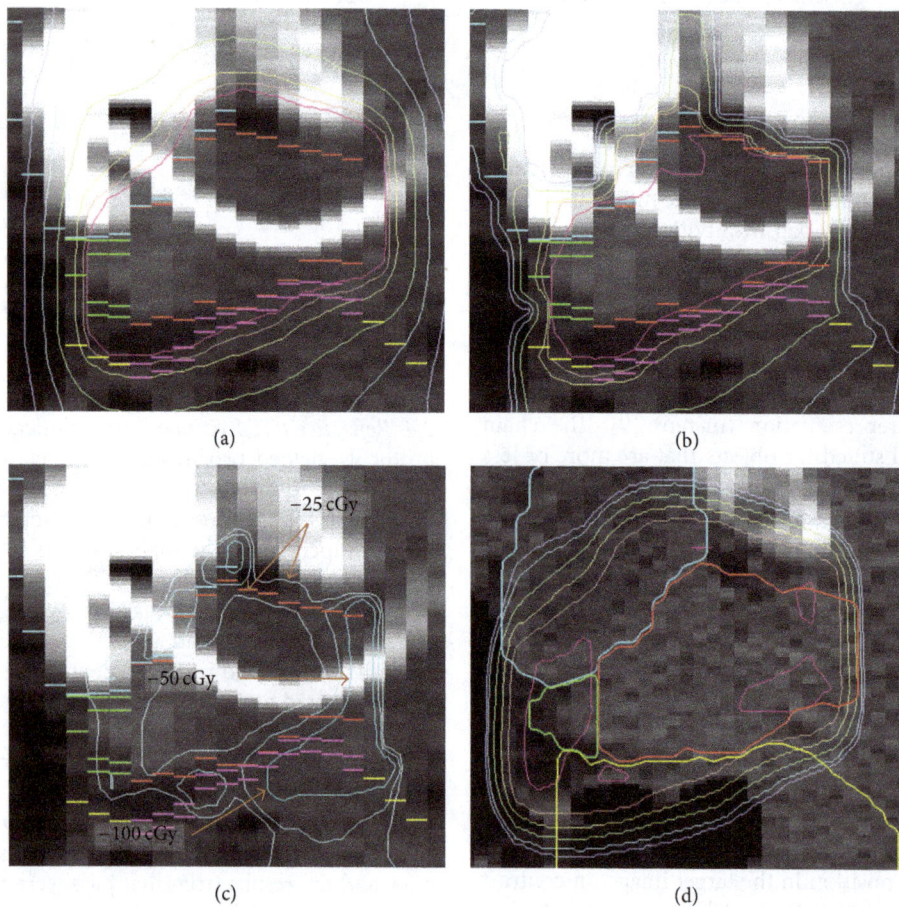

FIGURE 6: Organ contours and isodose curves on midsagittal slices for a typical case. Organs shown are the prostate (red), seminal vesicles (green), bladder (blue), rectum (yellow), and anterior rectal wall (purple). (a) Planned isodoses on pCT. (b) Cumulative isodoses on pCT. (c) Error dose on pCT. (d) Delivered isodoses computed from one tCT.

2.5. Calculation of Hypothetical Delivered Dose Distributions. Treatment dose distributions for each tCT and each mapped isocenter were computed using PlanUNC assuming all beams were delivered as planned for each of the three isocenters (Figure 6). This was accomplished by importing each tCT to PlanUNC, registering the ensemble of planned beams to each of the treatment isocenters in turn, and calculating

the delivered dose assuming all beams were delivered as planned. After dose calculation the DICOM-RT files for the planned and treatment dose distributions were imported to ARTSuite and dose distributions were mapped from tCTs to the pCT using (2) in the reverse direction. Except for a rind ~2–5 mm thick around the prostate, dose to interstitial tissues was not mapped since (2) applies only to modeled

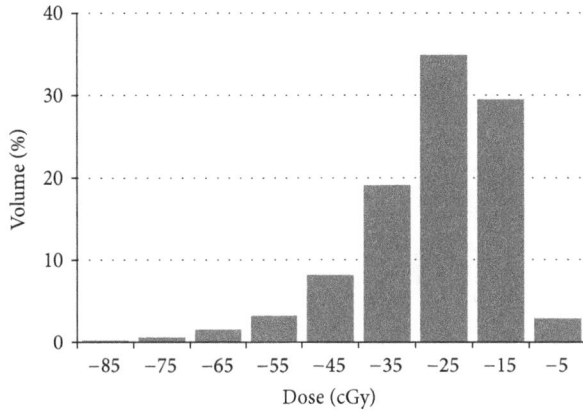

FIGURE 7: Prostate DVH for the error dose distribution shown in Figure 6(c). The bin size is 10 cGy.

tissues. Dose to the rind was mapped by extrapolating the skeletal framework a small distance beyond the prostate surface. The mapped treatment doses were summed over all tCTs and all isocenters and resampled to the grid of the planning dose to simplify comparison of planned and treatment dose distributions. Figure 6(a) shows the planned isodose curves for the 10, 25, 50, 85, 90, and 95% levels on the pCT for the initial (nonboost) portion. The proximal two slices (6 mm length) of the seminal vesicles were included in the PTV. Figure 6(b) shows the same isodose levels from the cumulative dose for the clinical protocol over 15 fractions. Error dose distributions (Figure 6(c)) were computed by subtracting the scaled planned dose distribution from the summed treatment dose distribution. The scaling factor was determined by the number of fractions contributing to the summed treatment dose. Isodose curves are shown for −100, −50, and −25 cGy. Figure 6(d) shows the same isodose levels as in Figure 6(a) computed from one of the 15 tCTs. The frequency distribution in Figure 7 illustrates the expected underdosing of the prostate due to differences between prostate shape and location at planning and treatment times.

For dose accumulation purposes, the spatial accuracy required for nonrigid registration of a point in the tCT with its corresponding point in the pCT depends on the tolerable dose error and the steepness of dose gradients near the points. Assuming that the spacing between calculation points in the dose grid is matched to the dose gradients [19, 20], correspondence errors should be small compared to the grid spacing. The clinical planning grid spacing was 5 mm in this study. Figure 8 shows color-coded maps of differences between the positions of two points, one point for each method, resulting from a single point in the tCT. The differences were ~1 mm along the x and y axes and ~2 mm along the z axis for the prostate ROI. The larger difference along the z axis is attributed to the 3 mm slice thickness. These findings support the use of m-reps for dose accumulation for this study.

3. Results

3.1. Distance Metrics.
Frequency histograms (Figure 9) were computed from the signed differences ($\Delta x, \Delta y, \Delta z$)

(Figure 10) between the reference isocenters and the clinical and automatic isocenters for all 243 tCTs. The bin width for Δx and Δy was 0.5 mm. To maintain comparable counts per bin, the width for Δz was chosen to be 1.0 mm. Summary statistics for all ten patients are given in Table 2. Figure 9 shows that the distributions for clinical and automatic isocenters are centered near the reference values in approximately Gaussian fashion, supporting the utility of the reference values.

Comparison of the frequency histograms for clinical and automatic protocols shows that automatic mapping is robust, as accurate as the clinical protocol along all three axes, and more precise than the clinical protocol, where accuracy is the average of the unsigned Δs compared to the reference values, and precision is the spread (standard deviation) for each axis. Even though the averages for the automatic method are smaller (closer to the references) than the clinical protocol, greater accuracy is not claimed because the references are not golden. On the other hand, the standard deviation is characteristic of the registration method and independent of the reference values. The ANOVA F-test is $<10^{-12}$ for all three axes, demonstrating that human and automatic variances are significantly different. As seen from Table 2, these observations apply for each individual patient. Moreover, the clinical protocol yielded 8 outliers, defined here as differences $>3\sigma_{clinical}$ ($\sigma_{clinical}$ = standard deviation of clinical protocol), with the largest being almost $5\sigma_{clinical}$. In comparison, the largest difference for the automatic approach is slightly less than $3\sigma_{clinical}$ along the x axis for patient 10, and for this case $\sigma_{clinical}$ is small ($\approx$1 mm).

Table 2 also gives results for Court and Dong [12] and Smitsmans et al. [13]. Both studies evaluated automatic localization of the prostate in tCTs via multiscale rigid registration with pCTs. The values given in Table 2 for these studies are differences in prostate position, as opposed to isocenter position, between automatic methods and manually prepared references. Court and Dong reported results for two patients: patient A had 22 tCTs and was considered less challenging than patient B, who had 21 tCTs. Smitsmans et al. looked at a collection of 19 patients with 8–13 tCTs each. The results in Table 2 are for 91% of the tCTs. The remaining 9% were considered outliers and quantitative results were not reported. The automatic rigid registration method presented in this paper appears qualitatively to be comparable in performance to both Court and Dong and Smitsmans et al. No direct quantitative comparisons are possible however due to differences in study designs.

3.2. Prostate DVHs

3.2.1. Initial Portion of Treatment Regimen.
Prostate DVHs for doses accumulated using the clinical, automatic, and reference isocenters for two typical patients are compared against the scaled planned DVHs in Figure 11. These cases illustrate (i) small differences among the three isocenters, (ii) degradation of the shoulder region, and (iii) a decrease in delivered versus planned dose of ~100–200 cGy scaled to the full nonboost portion. These general findings were consistent

TABLE 2: Summary statistics over all patients.

Patient	ΔX (mm) |Avg|† Clinic	Auto	Max, Min Clinic	Auto	Std Dev Clinic	Auto	ΔY (mm) |Avg|† Clinic	Auto	Max, Min Clinic	Auto	Std Dev Clinic	Auto	ΔZ (mm) |Avg|† Clinic	Auto	Max, Min Clinic	Auto	Std Dev Clinic	Auto
1	1.3	0.4	2.8, −3.0	1.7, −0.2	1.5	0.5	2.3	1.4	6.7, −6.0	0.2, −5.8	3.0	1.7	3.2	1.2	¥**12.9**, −2.2	3.5, −1.4	4.1	1.4
2	1.1	0.4	3.1, −1.6	1.2, −0.7	1.3	0.5	1.4	0.9	4.8, −4.2	2.0, −2.4	1.8	1.1	1.9	0.6	6.4, −6.6	2.5, −2.2	2.7	0.9
3	1.1	0.5	1.7, −3.4	1.7, −0.9	1.4	0.6	1.9	0.9	1.8, −6.1	2.0, −4.0	2.2	1.3	1.7	1.0	2.7, −4.9	3.5, −2.1	2.1	1.3
4	1.0	0.6	2.8, −3.6	2.8, −1.3	1.4	0.8	1.7	1.0	¥**11.7**, −6.8	0.5, −4.9	2.9	1.3	2.7	0.8	¥**18.4**, −6.5	1.1, −3.1	4.2	1.1
5	0.7	0.6	2.4, −1.5	1.2, −1.2	0.9	0.7	1.4	0.9	2.9, −4.4	0.8, −4.7	1.7	1.2	2.3	1.5	¥**11.2**, −2.2	4.5, −1.7	3.0	1.7
6	0.8	0.4	2.1, −1.6	0.6, −2.2	1.0	0.5	1.5	1.0	3.7, −4.3	2.5, −3.3	1.9	1.3	3.0	1.1	10.4, −4.8	3.3, −2.3	3.6	1.4
7	1.2	0.7	2.7, −3.5	0.2, −2.3	1.5	0.8	1.8	0.9	3.2, −5.2	2.1, −2.3	2.2	1.1	2.0	0.8	¥**11.8**, −1.4	2.8, −4.7	2.7	1.2
8	0.9	0.3	3.2, −1.8	0.9, −1.2	1.2	0.3	1.4	0.7	3.3, ¥**−6.2**	0.8, −2.4	1.8	0.8	1.8	0.8	¥**14.0**, −2.5	3.2, −1.9	2.8	1.1
9	0.9	0.6	3.3, 0.5	1.8, −0.4	1.0	0.6	1.4	0.8	3.0, −4.8	1.9, −1.3	1.9	0.9	2.9	0.8	4.4, −9.1	4.1, −1.3	3.6	1.1
10	0.7	0.6	2.9, −2.1	0.9, −3.1	1.0	0.8	1.0	0.8	4.6, −1.3	3.5, −2.0	1.3	1.2	2.0	1.3	5.3, −6.0	3.9, −1.6	2.6	1.5
All	1.1	0.6	3.3, −3.6	2.8, −3.1	1.4	0.8	1.8	1.1	11.7, −6.8	3.5, −5.8	2.3	1.5	2.5	1.1	¥**18.4**, −9.1	4.5, −4.7	3.5	1.4
Reference [12] Pat A	NA*	0.0#		1.0†			NA*	0.2#		1.1†		0.5	NA*	0.3#		2.4†		1.0
Reference [12] Pat B	NA*	0.3#		1.4†			NA*	−0.2#		1.9†		1.4	NA*	−0.1#		3.5†		1.9
Reference [13]	NA*	0.1					NA*	0.1				0.7	NA*	0.0				1.3

¥Bold values are outliers. †Average of unsigned differences. *Not applicable. +Maximum. #Average of signed differences.

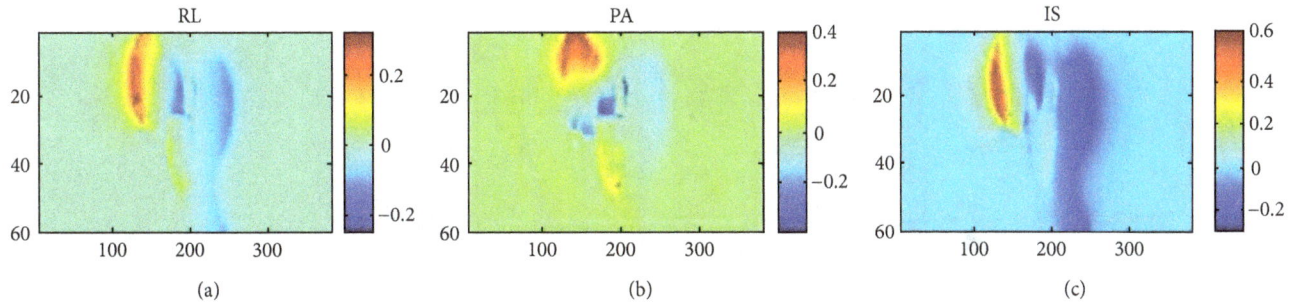

FIGURE 8: Color-coded difference maps for points in the tCT nonrigidly registered to the pCT using FEM and models. In the prostate ROI the agreement between the two methods is ~1 mm along the x and y axes and ~2 mm along the z axis. The larger difference along the z axis is attributed to the 3 mm slice thickness.

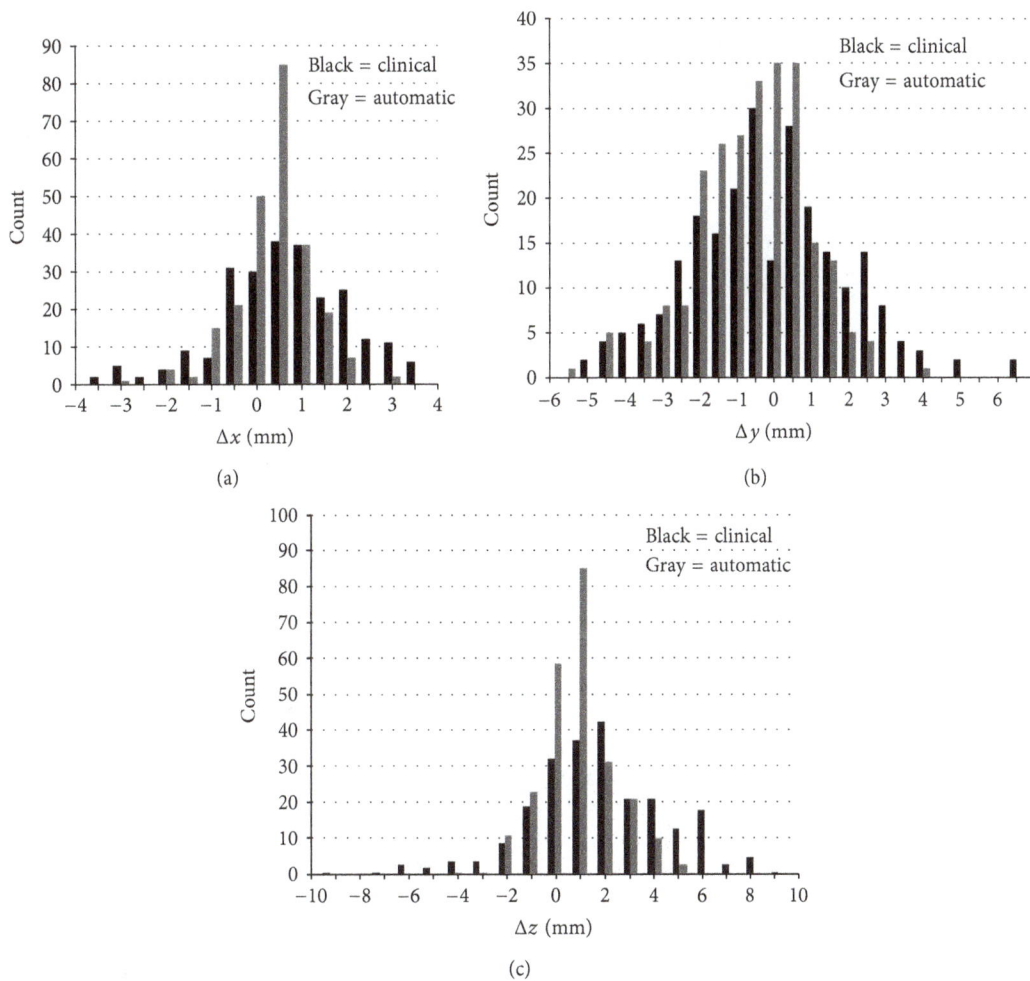

FIGURE 9: Frequency histograms for Δx, Δy, and Δz. The averages of the unsigned clinical values for Δx, Δy, and Δz, respectively, are 1.06 mm, 1.79 mm, and 2.54 mm. The averages of the automatic values are 0.58 mm, 1.14 mm, and 1.05 mm. Two clinical values are outside the Δy axis range and seven values are outside the Δz range. All of the automatic results are within the ranges of all axes.

across all ten patients, but the severity of shoulder degradation was patient specific. Automatic mapping performed better in the shoulder region (Figure 11(a)) than the clinical protocol in about half the cases and as well in the other half (Figure 11(b)). The absence of more significant differences is

attributed to margins (5 mm) that were relatively insensitive to isocenter mapping variations on the order of a few mm, a finding expected for properly designed margins.

Figure 7 shows the differential DVH for the error dose for the patient in Figure 11(a). Error isodose curves in Figure 6(c)

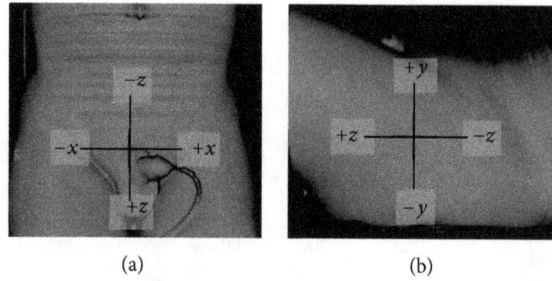

(a)   (b)

FIGURE 10: Coordinate system for calculating Δx, Δy, and Δz.

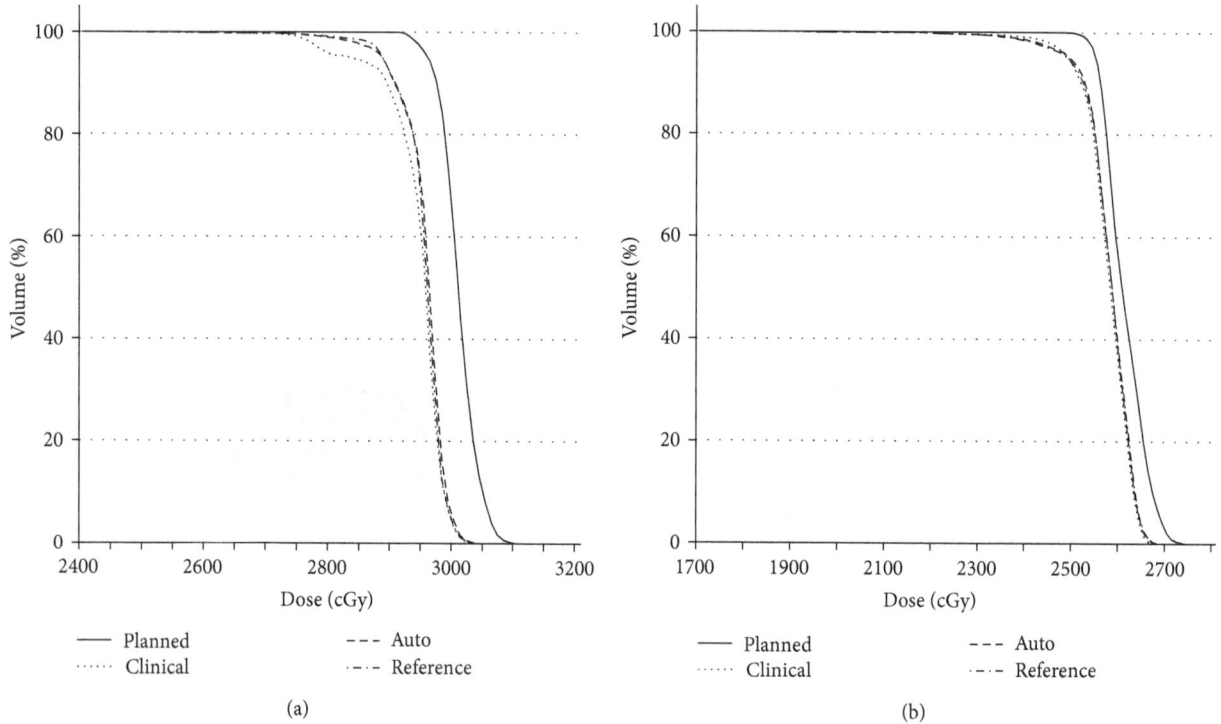

(a)   (b)

FIGURE 11: Prostate accumulated-dose DVHs for two patients. The planned doses have been scaled to the number of fractions accumulated for each patient.

show that the underdosed region occurs at the apex. The superior shift of the delivered dose distribution displayed on the tCT in Figure 6(d) was also present on other tCTs, explaining the origin of the under dose. Underdosing at the base was not observed for this patient because the planning target volume was enlarged superiorly to include the proximal SVs, providing extra protection at the base. However, underdosing was observed at both the base and apex for all patients whose SVs were not included in the target volume.

3.2.2. Boost Portion of Treatment Regimen. TCTs for boost fractions were available for only two patients. DVHs in Figure 12 were computed from tCTs acquired for four of twelve boost fractions. The DVHs for both patients show the same general trends observed for the initial treatment portion (Figure 11). However, the clear separation between the descending portions of the clinical and automatic isocenters

in Figure 12 suggests that automatic mapping may reduce the overall prostate under dose compared to the clinical protocol. If true, this finding would not be surprising since the boost margin (3 mm) would be expected to be more sensitive to image registration errors. However, further study is needed to test this finding.

4. Discussion and Conclusions

This work presents a formalism for mapping the planned isocenter to a tCT based on correspondence properties of a deformable prostate organ model that is used for registration of the pCT and tCT and for segmentation of the prostate in the tCT. The fully automatic mapping algorithm is as accurate as the clinical protocol but more precise. The algorithm had no failures or outliers for the tCTs studied. Better precision can be explained in terms of the robust properties of the algorithm and the absence of intra- and interuser variabilities. Moreover, human registrations were made under the pressure

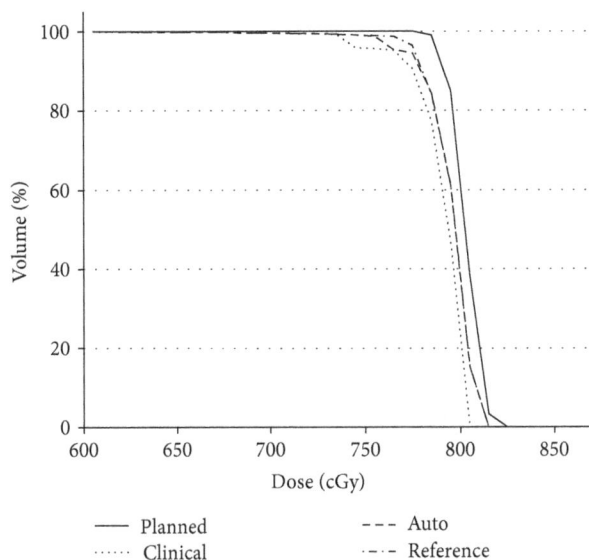

FIGURE 12: DVHs for a boost portion. The planned dose was scaled to four fractions.

of clinical time constraints that can hasten decisions and lead to suboptimal results.

In dosimetric comparisons for the prostate, automatic mapping showed less degradation in the shoulder region of DVHs for 50% of patients in this study. In the other 50%, degradation was no worse than the clinical protocol. The absence of large differences in dose-volume metrics is attributed to prostate margins that were relatively insensitive to variations in isocenter mapping on the order of a few mm.

The clinical significance of the observed dosimetric improvements was not addressed but appears to be modest for the patients in this study. This conclusion however depends on the prostate margin and dose fractionation scheme as suggested by Figure 12. In particular, dosimetric improvements might be significant for less forgiving forms of treatment delivery such as stereotactic body radiotherapy. Also the finding that accurate pCT and tCT image registration does not fully compensate for geometric variability supports conclusions of other studies [2, 3] that full compensation for patient-specific geometric changes requires off-line adaptive planning or online reoptimization.

The overall conclusion is that the automatic algorithm robustly maps the planned isocenter to a position close to the correct location in a tCT and thus is well suited to augment human judgment in the clinical setting. Furthermore, the algorithm offers the potential for reducing registration outliers. During the workflow for mapping the isocenter, all of the essential image processing steps for calculation of delivered dose and mapping the delivered dose to planning space are performed.

Conflict of Interests

Edward Chaney is an employee of Morphormics, Inc., and Principal Investigator of NIH Grant no. R44 CA141941 that

supported the research reported in this paper. Mark Foskey is an employee of Morphormics, Inc. Andrea Kress and An Qin were partially supported under subcontracts funded by NIH Grant no. R44 CA141941. The remaining authors declare no conflict of interests.

Acknowledgment

The research reported in this paper was supported by the National Cancer Institute of the National Institutes of Health under Award no. R44 CA141941. The content is solely the responsibility of the authors and does not necessarily represent the official views of the National Institutes of Health.

References

[1] W. Y. Song, B. Schaly, G. Bauman, J. J. Battista, and J. van Dyk, "Evaluation of image-guided radiation therapy (IGRT) technologies and their impact on the outcomes of hypofractionated prostate cancer treatments: a radiobiologic analysis," *International Journal of Radiation Oncology, Biology, Physics*, vol. 64, no. 1, pp. 289–300, 2006.

[2] D. Yan, D. Lockman, D. Brabbins, L. Tyburski, and A. Martinez, "An off-line strategy for constructing a patient-specific planning target volume in adaptive treatment process for prostate cancer," *International Journal of Radiation Oncology Biology Physics*, vol. 48, no. 1, pp. 289–302, 2000.

[3] D. Schulze, J. Liang, D. Yan, and T. Zhang, "Comparison of various online IGRT strategies: the benefits of online treatment plan re-optimization," *Radiotherapy and Oncology*, vol. 90, no. 3, pp. 367–376, 2009.

[4] P. Jannin, J. M. Fitzpatrick, D. J. Hawkes, X. Pennec, R. Shahidi, and M. W. Vannier, "Validation of medical image processing in image-guided therapy," *IEEE Transactions on Medical Imaging*, vol. 21, no. 12, pp. 1445–1449, 2002.

[5] J. R. Wong, Z. Gao, M. Uematsu et al., "Interfractional prostate shifts: review of 1870 computed tomography (CT) scans obtained during image-guided radiotherapy using CT-on-rails for the treatment of prostate cancer," *International Journal of Radiation Oncology, Biology, Physics*, vol. 72, no. 5, pp. 1396–1401, 2008.

[6] E. G. A. Aird and J. Conway, "CT simulation for radiotherapy treatment planning," *British Journal of Radiology*, vol. 75, no. 900, pp. 937–949, 2002.

[7] S. Sailer, E. L. Chaney, J. G. Rosenman, G. W. Sherouse, and J. E. Tepper, "Three dimensional treatment planning at the University of North Carolina at Chapel Hill," *Seminars in Radiation Oncology*, vol. 2, pp. 267–273, 1992.

[8] S. X. Chang, T. J. Cullip, J. G. Rosenman, P. H. Halvorsen, and J. E. Tepper, "Dose optimization via index-dose gradient minimization," *Medical Physics*, vol. 29, no. 6, pp. 1130–1146, 2002.

[9] S. M. Pizer, P. T. Fletcher, S. Joshi et al., "A method and software for segmentation of anatomic object ensembles by deformable m-reps," *Medical Physics*, vol. 32, no. 5, pp. 1335–1345, 2005.

[10] S. M. Pizer, R. E. Broadhurst, J. Y. Jeong et al., "Intra-patient anatomic statistical models for adaptive radiotherapy," in *Proceedings of the Medical Image Computing and Computer-Assisted Intervention Workshop (MICCAI '06)*, A. Frangi and H. Delingette, Eds., pp. 43–46, Copenhagen, Denmark, October 2006, From Statistical Atlases to Personalized Models: Understanding Complex Diseases in Populations and Individuals.

[11] D. Merck, G. Tracton, R. Saboo et al., "Training models of anatomic shape variability," *Medical Physics*, vol. 35, no. 8, pp. 3584–3596, 2008.

[12] L. E. Court and L. Dong, "Automatic registration of the prostate for computed-tomography-guided radiotherapy," *Medical Physics*, vol. 30, no. 10, pp. 2750–2757, 2003.

[13] M. Smitsmans, J. Wolthaus, X. Artignan et al., "Automatic localization of the prostate for on-line or off-line image-guided radiotherapy," *International Journal of Radiation Oncology, Biology, Physics*, vol. 60, no. 2, pp. 623–635, 2004.

[14] F. Maes, D. Vandermeulen, and P. Suetens, "Comparative evaluation of multiresolution optimization strategies for multimodality image registration by maximization of mutual information," *Medical Image Analysis*, vol. 3, no. 4, pp. 373–386, 1999.

[15] K. Siddiqi and S. Pizer, Eds., *Medial Representations: Mathematics, Algorithms and Applications*, vol. 37, chapter 8, Springer, Berlin, Germany, 2008.

[16] M. J. Murphy, F. J. Salguero, J. V. Siebers, D. Staub, and C. Vaman, "A method to estimate the effect of deformable image registration uncertainties on daily dose mapping," *Medical Physics*, vol. 39, no. 2, pp. 573–580, 2012.

[17] R. E. Broadhurst, J. Stough, S. M. Pizer, and E. L. Chaney, "A statistical appearance model based on intensity quantiles," in *Proceedings of the 3rd IEEE International Symposium on Biomedical Imaging*, pp. 422–425, April 2006.

[18] S. Frantz, K. Rohr, and H. Stiehl, "Localization of 3D anatomical point landmarks in 3D tomographic images using deformable models. Medical image computing and computer-assisted intervention," in *Medical Image Computing and Computer-Assisted Intervention*, vol. 1935 of *Lecture Notes in Computer Science*, pp. 492–501, 2000.

[19] A. Niemierko and M. Goitein, "The influence of the size of the grid used for dose calculation on the accuracy of dose estimation," *Medical Physics*, vol. 16, no. 2, pp. 239–247, 1989.

[20] J. F. Dempsey, H. E. Romeijn, J. G. Li, D. A. Low, and J. R. Palta, "A Fourier analysis of the dose grid resolution required for accurate IMRT fluence map optimization," *Medical Physics*, vol. 32, no. 2, pp. 380–388, 2005.

10

Comparison of Super Resolution Reconstruction Acquisition Geometries for Use in Mouse Phenotyping

Niranchana Manivannan,[1] **Bradley D. Clymer,**[1] **Anna Bratasz,**[2] **and Kimerly A. Powell**[2,3]

[1] *Department of Electrical and Computer Engineering, The Ohio State University, Columbus, OH 43210, USA*
[2] *Small Animal Imaging Shared Resources, The Ohio State University, Columbus, OH 43210, USA*
[3] *Department of Biomedical Informatics, The Ohio State University, Columbus, OH 43210, USA*

Correspondence should be addressed to Kimerly A. Powell; kimerly.powell@osumc.edu

Academic Editor: Anne Clough

3D isotropic imaging at high spatial resolution (30–100 microns) is important for comparing mouse phenotypes. 3D imaging at high spatial resolutions is limited by long acquisition times and is not possible in many *in vivo* settings. Super resolution reconstruction (SRR) is a postprocessing technique that has been proposed to improve spatial resolution in the slice-select direction using multiple 2D multislice acquisitions. Any 2D multislice acquisition can be used for SRR. In this study, the effects of using three different low-resolution acquisition geometries (orthogonal, rotational, and shifted) on SRR images were evaluated and compared to a known standard. Iterative back projection was used for the reconstruction of all three acquisition geometries. The results of the study indicate that super resolution reconstructed images based on orthogonally acquired low-resolution images resulted in reconstructed images with higher SNR and CNR in less acquisition time than those based on rotational and shifted acquisition geometries. However, interpolation artifacts were observed in SRR images based on orthogonal acquisition geometry, particularly when the slice thickness was greater than six times the inplane voxel size. Reconstructions based on rotational geometry appeared smoother than those based on orthogonal geometry, but they required two times longer to acquire than the orthogonal LR images.

1. Introduction

MRI is being used more frequently for evaluating morphological phenotypes in genetically engineered mouse models of disease [1]. 3D imaging at the highest spatial resolution is the preferred approach for comparing morphological phenotypes; however, it is not always possible in small animal *in vivo* imaging settings. This is due to the long acquisition times required to achieve high spatial resolution. Several factors limit obtaining high-resolution 3D isotropic images in the *in vivo* settings such as the length of time a mouse can be kept under anesthesia, motion artifacts that are likely to occur during long acquisition protocols that degrade image quality, and increased repetition times required at the high magnetic field strengths used for small animal imaging. Keeping animals under anesthesia for long periods of time (>2 hrs) is not desirable. MRI acquisition protocols with very long repetition times ($T_R > 1500$ ms), such as T2-weighted, diffusion-weighted (DW), and inversion recovery imaging are particularly affected by the long scan times required for 3D isotropic imaging. Thus, *in vivo* MR images in small animal studies are usually acquired using 2D multislice acquisitions with inplane resolutions (50–100 μm) which are 5–10 times greater than the resolution in the slice-select direction (500–1000 μm).

2D multislice images suffer from the effects of partial volume averaging due to their increased slice thickness, and when reformatted and viewed from a perspective other than the inplane acquisition direction, the features often appear blurry due to decreased resolution in the slice-select direction. Increasing the resolution in the slice-select direction comes at the expense of decreased signal-to-noise ratio (SNR) due to the smaller voxel size. Signal-to-noise ratio is directly proportional to voxel size and the square root of number of signal averages. Therefore, in order to compensate for a decrease in SNR due to a decrease in voxel size, the number of signal averages must be increased by a factor proportional to the decrease in voxel size and thus a proportional increase in acquisition time. Decreasing the slice thickness also requires increasing the number of slices in order to cover the same FOV which also results in increased acquisition time. This trade-off between spatial resolution, acceptable SNR, and image acquisition time is always a consideration when imaging live subjects. MRI acquisition techniques, such as parallel imaging [2] and partial Fourier imaging [3] have been proposed for speeding up acquisition times so that higher resolution images can be acquired. These techniques require specialized hardware and software for implementation and are not always available for small animal MRI applications. Super resolution reconstruction (SRR) is an image postprocessing approach that has been proposed to improve the resolution in the slice-select direction in 2D multislice MRI data set [4]. It is based on reconstructing a high-resolution (HR) image from a set of low-resolution (LR) image stacks that were obtained from different viewpoints of the same field-of-view (FOV). Its application is not limited by the availability of acquisition hardware or software and can be used in any multislice acquisition setting including those that utilize high-speed acquisition protocols, such as parallel or partial Fourier imaging.

The SRR approaches proposed this far for MRI have differed primarily in the orientation of the acquisition geometry of the set of LR image stacks and the iterative optimization technique used for SRR. Greenspan et al. [4] proposed collecting a set of LR image stacks by subpixel shifting the 2D multislice stack acquisitions in the slice-select direction. Irani and Peleg's iterative backprojection method (IBP) [5] was then used to reconstruct the HR image from the shifted LR stacks. For this method, the number of LR image stacks required to reconstruct an isotropic 3D HR image is directly related to the ratio of the slice thickness to the inplane resolution of the LR images. Thus, the more anisotropic the LR data acquisitions are the greater the number of LR image stacks are required. Shilling et al. [6] proposed acquiring a set of LR image stacks by rotating the slice-select direction in equal angle sampling intervals about a central axis. Six LR image stacks, obtained at 30° rotational increments, were used for SRR. Additive and multiplicative algebraic reconstructions were used to reconstruct the HR image from the LR image stacks. Additive correction was found to be better than the multiplicative method for high noise levels. Resolution enhancement was observed in phantom studies, ex vivo, and human brain scans. Souza and Senn [7] based their SR reconstructions on the acquisition of three orthogonal (i.e., coronal, sagittal, and axial) LR image stacks. IBP was also used for reconstructing HR images from the LR image stacks in this approach. Qualitative and quantitative evaluations indicated that SRR using LR image stacks acquired orthogonally might be useful for improving spatial resolution and contrast-to-noise ratios (CNR) similar to that observed using shifted and rotational geometries. Recently, Plenge et al. [8] evaluated the different optimization techniques used for SRR of MRI data. Their

results indicated that reconstruction methods based on IBP and least squares optimization techniques performed better than those based on algebraic reconstruction. Plenge's evaluation was performed using the rotational acquisition geometry proposed by Shilling et al. [6]. No evaluation of the effect of LR acquisition geometry on SRR has been performed.

Our overall goal was to determine whether SRR with a minimal number of LR views would be useful for morphological evaluations of in vivo animal models. In order for SRR to be applicable in small animal phenotyping applications, the LR image stacks must be acquired in significantly less time than a comparable HR 3D isotropic acquisition, and the SRR image should have comparable image quality to that observed in images obtained from a HR acquisition. To achieve this goal, we investigated the effect LR acquisition geometry (shifted, rotation, and orthogonal) and the number of LR image stacks with different voxel aspect ratios (AR) have on SRR. A voxel's AR refers to the proportional relationship of its size in each dimension (i.e., width : height : depth) and is directly related to SNR and acquisition time. For this study, quantitative and qualitative evaluations of SRR images were performed using a resolution (line pair) and a biological (ex vivo embryo) phantom. Image quality was assessed by comparing the SRR images to a HR 3D isotropically acquired image. SRR was also implemented for an in vivo animal imaging application.

2. Materials and Methods

2.1. Super Resolution Reconstruction Method. All SRR images were reconstructed using the IBP approach proposed by Irani and Peleg [5]. IBP was chosen because it has been widely used for super resolution reconstruction in the past and because of its easy implementation. A flowchart illustrating the IBP approach is provided in Figure 1. Initially, an HR image $\widehat{G}^{(0)}$ is approximated from the average of multiple LR images $\{f_k\}_{k=1}^{N}$ that have been geometrically transformed, T_k^{-1}, to the same orientation prior to averaging. A new set of LR images $\{\widehat{f}_k^{(0)}\}_{k=1}^{N}$, are obtained by simulating the imaging process (blurring h, and down sampling) in the predicted HR image $\widehat{G}^{(0)}$. For our case, a 1D Gaussian kernel with a FWHM equal to the LR slice thickness was used along the slice-select direction in the HR image for blurring because it closely matched the excitation profile used in the original image acquisition sequence. If the predicted HR image $\widehat{G}^{(0)}$ is the same as the true HR image G, then the simulated LR images $\{\widehat{f}_k^{(0)}\}_{k=1}^{N}$ should be equal to the observed LR images $\{f_k\}_{k=1}^{N}$. Therefore, the difference between the observed and simulated LR images $\{f_k - \widehat{f}_k^{(0)}\}_{k=1}^{N}$ is upsampled and backprojected on to $\widehat{G}^{(0)}$ using linear interpolation. This results in an updated HR image $\widehat{G}^{(1)} = \widehat{G}^{(0)} + (1/k) \sum_{k=1}^{N} (\text{upsample}\{f_k - \widehat{f}_k^{(0)}\})$ that can be downsampled and the simulated LR images $\{\widehat{f}_k^{(i)}\}_{k=1}^{N}$ are compared to the observed LR images $\{f_k\}_{k=1}^{N}$. These steps are iteratively repeated till the maximum error at the ith iteration according to $e^{(i)} = \text{Max}\{\| f_k - \widehat{f}_k^{(i)} \|\}_{k=1,2,...,N}$ is less

$$\boxed{\text{LR images } \{f_k\}_{k=1}^N}$$

$$\boxed{\text{HR image } \widehat{G}^{(0)} = \frac{1}{N}\sum_{k=1}^N T_k^{-1}[\text{upsample}\{f_k\}]}$$

$$\boxed{\begin{array}{c}\text{Simulated LR images}\\ \left\{\widehat{f}_k^{(i)}\right\}_{k=1}^N = [\text{downsample}\{T_k(G^{(i)}) * h\}]\end{array}}$$

$$\boxed{\begin{array}{c}\text{Error function}\\ e^{(i)} = \text{Max}\{\|f_k - \widehat{f}_k^{(i)}\|\}_{k=1,2,\dots,N} < \text{threshold}\end{array}}$$

$$\boxed{\text{Stop}} \quad \text{Yes}$$

$$\text{No}$$

$$\boxed{\begin{array}{c}\text{Upsampled difference}\\ d_k = \text{upsample}\left\{f_k - \widehat{f}_k^{(i)}\right\}\end{array}}$$

$$\boxed{\text{Updated HR image } \widehat{G}^{(i+1)} = \widehat{G}^{(i)} + \frac{1}{N}\sum_{k=1}^N T_k^{-1}(d_k)}$$

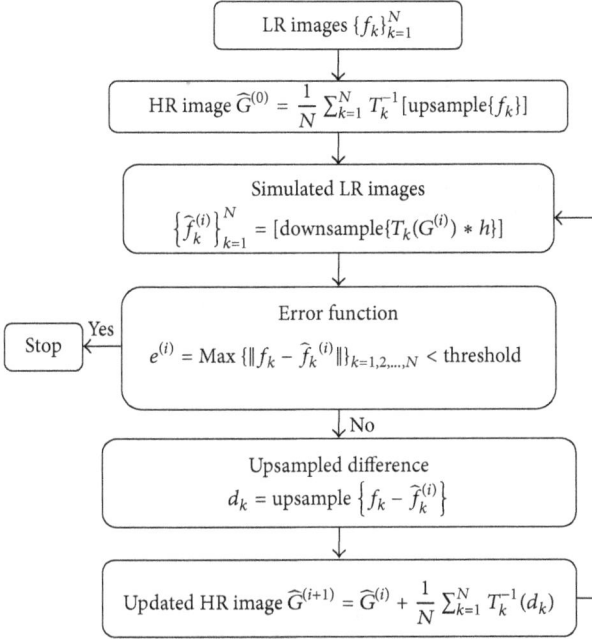

FIGURE 1: Block diagram of Irani and Peleg's IBP algorithm.

than a preset threshold. All SRR software was developed using Matlab v.2009a (MathWorks Inc., Mass, USA).

2.2. MR Image Acquisition

2.2.1. Resolution Phantom. A resolution phantom was constructed using five cylindrical quartz EPR tubes (0.5 mm ID, 0.7 mm OD). The tubes were cut into 2.5 cm lengths and were placed side-by-side with a known separation of 0.7 mm (see illustration in Figure 2(a)). The tubes were sealed with the air trapped inside them, resulting in a signal void within the tubes. They were then immersed in the center of a 15 mL tube (14 mm ID) filled with 1 : 30 (v : v) homogeneous mixture of gadopentetate dimeglumine (GD) Magnevist (Bayer Pharmaceutical, Wayne NJ) and water.

LR image stacks of the phantom were acquired using a Bruker Biospin Avance 500 MHz 11.7T magnet (Bruker Biospin, Karlsruhe, Germany) and a 25 mm diameter volume coil and a T1-weighted FLASH imaging sequence ($T_R = 348.2$ ms, $T_E = 6$ ms, FA = 90°, FOV = 2.6 × 2.6 cm, 1 mm slice thickness, navgs = 4, number of contiguous slices = 26, and acquisition time = 4 m 56 s). The phantom was imaged at two orientations relative to the slice-select direction of the three acquisition geometries. The first orientation was where the long axis of the tubes were positioned along the Y-axis as illustrated in Figures 2(a)–2(c). The second orientation was where the long axis of the tubes were positioned obliquely to the slice-select direction of the acquisition geometries as illustrated in Figure 2(d). For this orientation the tubes were rotated 40° in the XY-plane and 55° in the YZ-plane in the oblique orientation. The oblique orientation represents the most extreme case where edge reconstruction is affected due to partial volume averaging in the slice-select direction.

LR image stacks were collected using an inplane matrix size of 128 × 128 and 256 × 256 for voxel ARs of 1 : 1 : 5 and 1 : 1 : 10, respectively. For both orientations mentioned above, the stacks were obtained using the following three acquisition geometries: (1) five sets of LR image stacks were acquired using 0.20 mm subpixel shifts in the slice-select direction for voxel AR of 1 : 1 : 5 and ten sets were acquired using 0.10 mm subpixel shifts in the slice-select direction for voxel AR of 1 : 1 : 10 (shifted) (Figure 2(a)), (2) six sets were acquired with 30° angular rotations along the slice-select direction for both ARs of 1 : 1 : 5 and 1 : 1 : 10 (rotated) (Figure 2(b)), and (3) three sets were acquired orthogonally to one another in axial, coronal, and sagittal planes for both ARs of 1 : 1 : 5 and 1 : 1 : 10 (orthogonal) (Figure 2(c)). SRR images were calculated for each acquisition geometry using the SRR method described above.

The quality of the SRR was evaluated by visual inspection of the resolution phantom in the short axis view (i.e, short axis of the tubes) where blurring in the slice-select direction is expected to be the greatest due to the low resolution sampling in that direction. Intensity line plots were obtained to better visualize the effects of SRR on signal intensity and edge transitions. SRR images were compared to a high resolution image of the phantom acquired in the axial plane.

2.2.2. Biological Phantom. An *ex vivo* E17.5 wild type embryo was used as a biological phantom for evaluating the effects of SRR on live subject MRIs. It possesses anatomic structures similar to that observed in live animals and does not suffer from motion artifacts observed in *in vivo* imaging. It is also possible to obtain an isotropic high resolution volume image of the *ex vivo* embryo for comparison to the SRR images. The E17.5 embryo was fixed and stained for 2 hours using a 20 : 1 volume ratio of 4% paraformaldehyde and PBS : GD solution. It was then stabilized and stored in 15 mL of 200 : 1 PBS : GD solution prior to imaging. For MR imaging, the embryo was suspended in a 15 mL tube of Fluorinert FC-70(3M Company, St. Paul MN).

The LR image stacks of the *ex vivo* embryo were obtained using a Bruker Biospin Avance 500 MHz 11.7T magnet (Bruker Biospin, Karlsruhe, Germany) and a 25 mm diameter volume coil and T1-weighted FLASH imaging sequence ($T_R = 519.5$ ms, $T_E = 4$ ms, FA = 30.0, FOV = 2.2×2.2 cm, matrix = 512 × 512, navgs = 1, and acquisition time = 3 min) and two different slice thicknesses, 0.19 mm (voxel AR = 1 : 1 : 4, number of contiguous slices = 64) and 0.26 mm (voxel AR = 1 : 1 : 6, number of contiguous slices = 46). Two additional slice thicknesses were evaluated for the orthogonal acquisition geometry, 0.38 mm (voxel AR = 1 : 1 : 8, number of contiguous slices = 32) and 0.46 mm (voxel AR = 1 : 1 : 10, number of contiguous slices = 26). LR image stacks were obtained using the acquisition geometries outlined above: (1) four sets of LR image stacks were acquired using 0.0475 mm subpixel shifts in the slice-select direction for a voxel AR 1 : 1 : 4 and six sets were acquired using 0.0433 mm subpixel shifts in the slice-select direction for a voxel AR 1 : 1 : 6 (shifted), (2) six sets were acquired with 30° angular rotations along the slice-select direction for both ARs of 1 : 1 : 4 and 1 : 1 : 6 (rotated), and

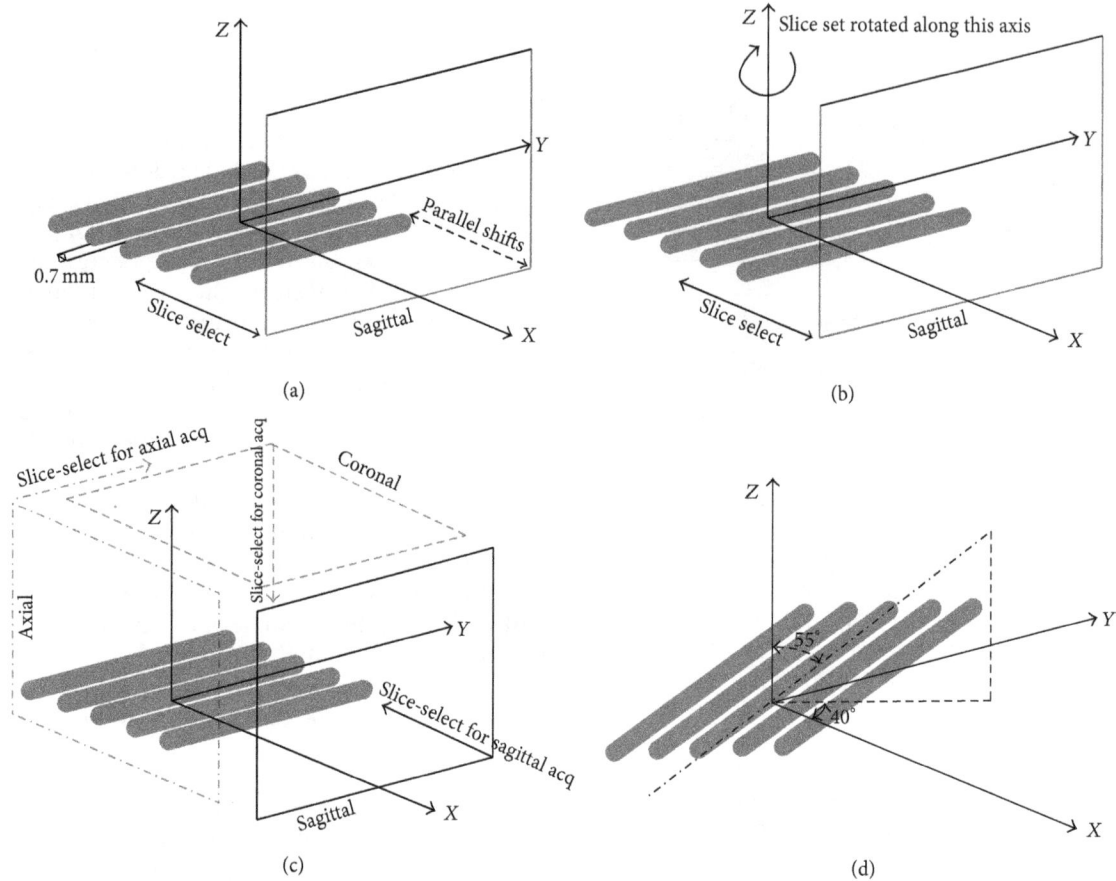

FIGURE 2: Schematic illustrating the orientation of the resolution phantom where the long axis of tubes were positioned orthogonally to the slice-select direction of the (a) shifted, (b) rotational, (c) orthogonal acquisition geometries, and (d) orientation of tubes in the resolution phantom for the oblique setup and the acquisition geometries shown in Figures 2(a), 2(b), and 2(c) were repeated for this oblique orientation. (Axes in this image represent physical coordinates and the main magnetic field is in Z direction).

(3) three sets were acquired orthogonal to another in axial, coronal, and sagittal planes for ARs of 1:1:4, 1:1:6, 1:1:8, and 1:1:10 (orthogonal). The embryo was positioned such that the subpixel shifts were done along the X axis for the shifted geometry and angular rotations were done around the Z axis for the rotational geometry (Figure 3). SRR images were calculated for each LR acquisition geometry using the SRR method described above.

3D isotropic volume images of the same embryo were acquired for comparison to the SRR images. A T1-weighted 3D FLASH sequence (T_R = 11.3 ms, T_E = 4.0 ms, FA = 20.0, FOV = 2.2 × 2.2 × 1.2 cm, matrix = 512 × 512 × 256, navgs = 1, acquisition time = 18.5 min) was used for the 3D imaging. The 3D image obtained from this acquisition protocol results in a high-quality image that is routinely used for biological phenotyping of *ex vivo* embryos in our laboratory.

2.2.3. Quantitative Measures. SRR images were qualitatively compared to the isotropically acquired 3D image of the biological phantom. SNR, contrast-to-noise ratio (CNR), and edge pixel width were used for quantitative evaluation of the SRR images. SNR and CNR were calculated using 9 × 9 × 9

voxel regions within homogenous regions of tissue illustrated in Figure 4. SNR was calculated using the following equation:

$$\text{SNR} = \frac{S}{\sigma_n}, \tag{1}$$

where S = mean signal intensity (regions selected in brain as shown in Figure 4) and σ_n = standard deviation of the noise (from background as shown in Figure 4). CNR was calculated using the following equation:

$$\text{CNR}_{hl} = \frac{|S_h - S_l|}{\text{Max}(\sigma_h, \sigma_l)}, \tag{2}$$

where S_l, S_h and σ_l, σ_h are mean signal intensity and standard deviation in low and high signal intensity ROIs.

Edge profiles were measured by nonlinear least-square fitting of a sigmoid function of the form [4, 6, 8]

$$f = a_1 + \frac{a_2}{1 + \exp(-a_3(x - a_4))}. \tag{3}$$

The edge width in high resolution pixels is computed by

$$\text{Edge Width [Pixels]} = \frac{4.4}{a_3}. \tag{4}$$

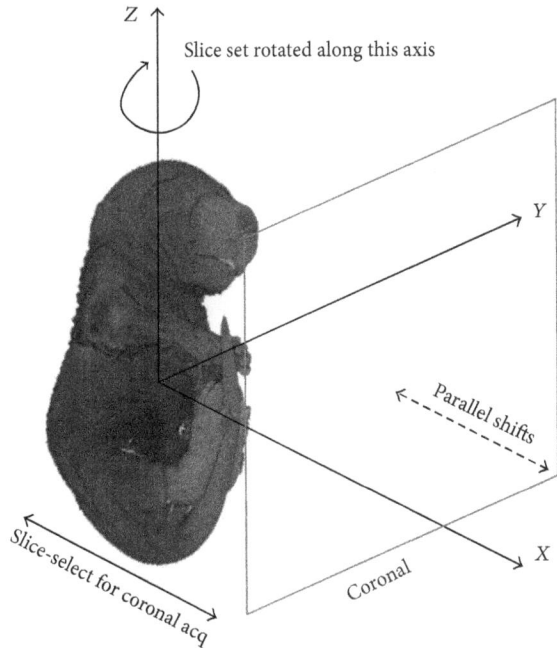

FIGURE 3: Schematic illustrating the orientation of the *ex vivo* embryo with respect to the slice-select direction of the acquisition geometries.

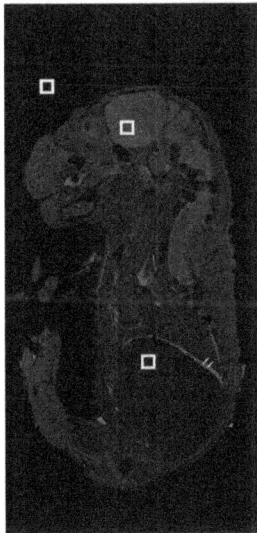

FIGURE 4: 2D slice image of the *ex vivo* embryo illustrating the location of $9 \times 9 \times 9$ voxel ROI chosen for SNR and CNR calculations and sample edge profiles chosen to calculate the edge width.

This corresponds to the rise length from 0.1 to 0.9 of the normalized values, when $a_3 = 4.4$, it corresponds to the rise length of one voxel. An estimate of resolution can be obtained from these edge widths. The mean edge width was calculated from 20 edge profiles obtained across the liver boundary as illustrated in Figure 4.

2.2.4. In Vivo Mouse. MR imaging of a live mouse was performed using a Bruker Biospin Avance 400 MHz 9.4T magnet (Bruker Biospin, Karlsruhe, Germany). All animal protocols were approved by the Institutional Laboratory Care and Use Committee of the Ohio State University. The mouse was placed prone on a temperature controlled mouse bed and inserted into the 35 mm diameter quadrature volume coil. The mouse was anesthetized with 2.5% isoflurane mixed with 1 liter per minute carbogen and maintained with 1–1.5% isoflurane during imaging. The respiration and temperature of the animal were monitored during the course of the experiment using a Small Animal Monitoring and Gating System (Model 1025, Small Animals Instruments, Inc. Stony Brook, NY). A bolus of 11 μL of 11.2 mg iron oxide I.V. (Feridex, AMAH Pharmaceuticals, Lexington MA) per 1 mL PBS was injected via tail vein approximately 20 min prior to imaging. An orthogonal set of LR image stacks (voxel AR of $1:1:10$) of the live mouse was acquired using a respiratory-gated T1-weighted FLASH imaging sequence (TR = 200 ms, TE = 2.72 ms, FA = 55.0, FOV = 2.5 cm × 2.5 cm, navgs = 8, FOV = 2.5 × 2.5, matrix = 256 × 256, 1 mm slice thickness, acqusition time = 15 min). Contiguous slices covering 25 mm of the upper abdominal region were acquired.

3. Results

3.1. Resolution Phantom. Short-axis images of the resolution phantom (voxel AR = $1:1:5$) where the long axis of the tubes were positioned along the Y-axis of Figure 2 are shown in Figures 5(a)–5(e). The lack of resolution in the slice-select direction is apparent in Figure 5(a), where the 2D images are acquired at a slice thickness greater than the distance between the tubes, and linear interpolation is used for reconstruction. Figures 5(b)–5(d) are the corresponding short axis images from the SRR images based on shifted, rotated, and orthogonal acquisition geometries, respectively. The five tubes are resolved in the SRR images based on all three acquisition geometries, however a significant blurring is observed in the slice-select direction for the SRR image based on parallel shifts (Figure 5(b)) and to a lesser extent for the SRR image based on rotational acquisition (Figure 5(c)). The SRR image based on orthogonal acquisition (Figure 5(d)) reproduced the five tubes with the least amount of blurring artifact and looked similar to that observed in the inplane short-axis image (Figure 5(e)), where the sampling rate is great enough to resolve the tubes in the image. The intensity line plot shown in Figure 5(f) illustrates a decrease in peak intensities in the SRR images relative to that observed for the inplane image, with the least amount of change observed in the SRR image based on the orthogonal acquisition geometry. Similar results were observed for the SRR HR images when the LR image stacks were collected with a voxel AR of $1:1:10$ (Figure 6).

Short axis images of the line pair phantom (voxel AR = $1:1:5$) where the long axes of the tubes were aligned oblique to the slice-select direction of the acquisition geometries are shown in Figures 5(g)–5(k). The lack of resolution in the slice-select direction is observed in Figure 5(g), where the 2D images are acquired at a slice thickness greater than the distance between the spaced tubes. The five tubes are not

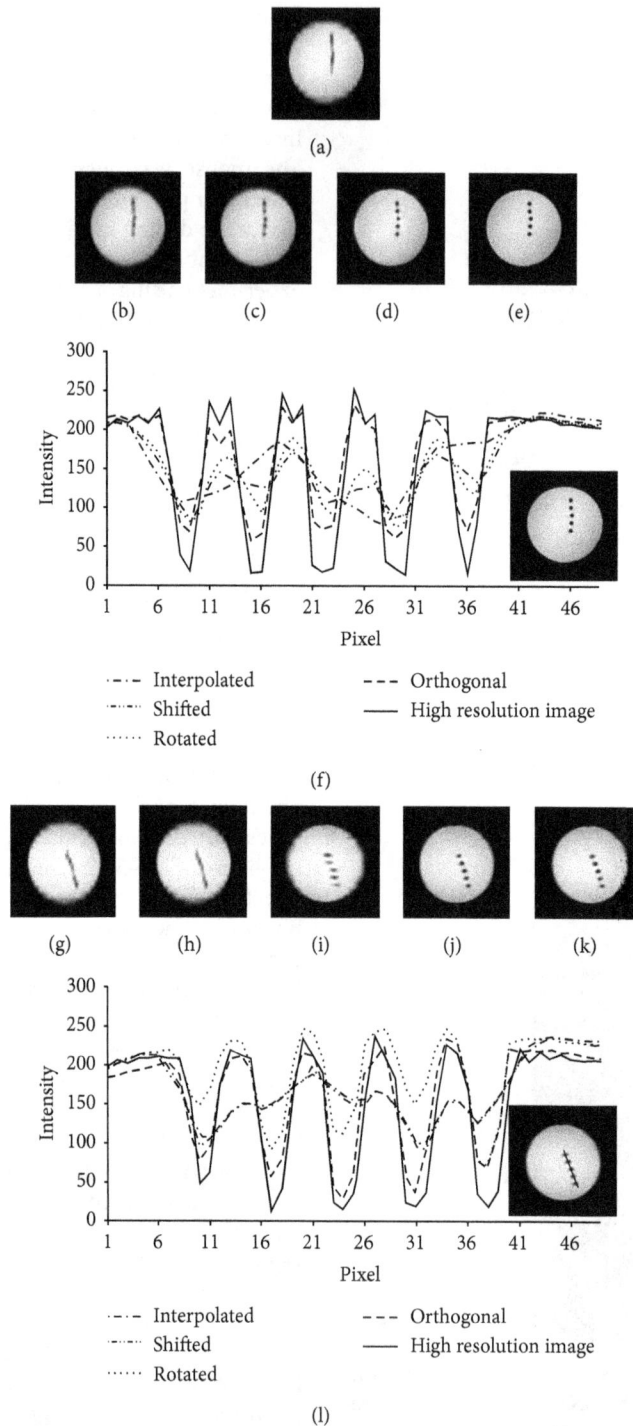

FIGURE 5: 2D slice images (image plane represented is orthogonal to the long axis of the tube which is placed along Y-axis in Figure 2(a)) of resolution phantom where the long axis of the tubes is orthogonal to the acquisition plane, and LR image stacks were collected with a voxel AR of $1:1:5$: (a) interpolated, (b) shifted, (c) rotational, (d) orthogonal, (e) inplane, and (f) line plot, and where the long axis of the tubes is oblique to the acquisition plane: (g) interpolated, (h) shifted, (i) rotational, (j) orthogonal, (k) inplane, and (l) line plot.

resolved in the reconstruction based on the parallel shift acquisition geometry (Figure 5(h)) but are resolved in the reconstructions based on rotational (Figure 5(i)) and orthogonal (Figure 5(j)) acquisition geometry. However, blurring is observed in the slice-select direction of the SRR image based on rotational acquisition geometry but not in the SRR image based on orthogonal acquisition geometry. This is better illustrated in the intensity line plot presented in Figure 5(l). Similar results were observed for low resolution data sets collected with a voxel AR of $1:1:10$ (Figure 6).

3.2. Biological Phantom. Increased resolution of biological structures in the *ex vivo* embryo was observed in the SRR images over a single LR image stack using straight linear interpolation (Figure 7). This was true for the SRR images based on LR image stacks acquired at both 0.19 mm (AR = 1:1:4) and 0.26 mm (AR = 1:1:6) slice thicknesses. Small structures (1-2 mm in width), such as those highlighted in the sinuses and the vertebrae, were not as clearly delineated in the SRR images as those observed in the isotropically acquired 3D image (Figure 7(e)).

The SRR image based on rotational geometry appeared more smooth than those based on the shifted and orthogonal geometries. This smoothing effect increased when the slice thickness of the LR images was increased from 0.19 (AR of 1:1:4) to 0.26 mm (AR of 1:1:6). Streaking artifacts were observed in uniform regions of the SRR images based on shifted (Figure 7(b)) and orthogonal (Figure 7(d)) geometries but were not as apparent in the SRR image based on rotational geometry (Figure 7(c)). These streaking artifacts were observed in the direction of linear interpolation used for upsampling in the LR direction.

The SRR images based on orthogonal acquisition for different voxel ARs are shown in Figure 8. The SRR images exhibited increased streaking artifacts with increasing slice thickness. Once the slice thickness was increased beyond a voxel AR of 1:1:6, we observed structures from adjacent slices that were not located in their proper through-plane location (Figure 8(d)). This artifact was not consistently observed with increasing slice thickness, as can be seen in Figure 8(e), suggesting the artifact is dependent upon where those structures are positioned in the original LR sampling.

SNR, CNR, mean edge width, and acquisition time for the SRR images and the isotropically acquired image of the *ex vivo* embryo are listed in Table 1. SNR and CNR increased for SRR images with increasing voxel AR. The SNR and the CNR for the SRR images were greater for the SRR images based on the orthogonal geometry followed by SRR images based on the rotated and shifted geometries. Mean edge width was similar for SRR images with voxel ARs of 1:1:4 and 1:1:6, but an increase was observed for the SR images based on orthogonal geometry at the increased voxel ARs of 1:1:8 and 1:1:10.

3.3. In Vivo Mouse. A 3D volume rendering of the SRR image of the live mouse is presented in Figure 9. Biological structures, such as the wall of the stomach, kidneys, and liver vasculature are clearly observed in all three image planes of the SRR image. A 3D volume rendering based on the sagitally acquired LR image with linear interpolation illustrates the loss of image quality in planes other than the primary HR acquisition plane. The streaking artifacts normally observed in the 2D slice view of the SRR images obtained from orthogonal acquisition are not observed in the volume rendered images. The total time to acquire all three LR image stacks used for the *in vivo* SRR was 45 minutes due to the respiratory and cardiac gating. A full 3D isotropic scan of this mouse would have taken more than 4 hrs with gating and would not be possible for live animal applications.

TABLE 1: Quantitative measures of image quality calculated from images of biological phantom.

AR	Int[b]	Shifted	Rotated	Orthogonal
SNR				
1:1:1[a]	26.8			
1:1:4	20.0	21.6	23.3	25.4
1:1:6	22.2	25.0	27.1	28.4
1:1:8				35.2
1:1:10				41.5
CNR				
1:1:1[a]	5.6			
1:1:4	5.1	5.3	6.0	6.9
1:1:6	5.8	6.8	7.2	8.0
1:1:8				7.9
1:1:10				7.9
Mean edge width (in HR pixels)				
1:1:1[a]	2.4			
1:1:4	5.9	4.2	3.7	3.2
1:1:6	6.1	4.1	3.8	3.5
1:1:8				3.9
1:1:10				4.4
Acquisition time (mins)				
1:1:1[a]	18.5			
1:1:4	3	12	18	9
1:1:6	3	18	18	9
1:1:8				9
1:1:10				9

[a]Isotropically acquired 3D image.
[b]Refers to linear interpolation from one LR image stack.

4. Discussion

The results from this study illustrate that SRR using multiple LR views improves image content and spatial resolution in the slice-select direction of 2D multislice acquisitions. Increased SNR and CNR were observed in the SRR images from the orthogonal acquisition compared to those reconstructed using shifted and rotational geometries. SRR images based on rotational acquisition geometry exhibited a smoothing of the edges in both the resolution and biological phantom. This was observed visually and in the mean edge width calculated from the SRR images. However, streaking artifacts were observed in the SRR images based on shifted and orthogonal geometries that became more pronounced at the higher ARs of 1:1:8 and 1:1:10. These streaking artifacts appear to be due to the linear interpolation used for upsampling the LR images and updated differences in LR and predicted HR images. The use of higher order or standard sigmoid-shaped interpolation kernels did not improve this streaking artifact.

Streaking artifacts may not be as apparent in the SRR images based on rotational geometry because the linear interpolation is occurring at oblique angles to the view plane or they may be averaged "out" due to the number of rotational angles used for the SRR. Streaking artifacts were only observed in 2D slice views of the SRR images and not in

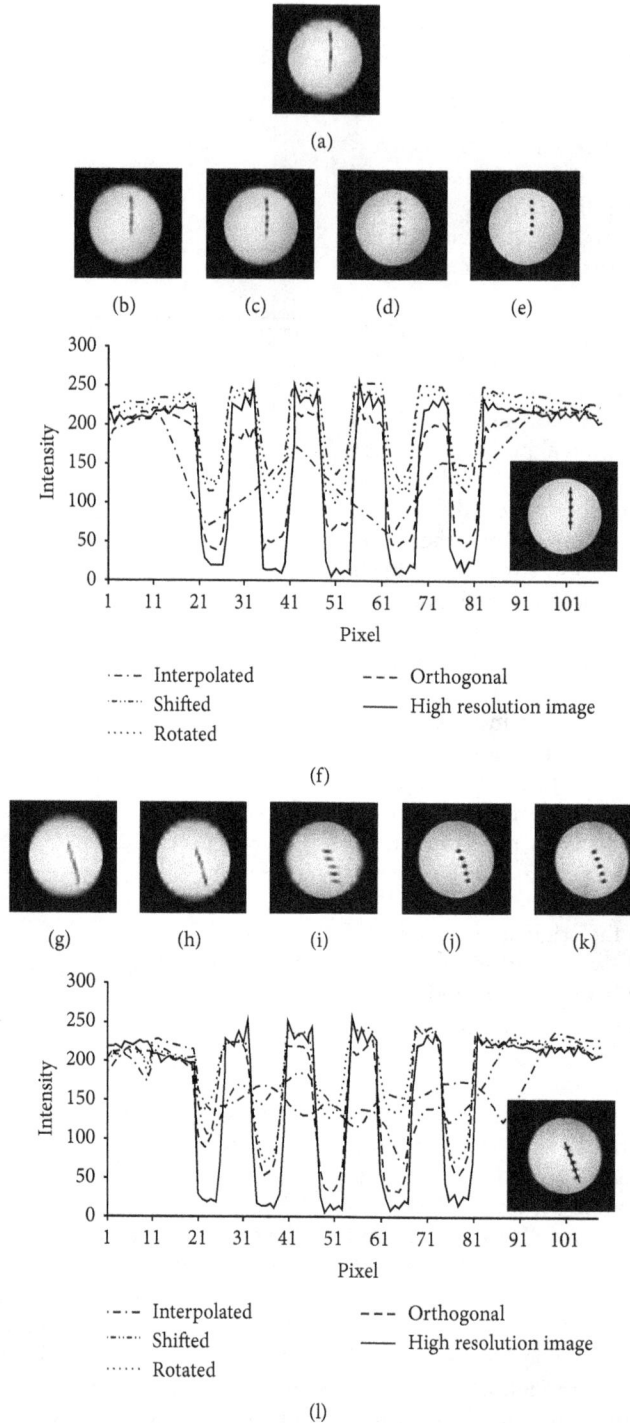

FIGURE 6: 2D slice images (image plane represented is orthogonal to the long axis of the tube which is placed along Y-axis in Figure 2(a)) of resolution phantom where the long axis of the tubes is orthogonal to the acquisition plane and LR image stacks were collected with a voxel AR of $1:1:10$: (a) interpolated, (b) shifted, (c) rotational, (d) orthogonal, (e) inplane, and (f) line plot, and where the long axis of the tubes is oblique to the acquisition plane: (g) interpolated, (h) shifted, (i) rotational, (j) orthogonal, (k) inplane, and (l) line plot.

the volume rendered images. This suggests that the ray tracing used for creating the volume rendered image is also averaging "out" the appearance of the streak artifacts.

The main advantage of using orthogonal acquisition for SRR over the other proposed acquisition geometries is that it requires the minimum number of views and thus the minimum amount of acquisition time. Additionally, orthogonal or nearly orthogonal acquisitions are typically acquired in most clinical and small animal imaging applications. SRR based on orthogonal views may result in better 3D volumes than

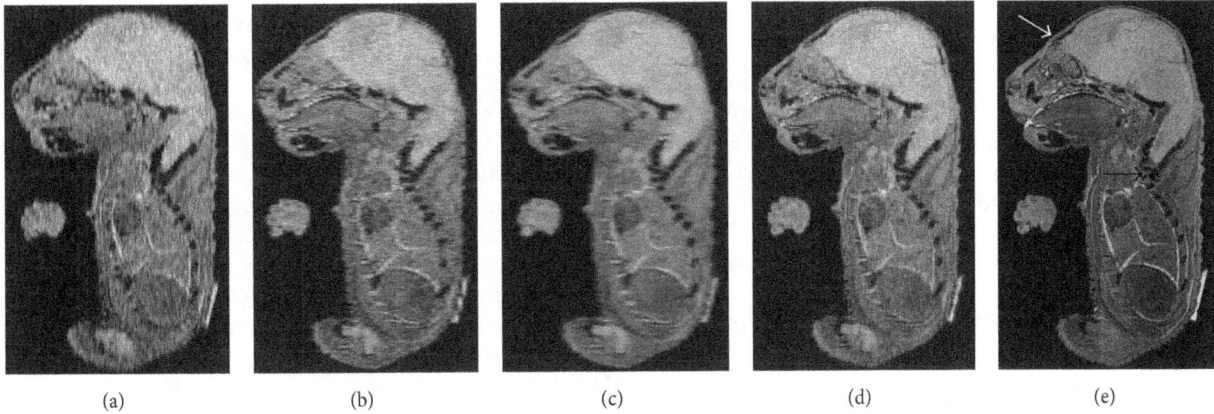

(a)   (b)   (c)   (d)   (e)

FIGURE 7: 2D sagittal view of SRR images of the *ex vivo* embryo based on different acquisition geometries: (a) interpolated, (b) shifted, (c) rotational, (d) orthogonal, and (e) isotropic. White arrow indicates structures in the nasal cavity not clearly observed in the corresponding SRR images.

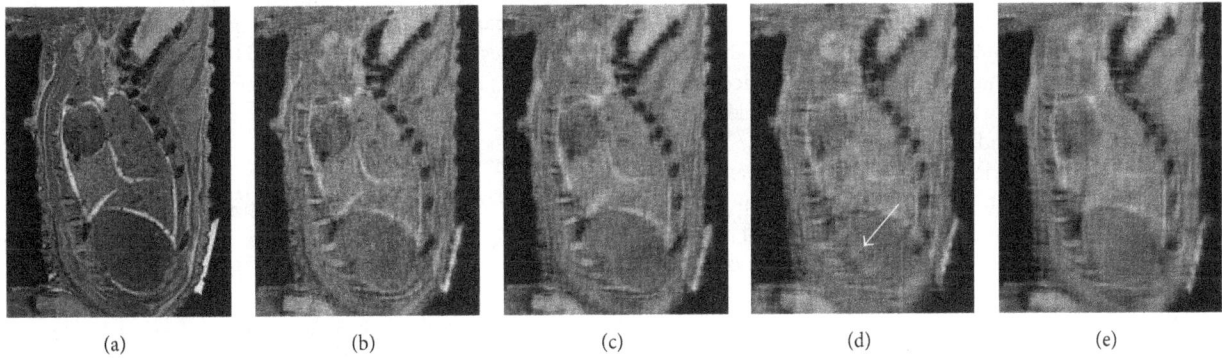

(a)   (b)   (c)   (d)   (e)

FIGURE 8: 2D sagittal view of the *ex vivo* embryo for (a) 3D isotropic acquisition and SRR images based on LR image stacks with AR equal to (b) $1:4$, (c) $1:6$, (d) $1:8$, and (e) $1:10$. White arrow highlights rib structures that are present in the SRR image but not present in the isotropic 3D image.

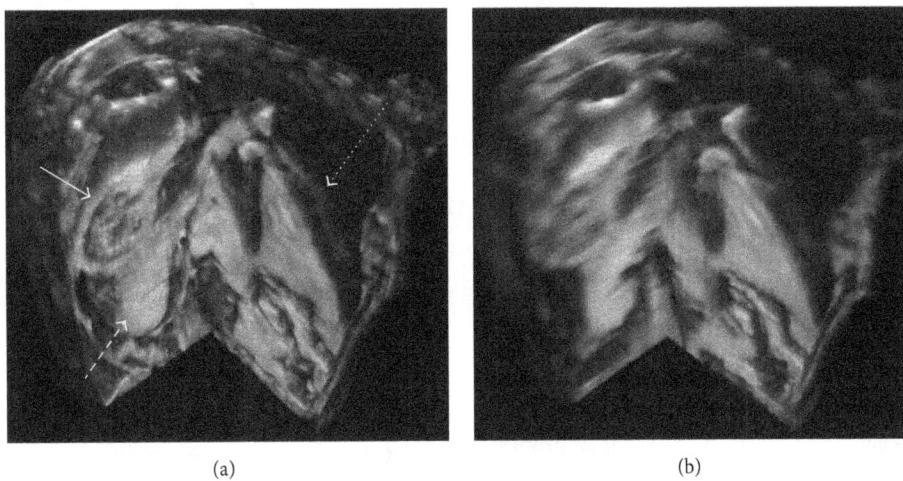

(a)   (b)

FIGURE 9: Cutaway section from 3D volume rendering of the *in vivo* mouse abdomen based on orthogonal SRR (a) with AR equal to $1:1:10$ and single interpolated view (b). The solid arrow points to the wall of the stomach, dashed arrow to the kidney, and dotted arrow to the liver vasculature. Biological structures can be observed clearly in any oblique cutting plane of the SRR image as opposed to single 2D multislice image with linear interpolation.

those based on the other two geometries because the high resolution volume space is more uniformly sampled in all three directions.

Theoretically, SRR images based on three views is an underdetermined problem when the slice thickness is three times greater than the inplane voxel size (AR = 1:1:3). Practically, the image quality of SRR images based on the orthogonal geometry and limited number of views was not significantly affected until the slice thickness of the LR image stacks was greater than six times the inplane voxel size (AR = 1:1:6). This was also observed in orthogonal super resolution reconstructions of a digital brain phantom by Gholipour et al. [9].

Whole body mouse phenotyping is typically performed in *ex vivo* specimens [1]. However, phenotyping in live animals has significant advantages in that you can observe structures in their native environment and monitor changes in structure and function over time. The main factors that affect the acquisition of HR images in live mice are the large field-of-view required for the whole body and the gated acquisitions required for respiratory and cardiac motion. We have successfully demonstrated that SRR can be implemented in a live animal model that requires respiratory- and ECG-gating to account for motion. A full 3D isotropic acquisition of the mouse used in this study would have taken more than 4 hrs with gating and would not be possible in a live animal imaging setting. This SRR acquisition was limited to an AR of 1:1:10 which is common for 2D multislice *in vivo* imaging applications. Visual comparison of different phenotypes using volume rendering would be possible at this resolution however image postprocessing such as object segmentation and quantitative analysis may suffer from the reconstruction artifacts observed in SRR images obtained at higher ARs.

SRR has been shown to be useful in clinical applications where images are corrupted by motion such as fetal brain imaging *in-utero* [10–12] and imaging of the tongue [13]. These approaches use registration to align the data to an anatomical model. Gholipour et al. [10] developed a model based super resolution reconstruction framework based on arbitrarily oriented slices in 3D acquisition space. This algorithm was applied to volume reconstructions from fetal brain MR images where interslice motion is prevalent. Rigid body registration was used to correct interslice motion using a slice-to-volume registration approach. Although this approach has shown to be effective using 2D acquisitions from arbitrary orientations, they have also suggested using multiple orthogonal or overlapped slice acquisitions for high resolution reconstructions. Woo et al. [13] used an orthogonal SRR approach to obtain high resolution 3D images of the tongue. Super resolution offered a viable alternative to obtain 3D volumes where acquisition time is limited by the involuntary motion of the tongue.

SRR has also recently been implemented for improving spatial resolution in DW imaging of the human brain using single-shot EPI acquisition protocols [14]. Spatial resolution in DW imaging is inherently low relative to the structures of interest and isotropic acquisition at high spatial resolution is virtually impossible due to the long scan times required for data acquisition. Although improvements to hardware and acquisition protocols have been implemented to address this problem, it still remains a challenge to obtain high resolution isotropic DW images.

In this work IBP was used for reconstructing the SRR images. More recently, regularized least square methods that incorporate prior knowledge as a regularization term have been proposed [15] for SRR implementation. These different optimization algorithms, such as LASR and Tikhonov regularization (TIK), have shown improved resolution over IBP optimization when the number of LR stacks used for reconstruction is greater than three (i.e., TIK) [8]. However, SNR was observed to be greater for IBP when a larger number of LR stacks was used for reconstruction. The results of Plenge's study suggest that different optimization schemes may perform better than others and may be dependent upon the application and the number of LR stacks used for reconstruction. Therefore, future work will focus on implementing these optimization schemes and testing them in our phenotyping models as well as developing techniques for reducing the streaking artifacts observed in the SRR images based on orthogonal acquisition geometry. These techniques should also help to reduce misregistration of structures observed in SRR images from higher ARs.

5. Conclusion

We have shown that the SRR images based on orthogonal acquisition geometry provide a better tradeoff between resolution, acquisition time, SNR, and CNR than those based on shifted and rotational acquisition geometries. This was observed for LR images with voxel ARs less than 1:1:6. However, for the orthogonal acquisition geometry, we observed when slice thickness was increased beyond a voxel AR of 1:1:6, artifacts resulted in the SRR image. As these artifacts were not consistently present in the same location with increasing voxel AR, we concluded that the artifact is dependent upon the sampling and where a specific slice occurs in the object being sampled. Finally, we demonstrated that SRR is applicable for *in vivo* gated acquisitions. This observation along with the possibility of applying the SRR algorithm with a higher voxel AR has the potential to make SRR a practical alternative for the acquisition of 3D HR isotropic images in small animal phenotyping applications.

Acknowledgments

The project described was supported in part by the National Center for Research Resources UL1RR025755 and the National Institutes of Health P30 CA16058.

References

[1] X. J. Chen and B. J. Nieman, "Mouse phenotyping with MRI," in *In Vivo NMR Imaging*, L. Schroder and C. Faber, Eds., pp. 595–631, Humana Press, 2011.

[2] J. F. Glockner, H. H. Hu, D. W. Stanley, L. Angelos, and K. King, "Parallel MR imaging: a user's guide," *Radiographics*, vol. 25, no. 5, pp. 1279–1297, 2005.

[3] S. Ljunggren, "A simple graphical representation of fourier-based imaging methods," *Journal of Magnetic Resonance*, vol. 54, no. 2, pp. 338–343, 1983.

[4] H. Greenspan, G. Oz, N. Kiryati, and S. Peled, "MRI inter-slice reconstruction using super-resolution," *Magnetic Resonance Imaging*, vol. 20, no. 5, pp. 437–446, 2002.

[5] M. Irani and S. Peleg, "Motion analysis for image enhancement: resolution, occlusion, and transparency," *Journal of Visual Communication and Image Representation*, vol. 4, no. 4, pp. 324–335, 1993.

[6] R. Z. Shilling, T. Q. Robbie, T. Bailloeul, K. Mewes, R. M. Mersereau, and M. E. Brummer, "A super-resolution framework for 3-D high-resolution and high-contrast imaging using 2-D multislice MRI," *IEEE Transactions on Medical Imaging*, vol. 28, no. 5, pp. 633–644, 2009.

[7] A. Souza and R. Senn, "Model-based super-resolution for MRI," in *Proceedings of the 30th Annual International Conference of the IEEE Engineering in Medicine and Biology Society (EMBS '08)*, pp. 430–434, August 2008.

[8] E. Plenge, D. H. J. Poot, M. Bernsen et al., "Super-resolution methods in MRI: can they improve the trade-off between resolution, signal-to-noise ratio, and acquisition time?" *Magnetic Resonance in Medicine*, vol. 68, no. 6, pp. 1983–1993, 2012.

[9] A. Gholipour, J. A. Estroff, M. Sahin, S. P. Prabhu, and S. K. Warfield, "Maximum a posteriori estimation of isotropic high-resolution volumetric MRI from orthogonal thick-slice scans," *Medical Image Computing and Computer-Assisted Intervention*, vol. 13, part 2, pp. 109–116, 2010.

[10] A. Gholipour, J. A. Estroff, and S. K. Warfield, "Robust super-resolution volume reconstruction from slice acquisitions: application to fetal brain MRI," *IEEE Transactions on Medical Imaging*, vol. 29, no. 10, pp. 1739–1758, 2010.

[11] F. Rousseau, K. Kim, C. Studholme, M. Koob, and J. L. Dietemann, "On super-resolution for fetal brain MRI," *Medical Image Computing and Computer-Assisted Intervention*, vol. 13, part 2, pp. 355–362, 2010.

[12] M. Kuklisova-Murgasova, G. Quaghebeur, M. A. Rutherford, J. V. Hajnal, and J. A. Schnabel, "Reconstruction of fetal brain MRI with intensity matching and complete outlier removal," *Medical Image Analysis*, vol. 16, no. 8, pp. 1550–1564, 2012.

[13] J. Woo, E. Z. Murano, M. Stone, and J. L. Prince, "Reconstruction of high-resolution tongue volumes from MRI," *IEEE Transactions on Biomedical Engineering*, vol. 59, no. 12, pp. 3511–3524, 2012.

[14] B. Scherrer, A. Gholipour, and S. Warfield, "Super-resolution reconstruction to increase the spatial resolution of diffusion weighted images from orthogonal anisotropic acquisitions," *Medical Image Analysis*, vol. 16, no. 7, pp. 1465–1476, 2012.

[15] D. H. J. Poot, V. Van Meir, and J. Sijbers, "General and efficient Super-resolution method for multi-slice MRI," in *Proceedings of the 13th International Conference on Medical Image Computing and Computer-Assisted Intervention—Part I*, pp. 615–622, Springer, 2010.

11

Robust Vessel Segmentation in Fundus Images

A. Budai,[1,2,3] **R. Bock,**[1,3] **A. Maier,**[1,3] **J. Hornegger,**[1,3] **and G. Michelson**[3,4,5]

[1] *Pattern Recognition Lab, Friedrich-Alexander University, Erlangen-Nuremberg, 91058 Erlangen, Germany*
[2] *International Max Planck Research School for Optics and Imaging (IMPRS), 91058 Erlangen, Germany*
[3] *Erlangen Graduate School in Advanced Optical Technologies (SAOT), 91052 Erlangen, Germany*
[4] *Department of Ophthalmology, Friedrich-Alexander University, Erlangen-Nuremberg, 91058 Erlangen, Germany*
[5] *Interdisciplinary Center of Ophthalmic Preventive Medicine and Imaging (IZPI), 91054 Erlangen, Germany*

Correspondence should be addressed to A. Budai; attila.budai@informatik.uni-erlangen.de

Academic Editor: Yue Wang

One of the most common modalities to examine the human eye is the eye-fundus photograph. The evaluation of fundus photographs is carried out by medical experts during time-consuming visual inspection. Our aim is to accelerate this process using computer aided diagnosis. As a first step, it is necessary to segment structures in the images for tissue differentiation. As the eye is the only organ, where the vasculature can be imaged in an in vivo and noninterventional way without using expensive scanners, the vessel tree is one of the most interesting and important structures to analyze. The quality and resolution of fundus images are rapidly increasing. Thus, segmentation methods need to be adapted to the new challenges of high resolutions. In this paper, we present a method to reduce calculation time, achieve high accuracy, and increase sensitivity compared to the original *Frangi* method. This method contains approaches to avoid potential problems like specular reflexes of thick vessels. The proposed method is evaluated using the *STARE* and *DRIVE* databases and we propose a new high resolution fundus database to compare it to the state-of-the-art algorithms. The results show an average accuracy above 94% and low computational needs. This outperforms state-of-the-art methods.

1. Introduction

In ophthalmology the most common way to examine the human eye is to take an eye-fundus photograph and to analyse it. During this kind of eye examinations a medical expert acquires a photo of the eye-background through the pupil with a fundus camera. The analysis of these images is commonly done by visual inspection. This process can require hours in front of a computer screen, in particular in case of medical screening. An example fundus image is shown in Figure 1.

Our goal is to speed up the diagnosis by processing the images using computer algorithms to find and highlight the most important details. In addition we aim to automatically identify abnormalities and diseases with minimal human interaction. Due to the rapidly increasing spatial resolution of fundus images, the common image processing methods which were developed and tested using low resolution images have shown drawbacks in clinical use. For this purpose, a new generation of methods needs to be developed. These methods need to be able to operate on high resolution images with low computational complexity. In this paper, we would like to introduce a novel vessel segmentation method with low computational needs and a public available high resolution fundus database with manually generated gold standards for evaluation of retinal structure segmentation methods. The proposed algorithms include modifications to the method proposed by Frangi et al. [1] to decrease the running time and to segment specular reflexes of thick vessels, which are not visible in lower resolution fundus images.

The structure of the paper is as follows. We describe the proposed methods in detail in Section 3. In Section 4, we present the evaluation methods and databases, including our proposed high resolution fundus database, while Section 5 presents the quantitative results. In Sections 6 and 7, the computational complexity and robustness of the proposed algorithm are analyzed. This is followed by a Discussion in Section 8 and the Conclusions in Section 9.

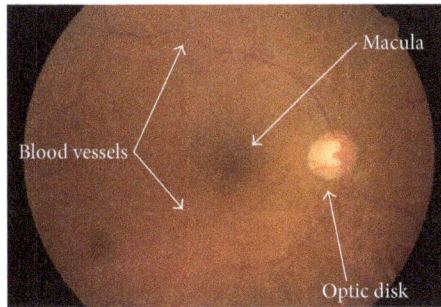

FIGURE 1: An example of eye-fundus image: the macula is shown in the middle, the optic disk is to the right, and the blood vessels are entering and leaving the eye through the optic disk.

2. Related Work

Retinal vessel segmentation is a challenging task and has been in the focus of researches all over the world for years. During this time many different algorithms were published [2]. The segmentation algorithms can be classified into two main groups: in unsupervised and supervised methods. Unsupervised methods classify vessels using heuristics, while supervised methods learn a criteria system automatically using prelabeled data as gold standard. We focus on heuristic methods, as supervised methods need a large training set for each camera setup. Heuristic methods instead require a set of parameters, which need to be adapted to the camera setup. Thus, they are much more independent from the test dataset during their development. A more detailed review of the segmentation and other retinal image processing algorithms can be found in the articles published by Kirbas and Quek [2] and Patton et al. [3].

Early, but one of the most common approaches for fundus images are the matched-filter approaches. One of the first methods was presented by Chaudhuri et al. [4]. It fits predefined vessel profiles with different sizes and orientations to the image to enhance vessels. Similar methods and improvements were published later on by different authors [5–8]. Early implementations of these methods were using a simple thresholding step to obtain a vessel segmentation. Sometimes these methods were combined with other approaches [9–12]. For example, Zhang et al. [12] combined matched filters with a method based on the Hessian matrix [1]. The matched filters provide high quality results, but the main disadvantage of these methods is their requirement for vessel profiles and comparisons of large regions for each pixel in the image, resulting in long computational time. The quality of the segmentation results heavily depends on the quality and size of the used vessel profile database. This can be specific towards ethnicity, camera setup, or even eye or vascular diseases, which reduces its applicability.

Some of the algorithms are specialized to segment only one or more objects, which are marked by a user or in a preprocessing step. These methods are usually not analyzing the whole image but the neighborhood of the already segmented regions. Region growing [13, 14] and tracking algorithms [15–18] are good examples for such kind of

segmentation methods. The region-growing approaches are trying to increase the segmented area with nearby pixels based on similarities and other criteria. These methods are one of the fastest approaches, while they may have problems at specific regions of the image, where the vessels have lower contrast compared to the nearby tissues, for example, vessel endings or thin vessels. In this case the region growing can segment large unwanted areas. Vessel tracking algorithms are more robust in those situations. They try to find a vessel-like structure in the already segmented region and track the given vessels. These algorithms can recognize vessel endings much easier, but they may have difficulties at bifurcations and vessel crossings, where the local structures do not look like usual vessels anymore. Hunter et al. [17] published a postprocessing step to solve some of these situations.

Other common segmentation approaches are model-based methods. The most known and commonly used ones are active contour-based methods, level-sets, and the so-called snakes [19]. The early snake-based algorithms start with an initial rough contour of the object, which is iteratively refined driven by multiple forces. In an optimal case, the forces reach their equilibrium exactly on the object boundaries. These methods are sensitive to their parameterization, while they may have problems if they have to segment thick and thin vessels in the same time. Thus, the parameters have to be set and refined manually by the user. The snakes in this form are mostly used in MR [20] or X-ray angiographic images [21] to segment pathologies and organs. The snake-based retinal vessel segmentation methods usually apply a vessel tracking framework to find the edges or the centerline of the vessels and track them using snakes [17, 22, 23]. This way the snakes are used to track only a vessel edge and the algorithm has less problems with vessel endings and different vessel thicknesses. Thus, their parameters are easier to optimize, but they inherit the problems of tracking algorithms with bifurcations and crossings.

Level-set methods provide a more robust solution than snakes. They are usually used in combination with other vessel enhancement techniques incorporating a smoothness constraint in their level set functions [24, 25].

For an automated segmentation method used in screening, the most important properties are robustness, efficiency, and the calculation time, because hundreds or thousands of images have to be processed each day. The state-of-the-art vessel segmentation methods [12, 22] usually have high computational needs and achieve an accuracy of 90% to 94% on eye-fundus images, with sensitivity of 60% to 70% and specificity above 99% on average [26]. This is due to the fact that approximately 85% of an image shows background structures. The high computational needs are due to multiple analysis of large regions to detect thick vessels. Thus, the computational needs of an algorithm is increasing exponentially with the diameter of the expected thickest vessel and the image resolution.

We present an algorithm based on the vessel enhancement method published by Frangi et al. [1] in combination with a multiresolution framework to decrease the computational needs and to increase the sensitivity by using a hysteresis thresholding. The method published by Frangi et al. [1] is a mathematical model-based approach and extracts vesselness features based on measurements of the eigenvalues of the Hessian matrix. The Hessian matrix contains the second-order derivatives in a local neighborhood. The method assumes that the vessels are tubular objects; thus, the ratio of the highest and lowest eigenvalue should be high, while this ratio is close to one in regions of constant values. The method was developed for CT angiography images, but it is applied in a wide variety of vessel segmentation algorithms and detection of tubular objects in different modalities [1, 27]. One of the disadvantages is the computational requirement. As Frangi et al. [1] proposed, the method calculates the Hessian matrix and the given measures for increasing neighborhood sizes, until the neighborhood is bigger than the expected thickest vessel. Given high resolution images, this can easily increase to 20 to 30 iterations per pixel.

3. Methods

All methods that were used to analyze the images are described in this section. First, we introduce the method proposed by Frangi et al. [1], which provides the basis of this work. This is followed by the description of the proposed method: the preprocessing steps in Section 3.2.1 and the used resolution hierarchy in Section 3.2.2. After that the vessel enhancement method is described to highlight the main differences to the Frangi method. We have chosen the method published by Frangi et al. [1] as a base for our own work, because it features some attractive properties.

(i) High accuracy is expected based on preliminary research [1, 27]. For further information please see Section 5.1. In comparison, our implementation of this method achieved a high accuracy.

(ii) No user interaction is required, except for setting a few parameters.

(iii) It is able to segment nonconnected objects without complex initialization steps. This is necessary in case of some abnormalities and in case of young patients, where reflections may disconnect vessels.

3.1. Frangi's Algorithm. To understand the proposed method, the reader should know the method by Frangi et al. [1]. Thus, in this section, we will introduce the method as it was published by Frangi et al. [1] in 1998.

The Hessian matrix of an n dimensional continuous function f contains the second-order derivatives. As we are working on a 2-dimensional image, our Hessian matrix is given as

$$H(f) = \begin{pmatrix} \dfrac{\partial^2 f}{\partial x^2} & \dfrac{\partial^2 f}{\partial x \partial y} \\ \dfrac{\partial^2 f}{\partial y \partial x} & \dfrac{\partial^2 f}{\partial y^2} \end{pmatrix}. \tag{1}$$

The Hessian matrix $H_{0,s}$ is calculated at each pixel position x_0 and scale s. Frangi used s as the standard deviation (σ) of Gaussians to approximate the second-order derivatives. A vesselness feature $V_0(s)$ is calculated at pixel position x_0

from the eigenvalues $\lambda_1 < \lambda_2$ of the Hessian matrix $H_{0,s}$ using equations of "dissimilarity measure" R_B and "second order structuredness" S

$$R_B = \frac{\lambda_1}{\lambda_2},$$

$$S = \sqrt{\lambda_1^2 + \lambda_2^2},$$

$$V_0(s) = \begin{cases} 0, & \text{if } \lambda_2 > 0, \\ \exp\left(-\dfrac{R_B^2}{2\beta^2}\right)\left(1 - \exp\left(-\dfrac{S^2}{2c^2}\right)\right), \end{cases} \tag{2}$$

where β and c are constants which control the sensitivity of the filter. R_B accounts for the deviation from blob-like structures, but can not differentiate background noise from real vessels. Since the background pixels have a small magnitude of derivatives and, thus; small eigenvalues, S helps to distinguish between noise and background.

The authors suggest to repeat the same calculations for varying sigma values from one to the thickest expected vessel thickness with an increment of 1.0 to enhance vessels with different thicknesses. The results are combined by a weighted maximum projection. In our implementation we added a thresholding step after the combination and optimized the parameters to reach the highest accuracy.

3.2. Proposed Method. After the preprocessing steps, we apply the same equations as described by Frangi et al. [1] for each resolution level with the same predefined sigma value.

Hence, we do not increase the sigma value linearly and apply the filter multiple times on the image as it was proposed by Frangi et al. [1]. In our case the sigma is always set to a small constant, while we apply the same method on copies of the input image with reduced resolutions. Thus, the parameter s of the original method corresponds to the resolution of the image, instead of the standard deviation of a Gaussian.

The proposed algorithm of our method is illustrated in Figure 2. Each of the steps will be discussed in detail in the next sections.

3.2.1. Preprocessing. The input images are digital color fundus photographs like the one in Figure 1. During the analysis we restrict ourselves to the green channel. It has the highest contrast between the vessels and the background, while it is not underilluminated or oversaturated like the other two channels, see Figure 3 for an example. Histogram stretching [28] and bilateral filtering [29] are applied to the green channel. The histogram stretching increases the contrast to make it easier for the algorithm to detect small changes and distinguish different tissues. The bilateral filtering [30] is a special denoising algorithm, which smooths intensity changes, while preserving the boundaries of different regions or tissues. This step reduces false positive detections caused by the texture of the background. After these modifications of the data, we can apply our resolution hierarchy described in the next section.

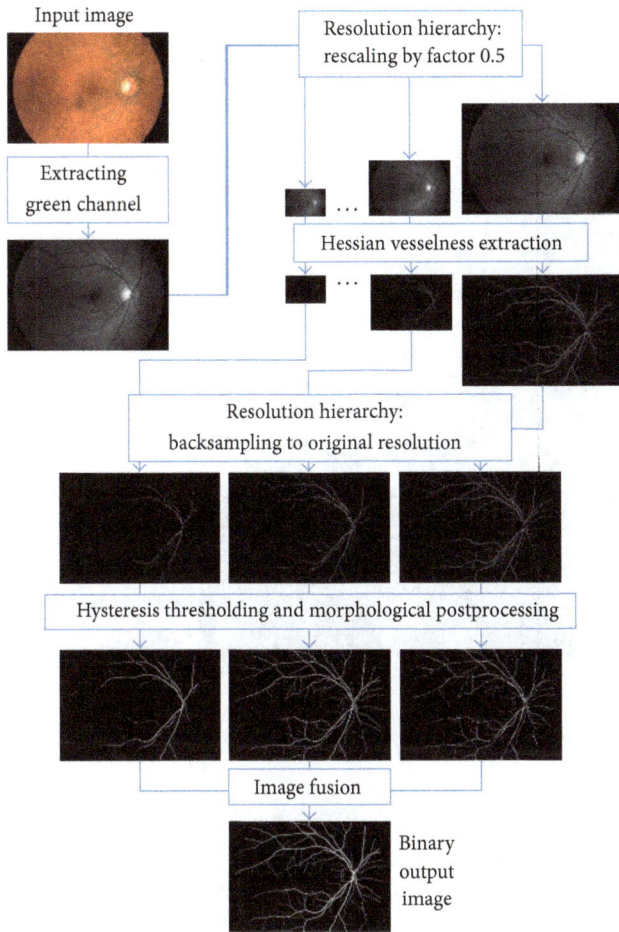

FIGURE 2: Pipeline of the proposed segmentation algorithm.

shows finer details, but the thickest vessels are not enhanced correctly. Figure 5(b) had a much lower resolution. Thus, the fine details disappeared, but the extraction of thick vessels were more accurate.

3.2.3. Specular Reflex Correction. As mentioned before, the flash of the camera may cause a bright specular reflex in the middle of thick vessels. Because of these reflections, the Hessian-based filter will have a much lower response. In our algorithm we developed a filter to be used on the highest level of our resolution pyramid to reduce the effect of these reflections. In this level only thick vessels are detected. We consider a 3×3 neighborhood for each pixel. If the center pixel has a lower value than two neighboring pixels in opposite directions in the vessel enhanced image, but higher value than the same two pixels in the fundus image of the same resolution level, then the center pixels are affected by specular reflex. In this case the two neighboring pixel's value will be interpolated to update the center pixel's value.

3.2.4. Hysteresis Threshold. After the vessel enhancement is completed in each resolution level and the results are resized to original resolution, all of them are binarized by a thresholding algorithm proposed by Canny [31]. The method performs better than a single thresholding in cases where the intensity of the objects is at some places high, but in certain positions the contrast between object and background falls under noise level. In our case this object is the vessel tree, where thin vessels and boundary pixel intensities can have extreme low intensity values. This method uses two thresholding values instead of one to binarize a gray-scale image. Both threshold values have different roles in the thresholding process.

(1) The first threshold is used to determine pixels with high intensities. It is required that this threshold is chosen in such a way that no background pixel can reach that value. Thus, we can label all the pixels above the threshold as "vessel pixels."

(2) We label all pixels below the second threshold value as "background pixel" and all pixels in between the two thresholds are considered "potential vessel pixels." These potential vessel pixels are labeled as vessels only if they are connected to a pixel labeled "vessel pixel" through other potential vessel pixels.

The thresholding values are computed for each image that a given percent of the pixels is segmented as "vessel pixels." Thus, the binarization is more robust to noise and intensity changes between images. They have to be optimized for each different protocol and field of view, where the ratio of vessel and background pixels is different in the resulting image. The binarization is used on each image separately.

3.2.5. Postprocessing. The final segmented image is generated by applying a pixel-wise OR operator on the binarized images originated from the different resolution levels. This way if a vessel was detected in one of the images, then it will be visible in the combined binary image.

3.2.2. Resolution Hierarchy. In a resolution hierarchy copies of the input image with reduced resolutions are generated; see Figure 4. By doing so, we calculate the Hessian matrix always for a small neighborhood which decreases the computational needs. The reduction is done by a subsampling followed by a low pass filtering to lower high jumps in intensities. The highest resolution level of the resolution hierarchy contains the original image, and all additional levels contain the image with a halved width and height compared to the previous level. For low resolution images, where the vessel thickness is not more than 5 to 10 pixels, 2 to 3 levels are sufficient, while images with higher resolutions may require additional levels. Compared to more than 20 iterations for the Frangi method, this means a speedup of a factor of 10. The vessel enhancement of the Frangi algorithm is applied on each resolution level with a standard deviation $\sigma = 1.0$.

Sometimes the flash of the camera causes a shining centerline on thick vessels. An additional correction method was developed to remove these specular reflection artifacts in the reduced resolution levels. The resulting images of the vessel enhancement are resized again using bilinear interpolation to the same resolution as the input image. Figure 5 shows the result of this resizing on two different resolution copies of the same region. Figure 5(a) had a high resolution and the result

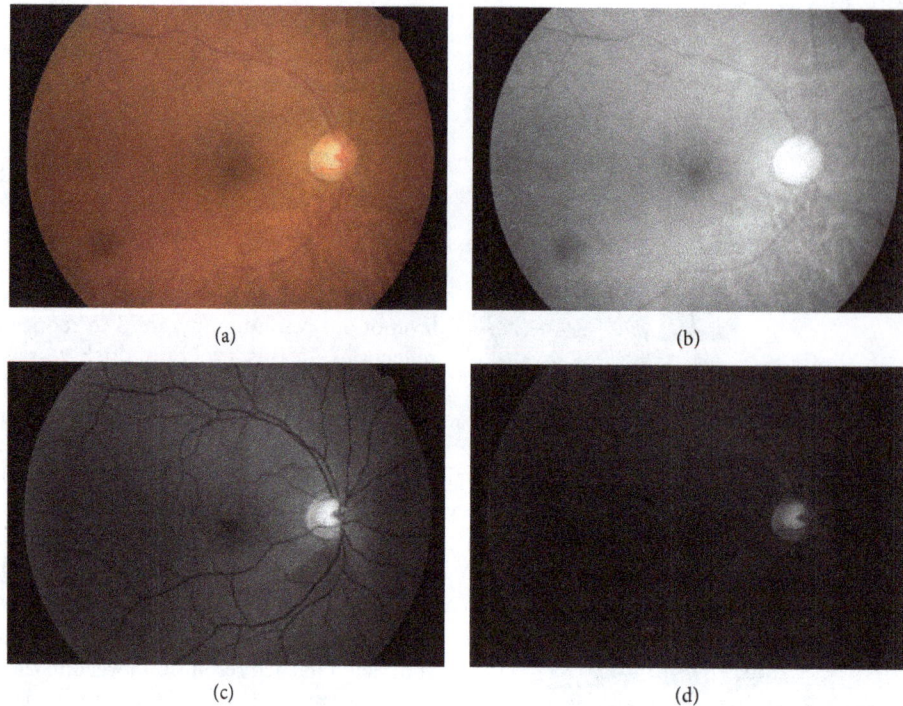

(a)

FIGURE 3: A fundus image (a) and its RGB decomposition showing the oversaturated red (b), the well-illuminated green (c), and the under-illuminated blue (d) channels.

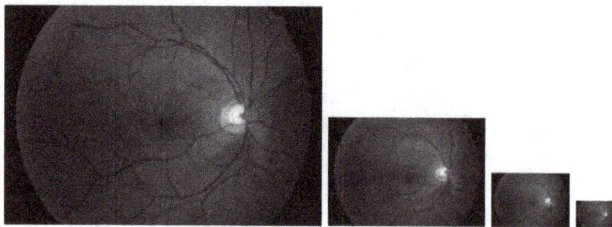

FIGURE 4: Example of a Gaussian resolution hierarchy using only the green channel of the input image and its three reduced resolution versions.

Afterwards a thinning function erodes the segmented region until it reaches the highest local gradient in the input image. This method avoids the slight oversegmentation in case that a thin vessel is detected in a higher level of the hierarchy.

As a last step a small kernel (3×3) morphological closing operator is used to smooth the boundaries and object size analysis algorithms are applied to fill small holes in the vessel tree and remove small undesired objects. Some example of input images and the calculated segmentations are presented in Figures 6 and 7.

4. Evaluation

We applied the original Frangi vesselness extraction and our proposed framework on the commonly used DRIVE [26] and STARE [32] databases and on our high resolution public database [33] to compare our framework to the state-of-the-art methods and to evaluate their effectivity. These databases contain manual segmentations of experts as gold standard. Based on these gold standards we calculated the sensitivity (Se), specificity (Sp), and accuracy (Acc) of each method. Both already existing databases contain an additional manual segmentation and the DRIVE database contains some measurements of multiple algorithms.

We compare the computation time of the proposed algorithm and an implemented Frangi vesselness algorithm as proposed by Frangi et al. [1]. The two public databases were used to evaluate the efficiency and for comparison to other state-of-the-art algorithms. These two databases suffer from containing only low resolution images, while the proposed method was developed for high resolution images. Thus, the benefit of the resolution hierarchy is only slightly noticeable. Since high resolution images are becoming more common in clinical use, we evaluated our methods on the high resolution $(3504 \times 2336$ pixels) images available [33], which were already used to evaluate other methods [6, 7]. The database contains 15 images of each healthy, diabetic retinopathy (DR), and glaucomatous eyes. The results of this evaluation are discussed in Section 5.2.

The technical details of the used image data are shown in Table 1. For each method, we applied the same parameter optimization process using a small subset of each database to assure that differences are not due to parameter settings. This algorithm sets the parameters to reach the highest possible accuracy without aiming at high sensitivity. Since the parameter is done using a small subset of the images, the results can be improved using a larger training set. Optimization based

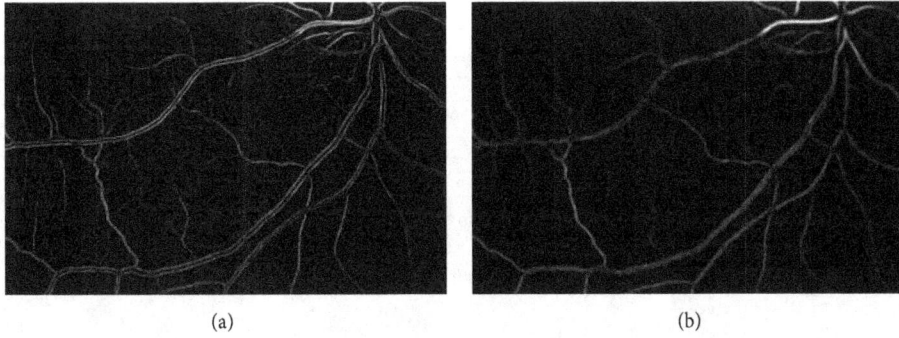

(a)   (b)

FIGURE 5: The resized vesselness images of two different resolution levels. In the highest resolution level (a) the enhanced image shows more details, while the result of a lower resolution level (b) shows a more accurate segmentation of thick vessels.

TABLE 1: Details of used databases.

Database	Images used	Resolution
DRIVE [26]	20	565×584
STARE [32]	20	700×605
High resolution fundus [33]	45	3504×2336

on a small subset may result in suboptimal settings for the whole dataset, but it shows the generalization capabilities of the method.

For the evaluation of computation times we always used the same common notebook equipped with a 2.3 GHz processor and 4 GB RAM and a single core implementation of the algorithms.

5. Results

5.1. Accuracy. The metrics calculated on the two public databases to analyze the effectivity of the algorithms are shown in Tables 2 and 3. During our development and in our comparisons we aimed at the highest possible accuracy. Therefore, we optimized the parameters of both—the proposed and the Frangi—methods. Thus, the parameters of the Frangi method and the proposed method are set to deliver the highest possible accuracy. This can result in a decreased sensitivity to gain specificity in order to increase the overall accuracy. This way the proposed method was able to reach the best accuracy using the DRIVE and high resolution fundus databases.

Both public databases contain a second manual segmentation made by a human observer, which was included in the comparison. We collected further results from published papers. For both databases the original method and the proposed method reached a high accuracy over 95% and 93%, respectively. As shown in Table 2, in case of the DRIVE database, this was enough to reach the highest accuracy. In case of the STARE database, as shown in Table 3, the sensitivity improved by 5% along with a slight increase in accuracy. Some examples of the segmentation results are shown in Figure 6.

The proposed algorithm and the original Frangi method were further tested on the three datasets of our own public

TABLE 2: Comparison of the results using the DRIVE [26] public database. The proposed methods achieved the best accuracy (Acc) compared to the state-of-the-art solutions.

Algorithm	Se	Sp	Acc
Proposed	0.644	**0.987**	**0.9572**
Frangi et al. [1]	0.660	0.985	0.9570
Marín et al. [34]	0.706	0.980	0.945
Human observer	0.776	0.972	0.947
Dizdaroglu et al. [24]	0.718	0.974	0.941
Soares et al. [35]	0.7283	0.9788	0.9466
Mendonça and Campilho [36]	**0.7344**	0.9764	0.9452
Staal et al. [37]	0.7194	0.9773	0.9442
Niemeijer et al. [38]	—	—	0.9416
Zana and Klein [39]	—	—	0.9377
Martinez-Perez et al. [40]	0.7246	0.9655	0.9344
Odstrčilík et al. [7]	0.7060	0.9693	0.9340
Espona et al. (subpixel accuracy) [41]	0.7313	0.9600	0.9325
Chaudhuri et al. [4]	0.6168	0.9741	0.9284
Al-Diri and Hunter [22]	—	—	0.9258
Espona et al. (pixel accuracy) [41]	0.6615	0.9575	0.9223
Jiang and Mojon [42]	—	—	0.9212
All background	—	—	0.8727

"—" indicates that this information was not available.

high resolution fundus database [33]. Figure 7 shows two examples of input images and segmentation results of this database. As these images have much higher resolutions, we use more resolution levels in the hierarchy and higher σ values in the original Frangi algorithm. This enables detection of vessels with a higher diameter, but also increases the computation times. Tables 4 and 5 show the sensitivity, specificity, and accuracy of these methods using the high resolution fundus dataset. Each datasets with manually segmented gold standard images is available online [33] for other researchers to test and compare their algorithms.

5.2. Performance. Tested on the two public databases, the proposed method has a reduced calculation time by 18% in case of the STARE database and 16% in case of the DRIVE database, as shown in Table 6. The computation

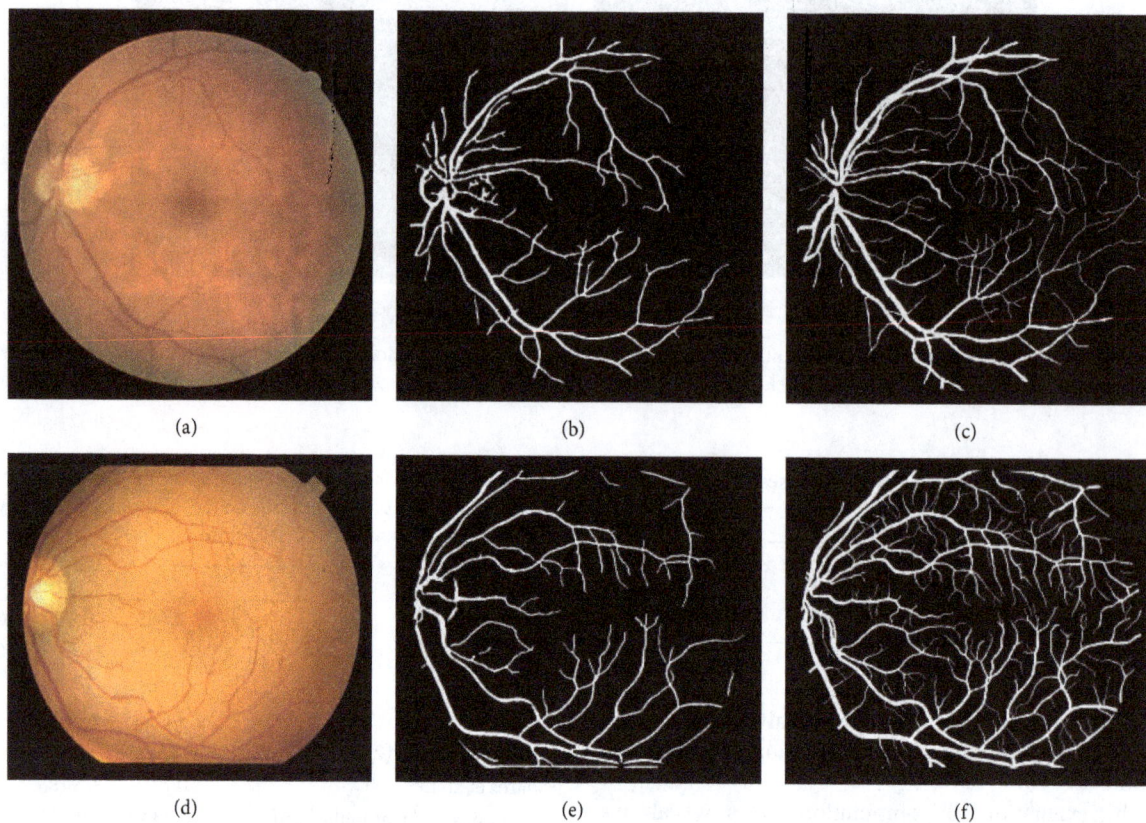

FIGURE 6: Example segmentation results on the DRIVE (upper row) and STARE (bottom row) public databases. From left to right: input fundus images, segmentation results, and gold standard images.

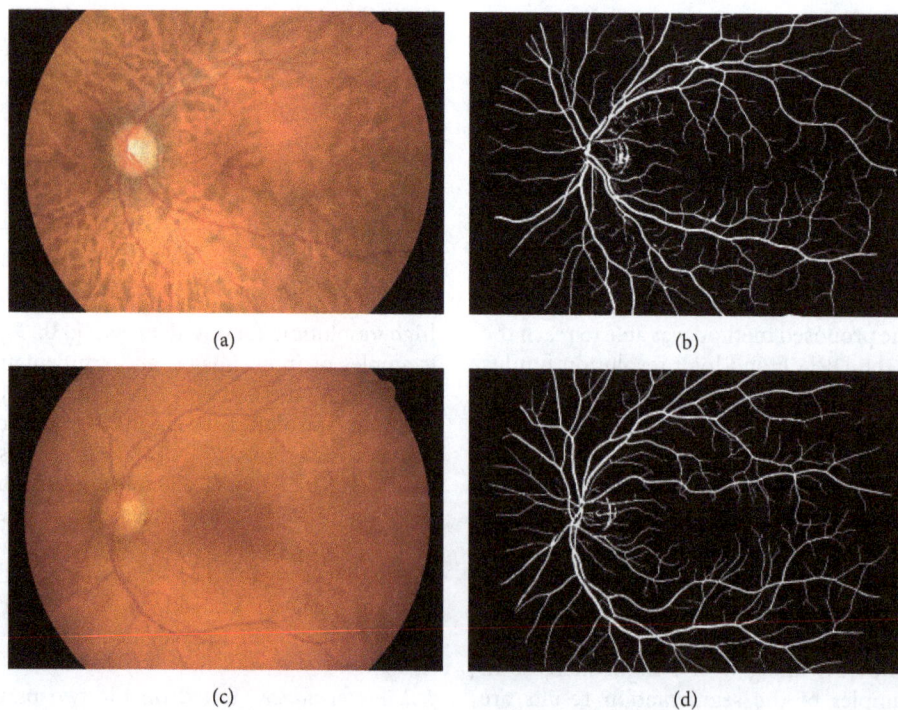

FIGURE 7: Example segmentation results on high resolution images with different illumination and background structures.

TABLE 3: Sensitivity (Se), specificity (Sp), and accuracy (Acc) of the methods measured on the STARE [32] database. The proposed modifications improved both the sensitivity and accuracy of the Frangi method.

Algorithm	Se	Sp	Acc
Proposed	0.58	0.982	0.9386
Frangi et al. [1]	0.529	**0.986**	0.9370
Marín et al. [34]	0.694	0.981	0.952
Staal et al. [37]	0.6970	0.9810	**0.9516**
Zhang et al. [12]	0.07177	0.9753	0.9484
Soares et al. [35]	0.7165	0.9748	0.9480
Mendonça and Campilho [36]	0.6996	0.9730	0.9440
Martinez-Perez et al. [40]	0.7506	0.9569	0.9410
Chaudhuri et al. [4]	0.6134	0.9755	0.9384
Human observer	0.8949	0.9390	0.9354
Odstrčilík et al. [7]	**0.7947**	0.9512	0.9341
Hoover et al. [9]	0.6751	0.9367	0.9267

TABLE 4: Overall sensitivity (Se), specificity (Sp), and accuracy (Acc) measured using our high resolution fundus database.

Algorithm	Se	Sp	Acc
Proposed	**0.669**	**0.985**	**0.961**
Frangi et al. [1]	0.622	0.982	0.954
Odstrčilík et al. [7]	0.774	0.966	0.949

TABLE 5: Sensitivity (Se), specificity (Sp), and accuracy (Acc) measured for the three datasets separately in our high resolution database.

Dataset	Algorithm	Se	Sp	Acc
Healthy	Proposed	0.662	**0.992**	**0.961**
Healthy	Frangi et al. [1]	0.621	0.989	0.955
Healthy	Odstrčilík et al. [7]	**0.786**	0.9750	0.953
Glaucomatous	Proposed	0.687	**0.986**	**0.965**
Glaucomatous	Frangi et al. [1]	0.654	0.984	0.961
Glaucomatous	Odstrčilík et al. [7]	**0.790**	0.964	0.949
Diabetic retinopathy	Proposed	0.658	**0.977**	**0.955**
Diabetic retinopathy	Frangi et al. [1]	0.590	0.972	0.946
Diabetic retinopathy	Odstrčilík et al. [7]	**0.746**	0.961	0.944

times were not available for most of the algorithms used for comparison in Section 5.1. Thus, these methods are excluded from the performance test. The resolution hierarchy made our proposed method faster on the low resolution images than the Frangi method. The speed improvement of the hierarchy is actually higher, but we used additional time for postprocessings and improvements, like filling the holes caused by central reflexes in the vessels and using a hysteresis thresholding in each resolution.

As the computation times of hysteresis threshold is rapidly increasing with the resolution, we tested the runtime using high resolution images to see if the gain using the resolution hierarchy is higher than the additional requirements of the thresholding. Table 7 shows the computation times for these images.

TABLE 6: Comparison of average runtime using two public databases. The effects of the proposed modifications on the calculation time in seconds as shown.

Algorithm	Runtime (in sec)		Accuracy	
	STARE	DRIVE	STARE	DRIVE
Frangi et al. [1]	1.62	1.27	0.9370	0.9570
Proposed	1.31	1.04	0.9386	0.9572
Espona et al. (subpixel accuracy)* [41]	—	31.7	—	0.9325
Mendonça and Campilho* [36]	—	150.0 [35]	0.9480	0.9466
Soares et al.* [35]	180.0	180.0	0.9480	0.9466
Staal et al.* [37]	—	900.0 [35]	0.9516	0.9442

Entries marked by "*" are results reported in the cited articles.

TABLE 7: Comparison of average runtime using high resolution (3504 × 2336) images.

Algorithm	Average runtime	Accuracy
Proposed method	26.693 ± 0.92 sec	0.961 ± 0.006
Original Frangi	39.288 ± 2.00 sec	0.954 ± 0.008
Odstrčilík et al. [7, 33]	18 minutes	0.949

The results show a calculation time difference of about 33.3%, which was less than 20% in case of low resolution images. This means that our proposed method performs the segmentation in higher resolution images faster in comparison to the original Frangi method.

6. Computational Complexity

To see the difference in computational complexity of both methods, we calculated the mathematical complexity of the Frangi method [1] and our proposed methods. As all segmentation methods need some pre- and postprocessing, we decided to calculate the mathematical complexity of the main vessel extraction only, plus our proposed direct modifications.

As a first step, we have to define the necessary parameters. Let n be the number of pixels in the input image, and define t as the highest expected vessel thickness which we would like to detect. With these two parameters, we can describe the complexity of the important components used in the algorithms:

(i) rescaling: $O(n)$ for each image;

(ii) calculating Hessian matrix: $O(t^2)$ for each pixel;

(iii) eigenvalue analysis: after calculating the Hessian matrix, it is independent of the parameters: $O(n)$ for each image;

(iv) postprocessing using mathematical morphology, and other operations: $O(n)$ for each image;

(v) maximum image calculation: $O(m \cdot n)$ where m is the number of images;

(vi) binarization by thresholding: $O(n)$ for each image.

In case of the original method, calculation of the Hessian matrix is done t times for each pixel, with increasing σ. After that all the images are summarized and thresholded. These methods result in a complexity of $O(t^3 \times n)$: $t \times n$ pixels, and $O(t^2)$ operations for each pixel, while the complexity of the other parts is neglectable.

The proposed method uses the rescaling. This results in a maximal pixel number of $1.5 \times n$ to work on instead of $t \times n$, and t is always set to one. Thus, the Hessian matrix calculation is done with a predefined $\sigma = 1.0$, which reduces the complexity to $O(n)$. After rescaling to the original resolution, postprocessing and binarization are done in linear complexity. This gives a computational complexity of $O(\log(t) * n)$: independently of the number of resolution levels, the maximal number of pixels is $1.5 \times n$, and σ is set to 1.0 which results in a computational complexity of $O(n)$ before fusing the binarized images. With $\log(t)$ number of rescaled images, after the fusion, the complexity is $O(\log(t) * n)$ with neglectable linear complexity of the postprocessing.

7. Robustness

To analyze the robustness and sensitivity of the method regarding changes in the parameters, we analyze it by further excluding some steps and changing the parameters.

As Table 8 shows, the algorithm is robust against changes in the parameters of pre- or postprocessing, except that not all of the processing steps are skipped. This increases the false positive values due to the appearance of small segmented noisy regions and also increases false negatives by not segmenting regions of vessels with specular reflexes.

The accuracy of the method improved surprisingly by increasing the σ to 2.0 for the vessel enhancement. Our analysis showed that the optimization using a small subset of images resulted in a suboptimal parameter set for the whole dataset. Changing the *sigma* value to 2.0 increased the sensitivity in multiple images, reaching an overall sensitivity over 0.7338 and accuracy over 0.9621.

8. Discussion

Our evaluation has shown that the proposed method not only has the highest accuracy using the high resolution images for which it was developed, but it has decent results using two lower resolution databases available online. This decrease is due to the slightly lower sensitivity caused by the lower image quality in the online databases. The proposed method has lower computational needs compared to the method proposed by Frangi et al. [1], as it was shown experimentally in Section 5.2 and mathematically proven in Section 6.

Furthermore, as shown in Section 7, the method is only slightly sensitive to the σ parameter of the vessel enhancement and the thresholding parameters. Changing σ can result in 5% change in sensitivity, while changing most of the other parameters resulted in a small variation in both sensitivity and specificity with an accuracy change under 0.1%.

Based on the results of Table 8, the pre- and postprocessing steps applied in the proposed method increased the

TABLE 8: Accuracy comparison of different settings using the high resolution fundus database.

Algorithm	Accuracy	Absolute change
Proposed method	0.9618 ± 0.0065	—
Without preprocessing	0.9558 ± 0.0064	0.62%
Thresholds decreased by 1%	0.9614 ± 0.0061	0.04%
Thresholds increased by 1%	0.9607 ± 0.0062	0.11%
Without postprocessing	0.9401 ± 0.0085	2.25%
Doubled morphology kernel size	0.9616 ± 0.0060	0.02%
$\sigma = 2.0$ for Hessian	$\mathbf{0.9621 \pm 0.0062}$	0.03%
$\sigma = 3.0$ for Hessian	$\mathbf{0.9621 \pm 0.0061}$	0.03%
$\sigma = 4.0$ for Hessian	0.9617 ± 0.0064	0.01%

overall accuracy of the segmentation by 1% to 2% by removing unwanted objects, filling some holes caused by specular reflexes, and smoothing the vessel edges.

9. Conclusion

In this paper we presented a multiresolution method for segmenting blood vessels in fundus photographs. The proposed method and the Frangi method were evaluated using multiple online available databases with diverging image resolution. The proposed algorithm shows in each case an increase both in sensitivity and accuracy to segment vessels compared to the Frangi method with a decreased computational complexity.

This gain in accuracy is mainly due to easier handling of central reflexes of thick vessels in lower resolution images, while the computational needs are significantly reduced by using the resolution hierarchy. This can be further improved by parallelization and implementation using a GPU.

With the proposed modifications the algorithm is more applicable in complex automatic systems, and the segmentation results can be used as a basis for other algorithms to analyze abnormalities of the human eye. Additionally we introduced a new high resolution fundus image database [33] to evaluate segmentation and localization methods, where our algorithm reached an accuracy of over 96% on average.

Acknowledgments

The authors gratefully acknowledge funding of the Erlangen Graduate School in Advanced Optical Technologies (SAOT) by the German National Science Foundation (DFG) in the framework of the excellence initiative. The authors gratefully acknowledge the aid and cooperation of the Department of Biomedical Engineering, FEEC, Brno University of Technology, Czech Republic.

References

[1] A. F. Frangi, W. J. Niessen, K. L. Vincken, and M. A. Viergever, *Multiscale Vessel Enhancement Filtering*, Springer, Heidelberg, Germany, 1998.

[2] C. Kirbas and F. Quek, "A review of vessel extraction techniques and algorithms," *ACM Computing Surveys*, vol. 36, no. 2, pp. 81–121, 2004.

[3] N. Patton, T. M. Aslam, T. MacGillivray et al., "Retinal image analysis: concepts, applications and potential," *Progress in Retinal and Eye Research*, vol. 25, no. 1, pp. 99–127, 2006.

[4] S. Chaudhuri, S. Chatterjee, N. Katz, M. Nelson, and M. Goldbaum, "Detection of blood vessels in retinal images using two-dimensional matched filters," *IEEE Transactions on Medical Imaging*, vol. 8, no. 3, pp. 263–269, 1989.

[5] M. Goldbaum, S. Moezzi, A. Taylor et al., "Automated diagnosis and image understanding with object extraction, object classification, and inferencing in retinal images," in *Proceedings of the IEEE International Conference on Image Processing (ICIP '96)*, pp. 695–698, September 1996.

[6] J. Odstrčilík, J. Jan, R. Kolar, and J. Gazarek, "Improvement of vessel segmentation by matched filtering in colour retinal images," in *Proceedings of the World Congress on Medical Physics and Biomedical Engineering (IFMBE '09)*, pp. 327–3330, 2009.

[7] J. Odstrčilík, R. Kolar, A. Budai et al., "Retinal vessel segmentation by improved matched filtering: evaluation on a new high-resolution fundus image database," *IET Image Processing*, vol. 7, no. 4, pp. 373–383, 2013.

[8] M. Sofka and C. V. Stewart, "Retinal vessel centerline extraction using multiscale matched filters, confidence and edge measures," *IEEE Transactions on Medical Imaging*, vol. 25, no. 12, pp. 1531–1546, 2006.

[9] A. Hoover, V. Kouznetsova, and M. Goldbaum, "Locating blood vessels in retinal images by piecewise threshold probing of a matched filter response," *IEEE Transactions on Medical Imaging*, vol. 19, no. 3, pp. 203–210, 2000.

[10] C.-H. Wu, G. Agam, and P. Stanchev, "A hybrid filtering approach to retinal vessel segmentation," in *Proceedings of the 4th IEEE International Symposium on Biomedical Imaging (ISBI '07)*, pp. 604–607, April 2007.

[11] G. B. Kande, P. V. Subbaiah, and T. S. Savithri, "Unsupervised fuzzy based vessel segmentation in pathological digital fundus images," *Journal of Medical Systems*, vol. 34, no. 5, pp. 849–858, 2010.

[12] B. Zhang, L. Zhang, L. Zhang, and F. Karray, "Retinal vessel extraction by matched filter with first-order derivative of Gaussian," *Computers in Biology and Medicine*, vol. 40, no. 4, pp. 438–445, 2010.

[13] R. Jain, R. Kasturi, and B. Schunk, *Machine Vision*, McGraw-Hill, New York, NY, USA, 1995.

[14] S. Eiho, H. Sekiguchi, N. Sugimoto, T. Hanakawa, and S. Urayama, "Branch-based region growing method for blood vessel segmentation," in *Proceedings of the International Congress for Photogrammetry and Remote Sensing*, 2004.

[15] M. J. Cree, D. Cornforth, and H. F. Jelinek, "Vessel segmentation and tracking using a two-dimensional model," in *Proceedings of the International Conference on Image and Vision Computing New Zealand (IVCNZ '05)*, pp. 345–350, Dunedin, New Zealand, 2005.

[16] F. K. H. Quek and C. Kirbas, "Vessel extraction in medical images by wave-propagation and traceback," *IEEE Transactions on Medical Imaging*, vol. 20, no. 2, pp. 117–131, 2001.

[17] A. Hunter, J. Lowell, and D. Steel, "Tram-line filtering for retinal vessel segmentation," in *Proceedings of the 3rd European Medical and Biological Engineering Conference*, 2005.

[18] O. Wink, W. J. Niessen, and M. A. Viergever, "Multiscale vessel tracking," *IEEE Transactions on Medical Imaging*, vol. 23, no. 1, pp. 130–133, 2004.

[19] M. Kass, A. Witkin, and D. Terzopoulos, "Snakes: active contour models," *International Journal of Computer Vision*, vol. 1, no. 4, pp. 321–331, 1988.

[20] D. Rueckert and P. Burger, "Contour fitting using stochastic and probabilistic relaxation for Cine MR Images," in *Computer Assisted Radiology*, pp. 137–142, Springer, Berlin, Germany, 1995.

[21] M. Hinz, K. D. Toennies, M. Grohmann, and R. Pohle, "Active double-contour for segmentation of vessels in digital subtraction angiography," in *Medical Imaging 2001 Image Processing*, Proceedings of SPIE, pp. 1554–1562, February 2001.

[22] B. Al-Diri and A. Hunter, "A ribbon of twins for extracting vessel boundaries," in *Proceedings of the 3rd European Medical and Biological Engineering Conference (EMBEC '05)*, 2005.

[23] R. Manniesing, M. A. Viergever, and W. J. Niessen, "Vessel axis tracking using topology constrained surface evolution," *IEEE Transactions on Medical Imaging*, vol. 26, no. 3, pp. 309–316, 2007.

[24] B. Dizdaroglu, E. Ataer-Cansizoglu, J. Kalpathy-Cramer, K. Keck, M. F. Chiang, and D. Erdogmus, "Level sets for retinal vasculature segmentation using seeds from ridges and edges from phase maps," in *Proceedings of the IEEE International Workshop on Machine Learning for Signal Processing*, IEEE, Santander, Spain, September 2012.

[25] J. Brieva, E. Gonzalez, F. Gonzalez, A. Bousse, and J. J. Bellanger, "A level set method for vessel segmentation in coronary angiography," in *Proceedings of the 27th IEEE Annual International Conference of the Engineering in Medicine and Biology Society (EMBS '05)*, pp. 6348–6351, IEEE, September 2005.

[26] J. Staal, M. D. Abramoff, M. Niemeijer, M. A. Viergever, and B. van Ginneken, DRIVE public online database, http://www.isi.uu.nl/Research/Databases/DRIVE/.

[27] L. Shi, B. Funt, and G. Hamarneh, "Quaternion color curvature," in *Proceedings of the 16th Color Imaging Conference: Color Science and Engineering Systems, Technologies, and Applications*, pp. 338–341, November 2008.

[28] M. Petrou and C. Petrou, *Image Processing: The Fundamentals*, John Wiley & Sons, Chichester, UK, 2nd edition, 2010.

[29] C. Tomasi and R. Manduchi, "Bilateral filtering for gray and color images," in *Proceedings of the 6th IEEE International Conference on Computer Vision (ICCV '98)*, pp. 839–846, January 1998.

[30] S. Paris, P. Kornprobst, J. Tumblin, and F. Durand, "Bilateral filtering: theory and applications," *Foundations and Trends in Computer Graphics and Vision*, vol. 4, no. 1, pp. 1–73, 2009.

[31] J. Canny, "A computational approach to edge detection," *IEEE Transactions on Pattern Analysis and Machine Intelligence*, vol. 8, no. 6, pp. 679–698, 1986.

[32] A. Hoover and M. Goldbaum, STARE public online database, http://www.ces.clemson.edu/~ahoover/stare/.

[33] A. Budai and J. Odstrčilík, High Resolution Fundus Image Database, September 2013.

[34] D. Marín, A. Aquino, M. E. Gegúndez-Arias, and J. M. Bravo, "A new supervised method for blood vessel segmentation in retinal images by using gray-level and moment invariants-based features," *IEEE Transactions on Medical Imaging*, vol. 30, no. 1, pp. 146–158, 2011.

[35] J. V. B. Soares, J. J. G. Leandro, R. M. Cesar Jr., H. F. Jelinek, and M. J. Cree, "Retinal vessel segmentation using the 2-D

Gabor wavelet and supervised classification," *IEEE Transactions on Medical Imaging*, vol. 25, no. 9, pp. 1214–1222, 2006.

[36] A. M. Mendonça and A. Campilho, "Segmentation of retinal blood vessels by combining the detection of centerlines and morphological reconstruction," *IEEE Transactions on Medical Imaging*, vol. 25, no. 9, pp. 1200–1213, 2006.

[37] J. Staal, M. D. Abràmoff, M. Niemeijer, M. A. Viergever, and B. van Ginneken, "Ridge-based vessel segmentation in color images of the retina," *IEEE Transactions on Medical Imaging*, vol. 23, no. 4, pp. 501–509, 2004.

[38] M. Niemeijer, J. Staal, B. van Ginneken, M. Loog, and M. D. Abràmoff, "Comparative study of retinal vessel segmentation methods on a new publicly available database," in *Medical Imaging 2004: Image Processing*, J. Michael Fitzpatrick and M. Sonka, Eds., vol. 5370 of *Proceedings of SPIE*, pp. 648–656, February 2004.

[39] F. Zana and J.-C. Klein, "Segmentation of vessel-like patterns using mathematical morphology and curvature evaluation," *IEEE Transactions on Image Processing*, vol. 10, no. 7, pp. 1010–1019, 2001.

[40] M. E. Martinez-Perez, A. D. Hughes, S. A. Thom, A. A. Bharath, and K. H. Parker, "Segmentation of blood vessels from red-free and fluorescein retinal images," *Medical Image Analysis*, vol. 11, no. 1, pp. 47–61, 2007.

[41] L. Espona, M. J. Carreira, M. G. Penedo, and M. Ortega, "Comparison of pixel and subpixel retinal vessel tree segmentation using a deformable contour model," in *Progress in Pattern Recognition, Image Analysis and Applications*, vol. 5197 of *Lecture Notes in Computer Science*, pp. 683–690, Springer, Berlin, Germany, 2008.

[42] X. Jiang and D. Mojon, "Adaptive local thresholding by verification-based multithreshold probing with application to vessel detection in retinal images," *IEEE Transactions on Pattern Analysis and Machine Intelligence*, vol. 25, no. 1, pp. 131–137, 2003.

12

Compressed Sensing-Based MRI Reconstruction Using Complex Double-Density Dual-Tree DWT

Zangen Zhu,[1] **Khan Wahid,**[1] **Paul Babyn,**[2] **and Ran Yang**[3]

[1] *Department of Electrical and Computer Engineering, University of Saskatchewan, Saskatoon, SK, Canada S7N 5A9*
[2] *Department of Medical Imaging, University of Saskatchewan and Saskatoon Health Region, Saskatoon, SK, Canada S7N 0W8*
[3] *School of Information Science and Technology, Sun Yat-Sen University, Guangzhou, Guangdong 510006, China*

Correspondence should be addressed to Khan Wahid; khan.wahid@usask.ca

Academic Editor: Koon-Pong Wong

Undersampling k-space data is an efficient way to speed up the magnetic resonance imaging (MRI) process. As a newly developed mathematical framework of signal sampling and recovery, compressed sensing (CS) allows signal acquisition using fewer samples than what is specified by Nyquist-Shannon sampling theorem whenever the signal is sparse. As a result, CS has great potential in reducing data acquisition time in MRI. In traditional compressed sensing MRI methods, an image is reconstructed by enforcing its sparse representation with respect to a basis, usually wavelet transform or total variation. In this paper, we propose an improved compressed sensing-based reconstruction method using the complex double-density dual-tree discrete wavelet transform. Our experiments demonstrate that this method can reduce aliasing artifacts and achieve higher peak signal-to-noise ratio (PSNR) and structural similarity (SSIM) index.

1. Introduction

Magnetic resonance imaging (MRI) is one of the major imaging modalities in use today. Compared to computed tomography (CT), MRI has advantages in imaging soft tissues. However, its relatively long imaging time remains a great challenge for clinical application, often limiting its application. Significant efforts have focused on faster data collection as well as reducing the amount of data required without degrading image quality. For example, parallel imaging [1–3] exploits redundancy in k-space by introducing multiple receiver channels, mitigating the aliasing artifacts caused by a reduced sampling rate. Recently, compressed sensing based MRI (CS-MRI) allows high quality reconstruction from undersampled data by enforcing the pseudo-sparsity of images in a predefined basis or dictionary, such as the traditional two-dimensional (2D) separable wavelet transform or total variation [4]. However, these basis sets may not provide sufficient sparse representation. The discrete wavelet transform (DWT), for example, has three major disadvantages: shift sensitivity [5], poor directionality [6], and lack of phase information [7, 8]. For these reasons, traditional DWTs fail to capture regularities of contours, since they are not able to sparsely represent one-dimensional singularities of 2D signals [9]. Therefore, improvements can be obtained by mitigating some of these disadvantages simultaneously.

In this paper, we propose an improved compressed sensing method for MR imaging by utilizing the double-density dual-tree DWT [10]. The use of complex wavelet transforms for compressed sensing was first proposed in [11]. The authors in [11] used dual-tree complex wavelet transform (DT-CWT) as a sparsifying transform, which only has wavelets oriented in six directions. But as natural images exhibit smooth regions that are punctuated with edges at several orientations, dual-tree complex wavelet transform may fail to sparsely represent the geometric regularity along the singularities, which require higher directional selectivity. Other contour-based transforms, such as contourlets [12], have also been investigated. But they can only sparsely represent the smooth contours but not the points in images [13, 14]. In this paper, we propose one possible solution by using a newly developed multiresolution tool, double-density dual-tree transform, which may provide sufficient sparse representation for MR images with different features. Total variation is also exploited as a penalty in the reconstruction formulation to suppress noise. Note that in [11], the authors applied their method to radial trajectories. In this paper, its variant on Cartesian sampling is used for comparison, namely, CS DT-CWT. To differentiate between the original compressed sensing based MRI algorithm [4] and the improved version, we will denote the original algorithm in [4] as CS and our proposed method as iCS (improved compressed sensing MRI).

The rest of this paper is organized as follows. In Section 2, we briefly review principles of MRI and then discuss the design of our proposed algorithm. In Section 3, we will present the experimental results of our algorithm in comparison with some other algorithms. Finally, a brief conclusion will be drawn.

2. Theory and Method

2.1. Magnetic Resonance Imaging (MRI). MRI signal is generated by the proton in hydrogen atoms, the main component of the human body. Each proton in an atomic nucleus possesses a fundamental spin. Since protons are charged particles, when a human body is placed in an strong static magnetic field B_0, protons will align themselves with the magnetic field, yielding a net magnetic moment precessing around B_0. This net magnetic precession is termed *Larmor precession*. The frequency of Larmor precession is proportional to the applied magnetic field strength as defined by

$$f = \gamma B_0, \qquad (1)$$

where γ is a constant (42.57 MHz/T) [15]. Next, a radiofrequency (RF) pulse is applied perpendicular to B_0. If the frequency of the applied pulse is equal to the Larmor frequency, the net magnetic moment will tilt away. Once the RF signal is removed, the protons realign themselves such that the net magnetic moment is again aligned around B_0. The protons return to equilibrium by emitting RF signal, which is then captured by a conductive field. This measurement is reconstructed to obtain gray-scale MR images.

To produce a 3D image, a gradient magnetic field, G_z, is added to B_0 so that the Larmor frequency changes linearly in the axial direction, z. Hence, an axial slice can be selected by choosing a specific Larmor frequency of that slice. Additionally, two gradient magnetic fields, G_x and G_y, are applied causing the resonant frequencies of the protons to vary according to their positions in the x-y plane. As a result, the signal is encoded in three dimensions. If the signal is fully sampled at the Nyquist rate, a 2D inverse Fourier transform is then used to transform the encoded image to the spatial domain. Consider the following:

$$x = F^{-1}y, \qquad (2)$$

where y is the measurements from scanner, which is also called k-space data, F is the Fourier transform matrix, and x is the desired MR image. But in the real world, downsampling may be needed for some applications, such as to fit the scans into one-breath hold or to enable real time-imaging.

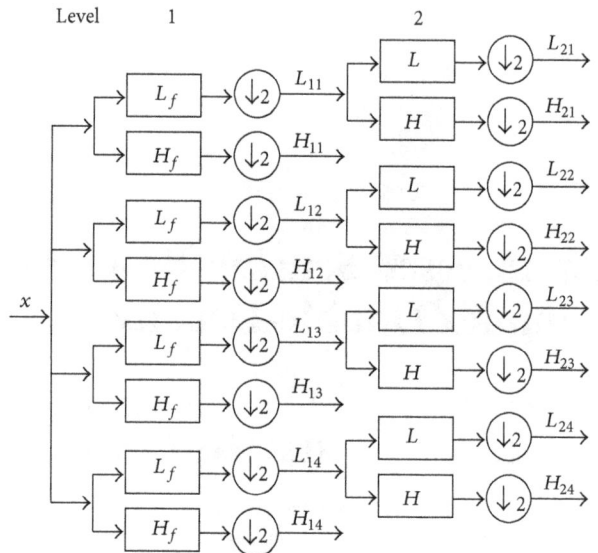

FIGURE 1: Two levels of 2D complex double-density dual-tree wavelet transform.

2.2. Features of Complex Double-Density Dual-Tree Wavelet. The 1D double-density discrete wavelet transform (DD-DWT) is based on one scaling function (i.e., low pass) and two different wavelets (i.e., high pass) where one wavelet is a half-sample shift of the other. The 2D transform applies the 1D transform alternately to the rows and column, giving nine subbands, where one is a low pass subband and the remaining eight subbands become eight wavelet filters. Thus, the 2D complex double-density dual-tree discrete wavelet transform (CDDDT-DWT) is implemented by using four 2D DD-DWT in parallel with different filter banks for rows and columns separately [10]. Figure 1 shows the process of two levels of the transform. L_f and H_f are the filter banks of the first level decomposition, which represent one scaling filter and eight wavelet filters. L and H are the filter banks for the second and remaining levels of decomposition. Therefore, four low pass subbands (L_{11}–L_{14}) and 32 high pass subbands (H_{11}–H_{14}) are produced after one level of the transform. As a result, 32 wavelets are created by the sum and difference on each pair of subbands.

Figure 2 shows the impulse responses of these transforms. The figures are obtained by setting all the wavelet coefficients to zero, for the exception of one wavelet coefficient in each of the high pass subbands of one level. We then take the inverse wavelet transform [16–18]. Therefore, if the transform has more directional wavelets, then fewer coefficients are needed to represent a given geometric object. Figure 2(a) shows the typical wavelets associated with the 2D wavelet transform. Obviously, 2D wavelet transform can resolve only three spatial-domain feature orientations: vertical, horizontal, and diagonal. In addition, the third wavelet does not have a dominant orientation, which is the main cause of artifact (checker board pattern). Therefore, traditional 2D separable wavelet fails to sparsely represent geometric structures, such as edges [19].

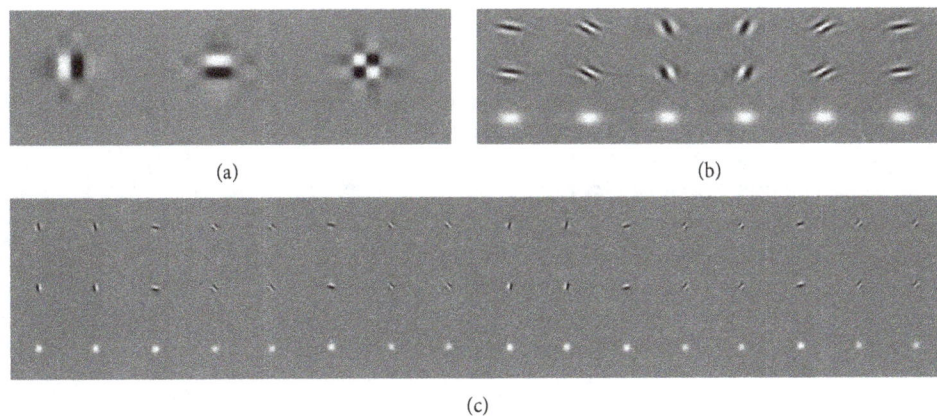

FIGURE 2: Impulse responses of (a) 2D DWT, (b) 2D DT-CWT, and (c) 2D CDDDT-DWT, as illustrated at level of 4 of the transforms.

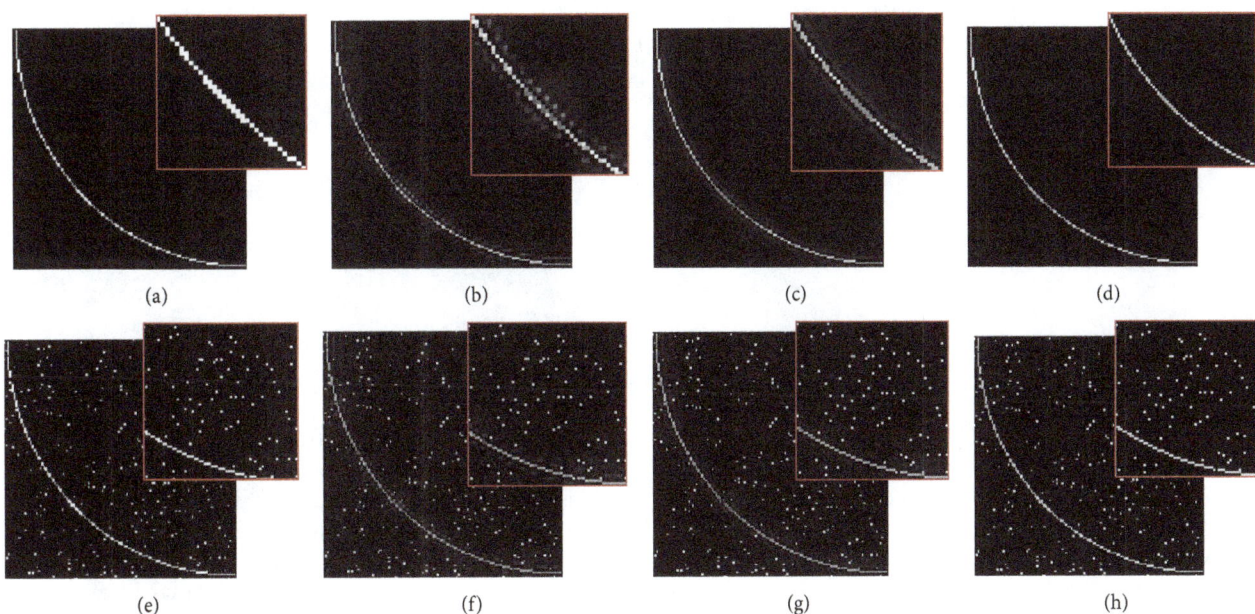

FIGURE 3: Improved directionality of complex double-density dual-tree wavelet transform: (a) original test image; reconstructed image using only the lowest level coefficients of (b) DWT; (c) DT-CWT; (d) CDDDT-DWT; (e)–(h) results of the same experiment with noisy image (zoomed-in at the right corner). Gray level is normalized between [0, 1] for all images and 4-level transform is used for all experiments.

In Figure 2(b), six orientations ($\pm15°$, $\pm45°$, $\pm75°$) are obtained by 2D DT-CWT. By contrast, complex double-density dual-tree wavelet transform has 32 wavelets oriented in 16 different angles (see Figure 2(c)). The 16 wavelets shown in the first (second) row can be interpreted as the real (imaginary) parts of the set of 16 complex wavelets and the third row are the magnitudes of the 16 complex wavelets. As we can see, the orientations are richer and finer. Additionally, all of the wavelets are free of checker board pattern. As a result, we can get more accurate representation for the geometric regions.

In Figure 3, we illustrate this benefit with two example images. The first image group only contains a curve purposely designed to demonstrate the improved directionality property of CDDDT-DWT. The second image group contains impulse (or salt and pepper) noise. We reconstruct the test images using the first stage of transform coefficients. As we can see from Figures 3(b) and 3(f), there are blocking artifacts

in DWT reconstructions since it can only accurately represent vertical and horizontal lines. Because DT-CWT has more directional wavelets, the reconstructed curve looks smoother and artifacts are reduced. But six orientations (Figure 2(b)) are not sufficient to accurately represent this curve as it contains all directions. The reconstructions from CDDDT-DWT are much closer to the original ones. This is because it has more wavelets which are strongly oriented at 16 different angles. One may also conclude that 16 orientations are sufficient to represent any geometric object with high precision. Compared to the curve, the points are better reconstructed by all the three transforms. As stated in the introduction section, wavelet transforms are good at capturing point singularities [20]. From this example, we can see that CDDDT-DWT can sparsely represent both contours and points, indicating its superiority for these tasks.

INPUTS:

y: undersampled k-space data

F_u: system matrix associated with the measurements

Φ: complex double-density dual-tree wavelet operator

λ_1, λ_2: tuning constants

OPTIONAL PARAMETERS:

Tol: stopping criteria by gradient magnitude (default 10^{-4})

Iter: stopping criteria by number of iterations (default 100)

α, ς: line search parameters (defaults $\alpha = 0.01, \varsigma = 0.6$)

OUTPUTS:

x: the numerical approximation to (6)

% Initialization

$k = 0; x_0; g_o = \nabla J(x_0); \Delta x_0 = -g_o$

% Iterations

$while\ (\|g_k\|_2 > \text{Tol})$

$\{$

% Backtracking line-search

$t = 5; while\ (J(x_k + t\Delta x_k) > J(x_k) + \alpha t \cdot Real(g_k^* \Delta x_k)$ and $k < \text{Iter})$

$\{t = \varsigma t\}$

$x_{k+1} = x_k + t\Delta x_k$

$g_{k+1} = \nabla J(x_{k+1})$

$\eta_k = g_{k+1} - g_k$

$\beta_{k+1} = \max\left\{0, \min\left\{\dfrac{g_{k+1}^T \eta_k}{\Delta x_k^T \eta_k}, \dfrac{\|g_{k+1}\|^2}{\Delta x_k^T \eta_k}\right\}\right\}$

$\Delta x_{k+1} = -g_{k+1} + \beta_{k+1}\Delta x_k$

$k = k+1$

$\}$

ALGORITHM 1

2.3. Reconstruction Algorithm Using Compressed Sensing.

The problem of undersampling k-space data actually leads to an underdetermined system of linear equations. One way to improve performance is to incorporate a prior knowledge into the reconstruction process which is based on the idea of sparsity in compressed sensing (CS) [21–23]. The essence of CS is that a signal, which in our case is the image x, can be completely reconstructed with a high probability with far less samples than required by conventional Nyquist-Shannon sampling theorem, if the image has a sparse/compressible representation in a transform domain Φ, such that most entries of the vector Φx are zero or close to zero.

The entire process consists of three steps [24]: encoding, sensing, and decoding. In the first step, the object image x of size n is encoded into a smaller vector $y = F_u x$ of a size m ($m < n$) by the system matrix. F_u denotes the Fourier matrix associated with some undersampled trajectory while y is the corresponding undersample k-space data. Directly solving the underdetermined linear system will yield numerous solutions. As we assume the image is approximately sparse in CDDDT-DWT, that is, $\alpha = \Phi x$, has few elements with relatively large magnitudes, a solution is possible. Then the second step is obtaining the undersampled k-space data y from the imaging system. Incorporating the sparsity prior knowledge into the process of image reconstruction, the third step is to recover α (and thus x) by solving the following constrained optimization problem:

$$\arg\min_x \|\Phi x\|_1 \quad \text{subject to } \|F_u x - y\|_2 < \varepsilon, \tag{3}$$

where ε is a parameter controlling the data consistency. It has been mathematically proven that if the image has only k entries with relatively large magnitudes, the order of $k \log(n)$ measurements is sufficient to accurately reconstruct x via the ℓ_1 norm minimization procedure with high probability. As we have noticed from Figure 3, noise may be also reconstructed by complex double-density dual-tree wavelet. Therefore, in our proposed algorithm, we include the total variation (TV) as a penalty because it was shown that it is efficient in suppressing the noise in the reconstructed image [24]. The constrained problem in (3) can also be converted into an unconstrained problem, giving rise to our proposed iCS model:

$$\arg\min_x \lambda_1 \|\Phi x\|_1 + \lambda_2 \|x\|_{\text{TV}} + \|F_u x - y\|_2^2, \tag{4}$$

where two regularization factors λ_1 and λ_2 are introduced to leverage the cost function's emphasis on the transform ℓ_1 penalty, TV penalty, and the data fidelity term. The selection of regularization factor has been an interesting area of research in the field of regularized iterative methods [25, 26]. A large λ_2 tends to suppress image gradient and make the reconstructed image look smooth, losing point-like features. In our study, we chose the optimized regularization parameters λ_1 and λ_2 for all methods for a fair comparison. The discussion will be given in next section. The TV term of an image in this work is defined as follows:

$$\|x\|_{\text{TV}} = \int |\nabla x| \, dx. \tag{5}$$

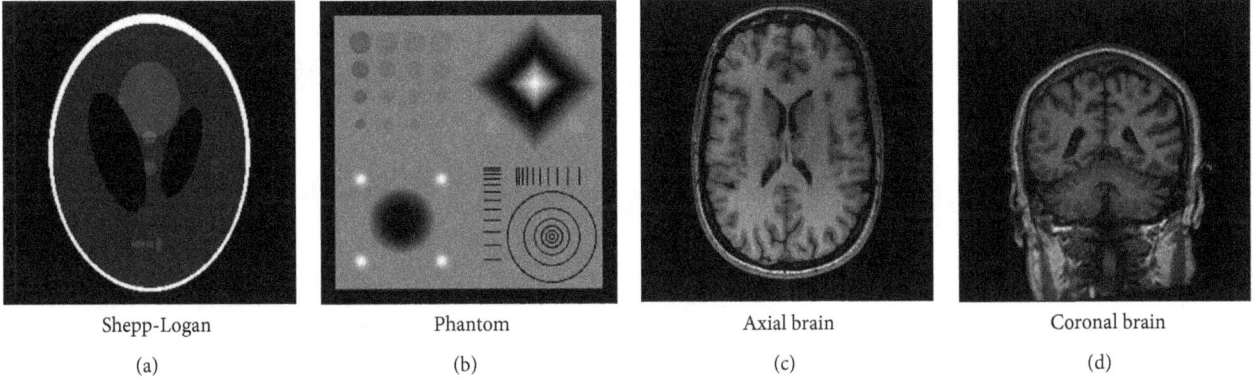

Shepp-Logan   Phantom   Axial brain   Coronal brain

(a)   (b)   (c)   (d)

FIGURE 4: Datasets in this study.

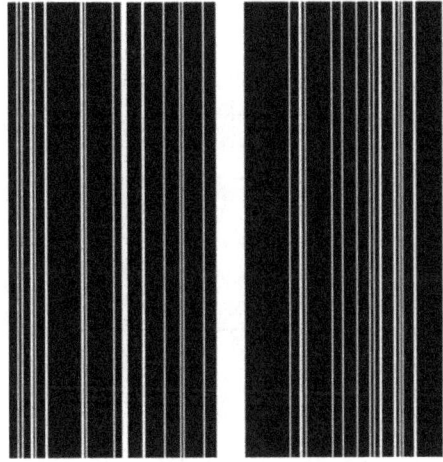

FIGURE 5: Sampling pattern at 0.2 sampling rate. Undersampling is done along the phase direction.

In a discrete version, (5) becomes

$$\|x\|_{\mathrm{TV}} = \sum_{i,j} \sqrt{\left(x_{i+1,j} - x_{i,j}\right)^2 + \left(x_{i,j+1} - x_{i,j}\right)^2}. \quad (6)$$

To speed up the implementation, we exploit a fast implementation of CDDDT-DWT [27]. Since (4) poses an unconstrained convex optimization problem, we propose solving it using a nonlinear conjugate gradient descent algorithm that is similar to [4]. It has been shown in [28] that the iterative algorithm in our study has better performance than the algorithm in [4]. $J(x)$ is the cost function as defined in (4). The iterative algorithm starts with a zero-filling Fourier reconstruction.

The conjugate gradient requires the computation of $\nabla J(x)$ which is

$$\nabla J(x) = \lambda_1 \nabla \|\Phi x\|_1 + \lambda_2 \nabla \|x\|_{\mathrm{TV}} + 2F_u^* \left(F_u x - y\right). \quad (7)$$

As the ℓ_1 norm and total variation term (5) is the sum of absolute values, the absolute values, however, are not smooth functions, and as a result (7) is not well defined. In [4],

Lustig et al. approximated the absolute value with a smooth function, $|x| \approx \sqrt{x^* x + \xi}$, where ξ is a positive smoothing param-eter. Then the gradient becomes $d|x| \approx x/\sqrt{x^* x + \xi}$.

We adopt this idea in our implementation. In particular, a smoothing factor $\xi = 10^{-15}$ is used. The algorithm of the proposed iCS method is shown in Algorithm 1.

3. Numerical and Experimental Results

In this section, we report our experiments to evaluate and validate the proposed algorithm. There are five sets of experiments. In the first two experiments, numerical phantoms and simulated k-space data were used to study the performance of our algorithm. The third and fourth experiments used real data collected from real scanners. In the fifth experiment, we manually add noise to the k-space data of the fourth data set. The first phantom that we consider is the discrete Shepp-Logan, which contains geometrical structure and directional-oriented curves. The second phantom is purposely designed to be nonsparse under total variation domain and contains features difficult to reproduce with partial Fourier sampling [29]. In such way, we can clearly see how the CDDDT-DWT affects the image quality. The third dataset was performed on

(a)

(b)

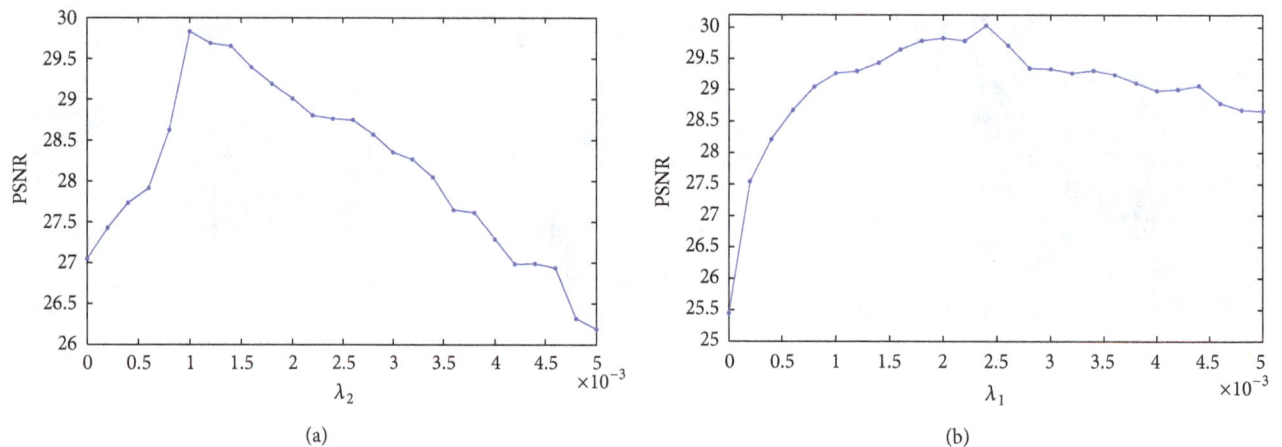

FIGURE 6: Analysis to find the optimum regularization parameters (for Coronal Brain data at sampling rate 0.25). (a) λ_2 when $\lambda_1 = 0.002$ for iCS method; (b) λ_1 when $\lambda_2 = 0.001$ for iCS method.

TABLE 1: Optimal parameter selections at 0.25 sampling rate for coronal brain data and 0.2 for other data.

Dataset	CS [4]		CS DT-CWT		iCS	
	λ_1	λ_2	λ_1	λ_2	λ_1	λ_2
Shepp-Logan	0.0014	0.0024	0.001	0.0026	0.0012	0.0024
Phantom	0.001	0.0016	0.001	0.0018	0.0016	0.0016
Axial brain	0.0014	0.001	0.0012	0.0012	0.0016	0.0008
Coronal brain	0.0014	0.0006	0.0014	0.0012	0.0024	0.001
Coronal brain with noise	0.0014	0.001	0.0012	0.0018	0.0018	0.0012

a 1.5T GE Signa Excite scanner. This T2-weighted dataset of the brain was acquired axially using a FSE sequence [30]. The final dataset was a coronal section of a brain obtained from a T1-weighted brain scan [31]. To have a clear differentiation between these datasets, we name these four datasets as Shepp-Logan, phantom, axial brain, and coronal brain, respectively, as shown in Figure 4. All images are of size 256×256.

Undersampling k-space is simulated with random phase encoding in Cartesian sampling. The sampling density decreases according to a power of distance from the origin. It should be pointed out that the proposed method also works with non-Cartesian sampling pattern, such as spiral and radial trajectories, although these are not shown. Reconstructions were performed at different sampling rates: 0.1, 0.15, 0.2, 0.25, 0.3, 0.35, and 0.4. A sampling pattern with sampling rate 0.2 is shown in Figure 5 where white bar means that the data is sampled and black means otherwise (i.e., not sampled).

The reconstructed data was quantitatively evaluated in terms of peak signal-to-noise rate (PSNR) and structural similarity (SSIM) index [32]. PSNR measures the difference between the reconstructed image $\hat{x}$ and original image x, which is defined by

$$PSNR = 20 \log_{10} \left(\frac{MAX}{\sqrt{MSE}} \right), \tag{8}$$

where $MSE = (1/n) \sum_{i=0}^{n} (x_i - \hat{x}_i)^2$ and MAX is the maximum possible pixel value of the image.

The structural similarity (SSIM) index is highly effective for measuring the structural similarity between two images.

Suppose ρ and t are local image patches taken from the same location of two images that are being compared. The local SSIM index measures three similarities of the image patches: the similarity of luminances $l(\rho, t)$, the similarity of contrasts $c(\rho, t)$, and similarity of structures $s(\rho, t)$. Local SSIM is defined as

$$S(\rho, t) = l(\rho, t) \cdot c(\rho, t) \cdot s(\rho, t)$$
$$= \left(\frac{2\mu_\rho \mu_t + C_1}{\mu_\rho^2 + \mu_t^2 + C_1} \right) \left(\frac{2\sigma_\rho \sigma_t + C_2}{\sigma_\rho^2 + \sigma_t^2 + C_2} \right) \left(\frac{2\sigma_{\rho t} + C_3}{\sigma_\rho \sigma_t + C_3} \right), \tag{9}$$

where μ_ρ and μ_t are local means, σ_ρ and σ_t are local standard deviations, and $\sigma_{\rho t}$ is cross-correlation after removing their means. C_1, C_2, and C_3 are stabilizers. The higher the value of SSIM, the higher image quality is delivered.

In this paper, three methods will be compared under identical conditions. These three methods have three different sparsity transforms Φ in (4). The first method uses the discrete wavelet transform (shown as CS) [4]; the second method uses dual-tree complex wavelet transform (shown as CS DT-CWT) [33]; the proposed method uses complex double-density dual-tree wavelet transform (CDDDT-DWT, denoted by iCS for the rest of the paper). A 4-level of Daubechies-4 wavelet transform was used for CS method. Reconstruction was done under the same conditions such as iterative algorithm and sampling pattern as the accuracy depends on the selection of optimum regularization parameters. We have used the last dataset, Coronal Brain, as an example to show the methodology of determining

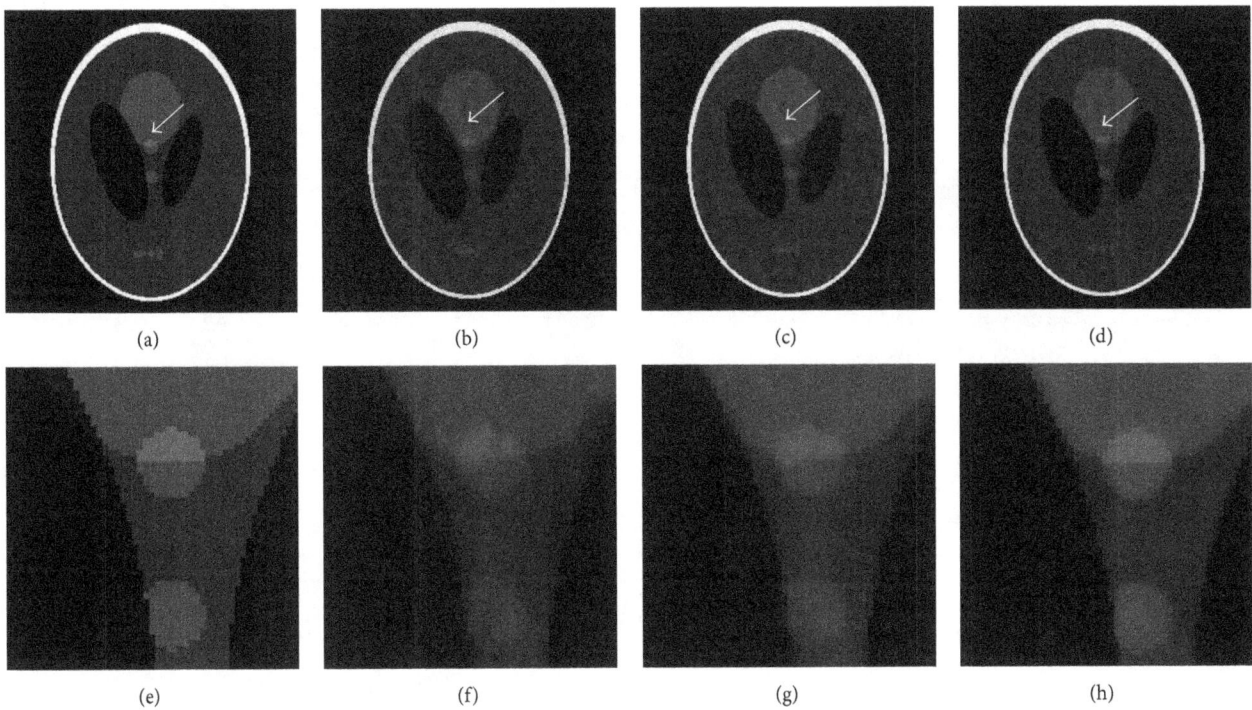

FIGURE 7: Original Shepp-Logan image and experimental results. (a) Original Shepp-Logan image. Reconstruction at sampling rate 0.2 by (b) CS; (c) CS DT-CWT; (d) iCS technique; (e), (f), (g), and (h) are detail views of region outlined by arrow in (a), (b), (c), and (d), respectively.

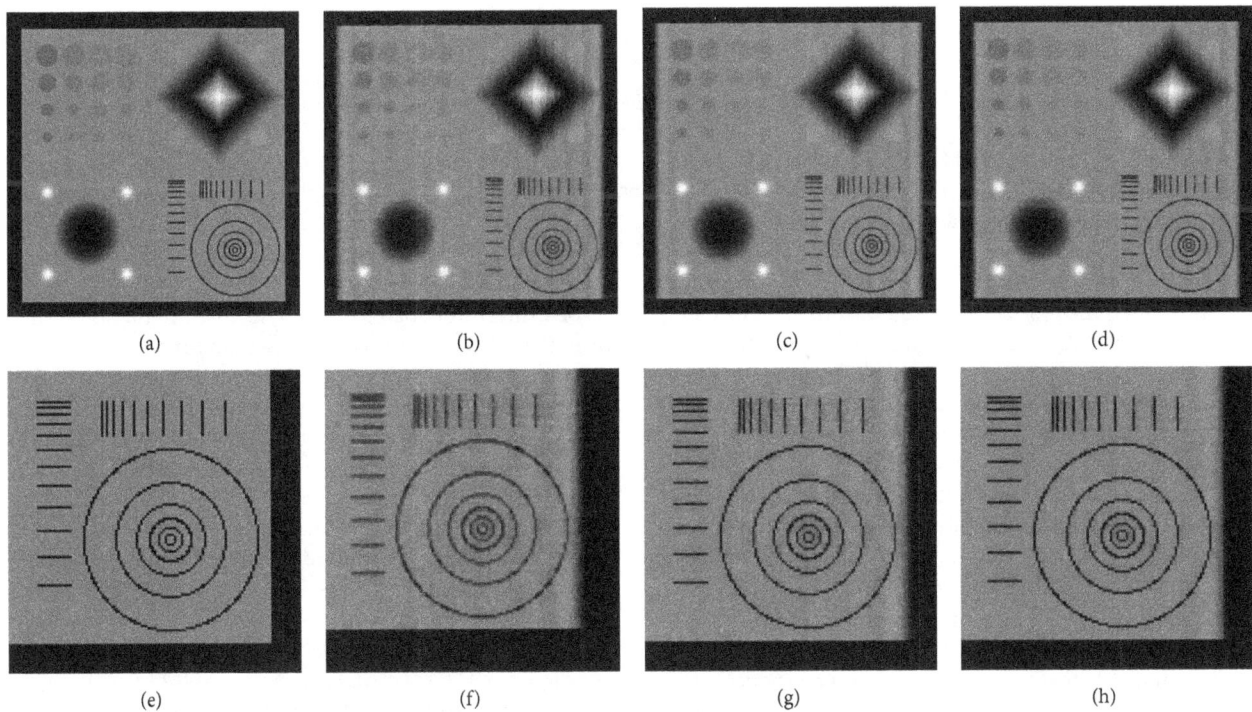

FIGURE 8: Original phantom image and experimental results. (a) Original phantom image. Reconstruction at sampling rate 0.2 by (b) CS; (c) CS DT-CWT; (d) iCS technique; (e), (f), (g), and (h) are detail views of region outlined by arrow in (a), (b), (c), and (d), respectively. Gray level is normalized in [0, 1].

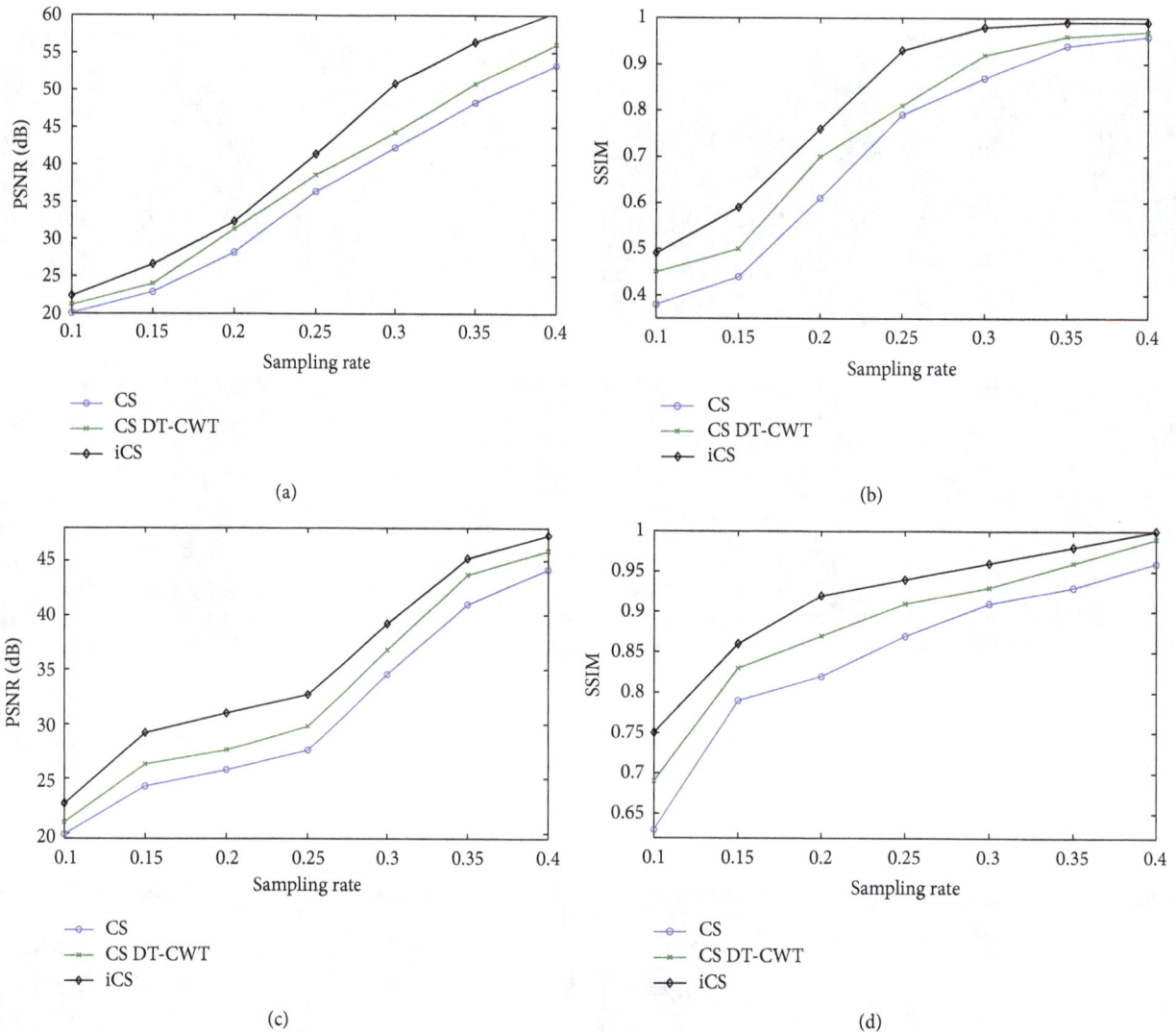

FIGURE 9: Plots of PSNR and SSIM versus different sampling rates. (a) PSNR of Shepp-Logan. (b) SSIM of Shepp-Logan. (c) PSNR of phantom dataset. (d) SSIM of phantom dataset.

the optimal parameters. For each algorithm, we alternately plotted the PSNR against one parameter keeping the other fixed. We started by setting $\lambda_1 = 0.002$. Figure 6(a) shows that the highest PSNR is obtained when λ_2 is 0.001. Then we set $\lambda_2 = 0.001$ and searched the optimal value for λ_1 that gives the highest PSNR, as shown in Figure 6(b). Thus, we used this recurring process to determine the optimum values of λ_1 and λ_2. Similar search was conducted for the other two compared methods and all datasets. The optimal values of these parameters are shown in Table 1.

We begin with the phantom experiments. Figure 7(a) is an image reconstructed from the fully sampled data. Figures 7(b), 7(c), and 7(d) are reconstructions by CS method, CS DT-CWT, and our proposed method iCS, respectively. The weakness of the traditional separable wavelet transform in representing two-dimensional singularities, for example, curves and edges, is visualized with the reconstructed Shepp-Logan images. As we have seen that separable wavelet transform can

resolve only three spatial-domain feature orientations. Therefore, the ellipses are not sparsely represented, causing substantial artifacts in the reconstructed images (Figure 7(b)). The artifacts become more serious when the size of ellipse is reduced. For example, two small ellipses around center (as indicated by white arrows) are faded away from the CS reconstruction. To see it clearly, detailed zoom-ins are shown in Figures 7(e)–7(h). Moreover, the CS reconstruction shows substantial artifacts in smooth region. By contrast, the proposed method reconstructs the image with higher visual image quality. From Figures 7(e) to 7(h), we can see that, with more directional wavelets, the ellipses are better reconstructed. The reconstruction by complex double-density dual-tree wavelet transform has the best visual image quality. Additionally, the two small ellipses could be clearly recognized; see Figure 7(h).

Similar results can be obtained from the second phantom experiment. From Figure 8(b), we can see significant aliasing

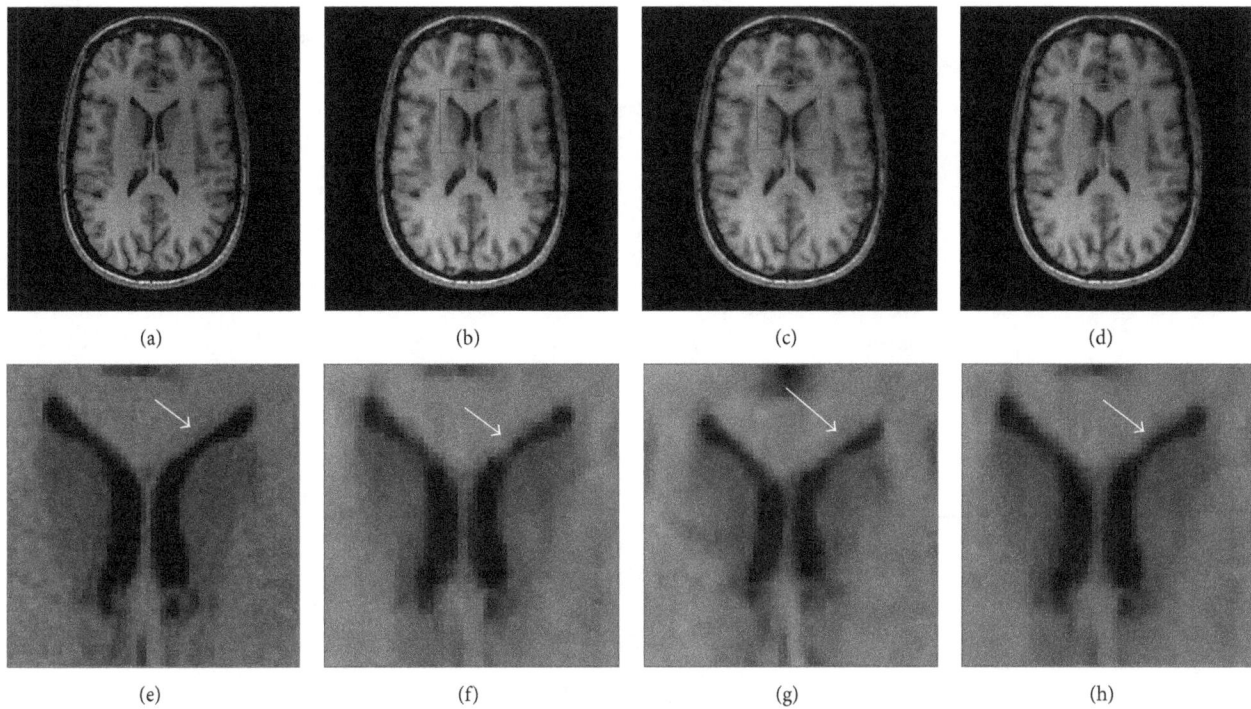

FIGURE 10: Original axial brain image and experimental results. (a) Original axial brain image. Reconstruction at sampling rate 0.2 by (b) CS; (c) CS DT-CWT; (d) iCS technique; (e), (f), (g), and (h) are detail views of region outlined by arrow in (a), (b), (c), and (d), respectively.

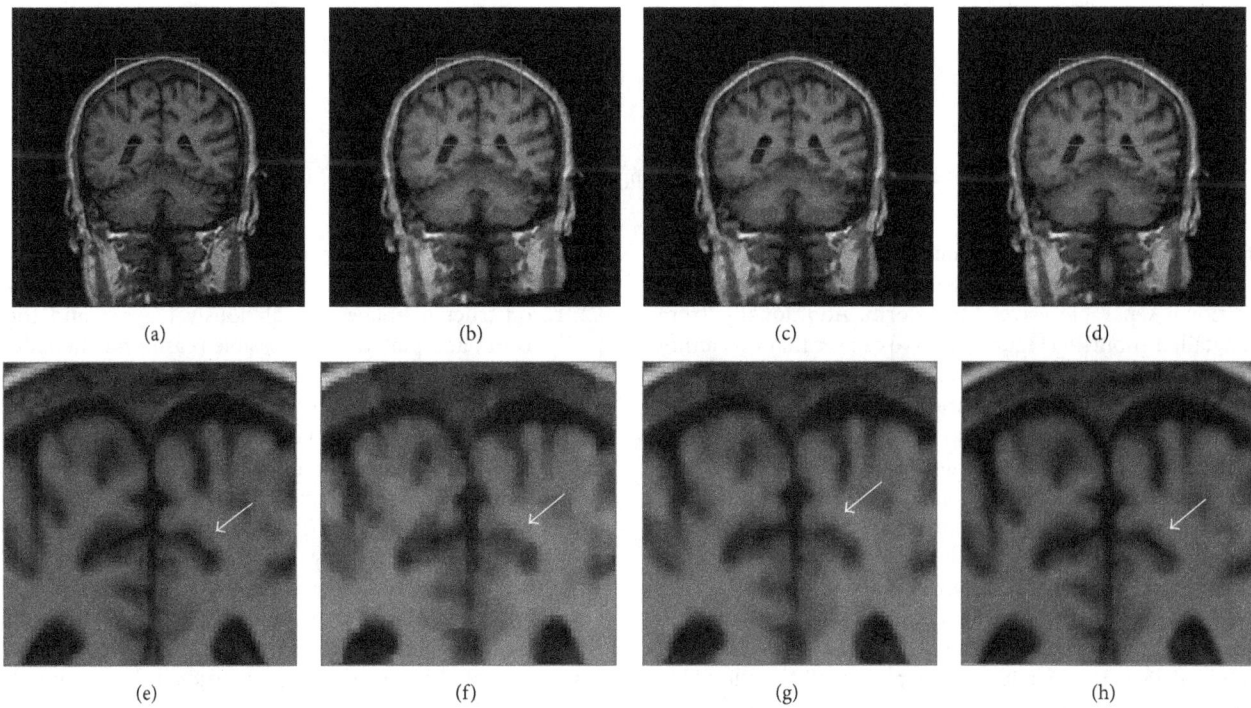

FIGURE 11: Original coronal brain image and experimental results. (a) Original coronal brain image. Reconstruction at sampling rate 0.25 by (b) CS; (c) CS DT-CWT; (d) iCS technique; (e), (f), (g), and (h) are detail views of region outlined by arrow in (a), (b), (c), and (d), respectively.

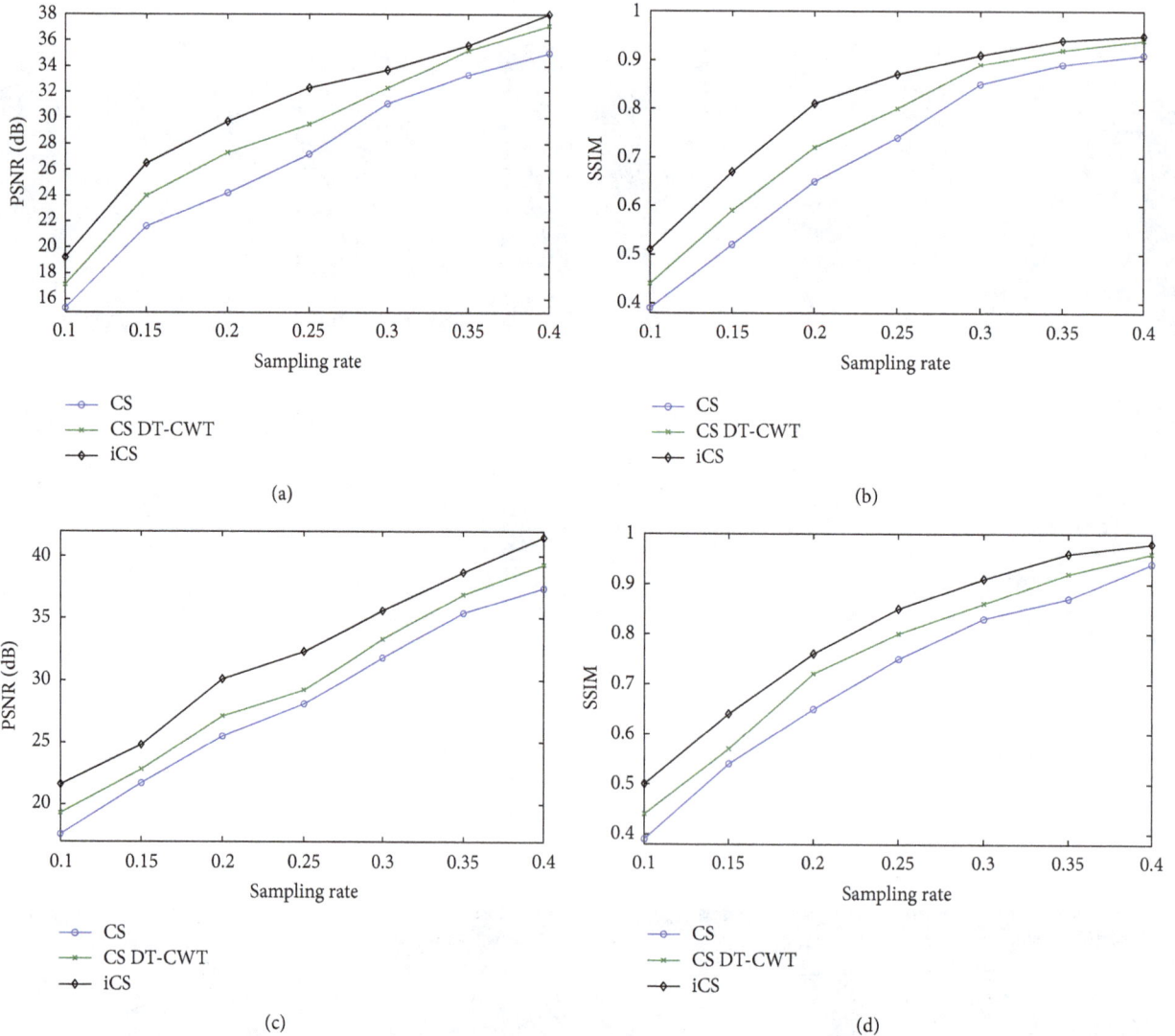

(a)

(b)

(c)

(d)

FIGURE 12: Plots of PSNR and SSIM for different sampling rates: (a)-(b) axial brain; (c)-(d) coronal brain.

artifacts in the CS reconstruction. These artifacts are caused by the use of nonideal low pass and high pass filters in the traditional separable wavelet transform. Additionally, from the detailed zoom-in (Figure 8(f)), we can see that CS cannot reconstruct those closely placed lines separately. By contrast, CS DT-CWT and iCS can separate these lines. One possible reason for this phenomenon may be that the wavelets of DW-CWT and CDDDT-DWT are finer than those of DWT see Figure 1. Therefore, small size objects are better reconstructed with finer wavelet filters. We can see reduced artifacts from Figures 8(f) to 8(g). This is evident that our method leads to a better reconstruction with higher spatial resolution.

In order to see how the results vary with the sampling rates, experiments were also performed at sampling rates of 0.1, 0.15, 0.25, 0.3, 0.35, and 0.4. The plots of PSNR and SSIM versus different sampling rates for the phantom simulations are shown in Figure 9. At sampling rate 0.25, the PSNRs and SSIMs increase dramatically. The PSNR of the Shepp-Logan image by our proposed method is 41.5 dB, and structural similarity is well above 0.93. There is no visual difference between

the reference and reconstructed images using the proposed method. On the other hand, reducing the sampling rate below 0.2, reconstructed images are obviously blurred and their quality is not acceptable. One possible reason for the failure of compressed sensing methods is that the initial image is too bad at such low sampling rates.

Next we consider the in vivo experiments without noise added purposely. Figures 10 and 11 show the reconstructed images where (a), (b), (c), and (d) are original images, CS reconstructions, CS DT-CWT reconstructions, and our iCS reconstructions, respectively. Note that although both CS reconstructions are able to reduce the undersampling artifacts significantly, the images obtained by CS contain significant blocking artifacts along directional edges. To emphasize this point, detail views of the reconstructed images are also displayed in these figures. This is because the diagonal wavelet of traditional wavelet transform does not have a dominant orientation see Figure 1(a). As a result, it can not represent the curves efficiently, leading to considerable artifacts along edges. Dual-tree complex wavelet transform can resolve six

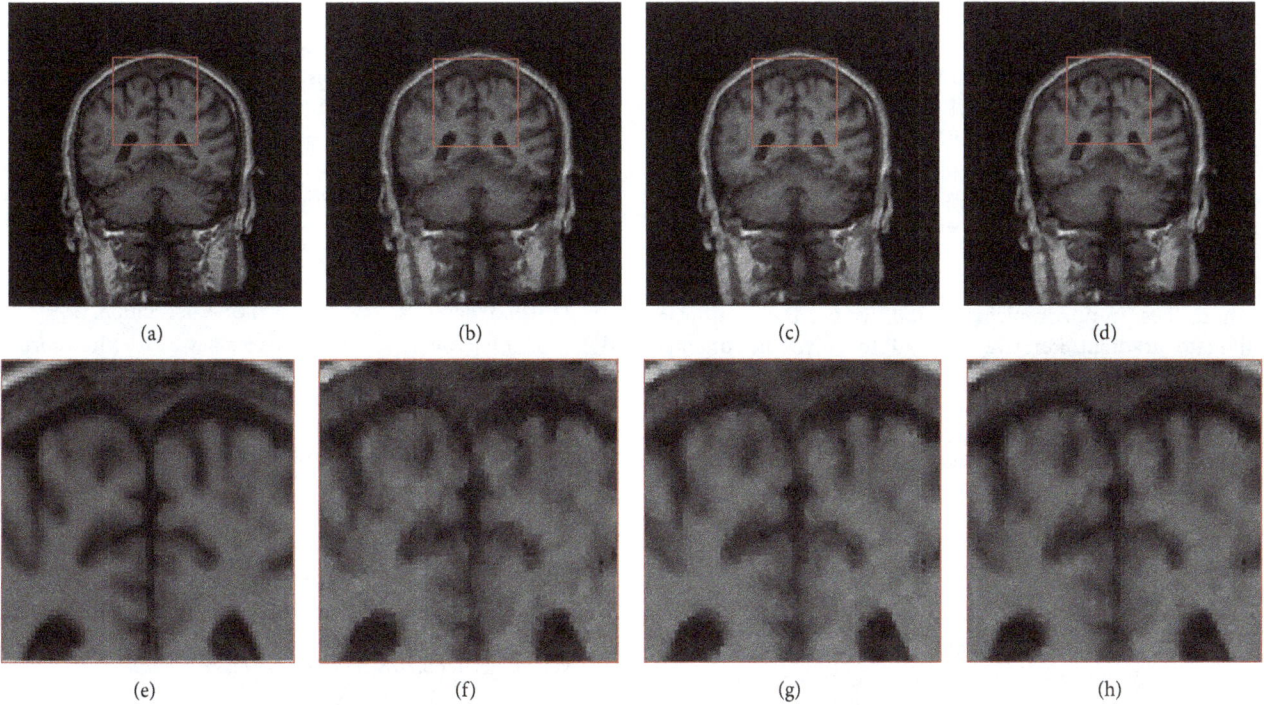

FIGURE 13: Original coronal brain image and experimental results with noisy data. (a) Original coronal brain image. Reconstruction at sampling rate 0.25 by (b) CS; (c) CS DT-CWT; (d) iCS technique; (e), (f), (g), and (h) are detail views of region outlined by arrow in (a), (b), (c), and (d), respectively.

TABLE 2: PSNR and SSIM of coronal brain image with noisy data at 0.25 sampling rate.

Image	Reconstruction methods	PSNR (dB)	SSIM
	CS [4]	24.9	0.61
Coronal brain	CS DT-CWT	27.1	0.69
	iCS	29.0	0.75

orientations, both of which have a dominant orientation, and thus the image quality is greatly improved by CS DT-CWT. In contrast, since complex double-density dual-tree wavelet has improved directional selectivity and finer wavelets than DWT and DT-CWT, the proposed method preserves more edges and small structures. Therefore, the images obtained using our proposed method are much closer to the original images. Figure 10(h) and Figure 11(h) indicate that edges are sharper in the reconstructed image using our proposed method.

The evaluation matrices (PSNRs and SSIMs) of the reconstructed images are also plotted against the sampling rates in Figure 12. Consistent increase of reconstruction accuracy using the proposed method is observed. Figure 12 also indicates that PSNRs and SSIMs of reconstructions by our proposed method in all cases are higher than those of other methods. One should also note that the original CS method can produce an accurate reconstruction given a sufficient sampling rate. For instance, the results in [4] showed that CS can produce high quality brain image without artifacts at sampling rate 0.42 (2.4 acceleration). This conclusion is confirmed by our in vivo experiments. Note that the PSNR of CS

method is well above 35 dB and SSIM is as high as 0.9 at sampling rate 0.4. But at low sampling rates, reconstructed image is not satisfactory. As a result, traditional wavelet transform fails to provide sparse representation, causing artifacts. Our proposed complex double-density dual-tree wavelet is able to capture those geometric features that are not captured by other transforms, producing a higher quality of image. The results of this test confirm that our proposed method outperforms the original CS method in preserving edges and suppressing undersampled artifacts.

Finally, we reconstructed the coronal brain image using imperfect k-space data to test the robustness of the proposed method. Additive Gaussian white noise e of relative magnitude $\|e\|_2/\|Fx_{\text{ture}}\|_2 = 0.05$ was purposely added to the k-space data. The results are shown in Figure 13. The optimum parameter selections are also shown in Table 1. From the table, we can see that the parameter λ_2 is bigger when noisy data is used for reconstruction for all the methods. This is because TV regularization is good at suppressing noise. Larger λ_2 can better suppress noise. But if λ_2 is too large, the reconstructed image will be oversmooth, losing low contrast or detailed information. The PSNR and SSIM are summarized in Table 2. Although the image quality is reduced, the proposed method can still maintain the best results.

From the various results presented in this section, proposed method delivers higher PSNR and SSIM than other methods. However, the computation time of CS-based methods including the proposed algorithm is about 70 seconds. Development of faster algorithms for solving problem (4) will be pursued in the future work.

4. Conclusion

In this paper, an improved compressed sensing MRI method is proposed. The directionality property of complex double-density dual-tree wavelet transform is investigated. Considering the edge features and quality, we employ objective measurements to evaluate the performance of our approach. Simulation results on phantom and in vivo data demonstrate that the proposed method can better reconstruct the edges and reduce undersampled artifacts than traditional CS-MRI method does. In our implementation, we use the nonlinear conjugate gradient iterative method to solve the unconstrained optimization problem. Further effort is needed to utilize a more advanced iterative method to improve reconstructed precision and reduce computational time for real time-imaging. Extension of this work with the nonconvex optimization is being considered to further improve the reconstruction.

References

[1] K. Pruessmann, M. Weiger, M. Scheidegger, and P. Boesiger, "SENSE: sensitivity encoding for fast MRI," *Magnetic Resonance in Medicine*, vol. 42, no. 5, pp. 952–962, 1999.

[2] M. A. Griswold, P. M. Jakob, R. M. Heidemann et al., "Generalized autocalibrating partially parallel acquisitions (GRAPPA)," *Magnetic Resonance in Medicine*, vol. 47, no. 6, pp. 1202–1210, 2002.

[3] D. K. Sodickson and W. J. Manning, "Simultaneous acquisition of spatial harmonics (SMASH): fast imaging with radiofrequency coil arrays," *Magnetic Resonance in Medicine*, vol. 38, no. 4, pp. 591–603, 1997.

[4] M. Lustig, D. Donoho, and J. M. Pauly, "Sparse MRI: the application of compressed sensing for rapid MR imaging," *Magnetic Resonance in Medicine*, vol. 58, no. 6, pp. 1182–1195, 2007.

[5] N. Kingsbury, "Complex wavelets for shift invariant analysis and filtering of signals," *Applied and Computational Harmonic Analysis*, vol. 10, no. 3, pp. 234–253, 2001.

[6] N. Kingsbury, "Image processing with complex wavelets," *Philosophical Transactions of the Royal Society of London A*, no. 357, pp. 2543–2560, 1999.

[7] F. Fernandes, *Directional, shift-insensitive, complex wavelet transforms with controllable redundancy [Ph.D. thesis]*, Rice University, 2002.

[8] P. Shukla, *Complex wavelet transforms and their applications [MPhil Thesis]*, University of Strathclyde, 2003.

[9] E. Candes and D. Donoho, "Curvelets—a surprisingly effective nonadaptive representation for objects with edges," in *Curve and Surface Fitting*, A. Cohen, C. Rabut, and L. L. Schumaker, Eds., Vanderbilt University Press, Nashville, Tenn, USA, 1999.

[10] I. W. Selesnick, "The double-density dual-tree DWT," *IEEE Transactions on Signal Processing*, vol. 52, no. 5, pp. 1304–1314, 2004.

[11] Y. Kim, M. Altbach, T. Trouard, and A. Bilgin, "Compressed sensing using dual-tree complex wavelet transform," *Proceedings of the International Society for Magnetic Resonance in Medicine*, vol. 17, p. 2814, 2009.

[12] M. N. Do and M. Vetterli, "The contourlet transform: an efficient directional multiresolution image representation," *IEEE Transactions on Image Processing*, vol. 14, no. 12, pp. 2091–2106, 2005.

[13] X. Qu, W. Zhang, D. Guo, C. Cai, S. Cai, and Z. Chen, "Iterative thresholding compressed sensing MRI based on contourlet transform," *Inverse Problems in Science and Engineering*, vol. 18, pp. 737–758, 2010.

[14] S. M. Gho, Y. Nam, S. Y. Zho, E. Y. Kim, and D. H. Kim, "Three dimension double inversion recovery gray matter imaging using compressed sensing," *Magnetic Resonance Imaging*, vol. 28, no. 10, pp. 1395–1402, 2010.

[15] E. Haacke, R. Brown, M. Thompson, and R. Venkatesan, *Magnetic Resonance Imaging: Physical Principles and Sequence Design*, Wiley-Liss, New York, NY, USA, 1st edition, 1999.

[16] N. G. Kingsbury, "The dual tree complex wavelet transform: a new efficient tool for image restoration and enhancement," in *Proceedings of the European Signal Processing Conference*, pp. 319–322, 1998.

[17] N. Kingsbury, "Complex wavelets for shift invariant analysis and filtering of signals," *Applied and Computational Harmonic Analysis*, vol. 10, pp. 234–253, 2001.

[18] http://eeweb.poly.edu/iselesni/DoubleSoftware/doubledual2D.html.

[19] E. Le Pennec and S. Mallat, "Sparse geometric image representations with bandelets," *IEEE Transactions on Image Processing*, vol. 14, no. 4, pp. 423–438, 2005.

[20] D. Donoho and X. Huo, "Combined image representation using edgelets and wavelets," in *Wavelet Applications in Signal and Image Processing*, vol. 3813 of *Proceedings of the SPIE*, pp. 468–476, Denver, Colo, USA, 1999.

[21] D. L. Donoho, "Compressed sensing," *IEEE Transactions on Information Theory*, vol. 52, no. 4, pp. 1289–1306, 2006.

[22] E. J. Candès, J. Romberg, and T. Tao, "Robust uncertainty principles: exact signal reconstruction from highly incomplete frequency information," *IEEE Transactions on Information Theory*, vol. 52, no. 2, pp. 489–509, 2006.

[23] Y. Tsaig and D. L. Donoho, "Extensions of compressed sensing," *Signal Processing*, vol. 86, no. 3, pp. 549–571, 2006.

[24] S. Ma, W. Yin, Y. Zhang, and A. Chakraborty, "An efficient algorithm for compressed MR imaging using total variation and wavelets," in *Proceedings of the 26th IEEE Conference on Computer Vision and Pattern Recognition (CVPR '08)*, June 2008.

[25] V. Agarwal, "Total variation regularization and L-curve method for the selection of regularization parameter," ECE599, 2003.

[26] M. Belge, M. E. Kilmer, and E. L. Miller, "Efficient determination of multiple regularization parameters in a generalized L-curve framework," *Inverse Problems*, vol. 18, no. 4, pp. 1161–1183, 2002.

[27] http://eeweb.poly.edu/iselesni/DoubleSoftware/index.html.

[28] W. Hager and H. Zhang, "A survey of nonlinear conjugate gradient methods," *Pacific Journal of Optimization*, vol. 2, pp. 35–58, 2006.

[29] D. S. Smith and E. B. Welch, "Non-sparse phantom for compressed sensing MRI reconstruction," in *Proceedings of the 19th Annual Meeting of International Society for Magnetic Resonance in Medicine (ISMRM '11)*, p. 2845, May 2011.

[30] http://www.eecs.berkeley.edu/~mlustig/Software.html.

[31] http://www.cma.mgh.harvard.edu/ibsr/data.html.

[32] Z. Wang, A. C. Bovik, H. R. Sheikh, and E. P. Simoncelli, "Image quality assessment: from error visibility to structural similarity," *IEEE Transactions on Image Processing*, vol. 13, no. 4, pp. 600–612, 2004.

[33] http://eeweb.poly.edu/iselesni/WaveletSoftware/dt2D.html.

13

Breast Tissue 3D Segmentation and Visualization on MRI

Hong Song,[1] Xiangfei Cui,[2] and Feifei Sun[2]

[1] *School of Software, Beijing Institute of Technology, 5 South Zhongguancun Street, Haidian District, Beijing 100081, China*
[2] *School of Computer Science & Technology, Beijing Institute of Technology, 5 South Zhongguancun Street, Haidian District, Beijing 100081, China*

Correspondence should be addressed to Hong Song; anniesun@bit.edu.cn

Academic Editor: Zhenming Yuan

Tissue segmentation and visualization are useful for breast lesion detection and quantitative analysis. In this paper, a 3D segmentation algorithm based on Kernel-based Fuzzy C-Means (KFCM) is proposed to separate the breast MR images into different tissues. Then, an improved volume rendering algorithm based on a new transfer function model is applied to implement 3D breast visualization. Experimental results have been shown visually and have achieved reasonable consistency.

1. Introduction

Recently, magnetic resonance imaging (MRI) technique has been widely used in diagnosing and detecting diseases. It provides an effective mean of noninvasively mapping the anatomy of a subject. It works better than X-ray computed tomography (CT) at soft tissue, such as breast. The three-dimensional segmentation and visualization of breast are useful for breast lesion detection and quantitative analysis.

Segmentation is applied to extract the interesting tissues in the breast. Several algorithms have been developed for segmenting the breast tissues. Threshold-based method, the gradient method, polynomial approximation method, the active contour models, and classifier segmentation are used in breast skin segmentation. Raba et al. [1] summarized that threshold-based method, the gradient method, polynomial approximation method, the active contour models, and classifier segmentation are the main methods commonly used in breast skin segmentation. Chen et al. [2] introduced the fuzzy clustering algorithm to the tumor region segmentation which had achieved better results. Kannan et al. [3] made the breast region segmentation by introducing new objective function of fuzzy c-means with the help of hypertangent function, Lagrangian multipliers method, and kernel functions. However, these studies did not separate the fat and fibroglandular tissues. Pathmanathan [4] suggested a region-growing method, which required the user to manually choose one or more seed points. This method got satisfying results, but it is inefficient and time consuming. Nie [5] used two steps to segment the breast: firstly, locating the skin border and lungs region by standard FCM algorithm and secondly, extracting the fibroglandular tissue by an adaptive FCM algorithm. However, it is a semiautomated method.

Two kinds of methods are mainly applied in volume visualization, which are surface rendering and volume rendering. For surface rendering, Marching Cubes (MC) algorithm [6] is usually used which was developed by Lorensen and Cline in 1987. MC represents 3D objects by surface representations such as triangular patches or polygonal meshes. However, MC algorithm suffered from a common problem of having to make a binary classification: either a surface passes through the current voxel or it does not [7]. Volume rendering addresses these defects, which can display the dataset by translucent images. By volume rendering, the internal structure can be seen and analyzed conveniently, which is useful for breast disease diagnosis. Most of the volume rendering algorithms are based on the optical theory [8]. The optical model can simulate the propagation of light in real world. Levoy [7] proposed ray-casting algorithm to display surfaces from volume data. Lacroute [9] improved ray casting with shear-warp algorithm. Maximum intensity projection (MIP) is a variant of volume rendering in which the color of the pixel in the final image is determined by the maximum value encountered along a ray.

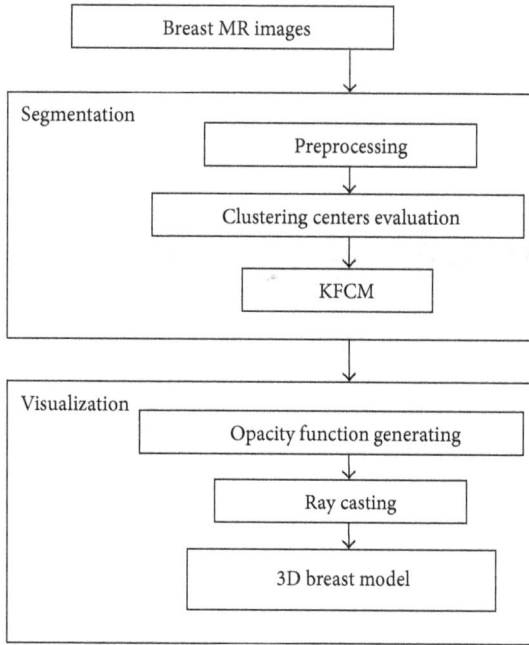

FIGURE 1: Overview of breast segmentation and visualization.

In this paper, firstly, an automatic segmentation algorithm based on KFCM is developed to separate breast images into different tissues. Secondly, an improved volume rendering algorithm based on a new transfer function model is proposed to visualize the breast on MRI. Figure 1 shows the procedure of the breast segmentation and visualization.

2. Breast Tissue Segmentation

Breast tissue segmentation is used to extract the interesting regions. It separates the breast into three parts: fat tissue, fibroglandular tissue, and air. In this paper, an automatic segmentation algorithm is developed, which consists of three steps described as follows.

2.1. Image Preprocessing. MR image has inhomogeneity, noise, and other factors which affect the continuity and accuracy of the images segmentation results. Therefore, the anisotropic diffusion filter [10] is introduced to reduce the image noise. And then binarization is performed on the image by using Otsu's thresholding algorithm. Since air produces almost zero MR signals, the background in MR images is virtually black, and the breast-skin boundary is relatively clear. Pectoral muscle appears dark gray in the axial T1-weighted breast images, and the grey level of this area is close to zero. So the direct threshold-based method is used to segment the breast region. Figure 2(a) is the original MR image that is partially enlarged. Figure 2(b) is the image that is processed by anisotropic diffusion filter which is smoother than the original image while the edges are well preserved.

2.2. Kernel-Based Fuzzy C-Means Clustering Algorithm. Typical Fuzzy C-Means (FCM) clustering algorithm is improved from C-means method, in which every iterative makes the sample belong to an exact cluster [11].

FCM introduces a fuzzy membership function which controls the degree of a sample belonging to different classes. The Kernel-based Fuzzy C-Means (KFCM) clustering method was proposed by Zhang [12, 13] based on FCM. It used a kernel function $\Phi(x)$ instead of the original Euclidian norm metric in typical FCM algorithm. The KFCM algorithm minimized the following objective function:

$$J_{kfcm} = \sum_{j=1}^{N} \sum_{i=1}^{c} p_{ij}^{m} \left\| \Phi\left(x_j\right) - \Phi\left(v_i\right) \right\|^2, \tag{1}$$

where p_{ij}^{m} is a fuzzy membership matrix. c is the number of clustering centers which is usually set by a priori knowledge. N is the number of sample points. v_i is the fuzzy center of the ith cluster. The parameter m is a constant which controls the fuzziness of the resulting partition. In the experiments, m is set as 2.

In this paper, the Gaussian function (see (2)) is selected as the kernel function:

$$K\left(x, y\right) = e^{-\|x-y\|^2/(2\sigma)^2}. \tag{2}$$

So the distance measure and the objective function can be redefined as

$$\left\| \Phi\left(x_j\right) - \Phi\left(v_i\right) \right\|^2 = K\left(x_j, x_k\right) + K\left(v_i, v_i\right) - 2K\left(x_j, v_i\right)$$
$$= 2 - 2K\left(x_j, v_i\right),$$
$$J_{kfcm} = \sum_{j=1}^{N} \sum_{i=1}^{c} 2p_{ij}^{m} \left(1 - K\left(x_j, v_i\right)\right). \tag{3}$$

The equations of clustering center and membership matrix are similar with FCM as follows:

$$p_{ij} = \frac{\left(1 - k(x_j - v_i)\right)^{1/(1-m)}}{\sum_{i=1}^{c} \left(1 - k(x_j, v_i)\right)^{1/(1-m)}},$$
$$v_i = \frac{\sum_{k=1}^{N} p_{ik}^{m} k\left(x_k, v_i\right) x_k}{\sum_{k=1}^{N} p_{ik}^{m} k\left(x_j, v_i\right)}. \tag{4}$$

Because the sum of every column value in the fuzzy membership matrix p_{ij}^{m} is 1,

$$\sum_{i=1}^{c} p_{ij} = 1 \quad (j = 1, 2, \ldots, N), \tag{5}$$

the result of KFCM is influenced by the number of the clustering centers. The result will be devious if the number is very different from the reality. However, the classification for breast using KFCM benefits from the good performance of convergence [11] because we know exactly the clustering number.

2.3. Evaluation of the Clustering Centers. The clustering centers of KFCM are initialized randomly without analyzing

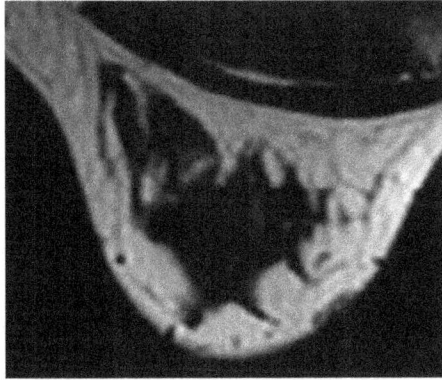

(a)

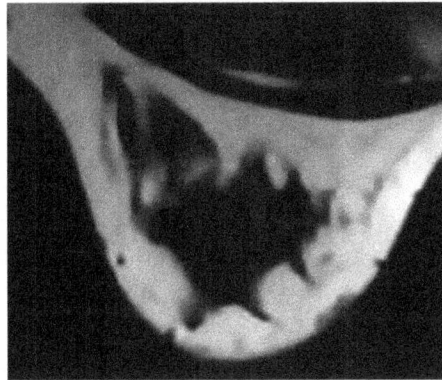

(b)

FIGURE 2: Breast image preprocessing ((a) original image; (b) after preprocessing).

the original dataset, which probably causes nonaccurate segmentation and needs more iteration times. So we utilize a boundary model to determine the rough boundary of breast tissues and then calculate more accurate clustering centers.

We assume that there are gradual changes in data value between different tissues. For scalar data, the gradient is a first derivative measure which describes the direction of greatest change. The gradient magnitude is a scalar quantity that represents the rate of change in the scalar field. Since precise boundary is unnecessary, the second directional derivative is abstained for reducing complexity. f' is used to represent the gradient magnitude, where f is the scalar function:

$$f' = \|\nabla f\| . \tag{6}$$

We assume that if we order the tissues by data value, then each type touches only types adjacent to it in the ordering [7]. The transition from one tissue to another is smooth. We create a 1D histogram of f' and find its peaks. The positions where peaks appear are approximately the boundary. We denote the boundary by

$$\Psi(x) \quad x = 1, 2, \ldots, N. \tag{7}$$

N is the number of positions whose gradient magnitude belongs to the peaks. There are three kinds of tissues in breast MR images (fat, fibroglandular, and air). So $\Psi_1(x)$, $\Psi_2(x)$, and

$\Psi_3(x)$ will be produced. And then compute the one moment of the discrete boundary points set [14]:

$$m_{pq} = \sum_{j=1}^{N} \sum_{i=1}^{N} i^p j^q f(i, j),$$

$$\mu_{pq} = \sum_{j=1}^{N} \sum_{i=1}^{N} (i - i_c)^p (j - j_c)^q f(i, j), \tag{8}$$

where $i_c = m_{10}/m_{00}$, $j_c = m_{01}/m_{00}$.

So the one moment can be used to initialize the clustering centers to perform the KFCM algorithm.

3. Breast Visualization

Volume rendering is useful for exploring the internal structure of the object such as breast. Most of the volume rendering algorithms are based on the optical theory. There are several different optical models for light interaction with volume densities of absorbing, emitting, reflecting, and scattering materials [8]. In this paper only absorption plus emission is considered in which voxel emits light itself and absorbs incoming light. It is the most common one in volume rendering [15]. Each pixel of the image casts a single ray into the dataset. The ray interacts with the scalar value of the dataset which has been virtually mapped to color and optical properties. The mapping is implemented through a transfer function. The optical properties then are used in compositing procedure which is known as the volume rendering integral. The integral is solved numerically to get the color of the pixel at last. This process continues until the color of all the pixels of the image is obtained, and then the final image will be displayed.

3.1. Optical Model and Composition. Every pixel casts a ray from viewing image to the volume, and then we resample the volume scalar data values at equispaced intervals through trilinear interpolation. The optical model and composition are not the main point of this paper and are presented here for completeness.

The process of the light propagation and the composition is parameterized. A ray cast into the volume is represented by $x(t)$, where t is the distance from the eye to the current position. The scalar value along $x(t)$ is denoted by $s(x(t))$. Since only absorption and emission are considered, the volume rendering equation integrates absorption coefficients and emissive colors:

$$c(t) = c(s(x(t))),$$

$$k(t) = k(s(x(t))). \tag{9}$$

Both $c(t)$ and $k(t)$ are functions of distance t instead of scalar s. We denote the energy which eventually reaches the eye from $t = d$ by c'. If $k(t)$ is constant along the ray,

$$c' = c \cdot e^{-kd} . \tag{10}$$

(a)

(b)

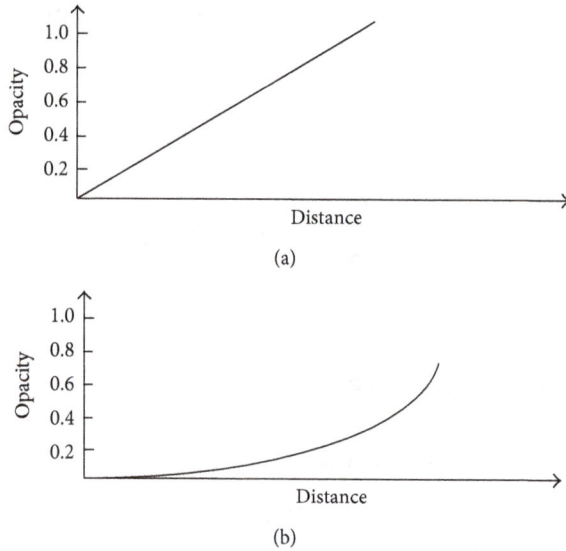

FIGURE 3: (a) Linear gradient. (b) Quadratic gradient.

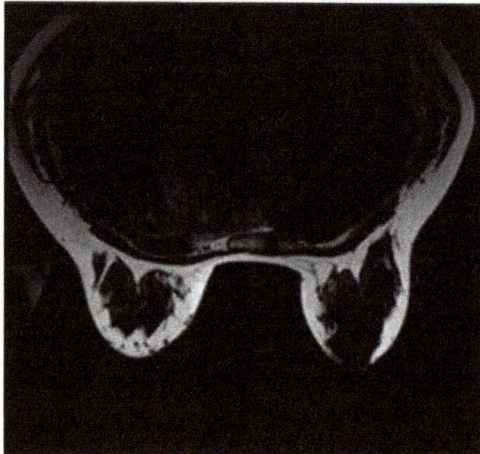

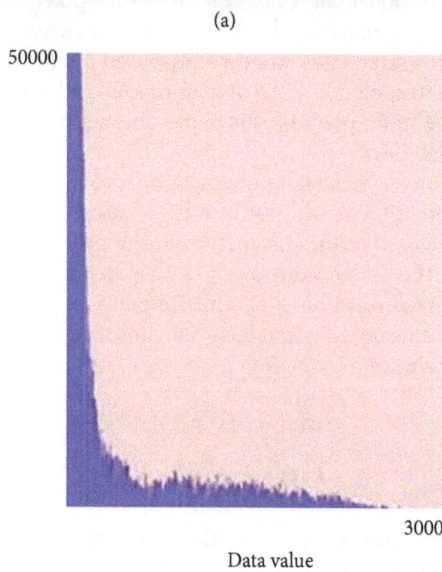

(a)

(b)

FIGURE 4: Breast MR image and its histogram. ((a) original MRI; (b) histogram).

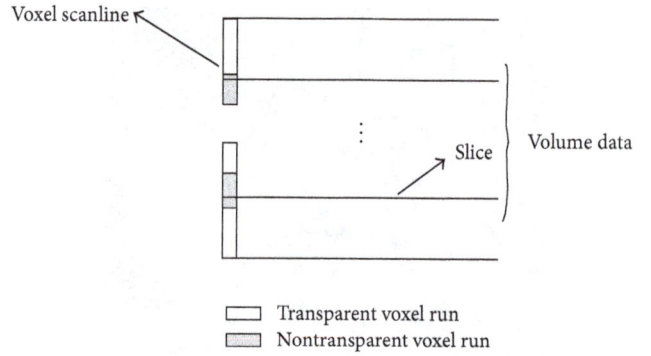

FIGURE 5: Scanline is perpendicular to the slices and skips the transparent region.

However, $k(t)$ is usually not constant. It depends on the distance from the eye, so

$$c' = c \cdot e^{-\int_0^d k(t)dt}. \tag{11}$$

So, the integral over the absorption coefficients in the exponent is

$$T(d_1, d_2) = \int_{d_2}^{d_1} k(t) \, dt, \tag{12}$$

which is also called the optical depth [15]. It is a single point. We should perform integral for all possible positions t along the ray to acquire the total amount of radiant energy C reaching the eye from direction:

$$C = \int_0^\infty c(t) \cdot e^{-T(0,t)dt}. \tag{13}$$

The integral of (12) can be approximated by a Riemann sum:

$$T(0, t) \approx \sum_{i=0}^{\lfloor t/\Delta t \rfloor} k(i \cdot \Delta t) \Delta t, \tag{14}$$

where Δt represents the distance between resampling points.

According to exponential formula, the component of (13) can be redefined as

$$e^{-T(0,t)} = \prod_{i=0}^{\lfloor t/\Delta t \rfloor} e^{-k(i \cdot \Delta t)\Delta t}. \tag{15}$$

The approximate evaluation of the volume rendering integral is

$$C = \sum_{i=0}^{n} C_i \prod_{j=0}^{i-1} (1 - A_j), \tag{16}$$

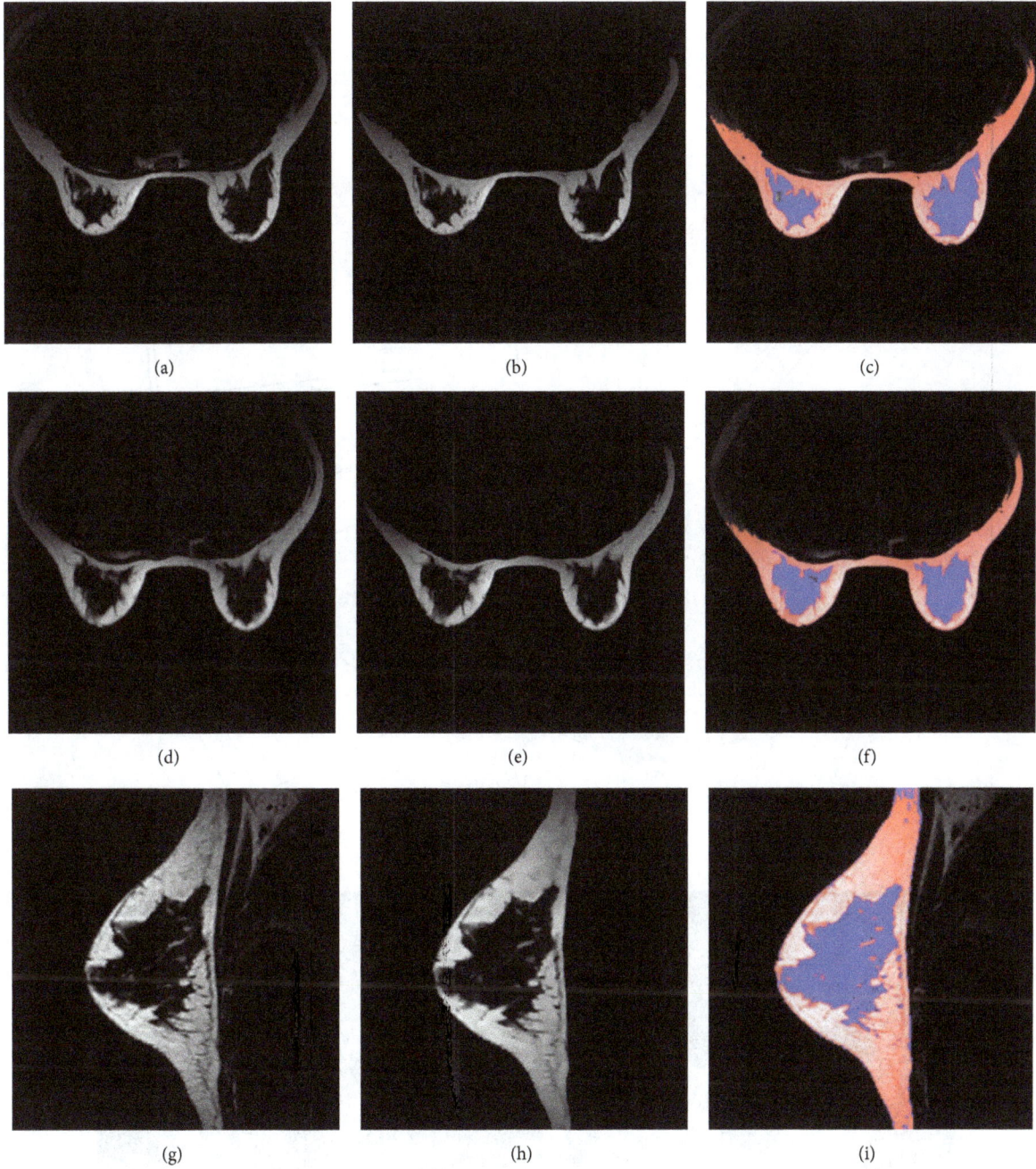

FIGURE 6: The results of segmentation in 2D field. ((a),(d), and (g) original images; (b), (e), and (h) the results of preprocessing; (c), (f), and (i) the result of KFCM.

where n is the number of samples, A_j is called opacity, and C_i is the emitted color of the ith ray segment:

$$A_i = 1 - e^{-k(i*\Delta t)\Delta t}, \tag{17}$$

$$C_i = c\,(i \cdot \Delta t)\,\Delta t. \tag{18}$$

In our case, the front-to-back order is applied by stepping i from 1 to n. The following iterative addresses (16):

$$\begin{aligned} C_i' &= C_{i+1}' + \left(1 - A_{i-1}'\right) C_i, \\ A_i' &= A_{i-1}' + \left(1 - A_{i-1}'\right) A_i \end{aligned} \tag{19}$$

So we can get one pixel of the final image. After all the pixels of the final image are integrated from all directions, the result of volume rendering will be displayed.

3.2. A New Transfer Function Model. Function $a(x)$ which is termed the opacity distribution function is introduced [16], which maps data value in an identical tissue to opacity. The independent variable is the Euclidean distance between data values and clustering centers, which are generated through KFCM. This function can be a piecewise function, polynomial function, or spline. In Figure 3, two opacity distribution

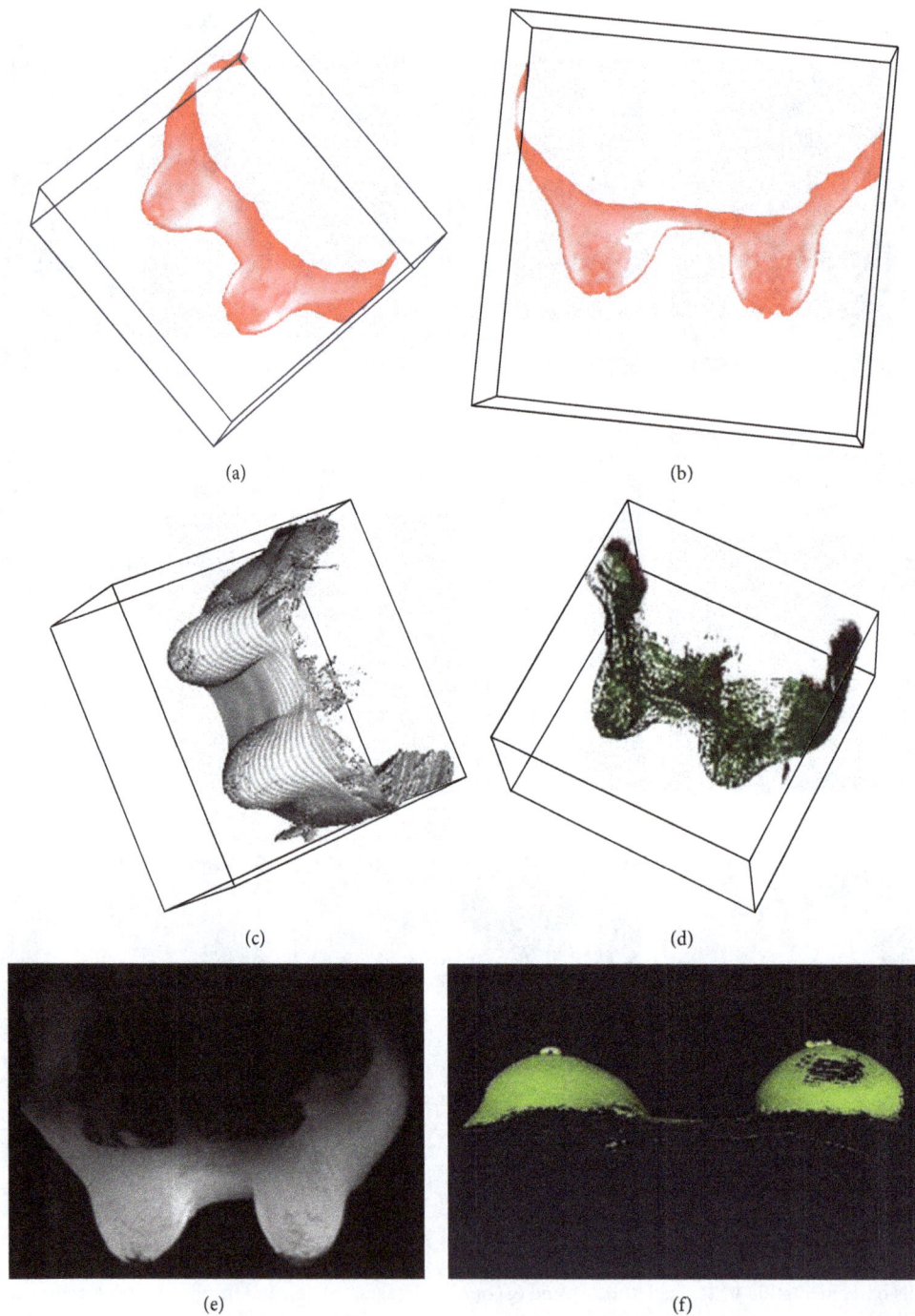

FIGURE 7: Results of 3D segmentation and visualization. ((a), (b) Results of segmentation and visualization based on proposed algorithms; (c) result of Marching Cubes; (d) result of ray casting with a linear transfer function; (e) result of MIP; (f) result of ImageVis3D).

functions are demonstrated. In Figure 3(a), the opacity has a linear gradient from the center of the sphere to the outline. In Figure 3(b), the opacity has a quadratic gradient in which we can largely concentrate on the boundary of the material.

3.3. *Performance Optimization.* According to Figure 4, the histogram of data values of one slice in the dataset implies that the data value of many points is zero. They should deserve

little attention. But in traditional ray-cast algorithm, we have to consider the voxels which contribute nothing to the final image. Therefore, a scanline that is perpendicular to the slices is introduced (Figure 5). The scanline consists of gray segments and white segments. The white segments represent transparent parts in the volume, which contribute little to the final image. So, the interpolation in preprocess and the iterative of (19) are abstained in transparent segments of the corresponding scanline. Therefore, the compositing speeds up.

4. Results and Discussion

The breast MR images we used in this paper were acquired from the Military General Hospital of Beijing PLA. There are 28 slices of 512×512 samples each. The procedure was implemented on a 3.4 GHz CPU, 2 G memory PC.

Figure 6 shows the results of KFCM algorithm of three slices in the dataset. This example indicates the effectiveness of KFCM algorithm in 2D field. Fibroglandular and fat tissues can be relatively separated precisely. The blue region is fibroglandular tissue. The shortcoming of KFCM is that the convergence time cannot be predicted and may be unacceptably long. However, through the initialization of clustering centers in Section 2.3, the convergence time can be made more acceptable.

Figure 7 shows the results of the breast visualization through various algorithms. In Figure 7(c), we can see that the result of Marching Cubes algorithm can well display the breast skin, but the internal structure cannot be seen. A simple linear transfer function was used to produce a result with misty fibroglandular tissue, as shown in Figure 7(d). The green regions represent fibroglandular tissue, and the white regions represent fat tissue. They are mixed together, so we could not easily distinguish them.

Figure 7(e) shows the result of MIP. MIP uses the maximum value encountered along a ray to determine the color, so it is difficult to design the transfer function. However, the region having the maximum value may not be the interested region, and furthermore it does not consider the contribution of the other points along the ray.

Figure 7(f) shows the results of ImageVis3D system which is developed by the Center for Integrative Biomedical Computing, University of Utah. This system can visualize the biological tissue well, but the transfer function should be adjusted manually, and the quality of the rendered image depends on the user's experience.

Figures 7(a) and 7(b) show the visualization of breast by KFCM algorithm. The number of clustering centers in KFCM is three: fat tissue, fibroglandular tissue, and air. The comparison of convergence time is shown in Table 1. We have tested a single dataset for three times. From Table 1, we can see that the convergence time is stably six minutes with the evaluation of the clustering center proposed in Section 2.3. It is faster and more predicable than KFCM with random clustering centers. Then, using the compositing algorithm described in Section 3.1 and the quadratic opacity distribution function described in Section 3.2, two views are computed. Comparing with the other results, Figures 7(a) and 7(b) show the fibroglandular more clearly. Fibroglandular tissue is separated from fat tissue well. The pink regions in the breast represent fibroglandular tissue, and the white regions in the breast represent fat tissue.

5. Conclusion

A 3D segmentation algorithm based on Kernel-based Fuzzy C-Means (KFCM) is presented to separate the breast images into different tissues. In the KFCM algorithm, we propose to evaluate the clustering centers through the rough boundary of breast tissues before clustering process. Then, an improved volume rendering algorithm based on a new transfer function model is applied to implement 3D breast visualization. Experimental results show that our algorithm can efficiently segment fibroglandular and fat tissues. Also, the visualization performance of our algorithm is better than ray-casting algorithm with a linear transfer function and MIP, which makes it useful for breast lesion detection and quantitative analysis.

TABLE 1: KFCM convergence time.

Test order	KFCM with evaluation of clustering center (mins)	KFCM with random clustering center (mins)
1	6	21
2	6	15
3	6	32

Acknowledgment

This project is supported by the National Natural Science Foundation of China (Grant no. 61240010).

References

[1] D. Raba, A. Oliver, J. Martí, M. Peracaula, and J. Espunya, "Breast segmentation with pectoral muscle suppression on digital mammograms," in *Proceedings of the 2nd Iberian Conference on Pattern Recognition and Image Analysis (IbPRIA '05)*, pp. 471–478, Estoril, Portugal, June 2005.

[2] W. Chen, M. L. Giger, and U. Bick, "A fuzzy c-means (FCM)-based approach for computerized segmentation of breast lesions in dynamic contrast-enhanced MR images," *Academic Radiology*, vol. 13, no. 1, pp. 63–72, 2006.

[3] S. R. Kannan, S. Ramathilagam, and A. Sathya, "Robust fuzzy C-means in classifying breast tissue regions," in *Proceedings of the International Conference on Advances in Recent Technologies in Communication and Computing (ARTCom '09)*, pp. 543–545, October 2009.

[4] P. Pathmanathan, "Predicting tumour location by simulating the deformation of the breast using nonlinear elasticity and the finite element method," Wolfson College University of Oxford, 2006.

[5] K. Nie, J.-H. Chen, S. Chan et al., "Development of a quantitative method for analysis of breast density based on three-dimensional breast MRI," *Medical Physics*, vol. 35, no. 12, pp. 5253–5262, 2008.

[6] W. E. Lorensen and H. E. Cline, "Marching Cubes: a high resolution 3D surface construction algorithm," *Computer Graphics*, vol. 21, no. 4, pp. 163–169, 1987.

[7] M. Levoy, "Display of surfaces from volume data," *IEEE Computer Graphics and Applications*, vol. 8, no. 5, pp. 29–37, 1988.

[8] N. Max, "Optical models for direct volume rendering," *IEEE Transactions on Visualization and Computer Graphics*, vol. 1, no. 2, pp. 99–108, 1995.

[9] P. Lacroute and M. Levoy, "Fast volume rendering using a shear-warp factorization of the viewing transformation," in *Proceedings of the ACM Computer Graphics (SIGGRAPH '94)*, pp. 451–458, July 1994.

[10] P. Perona and J. Malik, "Scale-space and edge detection using anisotropic diffusion," *IEEE Transactions on Pattern Analysis and Machine Intelligence*, vol. 12, no. 7, pp. 629–639, 1990.

[11] R. O. Duda, P. E. Har, and D. G. Stork, *Pattern Classification*, Wiley-Interscience, New York, NY, USA, 2nd edition, 2001.

[12] D. Zhang, "Kernel-based associative memories, clustering algorithms and their applications," Nanjing University of Aeronautics and Astronautics, 2004 (Chinese).

[13] D. Q. Zhang, "Kernel-based fuzzy clustering incorporating spatial constraints for image segmentation," in *Proceedings of the International Conference on Machine Learning and Cybernetics*, vol. 4, pp. 2189–2192.

[14] B. Wang, Q. Zhi, Z. Zhang, G. Geng, and M. Zhou, "Computation of center of mass for gray level image based on differential moments factor," *Journal of Computer-Aided Design and Computer Graphics*, vol. 16, no. 10, pp. 1360–1365, 2004 (Chinese).

[15] K. Engel, M. Hadwiger, and J. M. Kniss, "Real-time volume graphics," in *Proceedings of the ACM Computer Graphics (SIGGRAPH '04)*, article 29, 2004.

[16] G. Kindlmann and J. W. Durkin, "Semi-automatic generation of transfer functions for direct volume rendering ," in *Proceedings of the IEEE Symposium on Volume Visualization*, pp. 79–86, Research Triangle Park, NC, USA, 1998.

14

Contrast Improvement in Sub- and Ultraharmonic Ultrasound Contrast Imaging by Combining Several Hammerstein Models

Fatima Sbeity,[1] **Sébastien Ménigot,**[1,2] **Jamal Charara,**[3] **and Jean-Marc Girault**[1]

[1] Université François Rabelais de Tours, UMR-S930, 37032 Tours, France
[2] IUT Ville d'Avray, Université Paris Ouest Nanterre La Défense, 92410 Ville d'Avray, France
[3] Département de Physique et d'Électronique, Faculté des Sciences I, Université Libanaise, Hadath, Lebanon

Correspondence should be addressed to Jean-Marc Girault; jean-marc.girault@univ-tours.fr

Academic Editor: Guowei Wei

Sub- and ultraharmonic (SUH) ultrasound contrast imaging is an alternative modality to the second harmonic imaging, since, in specific conditions it could produce high quality echographic images. This modality enables the contrast enhancement of echographic images by using SUH present in the contrast agent response but absent from the nonperfused tissue. For a better access to the components generated by the ultrasound contrast agents, nonlinear techniques based on Hammerstein model are preferred. As the major limitation of Hammerstein model is its capacity of modeling harmonic components only, in this work we propose two methods allowing to model SUH. These new methods use several Hammerstein models to identify contrast agent signals having SUH components and to separate these components from harmonic components. The application of the proposed methods for modeling simulated contrast agent signals shows their efficiency in modeling these signals and in separating SUH components. The achieved gain with respect to the standard Hammerstein model was 26.8 dB and 22.8 dB for the two proposed methods, respectively.

1. Introduction

Introduction of contrast agents in ultrasound medical imaging has strongly improved the image contrast leading to a better medical diagnosis [1–3]. By adapting the transmitting ultrasound sequences composed of short wave trains to longer sinusoidal wave trains, it has been possible to enhance the harmonics detection witnessing of the presence of nonlinear explored media [3–5]. The most prominent example in echographic imaging is the second harmonic imaging (SHI) [3, 6] which consists to send a sinusoidal wave train of frequency f_0 and to receive the backscattered signal at twice the transmitted frequency, that is, $2f_0$ (see Figure 1).

Although the second harmonic imaging possesses undoubted advantages compared to standard echographic imaging, contrast harmonic imaging, however, has image contrast limitations related to the presence of harmonic components of nonlinear nonperfused tissues [7]. This contrast reduction can be overcome by proposing no more contrast harmonic imaging but rather contrast subultraharmonic (SUH) imaging [8, 9]. Under certain conditions of incident

frequency and pressure levels, this solution has been envisaged as a serious alternative [10, 11] since it has been shown that only contrast agent is capable of supplying SUH components sufficient to construct perfused tissue images with a strong contrast. Contrast SUH imaging consists to send a sinusoidal wave train of frequency f_0 and to extract from the backscattered signal only SUH frequencies at $f_0/2$, $(3/2)f_0, (5/2)f_0, \ldots$ (see Figure 2).

To extract such SUH components from the whole spectrum, a certain number of approaches called "black box methods" has been proposed such as those based on the multiple input and single output (MISO) Volterra filtering [12–14]. These recent methods are capable of accurately modeling the signal backscattered by the contrast agent with adequate values of order and memory of such models. However, these methods are quite complex methods, and they do not give an extraction of harmonic components $f_0, 2f_0$, $3f_0, \ldots$ and SUH components $(f_0/2)2, (3/2)f_0, (5/2)f_0, \ldots$ since they model all spectral components $(f_0/2)2, f_0, (3/2)f_0$, $2f_0, (5/2)f_0, 3f_0, \ldots$

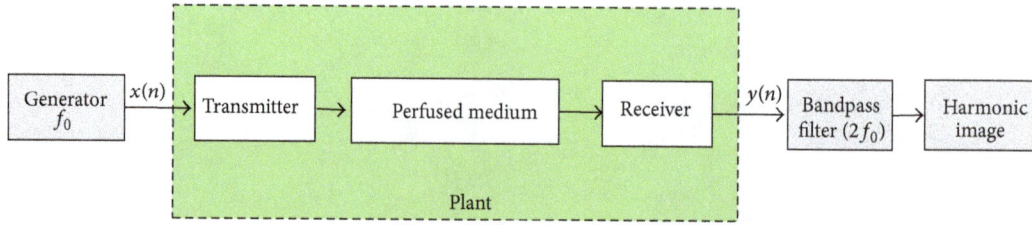

FIGURE 1: Block diagram of second harmonic imaging.

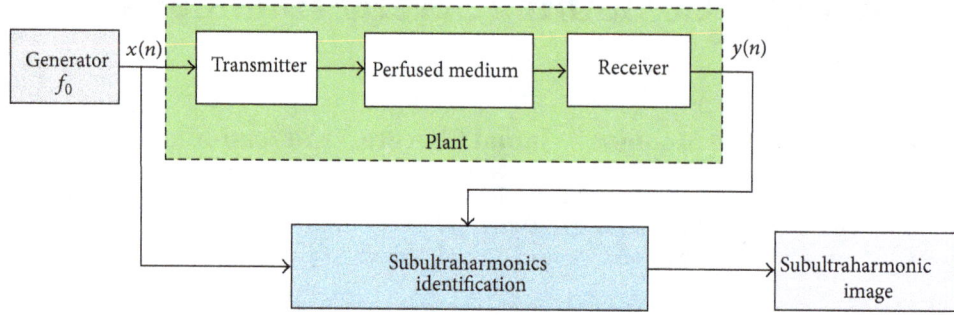

FIGURE 2: Block diagram of subultraharmonic imaging.

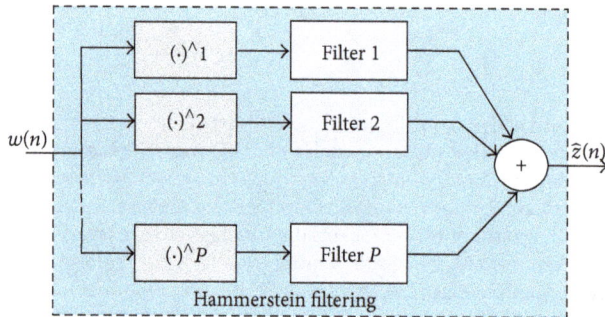

FIGURE 3: Block diagram of Hammerstein model.

In order to reduce the complexity of such methods and to extract SUH components from all spectral components, we propose two new original approaches neither based on the Volterra filtering but based on the Hammerstein filtering.

This paper is organized as follows: after recalling standard Hammerstein model, the new methods are presented. To validate our methods, we propose realistic simulations of contrast agents signals. Then a quantitative and qualitative comparison is made between the two proposed methods with respect to standard Hammerstein model. Finally a discussion completed by a conclusion closed the paper.

2. Methods

Polynomial Hammerstein model is a special type of nonlinear filters in which a static nonlinear system is followed by a dynamic linear system [15]. From this model, the nonlinear system is approximated by a polynomial function, and the linear part is a finite impulse response (FIR) filter. The block diagram of Hammerstein model is shown in Figure 3.

As for the Volterra decomposition, the Hammerstein decomposition is able to model harmonic components, but it was unable to model sub- and ultraharmonic (SUH) components. Before explaining how it was possible to model SUH components, we recall the Hammerstein decomposition.

2.1. Hammerstein Decomposition. The Hammerstein modeled signal $\widehat{z}(n)$ can be seen as the summation of P signals $z_p(n)$ coming from P parallel branches:

$$\widehat{z}(n) = \sum_{p=1}^{p} z_p(n). \tag{1}$$

In each branch, the signal $z_p(n)$ is the output of a linear filter $h_p(n)$ of input $w_p(n)$:

$$z_p(n) = \sum_{m=1}^{M} h_p(m) \cdot w^p(n-m) = \mathbf{w}_p(n)^T \mathbf{h}_p \tag{2}$$

with $\mathbf{h}_p = [h_p(1), \ldots, h_p(M)]^T$ and $\mathbf{w}_p(n) = [w^p(n-1), \ldots, w^p(n-M)]^T$. Note that the input filter signals $w_p(n) = w^p(n)$ are obtained from a polynomial function. Finally, $\forall n \in [M + 1, M + 2, \ldots, N]$, where N is the length of the input signal $w(n)$ and the vector signal of each branch p can be written by

$$\mathbf{Z}_p = \mathbf{W}_p^T \mathbf{h}_p \tag{3}$$

with $\mathbf{Z}_p^T = [z_p(M + 1), z_p(M + 2), \ldots, z_p(N)]$, and $\mathbf{W}_p = [\mathbf{w}_p(M), \mathbf{w}_p(M-1), \ldots, \mathbf{w}_p(N)]$. The output signal $\widehat{z}(n)$ of the model could be written in a vector form $\widehat{\mathbf{Z}}$ as follows:

$$\widehat{\mathbf{Z}} = \mathbf{W}\mathbf{H} \tag{4}$$

with $\mathbf{H} = [\mathbf{h}_1^T, \mathbf{h}_2^T, \ldots, \mathbf{h}_P^T]^T$ and $\mathbf{W} = [\mathbf{W}_1^T, \mathbf{W}_2^T, \ldots, \mathbf{W}_P^T]$. To determine directly the filter parameters $\mathbf{H}$ from (4), we have to minimize the mean square error given by

$$\arg \min_{h_p} \left(\mathbb{E} \left[(z - \hat{z})^2 \right] \right), \tag{5}$$

where z is the output signal of the non linear system and $\mathbb{E}$ is the symbol of the mathematical expectation. The corresponding solution is

$$\mathbf{H} = \left(\mathbf{W}^T \mathbf{W} \right)^{-1} \mathbf{W}^T \mathbf{Z}, \tag{6}$$

if $(\mathbf{W}^T \mathbf{W})$ is invertible. Otherwise, regularization techniques can be used.

Consequently, identifying a nonlinear system of input $x(n)$ and output $z(n)$ with an Hammerstein model is equivalent to calculate the signal $\hat{z}(n)$ using (4) and (5).

2.2. Sub- and Ultraharmonics Modeling.

As previously mentioned, Hammerstein model is able to model harmonic components only. This is justified by the steady state theorem reported in [16] which stipulates that the output response of the model to a periodic input of frequency f_0 is also a periodic signal of fundamental frequency f_0. Suppose that the transmitted signal $x(n)$ is periodic of frequency f_0, and that the signal backscattered by the contrast agent has the following spectral components $(f_0/2)2, f_0, (3/2)f_0, 2f_0, (5/2)f_0, 3f_0, \ldots$. Let $\hat{y}_{11}(n)$ be the output signal of the Hammerstein model of input $x(n)$ (see Figure 4). According to the theorem reported in [16], the spectral content of the output signal $\hat{y}_{11}(n)$ is composed of the following harmonic components $f_0, 2f_0, 3f_0, \ldots$ if and only if the input frequency is f_0.

Thus, modeling SUH components of frequency $f_0/2$, $(3/2)f_0, (5/2)f_0, \ldots$ using Hammerstein model is possible if and only if these components could be seen as integer multiples of the input frequency to the Hammerstein model. To do this, some modifications must be performed. Two types of modifications are proposed in this work, either at the input or at the output. Based on these two types of modifications, two methods for modeling and separating the sub- and ultraharmonic components using Hammerstein models are described in this section.

Each of the two proposed methods consists of two steps: one step for harmonic modeling and another step for SUH modeling. The first method is based on the modification of the input frequency, while the second one is based on modification of the output frequency.

2.2.1. Method 1: Modeling by Input Frequency Shifting.

As previously mentioned, this method consists of two steps; each step uses one Hammerstein model as presented in Figure 4.

(1) Harmonic modeling: harmonic modeling is done by identifying the system of input $x_{11}(n) = x(n)$ and output $y(n)$ with an Hammerstein model. The obtained signal $\hat{y}_{11}(n)$ has the harmonic components only. Referring to (4), the harmonic signal $\hat{y}_{11}(n)$ could be written as

$$\hat{Y}_{11} = X_{11} H_{11} \tag{7}$$

with X_{11} and H_{11} defined as in Section 1.

(2) sub- and ultraharmonic modeling: the SUH information is found in the difference signal $y_{21}(n)$ between the output signal $y(n)$ and the harmonic signal $\hat{y}_{11}(n)$:

$$y_{21}(n) = y(n) - \hat{y}_{11}(n). \tag{8}$$

The spectral content of $y_{21}(n)$ is composed of $f_0/2$, $(3/2)f_0, (5/2)f_0, \ldots$ by referring to the previous theorem; these components could be modeled using Hammerstein model if the input frequency is $f_0/2$. Consequently, the initial input signal $x(n)$ must be modified in such a way to bring up the subharmonic frequency $f_0/2$. To do this, the spectrum of $x(n)$ is downshifted by $f_0/2$ to shift the frequency f_0 toward the position of $f_0/2$. The modified input $x_{12}(n)$ is calculated according to the following equation:

$$x_{12}(n) = \mathfrak{R} \left((x(n) + j\tilde{x}(n,)) \cdot e^{-2\pi j(f_0/2)nT_s} \right)$$
$$= x(n) \cos \left(2\pi f_0 nT_s \frac{f_0}{2} \right) + \tilde{x}(n) \sin \left(2\pi nT_s \frac{f_0}{2} \right), \tag{9}$$

where $\mathfrak{R}$ is the real part, $\tilde{x}(n) = \mathcal{H}(x(n))$ is the Hilbert transform of $x(n)$, and T_s is the sampling frequency.

The modified input signal $x_{12}(n)$ could be written in the following vectorial form:

$$X_{12} = X_C + \widetilde{X}_C, \tag{10}$$

with

$$X_C = \left[x(1) \cos \left(2\pi \frac{f_0}{2} T_s \right) \quad x(2) \cos \left(2\pi 2 \frac{f_0}{2} T_s \right) \right.$$
$$\left. \cdots \quad x(N) \cos \left(2\pi N \frac{f_0}{2} T_s \right) \right],$$

$$\widetilde{X}_C = \left[x(1) \cos \left(2\pi \frac{f_0}{2} T_s \right) \quad x(2) \cos \left(2\pi 2 \frac{f_0}{2} T_s \right) \right.$$
$$\left. \cdots \quad x(N) \cos \left(2\pi N \frac{f_0}{2} T_s \right) \right]. \tag{11}$$

Then, the SUH signal $\hat{y}_{12}$ is the output of a Hammerstein model that identifies the system of input $x_{12}(n)$ and output $y_{12}(n)$. In the same way, $\hat{y}_{12}(n)$ is calculated according to the following equation:

$$\hat{Y}_{12} = X_{12} H_{12}. \tag{12}$$

Finally, the total modeled signal $\hat{y}(n)$ is the sum of the harmonic signal $\hat{y}_{11}(n)$ and the sub- and ultraharmonic signal $\hat{y}_{12}(n)$:

$$\hat{y}(n) = \hat{y}_{11}(n) + \hat{y}_{12}(n). \tag{13}$$

For this method, note that the maximal frequency that could be modeled is limited by the order P of the Hammerstein model. It is well known that the Hammerstein model of order P excited by a signal of frequency f_0 can model harmonic components until the Pth harmonic of

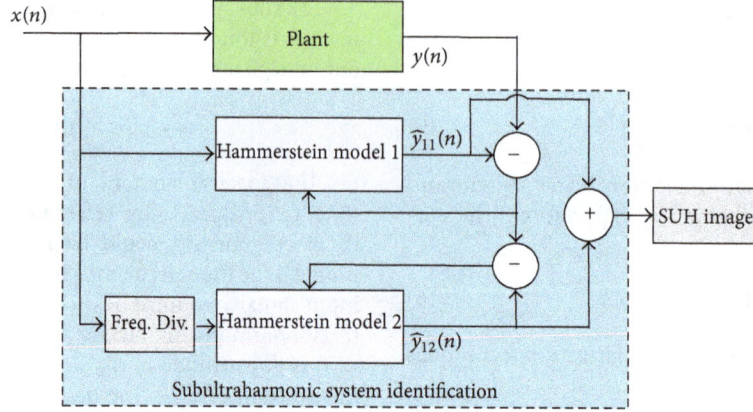

FIGURE 4: Block diagram of method 1, modeling by input frequency downshifting.

frequency Pf_0. In the case of ultrasound contrast agent and for some conditions explained later, the subharmonic component is $(f_0/2)$. In the second step of method 1, the Pth harmonic is $P(f_0/2)$. For example, modeling $y_{21}(n)$ with an Hammerstein model of order $P = 3$ and input $x_{mod}(n)$ of frequency $(f_0/2)$, calculated using (19), can model sub- and ultraharmonics until $(3/2)f_0$. Therefore, to model all the sub- and ultraharmonic components presented in the signal $y_{21}(n)$, the order of the Hammerstein model must be adjust by increasing to $P = 5$.

2.2.2. Method 2: Modeling by Output Frequency Shifting. This method also consists of two steps, on step dedicated for harmonic modeling and another step dedicated for SUH modeling. Each step uses one Hammerstein model as presented in Figure 5.

(1) Harmonic modeling: this step is the same as the first step of the method 1. The signal $y(n)$ is modeled with a Hammerstein model of input $x_{21}(n) = x(n)$. The obtained signal is the harmonic signal $\hat{y}_{21}(n)$ calculated according to

$$\hat{Y}_{21} = X_{21}H_{21}. \tag{14}$$

(2) Sub- and Ultraharmonic modeling: based on the same idea as reported in method 1, SUH components could be modeled when they are considered as integer multiples of the input frequency. In this method, we propose to keep the input signal $x(n)$ and to change the output signal $y(n)$ by upshifting its spectrum of $f_0/2$. Now, the SUH components are shifted toward the harmonics position, and then they could be modeled with a Hammerstein model. The modified output signal $y_{mod}(n)$ is calculated according to the following equation:

$$y_{mod}(n) = \Re\left((y(n) + j\tilde{y}(n)) \cdot e^{2\pi j(f_0/2)nT_s}\right)$$

$$= y(n)\cos\left(2\pi nT_s\frac{f_0}{2}\right) - \tilde{y}(n)\sin\left(2\pi nT_s\frac{f_0}{2}\right). \tag{15}$$

In vector form,

$$Y_{mod} = Y_C + \tilde{Y}_C, \tag{16}$$

with

$$Y_C = \left[\ y(1)\cos\left(2\pi\frac{f_0}{2}T_s\right)\ \ y(2)\cos\left(2\pi 2\frac{f_0}{2}T_s\right)\right.$$
$$\left.\cdots\ y(N)\cos\left(2\pi N\frac{f_0}{2}T_s\right)\ \right]$$

$$\tilde{Y}_C = \left[\ -\tilde{y}(1)\sin\left(2\pi\frac{f_0}{2}T_s\right)\ \ -\tilde{y}(2)\sin\left(2\pi 2\frac{f_0}{2}T_s\right)\right.$$
$$\left.\cdots\ -\tilde{y}(N)\sin\left(2\pi N\frac{f_0}{2}T_s\right)\ \right]. \tag{17}$$

Then the signal $y_{mod}(n)$ is modeled with a Hammerstein model of input $x(n)$. The obtained signal $\hat{y}_{22_{mod}}(n)$ is calculated according to the following equation:

$$\hat{Y}_{mod} = XH_{mod}. \tag{18}$$

has SUH components upshifted by $f_0/2$. To recover the sub- and ultraharmonic signal $\hat{y}_{22}(n)$, the signal $\hat{y}_{22_{mod}}(n)$ is downshifted of $f_0/2$ according to the following equation:

$$\hat{y}_{22}(n) = \Re\left(\left(\hat{y}_{mod}(n) + j\tilde{\hat{y}}_{mod}(n)\right) \cdot e^{-2\pi j(f_0/2)nT_s}\right)$$

$$= \hat{y}_{mod}(n)\cos\left(2\pi nT_e\frac{f_0}{2}\right)$$

$$+ \tilde{\hat{y}}_{mod}(n)\sin\left(2\pi nT_s\frac{f_0}{2}\right). \tag{19}$$

The final signal $\hat{y}(n)$ is the sum of the harmonic signal $\hat{y}_{11}(n)$ and the sub- and ultraharmonic signal $\hat{y}_{22}(n)$:

$$\hat{y}(n) = \hat{y}_{21}(n) + \hat{y}_{22}(n). \tag{20}$$

3. Simulations and Results

To validate the two proposed methods and to quantify their performance in ultrasound medical imaging, realistic simulations are proposed. To achieve these simulations, the free simulation program Bubblesim developed by Hoff [17] was used to calculate the scattered echoes for a specified

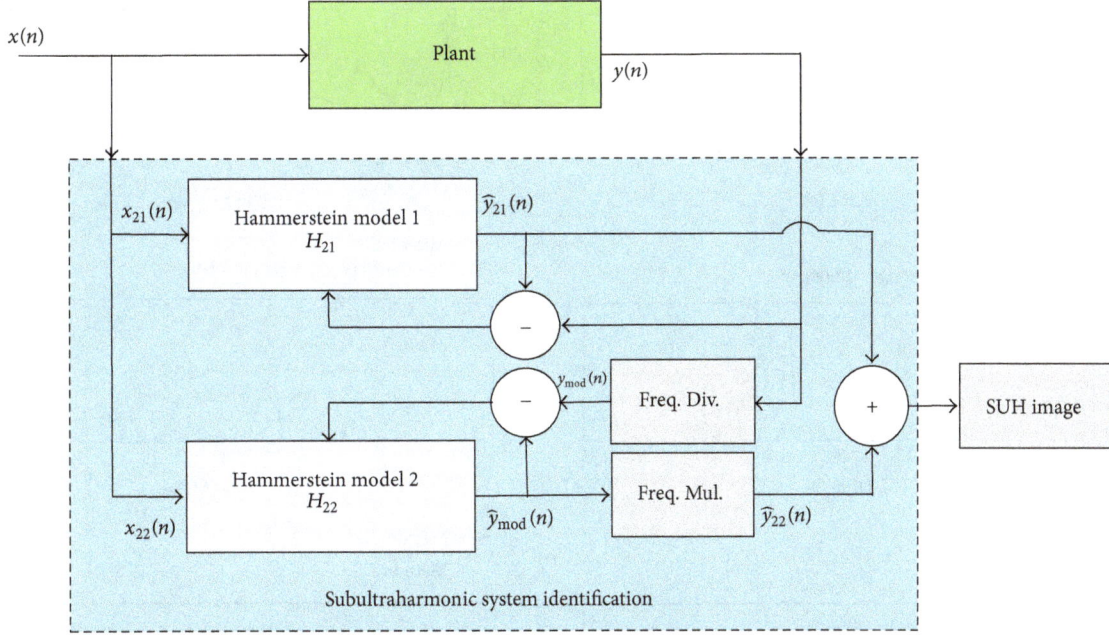

FIGURE 5: Block diagram of method 2: modeling by output frequency shifting.

TABLE 1: The parameters of contrast agent.

Resting radius	$r_0 = 1.5\,\mu m$
Shell thickness	$d_{Se} = 1.5\,nm$
Shear modulus	$G_s = 10\,MPa$
Shear viscosity	$\eta = 1.49\,Pa\cdot s$

contrast agent and excitation pulse. A modified version of Rayleigh-Plesset equation was chosen. The model presented by Church [18] and then modified by Hoff [17] is based on the theoretical description of contrast agents as air-filled particles with surface layers of elastic solids. In order to simulate the mean behavior of a contrast agent cloud, we hypothesized that the response of a cloud of N contrast agents was N times the response of a single contrast agent with the mean properties.

The incident burst is a sinusoidal wave composed of 18 cycles of frequency $f_0 = 4.5\,MHz$ and pressure of 0.6 MPa [13]. (The resonance frequency of the encapsulated contrast agent of 1.5 μm is about 2.5 MHz. The emission frequency at 4.5 MHz is nearly the double of the resonance frequency.) Under the previous conditions of frequency and pressure, the oscillation of the contrast agent is nonlinear with sub- and ultraharmonic generation. The sampling frequency is $f_s = 1/T_s = 60\,MHz$. The parameters of the contrast agent are given in the Table 1.

In this research work, the performances of the different methods are evaluated qualitatively and quantitatively.

3.1. Qualitative Evaluation.
Figure 6 represents a qualitative comparison in both time and frequency domains between the signal backscattered by the contrast agent $y(n)$ and the signal obtained with the standard Hammerstein model, method 1, and method 2. Method 1 is applied with a Hammerstein

model of order $P = 3$ and memory $M = 30$ for the first step and a Hammerstein model of order $P = 5$ and memory $M = 30$ for the second step. Method 2 is applied with a Hammerstein model of order $P = 3$ for the two steps and memory $M = 30$.

Figure 6(a) (top) shows that the modeled signal with the standard Hammerstein model does not describe correctly the signal backscattered by the contrast agent. Corresponding spectra in Figure 6(b) (top) show that the signal modeled with the standard Hammerstein model has the harmonic components only (f_0, $2f_0$, and $3f_0$). Figure 6(b) (middle, bottom) shows that the signals modeled with methods 1 and 2 perfectly describe the contrast agent signal. Corresponding spectra on Figure 6(b) (middle, bottom) show that all the frequency components are modeled: harmonics at ($f_0, 2f_0, 3f_0$), subharmonic $f_0/2$, and ultraharmonics ($(3/2)f_0, (5/2)f_0$).

Figure 7(a) (top) shows the different signal between $y(n)$ and the harmonic signal (in black) and the sub- and ultraharmonic signal obtained with method 1 (top) and method 2 (bottom). We can see the good agreement between the signals. Spectra on Figure 7(b). (top) confirms that subharmonic $f_0/2$, first ultra-harmonic $(3/2)f_0$, and second ultraharmonic $(5/2)f_0$ are well modeled and separated from other harmonic components. These results confirm the efficiency of the two proposed methods in modeling and separating the sub- and ultraharmonics present in contrast agent response.

3.1.1. Quantitative Evaluation.
To quantify the performance of each method and to know which method provides the best performance, a quantitative study is necessary. The relative mean square error EQMR defined as

$$\text{RMSE} = \frac{E\left[\left|\hat{y}(n) - y(n)\right|^2\right]}{E\left[\left|y(n)\right|^2\right]} \qquad (21)$$

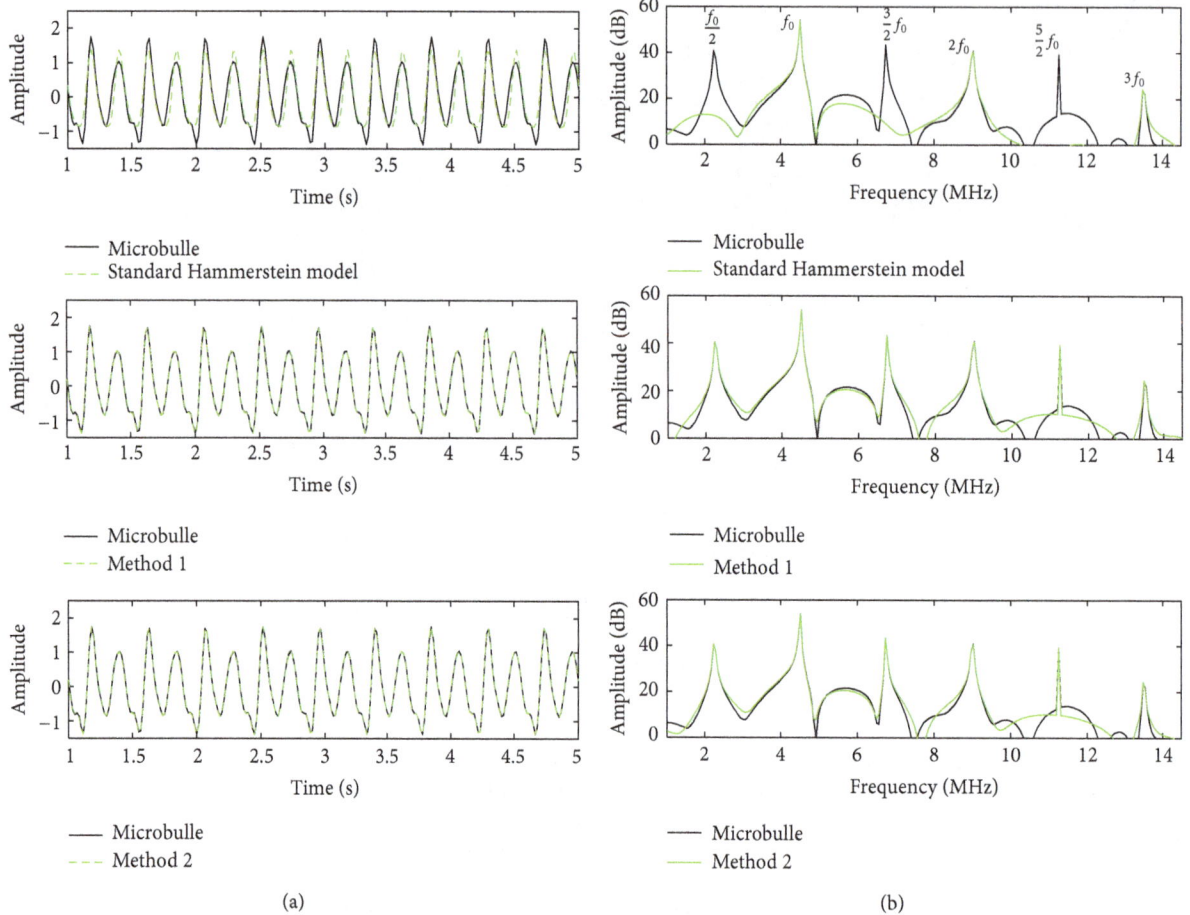

FIGURE 6: (a) Comparison between the signal backscattered by the contrast agent $y(n)$ (in black) and its estimation $\hat{y}(n)$ (in green): the signal modeled with (top) the standard Hammerstein model, (middle) method 1, and (bottom) method 2. (b) Spectra of different signals presented in (a). Here SNR = ∞ dB.

TABLE 2: RMSE between the signal backscattered by the contrast agent and that modeled with the Hammerstein model, method 1, and method 2.

	Standard Hammerstein	Method 1	Method 2
RMSE (dB)	−8.3	−30.5	−31.1

is evaluated for different noise levels at the system output. The noise level adjusted as the function of SNR (signal to noise ratio) is Gaussian and white. Ten realizations are made to evaluate the fluctuations of RMSE. RMSE for SNR = ∞, 20, 15, 10 dB is reported in Figure 8.

These simulations show that the RMSE achieved with the two proposed methods 1 and 2 is always less than the RMSE achieved with the standard Hammerstein model for the different SNR values.

The gap between the standard model and the two methods 1 and 2 decreases when the SNR value increases. A gap ranging from 4 to 26 dB could be obtained depending on the SNR conditions. These results confirm that the standard Hammerstein model is not adapted for sub- and ultra-harmonic modeling. A zoom on Figure 8(d) shows that the

RMSE varies slightly around a mean value. This result shows that the two methods 1 and 2 are robust toward noise. Note that the curves of variation of RMSE obtained with the two methods have the same trend, indicating that the two methods tend toward the optimal solution.

Table 2 sums up the RMSE values obtained with the standard Hammerstein model, method 1, and method 2 when the SNR = ∞.

4. Discussions and Conclusions

In this research work the problem of modeling sub and ultra-harmonics with Hammerstein model is presented. Usually, the standard Hammerstein model is able to model harmonics only, which are integer multiples of the input frequency. Sub and ultra-harmonics could not be modeled.

In this work, we propose for the first time two new methods that use Hammerstein filters that model sub and ultra-harmonics. The two methods are based on the same idea stipulating that modeling SUH with Hammerstein model is possible if the input signal or the output signal is modified In such a way that the SUH components become in the position of integer multiples of the input frequency.

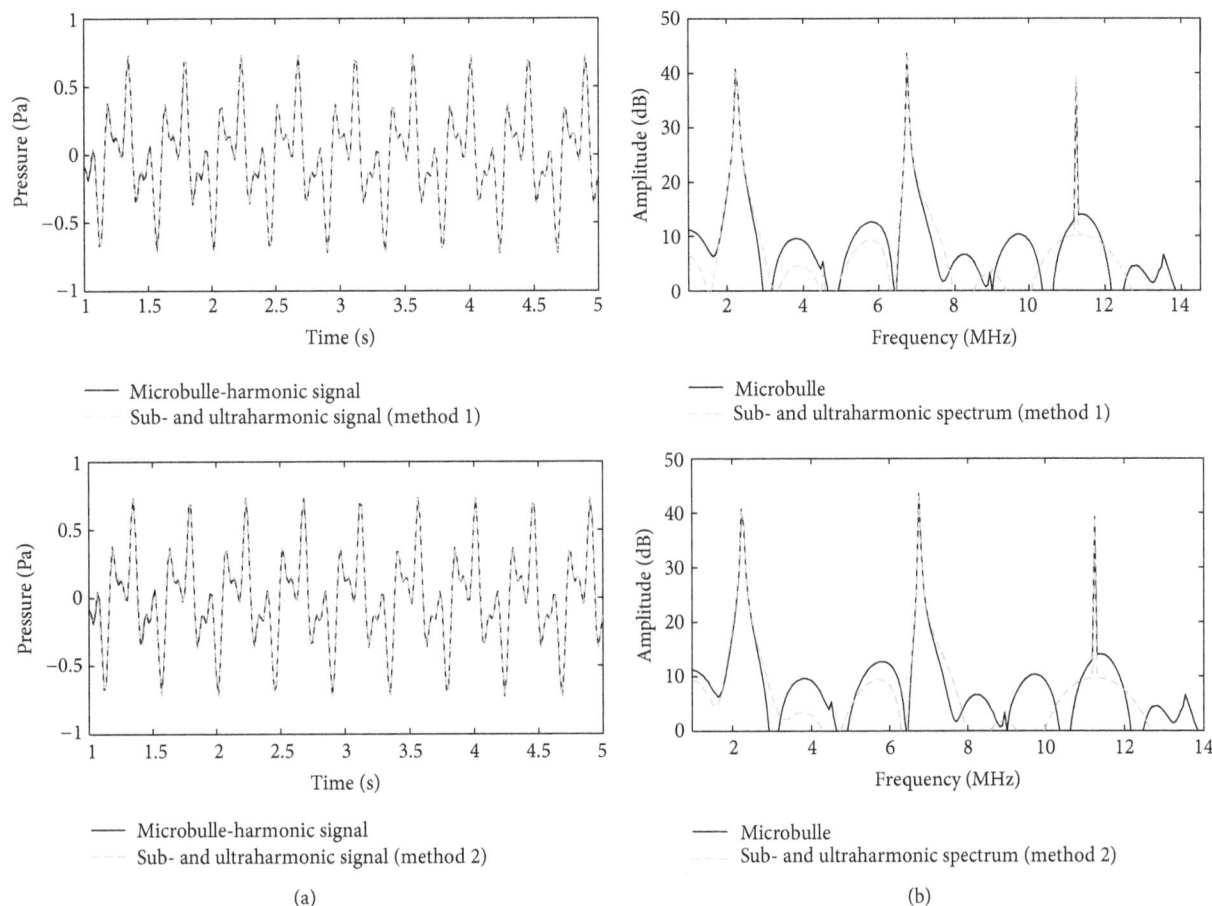

FIGURE 7: (a) Comparison between the backscattered difference signal between the backscattered signal by the contrast agent (black) and the SUH signal (green) modeled with (top) method 1 and (bottom) method 2. (b) Spectra of different signals presented in (a). Here SNR = ∞ dB.

Each method uses two Hammerstein models successively. The first one is dedicated to model harmonic components and the second one to model the SUH components.

The first method (method 1) applies a spectral down-shifting of $f_0/2$ on the input signal of the Hammerstein model. Now, SUH are seen as integer multiples of the input frequency, and therefore they can be modeled with Hammerstein model. In this step, the order of Hammerstein model is an important parameter that need to be adjusted to ensure the modeling of all SUH. For the second method (method 2), a spectral upshifting of $f_0/2$ is applied on the output signal to move the SUH components toward the harmonic positions. Then, SUH components can be modeled with Hammerstein model excited with the input signal of frequency f_0. Finally, a last spectral downshifting is performed to recover the SUH signal.

The two proposed methods are characterized by its simplicity. The originality of these methods is that they allow for the first time both the modeling of contrast agents signals and the separation of SUH components of the contrast agent response.

However, the two methods do not present the same advantages and disadvantages.

Method 1, which is based on the modification of the input signal, is less sensitive to the noise compared to method 2, which is based on the modification of the output signal. This is due to the fact that all the noise generated in the different parts of the non linear procedure are added to the output.

On the other hand, although method 1 has a more simple structure, it is slower than method 2. This is due to the fact that the second step of method 1 requires an order higher than method 2, the order of the first step being fixed. And as the computation time is related to the order of the model, higher the order, the slower the method.

The application of the proposed methods for modeling the contrast agents response shows their efficiency in modeling and in separating SUH components from other harmonic components. Gains of 25.8 dB and 22.8 dB in term of the RMSE are achieved with methods 1 and 2, respectively, compared to the standard Hammerstein model. The achieved error (RMSE) gain by the two methods is related to the sub and ultraharmonics energy initially presented in the output signal of the non linear system. The more important the energy of the sub- and ultraharmonics, the more important the gain. Although in this paper, the two methods works well

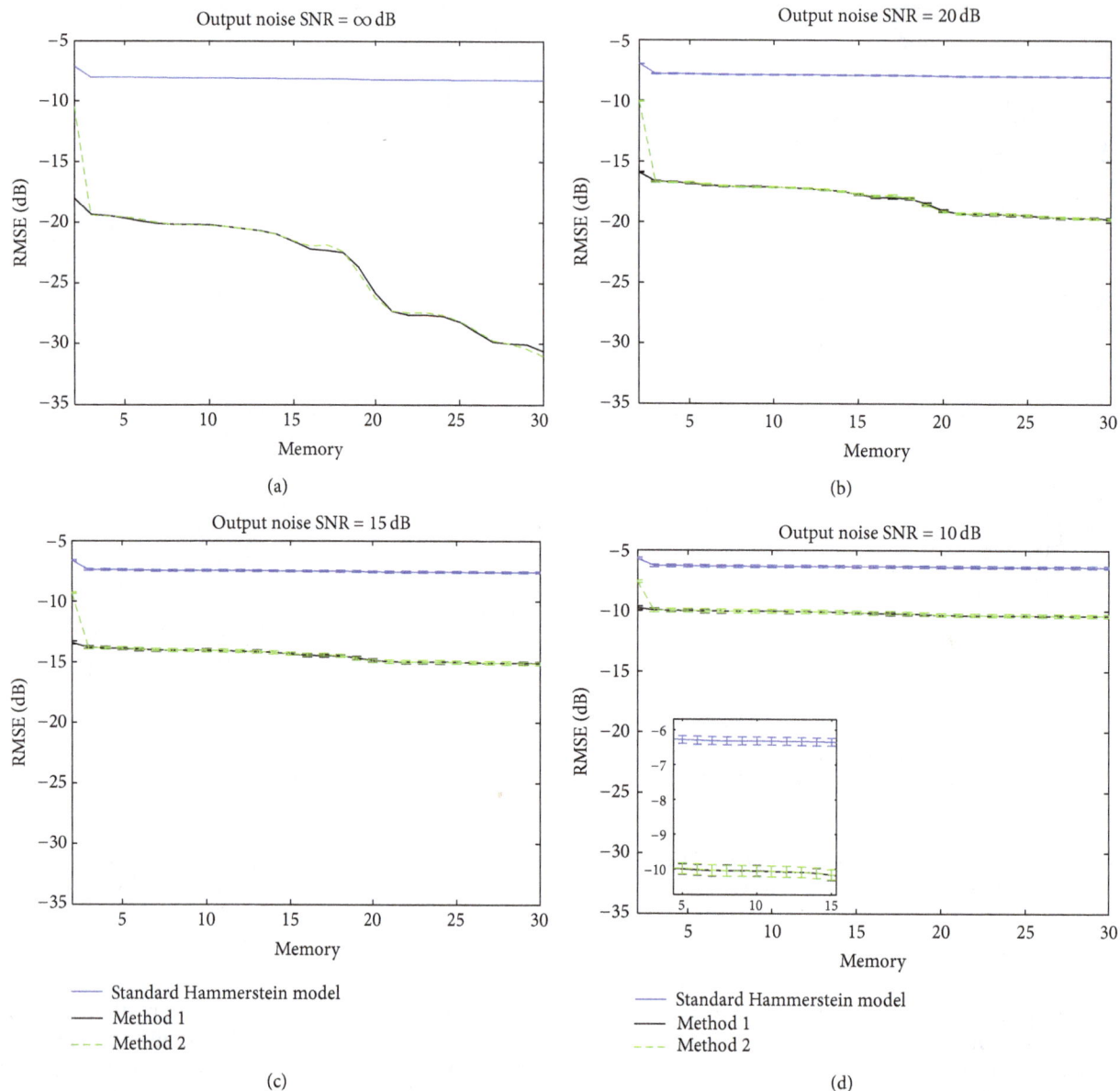

FIGURE 8: Variation of RMSE in dB between the backscattered signal by the contrast agent and that modeled with (blue) the standard Hammerstein model, (black) method 1, and (green) method 2 as a function of the memory of Hammerstein model in presence of output noise: SNR = ∞ dB, SNR = 20 dB, SNR = 15 dB, and SNR = 10 dB.

for $f_0/2$, $(3/2)f_0$, $(5/2)f_0$, these methods can be extended for other orders.

The two proposed methods find theirs applications in the field of sub and ultra-harmonic contrast imaging in order to produce high contrast images. This work opens a new research axis for new modeling techniques of SUH using Hammerstein model or any other non linear models.

Acknowledgment

The authors would to thank the Lebanese Council of Scientific Research (CNRSL) for financing this work.

References

[1] F. Calliada, R. Campani, O. Bottinelli, A. Bozzini, and M. G. Sommaruga, "Ultrasound contrast agents: basic principles," *European Journal of Radiology*, vol. 27, supplement 2, pp. S157–S160, 1998.

[2] F. Forsberg, D. A. Merton, J. B. Liu, L. Needleman, and B. B. Goldberg, "Clinical applications of ultrasound contrast agents," *Ultrasonics*, vol. 36, no. 1–5, pp. 695–701, 1998.

[3] P. J. A. Frinking, A. Bouakaz, J. Kirkhorn, F. J. Ten Cate, and N. De Jong, "Ultrasound contrast imaging: current and new potential methods," *Ultrasound in Medicine and Biology*, vol. 26, no. 6, pp. 965–975, 2000.

[4] N. de Jong, M. Emmer, A. van Wamel, and M. Versluis, "Ultrasonic characterization of ultrasound contrast agents," *Medical and Biological Engineering and Computing*, vol. 47, no. 8, pp. 861–873, 2009.

[5] T. G. Leighton, *The Acoustic Bubble*, Academic Press, London, UK, 1994.

[6] P. N. Burns, "Instrumentation for contrast echocardiography," *Echocardiography*, vol. 19, no. 3, pp. 241–258, 2002.

[7] M. A. Averkiou, "Tissue harmonic imaging," in *Proceedings of the IEEE Ultrasonics Symposium*, vol. 2, pp. 1563–1572, October 2000.

[8] P. M. Shankar, P. D. Krishna, and V. L. Newhouse, "Advantages of subharmonic over second harmonic backscatter for contrast-to-tissue echo enhancement," *Ultrasound in Medicine and Biology*, vol. 24, no. 3, pp. 395–399, 1998.

[9] R. Basude and M. A. Wheatley, "Generation of ultraharmonics in surfactant based ultrasound contrast agents: use and advantages," *Ultrasonics*, vol. 39, no. 6, pp. 437–444, 2001.

[10] F. Forsberg, W. T. Shi, and B. B. Goldberg, "Subharmonic imaging of contrast agents," *Ultrasonics*, vol. 38, no. 1, pp. 93–98, 2000.

[11] F. Forsberg, C. W. Piccoli, D. A. Merton, J. J. Palazzo, and A. L. Hall, "Breast lesions: imaging with contrast-enhanced subharmonic US: initial experience," *Radiology*, vol. 244, no. 3, pp. 718–726, 2007.

[12] O. M. Boaghe and S. A. Billings, "Subharmonic oscillation modeling and MISO Volterra series," *IEEE Transactions on Circuits and Systems I*, vol. 50, no. 7, pp. 877–884, 2003.

[13] C. Samakee and P. Phukpattaranont, "Application of MISO volterra series for modeling subharmonic of ultrasound contrast agent," *International Journal of Computer and Electrical Engineering*, vol. 4, no. 4, pp. 445–451, 2012.

[14] F. Sbeity, S. Ménigot, J. Charara, and J. M. Girault, "A general framework for modeling-sub and ultra-harmonics of ultrasound contrast agent signals with MISO volterra series," *Computational and Mathematical Methods in Medicine*, vol. 2013, Article ID 934538, 2013.

[15] A. Janczak, *Identification of Nonlinear Systems Using Neural Networks and Polynomial Models*, Springer, Berlin, Germany, 2005.

[16] S. Boyd, L. O. Chua, and C. A. Desoer, "Analytical foundations of volterra series," *IMA Journal of Mathematical Control and Information*, vol. 1, no. 3, pp. 243–282, 1984.

[17] L. Hoff, *Acoustic Characterization of Contrast Agents For Medical Ultrasound Imaging*, Kluwer Academic, Boston, Mass, USA, 2001.

[18] C. C. Church, "The effects of an elastic solid surface layer on the radial pulsations of gas bubbles," *Journal of the Acoustical Society of America*, vol. 97, no. 3, pp. 1510–1521, 1995.

15

Antenna Modeling and Reconstruction Accuracy of Time Domain-Based Image Reconstruction in Microwave Tomography

Andreas Fhager,[1] Shantanu K. Padhi,[2] Mikael Persson,[1] and John Howard[3]

[1] Biomedical Engineering Division, Department of Signal and Systems, Chalmers University of Technology, 41296 Gothenburg, Sweden
[2] Curtin Institute of Radio Astronomy (CIRA), ICRAR, Curtin University, Perth, WA 6102, Australia
[3] PRL, Research School of Physics and Engineering, Australian National University, Canberra, ACT 0200, Australia

Correspondence should be addressed to Andreas Fhager; andreas.fhager@chalmers.se

Academic Editor: Kenji Suzuki

Nonlinear microwave imaging heavily relies on an accurate numerical electromagnetic model of the antenna system. The model is used to simulate scattering data that is compared to its measured counterpart in order to reconstruct the image. In this paper an antenna system immersed in water is used to image different canonical objects in order to investigate the implication of modeling errors on the final reconstruction using a time domain-based iterative inverse reconstruction algorithm and three-dimensional FDTD modeling. With the test objects immersed in a background of air and tap water, respectively, we have studied the impact of antenna modeling errors, errors in the modeling of the background media, and made a comparison with a two-dimensional version of the algorithm. In conclusion even small modeling errors in the antennas can significantly alter the reconstructed image. Since the image reconstruction procedure is highly nonlinear general conclusions are very difficult to make. In our case it means that with the antenna system immersed in water and using our present FDTD-based electromagnetic model the imaging results are improved if refraining from modeling the water-wall-air interface and instead just use a homogeneous background of water in the model.

1. Introduction

Microwave imaging has received significant attention in the research community during the last couple of decades as a modality that potentially could improve the diagnostics of, for example, breast cancer tumors. Recent progress in the field has been reviewed in [1] and [2]. Today the research has come to the stage where early clinical trials have been and are being performed, [3–6]. The results from the clinical work are promising, but further development of the measurement systems as well as of the image reconstruction algorithms remains before the technique can be considered for daily clinical practice.

When performing microwave tomography the aim is to quantitatively reconstruct the dielectric parameters in the region under test. This involves solving a computationally challenging nonlinear and ill-posed optimization problem.

The image reconstruction algorithm utilizes measured data that are compared against a corresponding numerical simulation of the system, and the dielectric profile is iteratively updated based on the difference between the simulation and the measurement. Even though this comparison requires a realistic numerical model for the best accuracy, most of the published works have used 2D models together with a calibration procedure to enable the comparison with experimental data. Largely, this can be attributed to a significant increase in the computational load when moving from 2D to three-dimensional (3D) modeling. However the electromagnetic scattering and consequently the reconstruction problems are inherently a 3D problem. Furthermore it is usually not possible to create realistic antenna models in 2D, except for line source antennas. By using a 2D model to solve the inverse scattering problem inaccuracies will therefore inevitably be introduced in the reconstructed image. This problem has been identified by the research community, and, with the ever increasing computational resources available these days, the focus is now more and more turning to solving the full 3D problem. Recent works using 3D algorithm have been reported in [7–11].

In this paper we show several examples where images have been reconstructed from scattering data in order to discuss and illustrate the need for accurate modeling of the antenna system and its geometry to enable robust image reconstruction. The aim is also to get an understanding of what accuracy we could realistically expect in the reconstruction and how it is affected by various modeling errors. Examples of targets placed in a surrounding of air are studied, and in an effort to approach more biologically relevant settings we have studied examples where the antenna system was entirely immersed in water. The examples studied in this paper are entirely based on experimental measurement data. Our reconstruction algorithm, described in [12], is based on FDTD modeling to solve the forward scattering problem and the adjoint Maxwell's equations to compute gradients used in an iterative optimization procedure.

The paper is organized as follows. In Section 2, the theoretical background of our work is described including FDTD methods with the minimization procedure. The experimental prototype is described in Section 3. In Section 4, the forward modeling is investigated, and the corresponding imaging results originating from experimental data are presented and discussed. And finally the conclusions are drawn in Section 5.

2. Theoretical Background

An iterative electromagnetic time-domain inversion algorithm has been used and applied in estimating the dielectric parameters of different test objects. The foundation of the algorithm is an electromagnetic solver based on the FDTD method, [13], is used to numerically model the antennas and to simulate the field propagation inside the system. The same solver is used to compute the adjoint Maxwell problem which is required for the gradient computation in the optimization algorithm. The adjoint field is used extensively elsewhere in various types of inverse problems see, for example, [14, 15]. The algorithm used here is described in [12]. A corresponding 2D version has also been described in detail in [16, 17].

Our basic idea for solving the inverse electromagnetic problem is to use scattering measurements of wideband pulses for several transmitter/receiver combinations surrounding a region of interest and thereafter to compare the measured data in the time domain with a corresponding numerical simulation of the system. In the first iteration one starts with comparing the measurement with a simulation of an empty antenna system. Thus there is a difference between the measured and the simulated data, and this difference is used to update the dielectric properties inside the region of interest. In this way the dielectric distribution is iteratively refined until the desired agreement between the simulated and measured signals has been achieved. The underlying assumption for this approach is that as the difference between

the simulated and measured data is decreasing, the reconstruction is also converging. In other words, the aim of the reconstruction procedure is to minimize the objective functional, F, defined as

$$F(\epsilon, \sigma) = \int_0^T \sum_{m=1}^M \sum_{n=1}^N |\mathbf{E}_{mn}(\epsilon, \sigma, t) - \mathbf{E}_{mn}^m(t)|^2 dt, \quad (1)$$

where $\mathbf{E}_{mn}(\epsilon, \sigma, t)$ is the calculated field from the computational model and $\mathbf{E}_{mn}^m(t)$ is the corresponding measured data when antenna number m has been used as transmitter and antenna n as receiver. M is the number of transmitters, N is the number of receivers, and T is the duration of the pulse. In a 2D TM-mode formulation only one spatial field component is used in (1), but for the 3D formulation it is necessary to include all three spatial components.

In search for the minimum of the objective functional it is differentiated with respect to the dielectric components by a first order perturbation analysis. In this way the Fréchet derivatives with respect to the conductivity and the permittivity of the functional are used to define gradients, in every grid point, inside the region. The gradients are used with the conjugate-gradient method together with the successive parabolic interpolation line search to minimize the objective functional. The reconstruction procedure is then iterated with the objective functional as a measure to monitor the convergence and to determine when the reconstruction is completed. Usually the minimization procedure converges within 10–20 iterations.

In the 2D simulations it is not possible to construct a realistic antenna model, but the transmitter is only modeled with a hard point source, in which the field strength is prescribed at the source position. At the receiver locations the field values are sampled directly from the corresponding E-field component in the grid. By contrast, the 3D algorithm allows for realistic antenna models. We are using the thin-wire approximation to model the monopoles, [18], and the RVS with 50 Ω impedance to model the feed at the transmitting, receiving, and inactive antennas, [19, 20]. Furthermore the ground plane in our experimental system is modeled as a perfect electric conductor; that is, the corresponding field components in the FDTD grid are set to zero. The walls of the tank have dielectric properties close to those of air and are therefore neglected in the numerical model. Outside the antenna system the computational grid is truncated by the CPML absorbing boundary condition implying that the region outside the antenna array is treated as open empty space. In the case where the tank is filled with a liquid it has been modeled as a cubic volume with side lengths equal to the inner measures of the tank and a height equal to the level of the liquid. Even in this case we have not modeled the tank material but instead treated everything outside as empty space and terminated the computation domain with CPML. A more detailed discussion and validation of the FDTD antenna array model with a comparison against experimental data measured with the antennas in air can be found in our previous work [21].

As already mentioned the solution of the inverse problem heavily relies on the comparison between the measured and the simulated scattering data. To compensate for systematic modeling errors a calibration procedure of the measured data is used such that

$$E_{\text{cal}}^{m}(f) = \frac{S_{\text{scat}}^{m}(f)}{S_{\text{ref}}^{m}(f)} E_{\text{ref}}^{s}(f). \tag{2}$$

S_{scat}^{m} is the measured reflection and transmission coefficients of the test object, $S_{\text{ref}}^{m}(f)$ is a reference measurement of an empty system, and $E_{\text{ref}}^{s}(f)$ is a corresponding reference simulation. Finally $E_{\text{cal}}^{m}(f)$ is the calibrated data used for comparing the FDTD simulations in the reconstruction process. This calibration procedure has been applied to the measured data for both the 2D and the 3D imaging examples in this paper.

In our experimental prototype the antennas are positioned in a plane. The possibility to accurately reconstruct out-of-plane objects is thus very limited: to do so it would be necessary also to make additional measurements outside the antenna plane. To allow imaging with the 3D algorithm of a test object with finite height, we implemented a heuristic pseudo-3D technique that assumed constant properties of the test object as a function of height, z, above the ground plane. The gradients computed in the grid cell plane immediately above the ground plane were copied upwards to the height of the test object. This method needs a priori information about the height of the reconstructed target. Since the reconstruction problem is both nonlinear and ill-posed, the resulting image strongly depends on the adopted regularization technique, the initialization of the reconstruction, and also the spectral content of the pulse. Here we used the same techniques as described in [12] to overcome these challenges.

3. Experimental Setup

The measurement strategy is to measure the multistatic scattering matrix at a large number of frequencies and to use that data to generate a time-domain pulse via an inverse Fourier transformation. In the experimental system 20 monopole antennas, each of length 19.5 mm and diameter 0.8 mm, are arranged evenly distributed on a circle with radius 100 mm. The circle of antennas is centered on a square ground plane with side length 250 mm mounted at the bottom of a tank, made of 1 cm thick perspex sheets with inner measures 350×350 mm^2. To measure the multistatic matrix each antenna is operated as a transmitter as well as a receiver. The microwave measurements are made with network analyzer Agilent E8362 B PNA which is a two-port network analyzer. To fully control the experiment a 2:32 switch multiplexer module, Cytec CXM/128-S-W, is used to automatically connect and disconnect the different combinations of antenna pairs to the network analyzer. Figure 1 shows a photograph of the antenna array.

4. Results and Discussion

In our previous publication, [21], a detailed study was made of the FDTD modeling compared to measured data of an empty system, and the accuracy of the modeling was verified. One

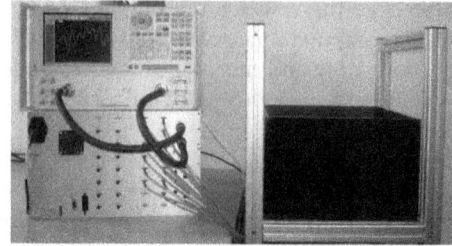

(a) The measurement system

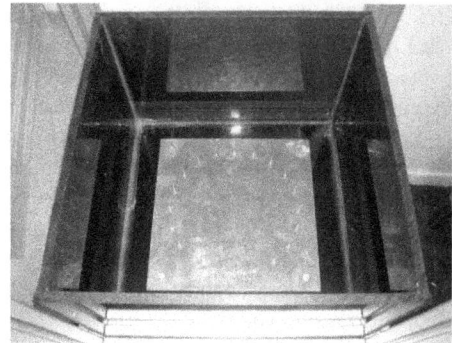

(b) The antenna array

FIGURE 1: (a) The system consists of a VNA, a switch, and an antenna array. (b) Closeup of the antenna array placed inside a tank. The monopoles are seen mounted in a circle over the ground plane. The entire antenna system is mounted inside a tank made of perspex sheets.

of the aims of the present paper is to study how errors in the antenna model, for example, the monopole length, of the FDTD model impact the reconstruction. To do so we study the antenna modeling and image reconstruction both when the tank is empty and when it is filled with water. The reason why it is interesting to study the antenna system immersed in water is that water is a good model for the matching medium that has to be used when applying microwave tomography to imaging the interior of the human body. Without a matching medium the majority of the irradiated energy would be reflected from the skin, thereby never penetrating into the body and producing useful data.

To enable a quantitative evaluation of the accuracy of the reconstructed images we have adopted the relative squared error of the image, and for the permittivity image it is defined in (3), and analogously for the conductivity image. The integration of the relative squared error is made over the reconstruction domain Ω where $r < R_{\text{rd}}$,

$$\delta = \frac{\int_{\Omega} \left| \epsilon_{\text{original}} - \epsilon_{\text{reconstructed}} \right|^{2} dS}{\int_{\Omega} \left| \epsilon_{\text{original}} - \epsilon_{\text{background}} \right|^{2} dS}. \tag{3}$$

4.1. Reconstruction of a Single Dielectric Target in Air. With the purpose to study how the reconstructed image is affected by errors in the length of the monopole antenna model, we first studied a single dielectric target in an otherwise empty antenna array. The imaging situation was the same as in our previous publication, [12], that is, a single target made of sunflower oil surrounded by air. The dielectric properties of the target were ϵ_r = 2.7 and σ = 0.015 S/m at 2.3 GHz. It was shaped like a cylinder with diameter 56 mm and height 20 mm and was placed at 14 mm offset in the y direction from the center of the antenna array. It had constant properties along its height in the z direction, and thus it is only necessary to show a cross-sectional slice of the dielectric profile. The FDTD model data is summarized in Table 1. A cylindrical volume of height 20 mm and radius R_{rd} = 90 mm centered in the antenna array was used as the reconstruction domain together with the pseudo-3D approach described earlier. To investigate the accuracy of the reconstructed image with respect to the modeling, different lengths of the monopoles were used in the numerical electromagnetic model. The length of the monopoles in the antenna system is 19.5 mm, but images were reconstructed modeling the length as 16, 18, 20, 22, and 24 mm, respectively. This resulted in a change in the computed resonance frequency and the associated signal strength. The reconstruction results together with an illustration of the original dielectric distribution are shown in Figure 2. The results obtained with 20 mm monopole length in Figures 2(d) and 2(j) are identical to what was published earlier [12] and represent a scenario where the numerical modeling at the given grid size is as close as possible to the experimental system. As a measure of reconstruction accuracy the relative error as defined in (3) has been calculated for each reconstructed image, and it is shown in the figure below the respective reconstruction. The reconstructed object permittivities are on average about ϵ_r = 2.1, 2.2, 2.4, 2.7, 3.0, respectively, for the various monopole lengths. The minimum value is 12.5% smaller and the maximum value is 25% larger than what was obtained for the 20 mm monopole length. The recontructions of the conductivity are, however, not accurate, but it is clearly evident that the artifacts increase the more the monopole lengths deviate from the real value. The reason why the reconstruction is less accurate is that the difference in the imaginary part of the complex dielectric permittivity between the object and background is only a fraction in comparison with the difference in the real part. Reconstruction errors in the real part therefore overwhelm attempts to reconstruct the imaginary part, and consequently the accuracy is reduced. Compared to the original dielectric profile, however, the most accurate reconstruction of the permittivity is obtained for the 18 mm monopole. This reflects the deviaton of half a grid cell between the 20 mm antenna model and the precise length of the monopole with the real length being 19.5 mm. But also there is a tolerance in the cutting of the monopoles of about 0.5 mm. Numerical uncertainties in the FDTD solution and errors in the dielectric measurement of the sunflower oil are other reasons.

In Figure 3 the functional values of the reconstructions have been plotted. In all cases the starting values have been normalized to one. Firstly these plots illustrate the convergence of the reconstruction process, but it also shows that the lowest functional value was obtained for the reconstruction with the 20 mm monopole. A nice illustration of the ill-posedness of the problem is that the difference between the 20 mm and the 22 mm case is on the verge of being negligible even if the difference in the reconstructed image

TABLE 1: Specifications of the 3D FDTD modeling and reconstruction parameters for the sun flower oil target in an otherwise empty antenna system.

FDTD grid	$149 \times 149 \times 38$
Grid size length	2 mm
CPML	7 layers
Pulse center frequency	2.3 GHz
Pulse FWHM bandwidth	2.3 GHz
Water level	No water in tank
Background properties	ϵ_r = 1.0, σ = 0.0 S/m
Antenna model	Thin wire
Feed model	50 Ω RVS

is certainly not. Another conclusion from this result is that a model error in the antenna length of only one grid cell resulted in a considerable change in the reconstructed image. In summary these results clearly show the need of using an accurate antenna length in order to maximize the accuracy of the reconstructed image.

4.2. Evaluation of the Forward Simulation with the Antenna Array Immersed in Water. In this section we study the situation when the antenna array tank was filled with tap water, having dielectric properties ϵ_r = 77.5, σ = 0.05 S/m at 0.5 GHz. We also present a comparison between measured data and corresponding computed reflection and transmission coefficients. By replacing the air in the tank with water we further approach biologically relevant imaging scenarios. With the aim to study how modeling errors affect the reconstructed images we first studied how the forward modeling of the antenna system was affected by different antenna modeling errors.

4.2.1. Full 3D Model. The experimental situation was such that the tank was filled with ordinary tap water up to a level of 50 mm above the ground plane. In the FDTD model measured dielectric values of the water at 0.5 GHz were used as this was in the center of the frequency spectrum used for the imaging. In the FDTD modeling care was also taken to represent the physical reality as accurately as possible, and the corresponding settings are summarized in Table 2. Modeling errors were introduced by varying some of the parameters in this table. Unfortunately it is not viable to show scattering data for all antenna combinations, but instead only a few representative cases are shown. Measured and simulated reflection and transmission coefficients between two adjacent antennas using the model parameters from Table 2 are shown in Figure 4. As can be seen, the agreement between the calculated and the measured data is very close. The calculated resonant frequency is 0.70 GHz compared with the measured resonant frequency of 0.67 GHz. There are ripples with approximately the same magnitude both in calculated and measured data and where some ripples agree with each other and some do not. The details about these ripples are further discussed in the following sections. The measured transmission coefficients are on average below

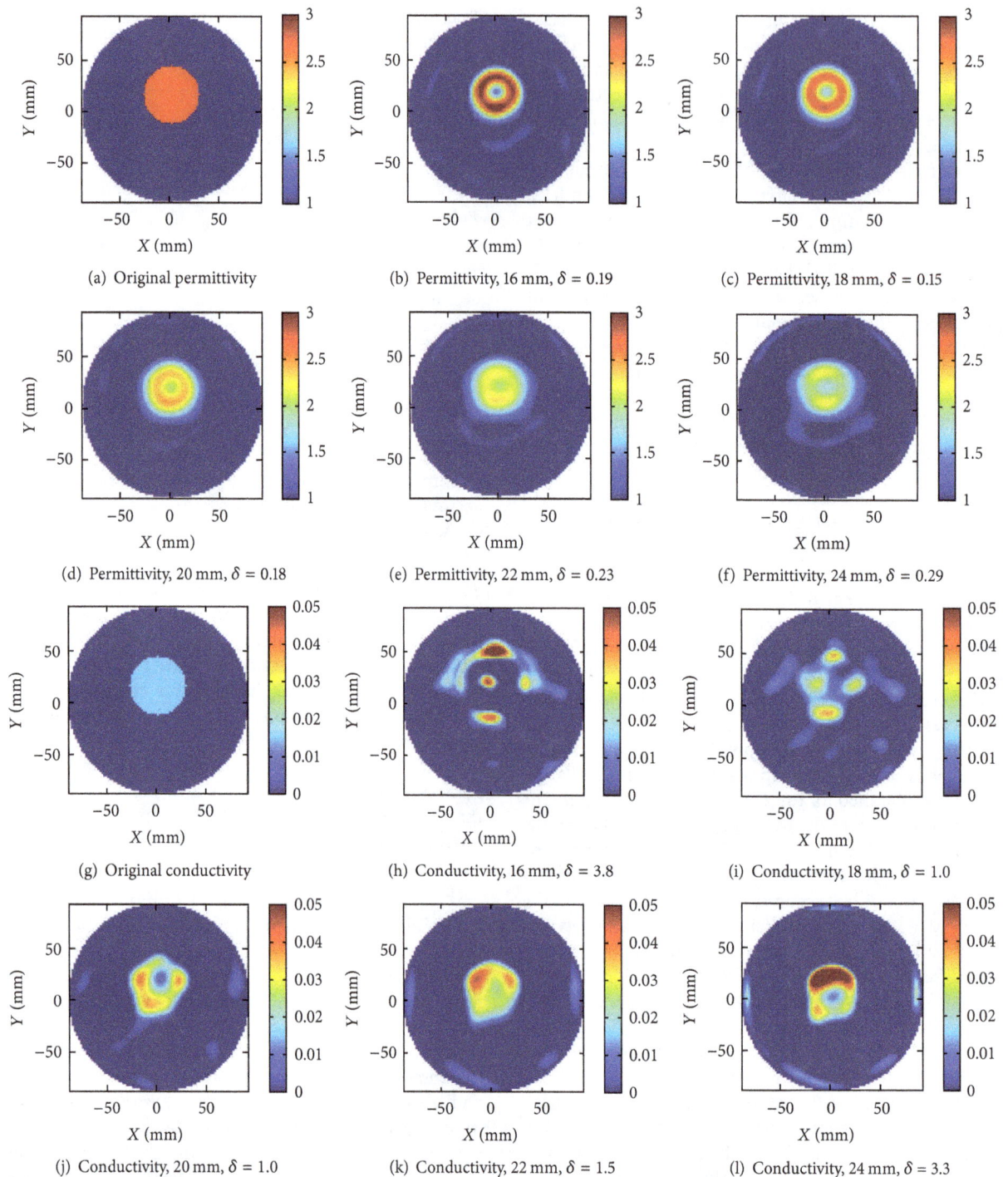

FIGURE 2: Reconstructed images of the sunflower oil target using monopole lengths 16, 18, 20, 22, and 24 mm, respectively. Both permittivity and conductivity images are shown, and in (a) and (g) the original dielectric distribution has been illustrated. The original target had $\epsilon_r = 2.7$ and $\sigma = 0.015$ S/m at 2.3 GHz and had diameter 56 mm.

−15 dB compared to the calculated transmission coefficient below −12 dB.

4.2.2. Hard Source Feed Model. Due to its simplicity, the hard source model is very appealing to use in FDTD simulations. However, it is not as accurate as the RVS when modeling

the monopole feed. To quantify the errors associated with a hard source we investigate its applicability to model the monopole feed. In the first example, we replaced the RVS feed model with a hard source. In the second example, we used the hard source and completely removed the modeling of the rest of the monopole. The use of a hard source also implied that we could not use the transmitting antenna in the

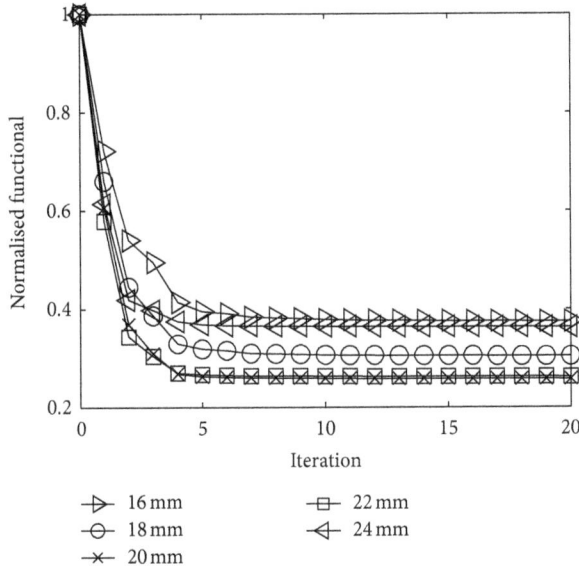

FIGURE 3: Normalized functional values as a function of the iteration number for the reconstructions of the sunflower target.

TABLE 2: Specifications of the 3D FDTD modeling when the antenna system was filled with water.

FDTD grid	$179 \times 179 \times 35$
Grid size length	2 mm
CPML	7 layers
Pulse center frequency	0.5 GHz
Pulse FWHM bandwidth	0.5 GHz
Water level in tank	50 mm
Water properties	$\epsilon_r = 77.5, \sigma = 0.05\,\text{S/m}$
Background properties	$\epsilon_r = 1.0, \sigma = 0.0\,\text{S/m}$
Antenna model	Thin wire
Feed model	50 Ω RVS

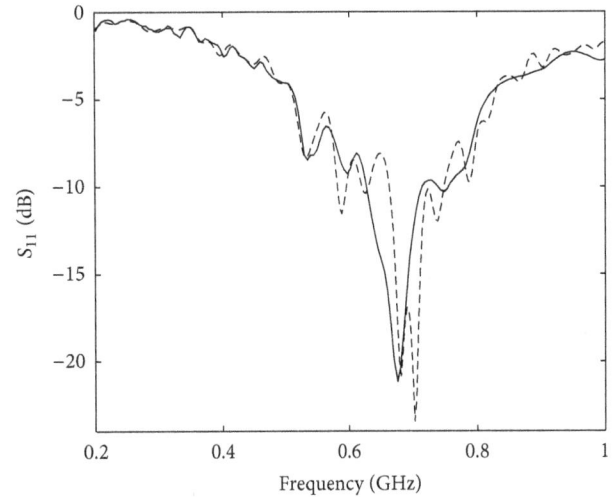

(a) Reflection coefficient, S_{11}

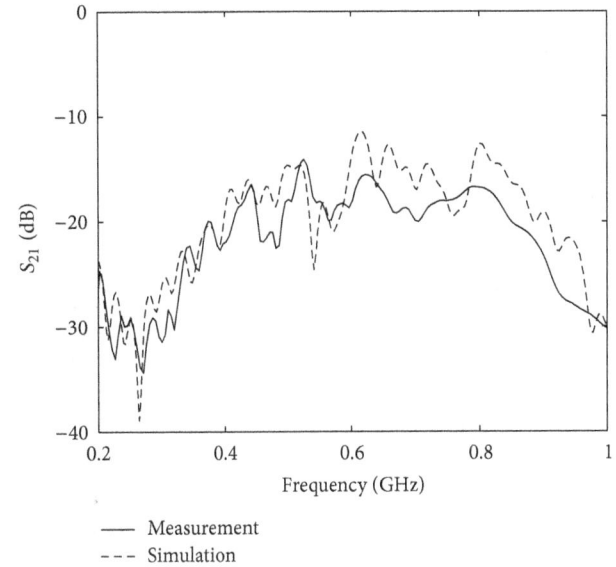

—— Measurement
--- Simulation

(b) Transmission coefficient, S_{21}

FIGURE 4: Comparison between measured and simulated reflection (S_{11}) and transmission (S_{21}) coefficients over the frequency range of interest for the imaging examples.

gradient computation as we do not calculate the reflection coefficient with the hard source model. Calculation of the reflection coefficient requires knowledge of the reflected wave, but since the E-field is directly set in the source cell, no update of the field will be made due to reflected waves. Instead we used only transmission data for the following reconstructions. As an illustration of the impact of the hard source on the simulated scattering data S_{21} for adjacent antennas has been plotted in Figure 5. For convenience the same measured and simulated data for the full 3D model as in Figure 4 has also been replotted in the same graph. As can be seen, in the first example, the RVS feed model improves the transmission coefficient data over the hard source model, and, in the second example, the system becomes very lossy due to the inaccurate model, and therefore the deviation from the measured data increases.

4.2.3. Open Water Model. Solving the reconstruction problem is a computationally very demanding problem, and one strategy to reduce the simulation time is to reduce the size of the computational domain. Therefore we have investigated the need for modeling the exact volume of the water in the tank and instead modeled the water as a background directly terminated by CPML. The CPML is absorbing any outgoing wave and the result inside the computation domain is the same as if the simulation was made in an infinitely large space. In this FDTD simulation the entire computational grid was therefore assigned the properties of water, and as there were no need to model the water-air interface in the computational domain, the CPML could be moved closer to the antennas and thus the computational domain reduced. In Figure 6 the corresponding reflection, S_{11}, and transmission, S_{21}, coefficients have been plotted. For comparison the figures also contain the measured data and the data simulated with

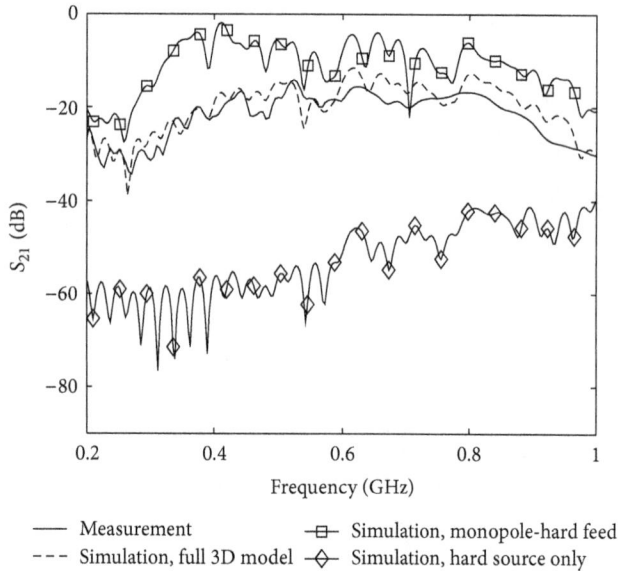

— Measurement   —□— Simulation, monopole-hard feed
--- Simulation, full 3D model   —◇— Simulation, hard source only

FIGURE 5: Measurement and simulations of the transmission coefficients S_{21} between two adjacent antennas. For ease of comparison the transmission data from Figure 4 has been kept and plotted together with the case when (1) The RVS has been replaced by a hard source and (2) the wire model has been removed and only a hard source has been used as transmitter.

the full 3D FDTD model from Figure 4. The S_{11} data show how the computed resonance frequency has increased about 0.5 GHz, and we can also see how the fast varying ripple due to the water-air interface reflections has vanished. Similar changes can also be seen in the S_{21} data.

4.2.4. 2D Model. We have also made a comparison with a 2D computational model. The reason is that the computation time is significantly reduced compared to the 3D case. Therefore a good understanding is desired of when the 2D approximation is applicable for imaging. In this section we show computed transmission data obtained with a 2D model, and also here two examples are considered. The first is the modeling of the volume of water in the tank as a 350×350 mm square in the 2D FDTD grid. In Table 3 the corresponding FDTD model parameters are summarized. In analogy with the 3D open water background model the second example was a 2D homogeneous background of water terminated with CPML. In Figure 7 transmission data is plotted for these two cases and again the measured data and the full 3D model data are shown. For the simulation data with the 2D square tank model the deviation from the measured data is of similar magnitude as for the case as with the hard source feed in Figure 5, at least around the center frequency 0.5 GHz. However, the amplitude of the ripple is larger and the deviation is much more significant. The fast varying ripple is clearly seen and is primarily due to the reflections from the water-air interface in the model. For the simulation in the homogeneous background this ripple is vanished, but in this case the computed data do not show much resemblance at all to the measured data.

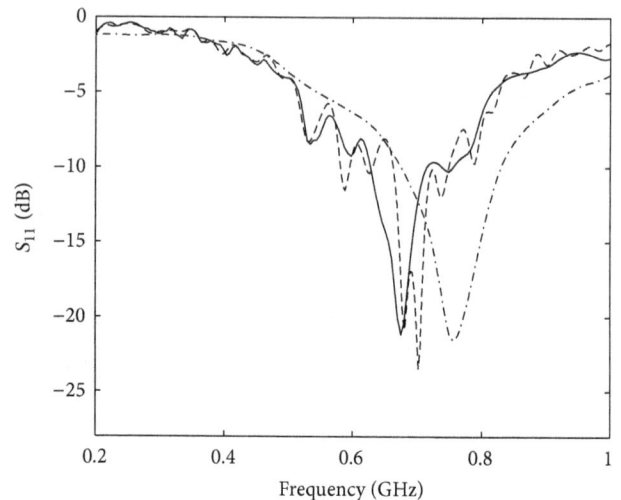

(a) Reflection coefficient, S_{11}

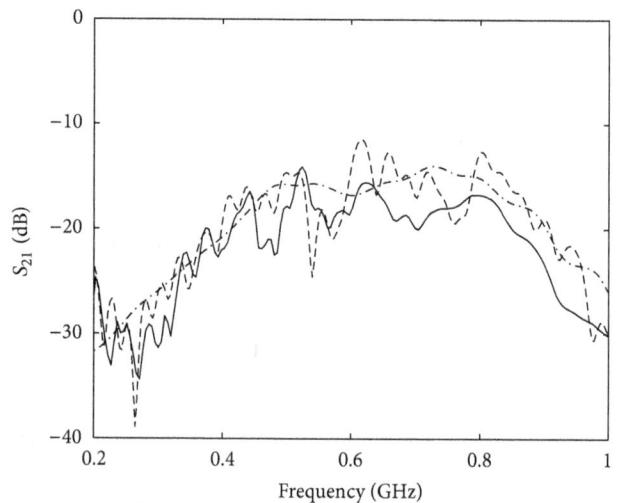

— Measurement
--- Simulation, full 3D model
-·-· Simulation, open water model

(b) Transmission coefficient, S_{21}

FIGURE 6: (a) Reflection coefficients with the antennas modeled in an infinite water background. For comparison the original measured and simulated data is shown. (b) Corresponding transmission coefficients for two adjacent antennas.

4.3. Reconstruction of Targets Immersed in Water. In the following section, we show the reconstructed images from experimental scattering data. Two different target models were used and reconstructed using the various antenna array models discussed above. The aim was to investigate the impact on the reconstruction caused by the different modeling introduced in Section 4.2.

We have performed image reconstruction of targets immersed into ordinary tap water. In comparison to air a FDTD simulation of water is more time consuming due to the higher permittivity and the corresponding need for shorter time stepping in the FDTD algorithm. To save some computation time the reconstructions were therefore made using

TABLE 3: Specifications of the 2D FDTD modeling when the antenna system was filled with water.

FDTD grid	179×179
Grid size length	2 mm
CPML	7 layers
Pulse center frequency	0.5 GHz
Pulse FWHM bandwidth	0.5 GHz
Water properties	$\epsilon_r = 77.5, \sigma = 0.05$ S/m
Background properties	$\epsilon_r = 1.0, \sigma = 0.0$ S/m
Transmitting antenna model	Hard source
Receiving antenna model	Field is sampled

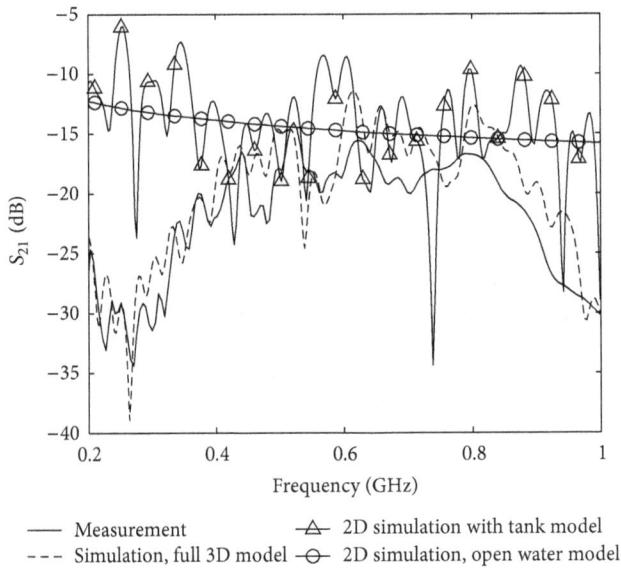

— Measurement —△— 2D simulation with tank model
--- Simulation, full 3D model —⊖— 2D simulation, open water model

FIGURE 7: Transmission coefficients for the 2D FDTD model with the tank model and with the homogeneous background of water. For ease of comparison both the measured data and the simulation with the full 3D model are also shown.

a multigrid technique where 10 iterations where performed on a $(90 \times 90 \times 16)$ computational domain with grid size length 4 mm. The final reconstruction of the $10'$th iteration was then taken as a starting point for 10 additional iterations on a $(179 \times 179 \times 31)$ domain with grid size length 2 mm. The electromagnetic pulse had center frequency 0.5 GHz and FWHM bandwidth 0.5 GHz. The same pseudo-3D approach as previously described was used in a reconstruction domain of height 50 mm and radius $R_{rd} = 80$ mm. Two different targets were used in the reconstructions. The first was made of a mixture of deionized water and ethanol resulting in permittivity $\epsilon_r = 57$ and conductivity $\sigma = 0.11$ S/m at the frequency 0.5 GHz. The mixture was filled up to height 50 mm in a thin-walled plastic cup with diameter 42 mm and immersed into the water for the measurement. The second target was a plastic rod with permittivity $\epsilon_r \approx 2.5$, conductivity $\sigma \approx 0$ S/m, and diameter 15 mm.

4.3.1. Full 3D Model.
Two different scenarios were reconstructed, the first with the center of the water/ethanol target

positioned 39 mm from the center point of the antenna array. In Figure 8 an illustration of the original target is shown together with the reconstructed images.

The second scenario that was reconstructed included both targets, the water/ethanol mixture and the plastic target, and these results are shown in Figure 9. In both cases we see that in the permittivity both size and position of the targets have been accurately reconstructed. The relative error for this second example with the two targets was computed to be $\delta = 0.42$. In the conductivity we can perhaps see an indication of a target in the appropriate positions, but the image region is also cluttered with other artifacts, and comparison with the relative error is not meaningful. Furthermore the absolute values of the permittivity are not in total agreement with the original values, especially not for the small plastic target. With the same arguments as for the previous object in air where the conductivity also was badly reconstructed, it is not to expect anything else in this case. The difference between the background and the target made of water/ethanol mixture is about $\Re\{\Delta\epsilon_r^*\} = 20$ in the real part but for the imaginary part only $\Im\{\Delta\epsilon_r^*\} = 2$. For the plastic rod the difference is $\Re\{\Delta\epsilon_r^*\} = 75$ and $\Im\{\Delta\epsilon_r^*\} = 2$.

4.3.2. Hard Source Feed Model.
To assess the question of how the reconstructed image is affected by inaccuracies in the forward modeling we have taken the example with the two targets, the plastic rod, and the water/ethanol mixture and performed reconstructions with distorted electromagnetic models.

Using the two altered antenna models with hard source feed new images of the original targets from Figures 9(a) and 9(b) have been reconstructed and shown in Figure 10. In (a) and (b) in this figure the RVS was replaced with the hard source feed, and in (c) and (d) the model of the monopole wire was completely removed and only the hard source was used as transmitter model. The relative errors in the permittivity images were computed to be $\delta = 0.54$ and $\delta = 0.58$, respectively. One can clearly see that, for the case where only the hard source was used to model the transmitter, the distortions of the reconstructed images are also the largest. This also corresponds to the case where the S-parameter data deviate the most from the measured data in Figure 5. However one should not believe that there exists a simple relation between the deviation between the measured and simulated data on one hand and the errors in the reconstructed images on the other hand. It is instead a highly nonlinear relation and a balance between the measurement, the reconstruction algorithm, the regularization, the modeling accuracy, and the calibration procedure. To summarize, so far the results shown indicate that the accuracy of the reconstructed image is highly influenced by the details in the antenna models and in the propagation model. So far we have also modeled the volume of water according to measurements of the level in the tank.

4.3.3. Open Water Model.
We have investigated the need of actually modeling the exact extent of the water volume in the tank. For this experiment we used the RVS feed thin-wire monopole model, and the algorithmic settings were

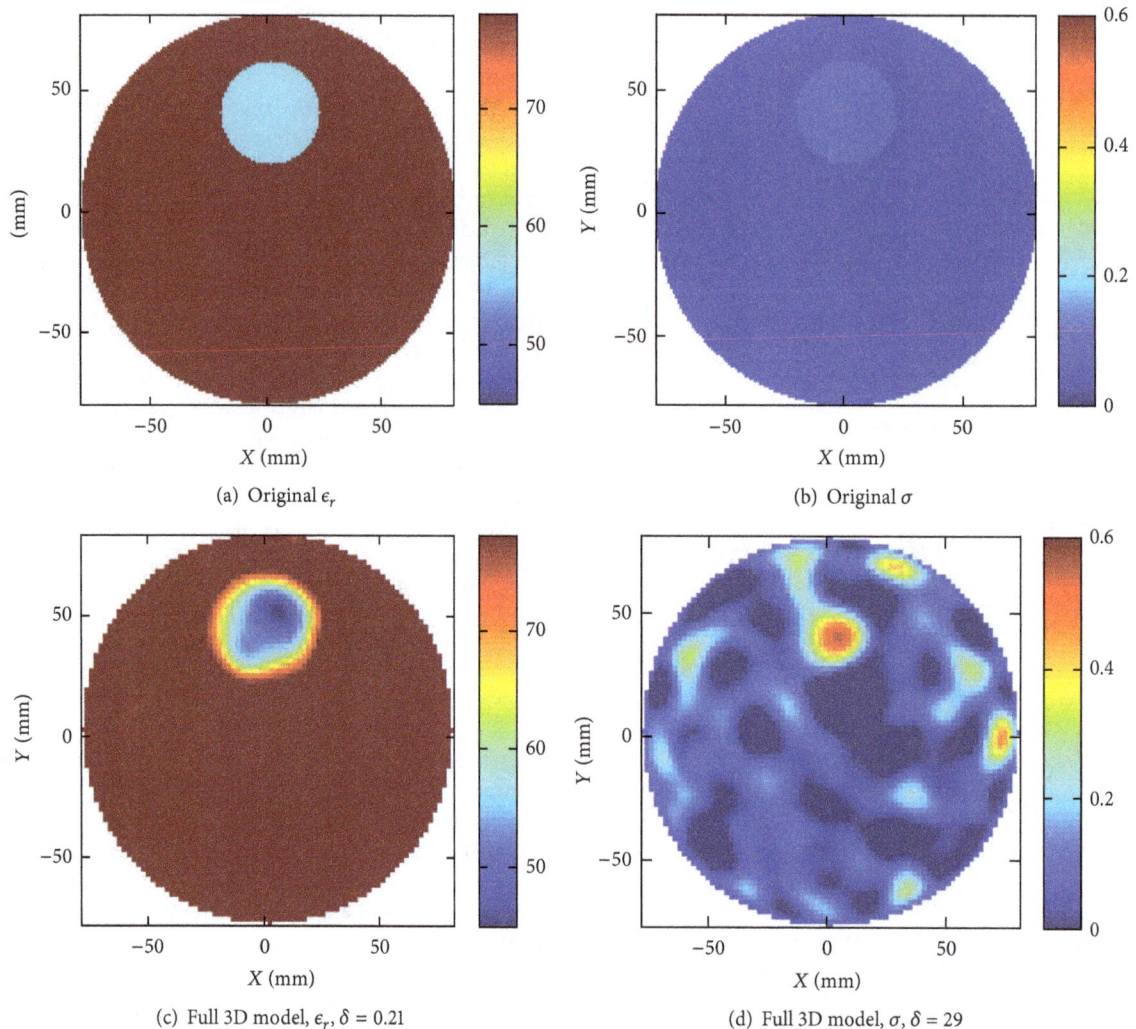

(a) Original ϵ_r

(b) Original σ

(c) Full 3D model, ϵ_r, $\delta = 0.21$

(d) Full 3D model, σ, $\delta = 29$

FIGURE 8: (a and b) Original configuration of the water/ethanol target immersed in water. (c and d) Reconstructions using the 3D algorithm.

otherwise identical to the previous examples but with the dielectric properties of water assigned to all the grid cells in the computational domain which was then terminated by seven layers of CPML. The reconstruction can be seen in Figure 11. Interestingly the results are improved over the reconstructions made with the tank model, and, for example, the absolute values of the objects are better estimated with the 3D algorithm. The improvement is confirmed by the relative error which was calculated to be $\delta = 0.36$ for the permittivity image, a decrease of about 14% compared to the reconstruction with the full 3D model in Figure 9. These results might be a bit surprising and contradictory to the idea that the better the forward model the better the reconstruction. However, we do not believe that it is the case. If we examine the scattering data in Figure 6 carefully, we see that even if the data simulated with the numerical tank model contains a similar ripple of the same magnitude as the measured data, the agreement in the details is not perfect. On average one can however approximately estimate the modeling errors in the two cases to be of similar magnitude in comparison to the measured data. Even if we have carefully

created the model, the numerical grid is ultimately limiting the resolution and causing simulation errors. A refined grid should improve the modeling accuracy but that would also imply that the problem size increases beyond what can be practically handled by our computer cluster due to memory and simulation time requirements. These results suggest that we in this situation are better off by using the simpler open water model and relying on the calibration to resolve the remaining discrepancy between the simulated and the measured data. This is not a result that is obvious to predict but instead a result of the nonlinear property of the problem. In practice the optimal numerical model would thus have to be determined from case to case in different imaging situations and with different imaging systems.

4.3.4. 2D Model.
For comparison we have also performed image reconstruction of the same targets using a 2D version of the algorithm. The first reconstruction made with the water tank modeled as a square of the single target as shown in Figures 8(a) and 8(b), and the reconstructed images

(a) Original ϵ_r

(b) Original σ

(c) Full 3D model, ϵ_r, $\delta = 0.42$

(d) Full 3D model, σ, $\delta = 29$

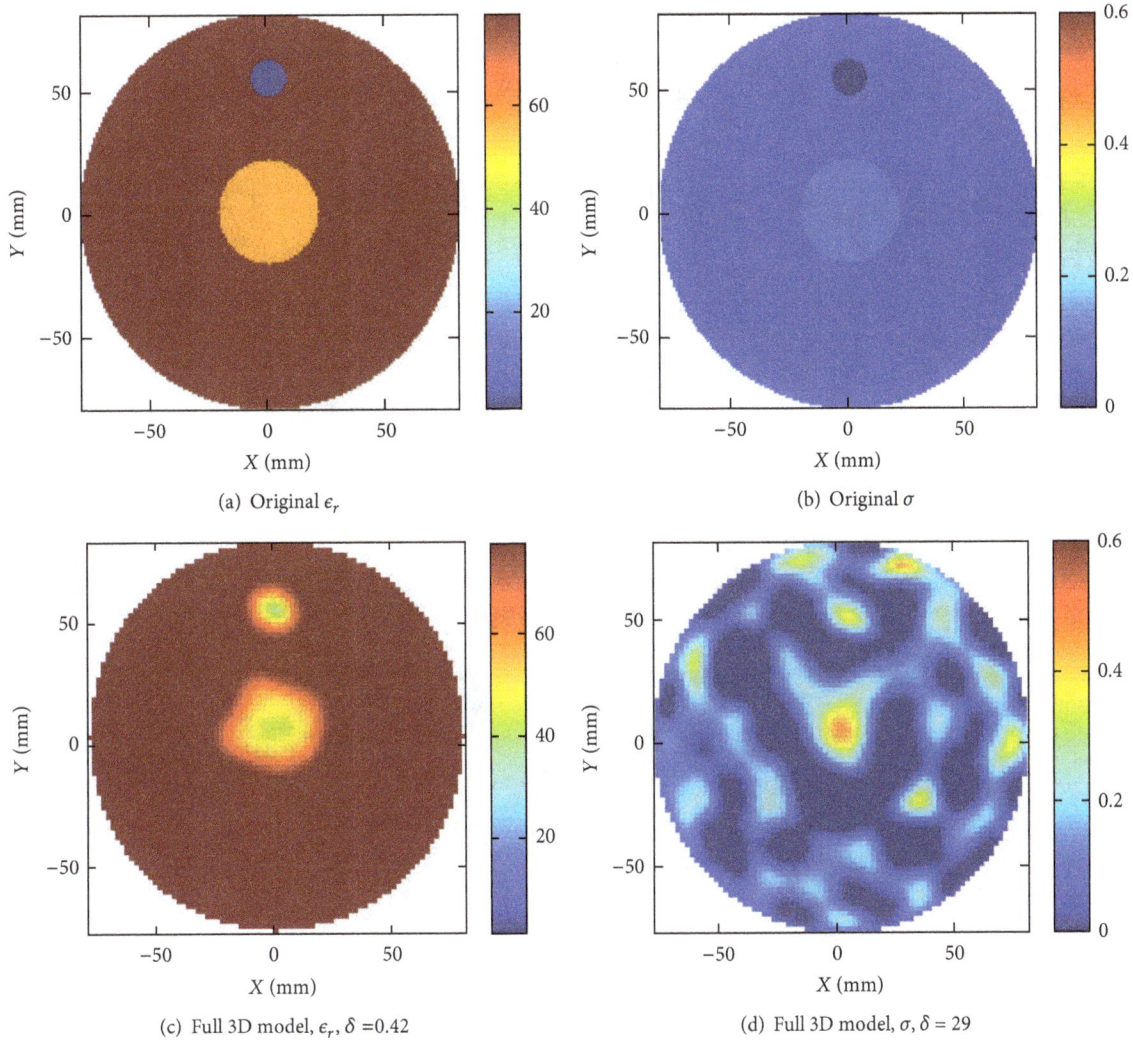

FIGURE 9: (a and b) Original configuration of the water/ethanol and plastic targets immersed in water. (c and d) Reconstructions using the 3D algorithm.

are shown in Figures 12(a) and 12(b). The corresponding reconstruction of the scenario with two objects as shown in Figures 9(a) and 9(b) is shown in Figures 12(c) and 12(d). In these reconstructions we hardly see any object at all. Previous reconstructions made in air of sunflower oil targets with the 2D algorithm published in [12] showed a serious distortion of the size and dielectric values of the targets but a qualitatively correct image could usually be obtained. The reason for the distortion of the reconstructed objects could be attributed to 2D approximation errors as the targets only had the same height as the monopoles. It is a bit surprising that the reconstructed images shown in this paper of targets immersed in water hardly shows anything at all as the electromagnetic waves now in fact should be better confined inside the layer constituted by the water and therefore better conforming to the 2D approximation. Enclosure is provided by the ground plane on the bottom and the impedance step in the water-air interface. However these images are representative for our results showing that robust

image reconstruction is not possible to achieve in water using this 2D algorithm. The situation can be somewhat improved by employing the open water modeling also in 2D; that is, we replace the square water tank model in the background of air with a modeling of a homogeneous background of water to simulate an open domain. The corresponding reconstruction is plotted in Figure 13. In this reconstruction we clearly see the two objects appearing, where the large object contains a spurious hole and the dielectric values are not quite close to the original values. Even if the situation is improved, this reconstruction cannot be considered satisfactory. A similar spurious hole in the reconstruction can be seen also in the reconstructions from short monopole lengths in Figure 2 and arises due to the modeling errors of the antenna. Furthermore associated with every target object is an optimal spectral content that will produce an optimal image [17], and holes usually appear when the spectral content is moved towards higher frequencies. With these two causes for the inaccuracy in the image we have not been able to improve the outcome

(a) Thin-wire with hard feed, ϵ_r, $\delta = 0.54$

(b) Thin-wire with hard feed, σ, $\delta = 30$

(c) Hard source transmitter, ϵ_r, $\delta = 0.58$

(d) Hard source transmitter, σ, $\delta = 87$

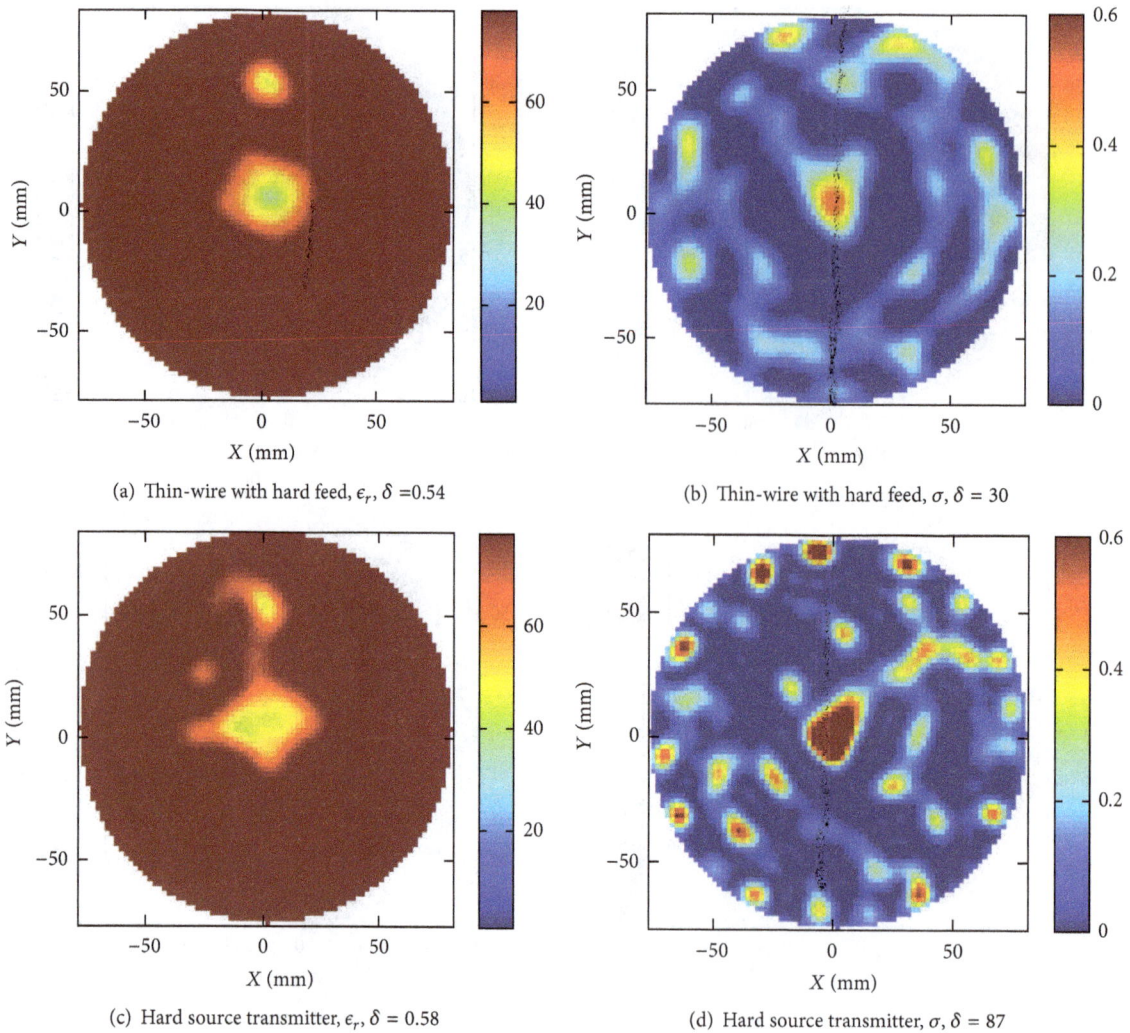

FIGURE 10: Reconstructions of the two target model from Figures 9(a) and 9(b). Here (a) and (b) show the reconstructed result when replacing the RVS feed of the monopole with a hard source. In (c) and (d) the results when removing the wire model of the antenna and using only a hard source as the transmitter model, and on the receiver side the field was directly sampled in the corresponding grid point.

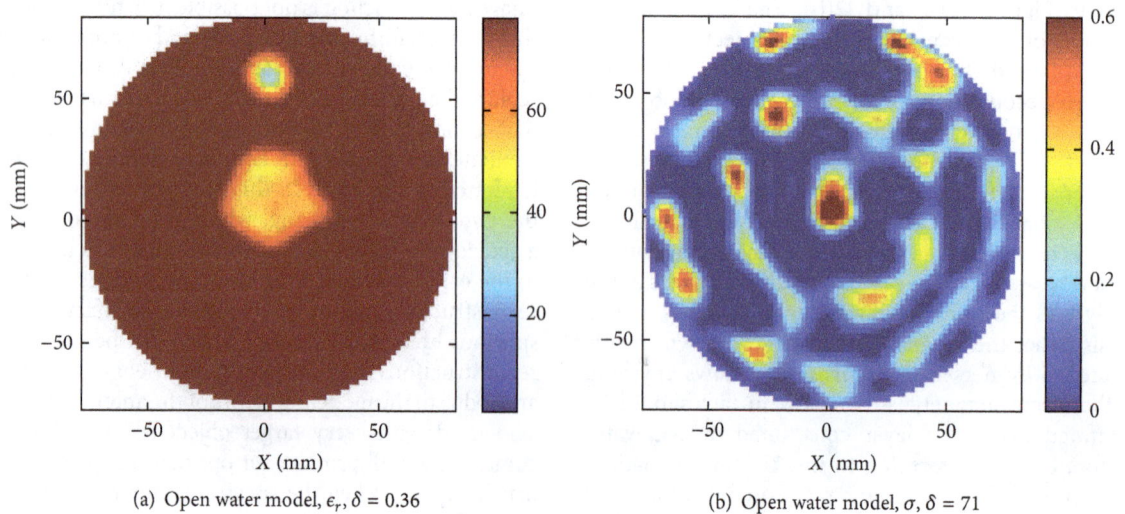

(a) Open water model, ϵ_r, $\delta = 0.36$

(b) Open water model, σ, $\delta = 71$

FIGURE 11: For an open space of water (a) and (b) show the dielectric distribution reconstructed with the 3D model.

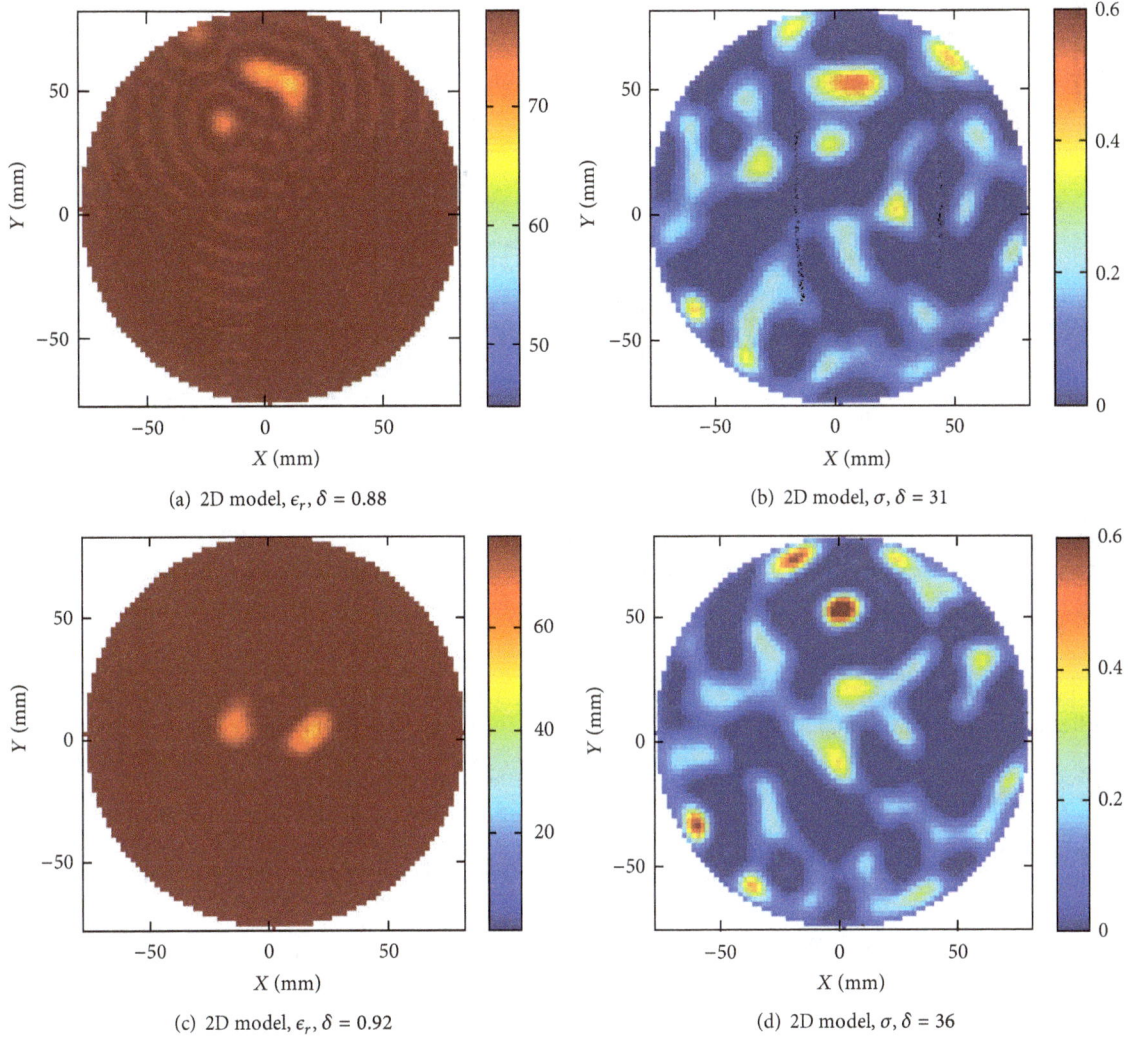

(a) 2D model, ϵ_r, $\delta = 0.88$

(b) 2D model, σ, $\delta = 31$

(c) 2D model, ϵ_r, $\delta = 0.92$

(d) 2D model, σ, $\delta = 36$

FIGURE 12: Reconstructed images using the 2D model. The water tank was modeled as a square in a background medium consisting of air. (a) and (b). Reconstruction of the original target from Figures 8(a), 8(b), 8(c), and 8(d). Reconstruction of the original target from Figures 9(a) and 9(b).

any further by tuning the parameters in the reconstruction algorithm.

5. Conclusion

We have shown successful reconstruction of single and multiple targets immersed in water using a FDTD-based 3D reconstruction algorithm. By investigating various imaging scenarios we have also assessed the question of how the accuracy in the numerical forward model affects the reconstructed image. The results show that a realistic model of the antennas is necessary to achieve robust and reliable imaging. The same results also indicate that small modeling errors, such as in the length of the monopole, can have a clearly evident impact on the resulting image. For a simple antenna such as a monopole the modeling is very simple, and it is not difficult to produce a reasonably accurate numerical model using the thin-wire approximation and the RVS. However

there is always an inherent limitation due to the finite grid size, and, when moving to more advanced antennas, such as patch antennas, modeling accuracy will become a more challenging task. Accurate antenna modeling requires a fine FDTD grid, but at the same time we must keep the grid as coarse as possible to lower the simulation time and memory requirement. Furthermore we have seen that when filling the tank containing the antenna system with normal tap water, the water-air interface causes significant reflections that are clearly identified in the scattering data. Despite this effect the accuracy of the reconstructed results is in fact improved when we instead use an open water model. This result shows that an apparent improvement in the antenna modeling and the corresponding computed scattering data is in fact not beneficial when it comes to imaging. One possible explanation could be that when comparing different models with similar modeling errors the nonlinearity of the reconstruction problem makes it impossible to predict the outcome. Instead the result will be strongly case dependent

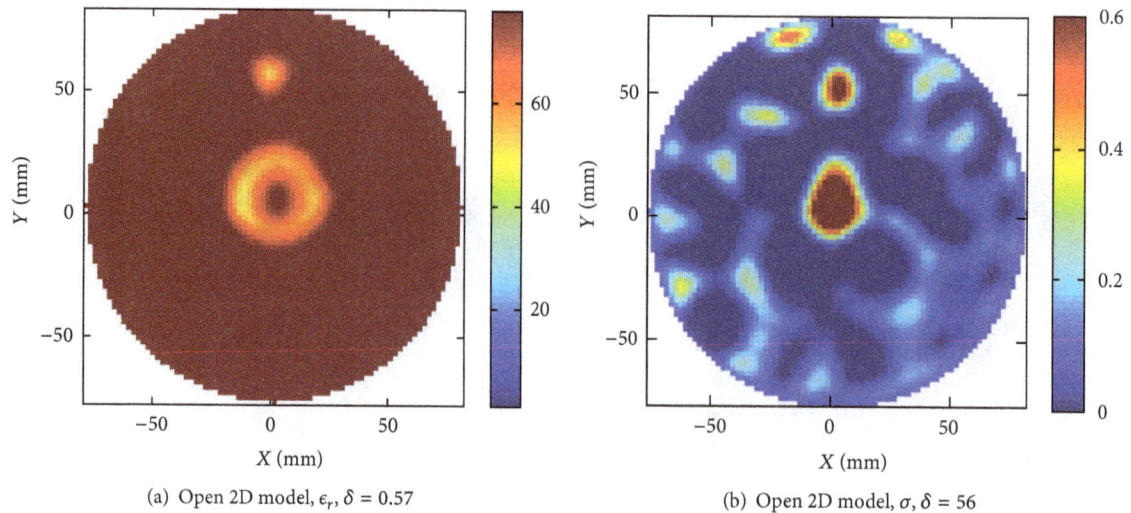

(a) Open 2D model, ϵ_r, $\delta = 0.57$

(b) Open 2D model, σ, $\delta = 56$

FIGURE 13: Reconstructed images using the open water 2D model. The water tank was modeled as a homogeneous background of water where the computation domain was terminated by CPML to model an open domain. (a) and (b) Reconstruction of the original target from Figures 9(a) and 9(b).

and to fully predict the result one would have to perform detailed studies of the particular imaging scenario.

Acknowledgments

This work was supported in part by VINNOVA within the VINN Excellence Center Chase and in part by SSF within the Strategic Research Center Charmant, and by the Australian Research Council (ARC) Australia, under Grant DP-0667064.

References

[1] E. C. Fear, P. M. Meaney, and M. A. Stuchly, "Microwaves for breast cancer detection?" *IEEE Potentials*, vol. 22, no. 1, pp. 12–18, 2003.

[2] N. K. Nikolova, "Microwave imaging for breast cancer," *IEEE Microwave Magazine*, vol. 12, no. 7, pp. 78–94, 2011.

[3] M. Klemm, I. Craddock, J. Leendertz, A. Preece, and R. Benjamin, "Experimental and clinical results of breast cancer detection using UWB microwave radar," in *Proceedings of the IEEE Antennas and Propagation Society International Symposium*, vol. 1–9, pp. 3014–3017, July 2008.

[4] P. M. Meaney, M. W. Fanning, T. Raynolds et al., "Initial clinical experience with microwave breast imaging in women with normal mammography," *Academic Radiology*, vol. 14, no. 2, pp. 207–218, 2007.

[5] S. P. Poplack, T. D. Tosteson, W. A. Wells et al., "Electromagnetic breast imaging: results of a pilot study in women with abnormal mammograms," *Radiology*, vol. 243, no. 2, pp. 350–359, 2007.

[6] M. Shere, A. Preece, I. Craddock, J. Leendertz, and M. Klemm, "Multistatic radar: first trials of a new breast imaging modality," *Breast Cancer Research*, vol. 11, supplement 2, article 05, 2009.

[7] Q. Fang, P. M. Meaney, and K. D. Paulsen, "Viable three-dimensional medical microwave tomography: theory and numerical experiments," *IEEE Transactions on Antennas and Propagation*, vol. 58, no. 2, pp. 449–458, 2010.

[8] T. Rubæk, O. S. Kim, and P. Meincke, "Computational validation of a 3-D microwave imaging system for breast-cancer screening," *IEEE Transactions on Antennas and Propagation*, vol. 57, no. 7, pp. 2105–2115, 2009.

[9] S. Y. Semenov, A. E. Bulyshev, A. Abubakar et al., "Microwave-tomographic imaging of the high dielectric-contrast objects using different image-reconstruction approaches," *IEEE Transactions on Microwave Theory and Techniques*, vol. 53, no. 7, pp. 2284–2293, 2005.

[10] D. W. Winters, J. D. Shea, P. Kosmas, B. D. van Veen, and S. C. Hagness, "Three-dimensional microwave breast imaging: dispersive dielectric properties estimation using patient-specific basis functions," *IEEE Transactions on Medical Imaging*, vol. 28, no. 7, pp. 969–981, 2009.

[11] Z. Q. Zhang and Q. H. Liu, "Three-dimensional nonlinear image reconstruction for microwave biomedical imaging," *IEEE Transactions on Biomedical Engineering*, vol. 51, no. 3, pp. 544–548, 2004.

[12] A. Fhager, S. K. Padhi, and J. Howard, "3D image reconstruction in microwave tomography using an efficient FDTD model," *IEEE Antennas and Wireless Propagation Letters*, vol. 8, pp. 1353–1356, 2009.

[13] A. Taove and S. C. Hagness, *Computational Electrodynamics: The Finite-Difference Time-Domain Method*, Artech House, Boston, Mass, USA, 3rd edition, 2005.

[14] Q. Fang, P. M. Meaney, S. D. Geimer, S. Y. Streltsov, and K. D. Paulsen, "Microwave image reconstruction from 3D fields coupled to 2D parameter estimation," *IEEE Transactions on Medical Imaging*, vol. 23, pp. 475–484, 2004.

[15] C. T. Liauh, R. G. Hills, and R. B. Roemer, "Comparison of the adjoint and influence coefficient methods for solving the inverse hyperthermia problem," *Journal of Biomechanical Engineering*, vol. 115, no. 1, pp. 63–71, 1993.

[16] A. Fhager and M. Persson, "Comparison of two image reconstruction algorithms for microwave tomography," *Radio Science*, vol. 40, no. 3, Article ID RS3017, 2005.

[17] A. Fhager, P. Hashemzadeh, and M. Persson, "Reconstruction quality and spectral content of an electromagnetic time-domain

inversion algorithm," *IEEE Transactions on Biomedical Engineering*, vol. 53, no. 8, pp. 1594–1604, 2006.

[18] R. M. Mäkinen, J. S. Juntunen, and M. A. Kivikoski, "An improved thin-wire model for FDTD," *IEEE Transactions on Microwave Theory and Techniques*, vol. 50, no. 5, pp. 1245–1255, 2002.

[19] J. Juntunen, "Note on the S-parameter and input impedance extraction in antenna simulations using FDTD," *Microwave and Optical Technology Letters*, vol. 28, pp. 8–11, 2001.

[20] O. P. M. Pekonen and J. Xu, "Rigorous analysis of circuit parameter extraction from an FDTD simulation excited with a resistive voltage source," *Microwave and Optical Technology Letters*, vol. 12, no. 4, pp. 205–210, 1996.

[21] S. Nordebo, A. Fhager, M. Gustafsson, and M. Persson, "Measured antenna response of a proposed microwave tomography system using an efficient 3-D FDTD model," *IEEE Antennas and Wireless Propagation Letters*, vol. 7, pp. 689–692, 2008.

16

Using Dynamic Contrast-Enhanced Magnetic Resonance Imaging Data to Constrain a Positron Emission Tomography Kinetic Model: Theory and Simulations

Jacob U. Fluckiger,[1] **Xia Li,**[2,3] **Jennifer G. Whisenant,**[2,4] **Todd E. Peterson,**[2,3,5] **John C. Gore,**[2,3,4,5,6,7] **and Thomas E. Yankeelov**[2,3,4,5,6,8]

[1] *Department of Radiology, Northwestern University, Chicago, IL 60611, USA*

[2] *Institute of Imaging Science, Vanderbilt University, Nashville, TN 37212, USA*

[3] *Department of Radiology and Radiological Sciences, Vanderbilt University, Nashville, TN 37212, USA*

[4] *Program in Chemical and Physical Biology, Vanderbilt University, Nashville, TN 37212, USA*

[5] *Department of Physics and Astronomy, Vanderbilt University, Nashville, TN 37212, USA*

[6] *Department of Biomedical Engineering, Vanderbilt University, Nashville, TN 37212, USA*

[7] *Department of Molecular Physiology and Biophysics, Vanderbilt University, Nashville, TN 37212, USA*

[8] *Department of Cancer Biology, Vanderbilt University, Nashville, TN 37212, USA*

Correspondence should be addressed to Thomas E. Yankeelov; thomas.yankeelov@vanderbilt.edu

Academic Editor: Guowei Wei

We show how dynamic contrast-enhanced magnetic resonance imaging (DCE-MRI) data can constrain a compartmental model for analyzing dynamic positron emission tomography (PET) data. We first develop the theory that enables the use of DCE-MRI data to separate whole tissue time activity curves (TACs) available from dynamic PET data into individual TACs associated with the blood space, the extravascular-extracellular space (EES), and the extravascular-intracellular space (EIS). Then we simulate whole tissue TACs over a range of physiologically relevant kinetic parameter values and show that using appropriate DCE-MRI data can separate the PET TAC into the three components with accuracy that is noise dependent. The simulations show that accurate blood, EES, and EIS TACs can be obtained as evidenced by concordance correlation coefficients >0.9 between the true and estimated TACs. Additionally, provided that the estimated DCE-MRI parameters are within 10% of their true values, the errors in the PET kinetic parameters are within approximately 20% of their true values. The parameters returned by this approach may provide new information on the transport of a tracer in a variety of dynamic PET studies.

1. Introduction

There is an extensive literature on the use of compartmental modeling to understand the distribution and retention of various positron emission tomography (PET) radiotracers (see, e.g., [1, 2]). A series of ordinary, first-order, linear differential equations are often used to model the body as a series of well-mixed "compartments," between which a tracer may be transported. Solving the differential equations and then fitting those solutions to measured tissue time activity curves (TACs) return estimates of a number of relevant physiological parameters. Typical dynamic PET models return parameters describing the metabolic rates of tracer utilization. The models used to extract these parameters have several free parameters and the measured TAC is, in practice, a weighted sum of unknown TACs from multiple compartments. This results in the introduction of extra assumptions into the analysis. Another central issue in standard dynamic PET modeling is the difficulty of obtaining a reasonable time course of the concentration of the injected tracer in the blood plasma (i.e., the arterial input function), especially for small animal studies. Thus, the current state-of-the-art in PET kinetic modeling typically requires simplifying assumptions to reduce the number of free parameters and/or nonlinear fitting methods which are well known to be sensitive to measurement noise [1]. Here, we introduce a method that exploits the data available from dynamic contrast-enhanced magnetic resonance imaging (DCE-MRI) studies to constrain the kinetic modeling of nuclear measurements and potentially provide new insight into the physical distribution and transfer of PET radiotracers.

Similar to a kinetic PET study, DCE-MRI involves the serial acquisition of images before, during, and after the injection of a contrast agent [3]. As the contrast agent perfuses into the voxel (or region) of interest, it changes the tissue's native relaxation rates to an extent determined by the concentration of the contrast agent. By following the image sequence and fitting the resulting signal intensity with an appropriate mathematical model, various parameters related to blood vessel perfusion and permeability and tissue volume fractions (i.e., the blood fraction, extravascular-extracellular space (EES), and extravascular-intracellular space (EIS)) can be extracted. The three volume fraction parameters can potentially be used to constrain the modeling of kinetic PET data; that is, the formalism below allows the separation of the overall tissue TAC into TACs associated with the blood, EES, and EIS compartments. This enables access to compartments that are not typically accessible in dynamic PET studies.

It is important to note that there exists a subtle, though fundamental, difference between the compartmental models employed in quantitative DCE-MRI and dynamic PET analyses. The compartments in kinetic PET modeling typically (^{15}O labeled H$_2$O is one notable exception) refer to biochemical compartments (e.g., bound or free), whereas the compartments in kinetic MRI modeling refer to physical compartments (e.g., the blood, EES, or EIS). Thus, when the compartments extracted from a DCE-MRI analysis are used to separate the PET TAC into different compartments, the TAC is separated into the compartments determined from the DCE-MRI data—and these compartments are fundamentally different than the biochemical compartments. This means that the TACs associated with these compartments, as well as the kinetic parameters describing the movement of the tracer between these compartments, are not the same as those reported in the existing PET literature. More specifically, in this contribution, we develop the formalism required to use DCE-MRI data to extract separate TACs for the blood pool (i.e., the input function), EES, and EIS and then show how these time courses can be used to fit simplified versions (i.e., fewer free parameters with known TACs) of a PET compartmental model to extract kinetic parameters related to the delivery and retention of PET tracer that is distributed amongst the blood space, EES, and EIS. We conclude by discussing how the access to these new physiological parameters may be of use in future dynamic PET studies.

2. Materials and Methods

2.1. PET Kinetic Modeling. Figure 1 depicts the compartmental model that we will use for this study; from left

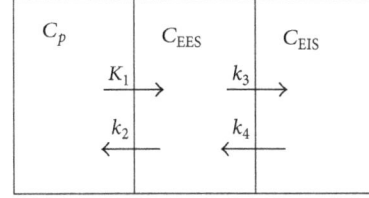

FIGURE 1: A schematic representation of the three-compartment model used with the dynamic PET imaging. From left to right, the three compartments represent the blood plasma, the extracellular-extravascular space, and the extracellular-intravascular space.

to right, the compartments are the plasma, extravascular-extracellular space, and extravascular-intracellular space, respectively. We again note that these compartments are not those identified in a typical PET kinetic modeling, which consider the three (biochemical) compartments of radiotracer distribution as plasma, free and nonspecifically bound in tissue, and specifically bound [1]. Rather, the (physical) compartments chosen here reflect those typically identifiable in a dynamic contrast-enhanced MRI acquisition described below. The set of compartments described by this model provides access to other potentially useful compartments and rate constants. Thus, while the mathematical description of the tracer concentrations is unchanged, it does change the interpretation of the parameter values; we return to this important point in Section 4. The following set of first-order, ordinary, linear differential equations describe the system depicted in Figure 1:

$$\frac{dC_p(t)}{dt} = k_2 C_{\text{EES}}(t) - K_1 C_p(t),$$

$$\frac{dC_{\text{EES}}(t)}{dt} = K_1 C_p(t) - k_2 C_{\text{EES}}(t) - k_3 C_{\text{EES}}(t) + k_4 C_{\text{EIS}}(t),$$

$$\frac{dC_{\text{EIS}}(t)}{dt} = k_3 C_{\text{EES}}(t) - k_4 C_{\text{EIS}}(t),$$

$$(1)$$

where C_p, C_{EES}, and C_{EIS} are the concentrations of the tracer in the blood plasma, extravascular-extracellular, and extravascular-intracellular spaces, respectively. There are four unknown rate constants and three unknown concentration-of-tracer time courses. The problem is compounded by the fact that a typical PET study measures only the total concentration of the tracer in a given voxel or region of interest, C_{tissue}, which is determined by the concentration of the tracer in each compartment and the relative volume contributions of each compartment:

$$C_{\text{tissue}}(t) = v_b C_b(t) + v_{\text{EES}} C_{\text{EES}}(t) + v_{\text{EIS}} C_{\text{EIS}}(t), \quad (2)$$

where v_b, v_{EES}, and v_{EIS} are the blood, extravascular-extracellular, and extravascular-intracellular volume fractions, respectively. Solving the second two relations in (1) yields

$$C_{\mathrm{EES}}(t) = \frac{K_1}{\alpha_2 - \alpha_1} C_p(t) \otimes \left[(k_4 - \alpha_1) e^{-\alpha_1 t} + (\alpha_2 - k_4) e^{-\alpha_2 t} \right],$$

$$C_{\mathrm{EIS}}(t) = \frac{K_1 k_3}{\alpha_2 - \alpha_1} C_p(t) \otimes \left[e^{-\alpha_1 t} - e^{-\alpha_2 t} \right],$$

$$\alpha_{1,2} = \frac{(k_2 + k_3 + k_4) \pm \sqrt{(k_2 + k_3 + k_4)^2 - 4k_2 k_4}}{2}. \tag{3}$$

If we note that $v_b + v_{\mathrm{EES}} + v_{\mathrm{EIS}} = 1$, $v_p = v_b \cdot (1 - \mathrm{hematocrit})$ and assume that the plasma free fraction is 1, then the solution (i.e., (2) and (3)) has six unknown parameters and three unknown concentration-of-tracer time courses. If the arterial input function can be measured reliably, this is reduced to two unknown concentration time courses. After briefly introducing the relevant aspects of DCE-MRI modeling, we proceed to show how DCE data can constrain this PET model by eliminating unknown parameters and determining unknown concentration-of-tracer time courses.

2.2. DCE-MRI Kinetic Modeling. A typical DCE-MRI study employs an untargeted contrast agent that is distributed from blood into tissue, but is unable to appreciably penetrate cells, so the compartmental model is considerably simpler than the above model for PET tracer kinetics and is given as:

$$\frac{dC_{\mathrm{tissue}}(t)}{dt} = K^{\mathrm{trans}} C_p(t) - \frac{K^{\mathrm{trans}}}{v_{\mathrm{EES}}} C_{\mathrm{tissue}}(t), \tag{4}$$

where C_{tissue} and C_p are the concentration of an MRI contrast agent in the tissue and plasma space, respectively, K^{trans} represents the volume transfer constant for the agent between the blood plasma (in units of mL (blood)/mL (tissue)/min) and the extravascular-extracellular space, and v_{EES} are as above. This corresponds to the first two compartments in Figure 1. The intracellular compartment concentration C_{EIS}, along with the rate constants k_3 and k_4, is zero since standard, clinically approved MRI contrast agents remain extracellular. The solution to (4) is given as follows:

$$C_{\mathrm{tissue}}(t) = K^{\mathrm{trans}} \exp\left(\frac{-K^{\mathrm{trans}} t}{v_{\mathrm{EES}}} \right) \otimes C_p(t). \tag{5}$$

Many have noted that this model does not explicitly account for the plasma fraction, and thus (5) is frequently amended to include a blood plasma component as follows:

$$C_{\mathrm{tissue}}(t) = K^{\mathrm{trans}} \exp\left(\frac{-K^{\mathrm{trans}} t}{v_{\mathrm{EES}}} \right) \otimes C_p(t) + v_p C_p(t), \tag{6}$$

where v_p is the blood plasma fraction. By measuring heavily T1-weighted DCE-MRI data in the tissue of interest (e.g., a tumor) and a feeding vessel before, during, and after the injection of a standard extracellular contrast agent, the

$C_{\mathrm{tissue}}(t)$ and $C_p(t)$ time courses can be estimated and fit to (6) to extract K^{trans}, v_{EES}, and v_p; the latter two can be used to assign v_{EES}, v_b ($= v_p/(1-\mathrm{hematocrit})$), and v_{EIS} ($= 1-v_b-v_{\mathrm{EES}}$) in the PET model.

2.3. Constraining PET Kinetic Modeling. We now show how DCE-MRI data can be used to eliminate a number of the unknown quantities in (2) and (3). The method adapts the approach developed by Asllani et al. [4] for partial volume corrections in MRI studies of blood flow.

If we take the v_p ($= v_b \cdot (1 - \mathrm{hematocrit})$) and v_{EES} values returned from a typical DCE-MRI study as *a priori* knowledge for the PET analysis, then this reduces the number of unknowns to four rate constants (K_1–k_4) and three concentration time courses (C_p, C_{EES}, and C_{EIS}). We then consider a DCE-MRI scan and a PET study that have been spatially registered such that they have the same voxel sizes. This implementation differs from the one given in [4] which does not incorporate spatial registration; we return to this point in Section 4. Next we take advantage of the differences in spatial resolution between the acquired MRI and PET data and define a small region of tissue, a 5×5 voxel window centered on a particular voxel of interest, from both the DCE-MRI and PET studies. If we assume that the tissue PET tracer concentration (the left hand side of (2)) in each voxel of the 5×5 window is equal to the *measured* tissue concentration in the central (particular) PET voxel and assume that the C_b, C_{EES}, and C_{EIS} are identical in each MRI voxel—reasonable assumptions for a small window—then we can write a system of equations in the three unknowns. In particular, for the *i*th voxel within the window, we have

$$C_{\mathrm{tissue}}(t) = v_{i,b} C_b(t) + v_{i,\mathrm{EES}} C_{\mathrm{EES}}(t) + v_{i,\mathrm{EIS}} C_{\mathrm{EIS}}(t), \tag{7}$$

where i runs from 1 to N, the number of voxels in the search window. If we define the matrix A to be

$$A = \begin{vmatrix} v_{1,b} & v_{1,\mathrm{EES}} & v_{1,\mathrm{EIS}} \\ v_{2,b} & v_{2,\mathrm{EES}} & v_{2,\mathrm{EIS}} \\ \cdots & \cdots & \cdots \\ v_{N,b} & v_{N,\mathrm{EES}} & v_{N,\mathrm{EIS}} \end{vmatrix} \tag{8}$$

and the column vector C to be

$$C = \begin{bmatrix} C_b \\ C_{\mathrm{EES}} \\ C_{\mathrm{EIS}} \end{bmatrix}, \tag{9}$$

then we can rewrite the system in (7) as

$$C_{\mathrm{tissue}} = A_{ij} C_i, \tag{10}$$

where C_{tissue} is a column vector of length N. The optimal least-squares solution to (10), which is an overdetermined problem (5), is given by

$$C = \left(A^T \cdot A \right)^{-1} A^T \cdot C_{\mathrm{tissue}}, \tag{11}$$

where $(A^T \cdot A^{-1}) A^T$ is the pseudoinverse and every term on the right-handside is known. In principle, this analysis should

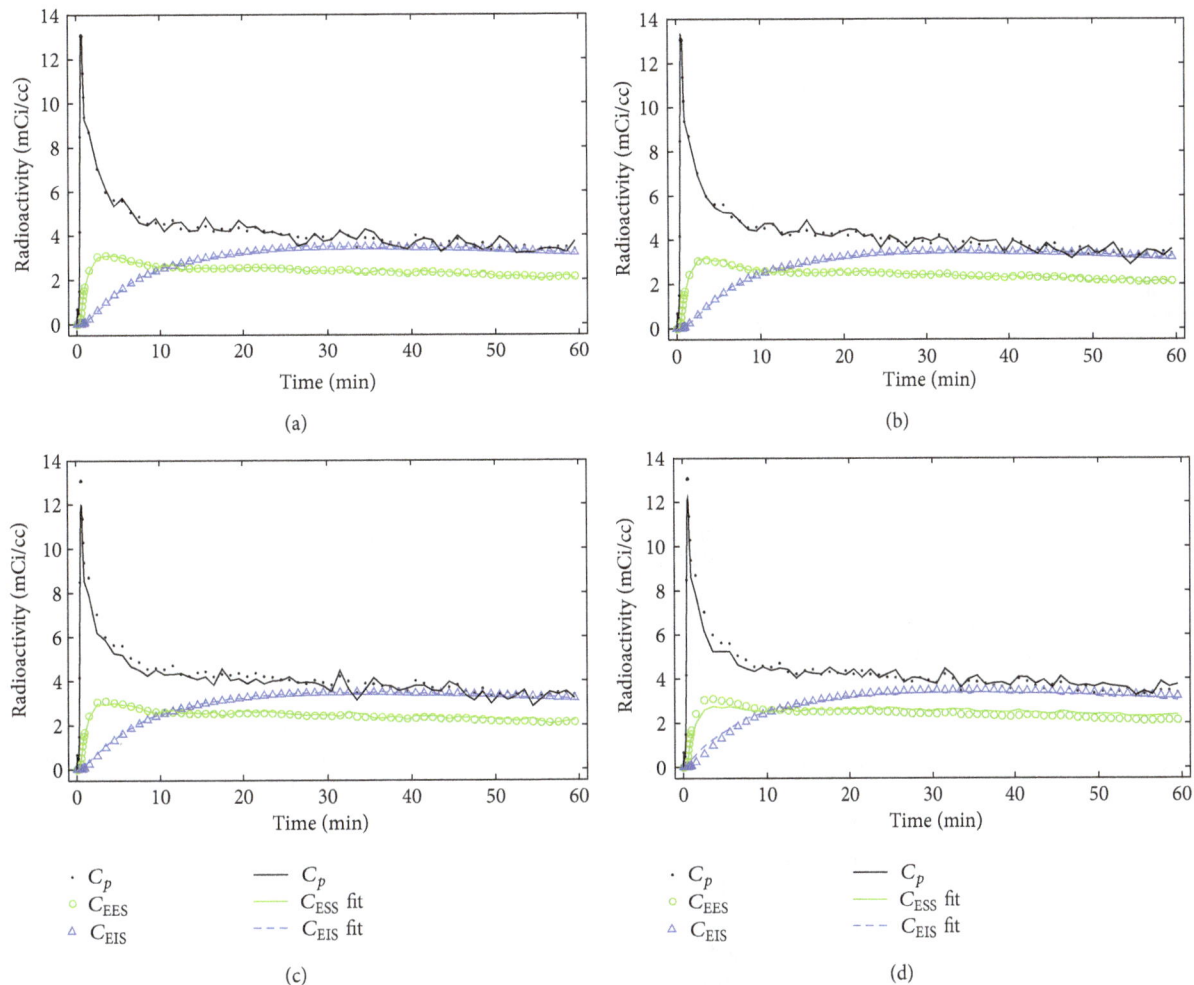

FIGURE 2: An example of simulated tissue curves and the fits provided by (11). These panels represent 25 voxels with (a) no error in the DCE-MRI parameters, (b) 5% error, (c) 10% error, and (d) 15% error. The AIF used in these simulations was measured from the left ventricle of a mouse, which results in some noise even with no error in the DCE-MRI parameters (see panel (a)).

return time courses for C_b (and thus $C_p(t)$), C_{EES}, and C_{EIS}, which can then be used to drive the PET kinetic analysis described by (3) to return the k_i. This approach also solves the problem of not knowing how to separate the measured whole tissue PET signal into C_{EES}, C_{EIS}, and C_p components.

2.4. Simulations. To evaluate the theory above, we simulated kinetic PET data over a range of parameter combinations. The simulations were initialized with an arterial input function $C_p(t)$ measured from a dynamic ^{18}F-fluorothymidine (FLT) PET scan (data not shown as the particular tracer employed is not central to this paper; that is, all that is needed is a reasonable, experimentally measured input function). This time course was then used to drive (2)-(3) with k_i values that were randomly selected from uniform distributions. The range of the distribution of the parameters used here was chosen to be of the same order as those given in the literature [5, 6], though we again note that the parameters listed in (2)-(3) are not the same as those in the references. Experimental

noise was simulated in two ways. For each time point, the standard deviation of the noise level was set to 1, 10, 20, 30, 40, and 50 times the square root of the whole tissue concentration simulated at that time point [7]. A second source of systematic error was included by varying the accuracy of the parameters extracted from the DCE-MRI analysis and used as *a priori* data for (11). As indicated by (8), 25 sets of values of v_b, v_{EES}, and v_{EIS} are required per PET voxel. Reliable values are available for v_b and v_{EES} so we assigned the 25 voxel values randomly selected from uniform distributions with ranges from 0.04 to 0.12 and 0.25 to 0.45, respectively [8–10]. Each v_{EIS} value was assigned according to $v_{EIS} = 1 - (v_b + v_{EES})$. For each noise realization, the simulated whole tissue data were first analyzed *via* (11) to extract estimates of the C_{EES}, C_{EIS}, and C_b time courses. After the first step, we computed the concordance correlation coefficient (CCC) between the extracted C_{EES}, C_{EIS}, and C_b and the true C_{EES}, C_{EIS}, and C_b time courses. The CCC tests the strength of the correlation, as well as the deviation of the correlation from the line of unity. The extracted time courses were then analyzed with (2) and (3) to return estimates of the kinetic PET parameters. While there are several ways to execute this fitting, we elected to perform a procedure whereby C_b and C_{EES} were combined with the first expression in (3), C_b and C_{EIS} were combined with the second expression in (3), and the residuals for both sets of data were optimized simultaneously. This procedure was performed 1000 times with different combinations of parameters and realizations of noise, and the extracted PET parameters were then compared to their actual values and the mean ± the 95% confidence interval was computed. We then performed a second set of simulations to examine the effect of error in the DCE-MRI parameters on the accuracy of the kinetic PET parameters. The noise level in the simulated TACs was set to the square root of the whole tissue concentration and an error was added to the DCE-MRI parameters such that the 95% confidence interval of the assigned parameter value was 0%, 5%, 10%, and 15% of the mean value. Higher errors in the DCE-MRI parameters yielded unreliable results in the PET kinetic analysis. As before, this procedure was performed 1000 times and both the CCC values between the true and extracted time courses and the error in the extracted PET parameters were computed.

3. Results

Figure 2 shows the ability of the algorithm to correctly separate the C_{EES}, C_{EIS}, and C_b time courses from one simulated, whole tissue dataset. The parameter values were $K_1 = 0.3$ (mL/min/g), $k_2 = 0.5$ (min^{-1}), $k_3 = 0.15$ (min^{-1}), and $k_4 = 0.1$ (min^{-1}). The solid lines indicate the extracted curves, while the individual points correspond to the true (simulated) data; the filled circles in each panel depict the measured C_b time course used to drive all the simulations. The four panels correspond to time courses extracted when the DCE-MRI parameters have errors of 0%, 5%, 10%, and 15%. In all four panels, the error in C_{EIS} is less than 5%. C_{EES} is extracted with an error of less than 5% when the DCE-MRI parameters have errors of 10% or less (panels (a)–(c)). The maximum error in C_{EES} when the DCE-MRI parameters have errors of 15% is approximately 10%. For the C_b component, the maximum error in the extracted time course increases with the errors in the DCE-MRI parameters.

As stated above, two sets of noise realizations were performed. Figures 3 and 4 display results of simulations done with varying levels of noise added to the simulated C_{tissue} curves, and with no error in the DCE-MRI parameters. Figure 3 shows the CCC (vertical axis) between the extracted and true C_{EES}, C_{EIS}, and C_b time courses as a function of increasing C_{tissue} noise for one combination of PET kinetic parameters. The results are presented as the mean ± the minimum and maximum CCC values obtained over the 1000 noise realizations. The results from the other seven combinations of PET kinetic parameters are similar. In all cases, when no noise is added to the simulated C_{tissue} curves, the CCC values are uniformly 1.00. The mean CCC values decrease with increased noise, with the CCC for C_b and C_{EES} decreasing to 0.2 at the maximum level of noise tested here.

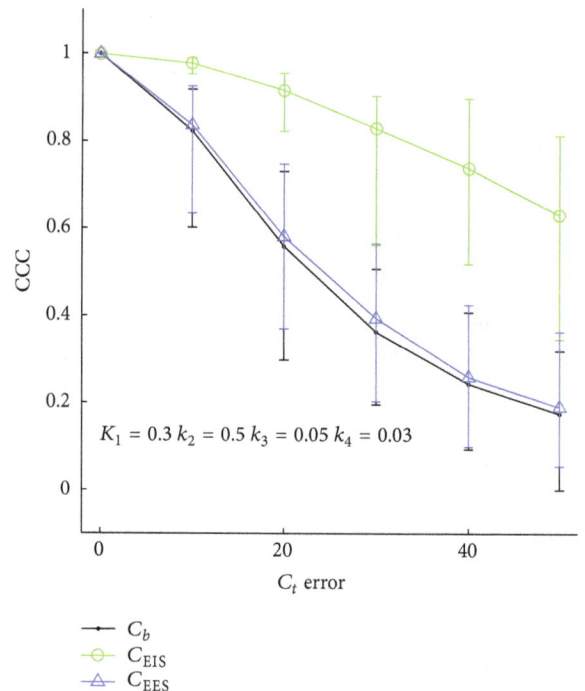

Figure 3: The concordance correlation coefficient between the estimated and true values of the time courses as a function of noise in the tissue curves for a single set of PET kinetic parameters. If the C_t error is less than 10 times the square root of activity level, then the CCC is greater than 0.75. Once C_t error is greater than this, the ability to faithfully reconstruct the time courses is substantially reduced.

For all combinations of PET kinetic parameters, the C_{EIS} time courses are the least affected by noise in the tissue curves.

Figure 4 presents four panels showing the error in the extracted k_i as a function of the error in the DCE-MRI kinetic parameters. Each panel corresponds to a different combination of k_i values that are listed at the bottom of each panel. The data are presented as mean ± one standard error. The error trends in the other sets of PET kinetic parameters is similar to those shown. Across all parameter combinations, the error in the extracted PET kinetic parameters is below 50% provided that the error in the simulated C_t curves is below 20 times the square root of the concentration. However, as the noise continues to increase, the error in the k_3 and k_4 parameters increases rapidly to above 100%. The error in K_1 and k_2 parameters increases less rapidly than that for k_3 and k_4.

Figures 5 and 6 display similar results as those in Figures 3 and 4. These two figures display the results from the simulations where the error in the DCE-MRI parameters increased from 0 to 15%. As stated above, in these simulations, the error in the C_t time course was fixed to the square root of the concentration in the tissue. Figure 5 shows the CCC between the extracted and true C_{EES}, C_{EIS}, and C_b time courses as a function of percent error in the DCE-MRI parameters for a single set of PET kinetic parameters. The mean CCCs are all above 0.9 across all parameter combinations and noise realizations. The minimum CCC

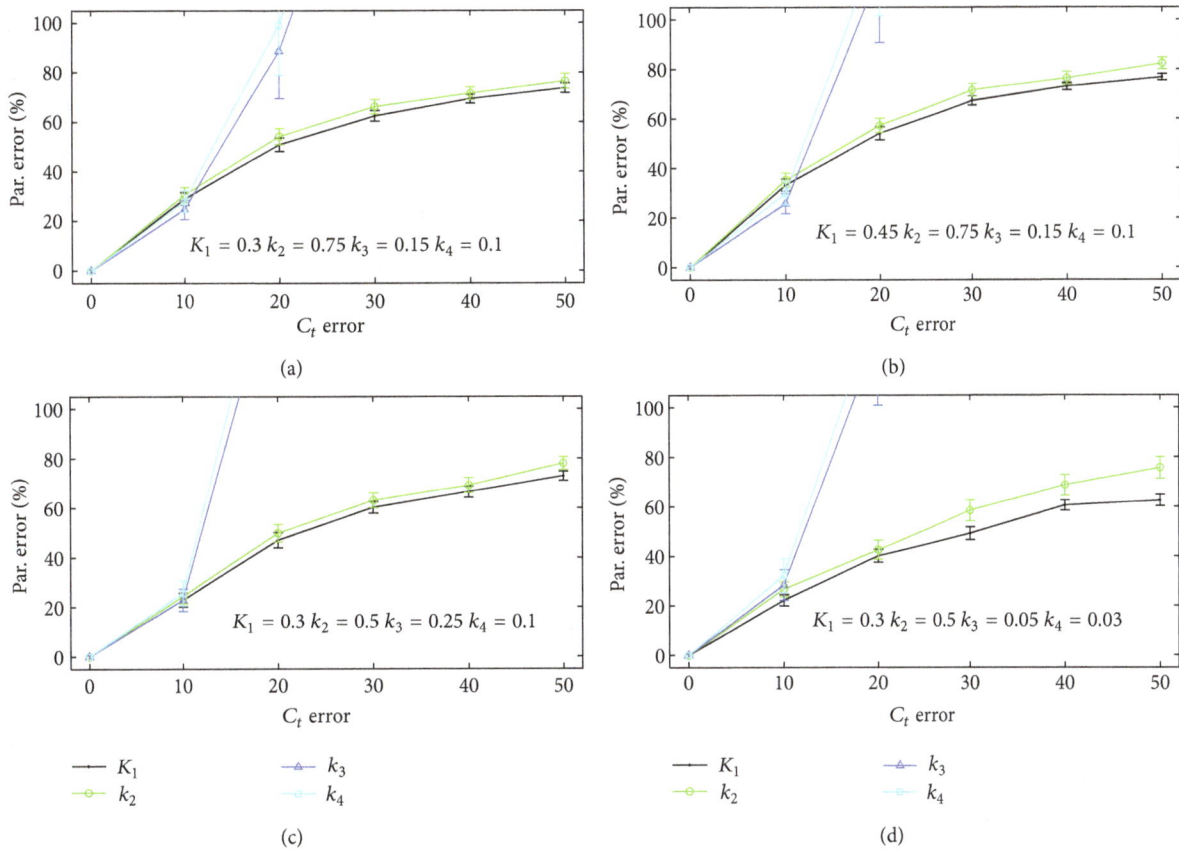

FIGURE 4: The error in the estimated PET kinetic parameters as a function of the noise in the tissue curves. Each panel corresponds to a different set of PET kinetic parameters. For each set of parameters, when the error in C_t is less than 10 times the square root of the activity level, the parameter error is less than 50. As the error in C_t continues to increase, the error in k_3 and k_4 increases rapidly. The error in K_1 and k_2 also continues to increase, but less rapidly.

over all the realizations was 0.6, which occurred when the error in the DCE parameters is 15%.

Figure 6 again presents four panels showing the error in the extracted k_i as a function of the error in the DCE-MRI kinetic parameters. The range and combinations of the k_i are the same as in Figure 5. The data are presented as mean ± one standard error. Across all eight parameter combinations tested, the errors in the extracted PET kinetic parameters are below 25% provided that the error in the DCE-MRI parameters is below 10%. However, once the DCE-MRI error approaches 15%, there are certain combinations of kinetic PET parameters that lead to errors as high as 50% in the extracted parameters; one example can be seen in panel (d).

4. Discussion

Since the advent of the first prototype SPECT-CT system in 1990 [11, 12], multimodality imaging has been largely focused on combining form and function. In particular, SPECT-CT and PET-CT systems have combined the high-resolution anatomical images available through CT imaging with the molecular information provided by nuclear medicine [13, 14]. New developments in multimodality imaging are increasingly focused on combining data sets to enable

new measurements not previously possible. One example of this new type of functional imaging is the combination of dynamic PET imaging with dynamic MR imaging. The introduction of PET/MR hybrid scanners [15–17] makes the approach outlined here practical. With these scanners, the data could be acquired at nearly the same time and would be readily registered.

The results from the simulations show that the method returns good estimates for the time courses C_b, C_{EES}, and C_{EIS} as well as the PET kinetic parameters k_i when the noise in the tissue curves and the error in the volume fractions measured by DCE-MRI are both small. The method is highly sensitive to increased noise in the TACs, as seen in Figures 3 and 4. This is a potential limitation of the proposed method. More sophisticated imaging or postprocessing techniques focusing on reducing the noise in the measured PET data would allow for higher accuracy in the estimated PET kinetic parameters.

As seen in Figures 5 and 6, the accuracy of the PET parameters also depends on how well the DCE-MRI parameters are known. The dependence of the PET parameter estimates on the error in the DCE-MRI parameters is smaller than the dependence on the noise in the tissue concentration curves. Other studies have shown that the error in the DCE-MRI parameters depends on several factors, including the

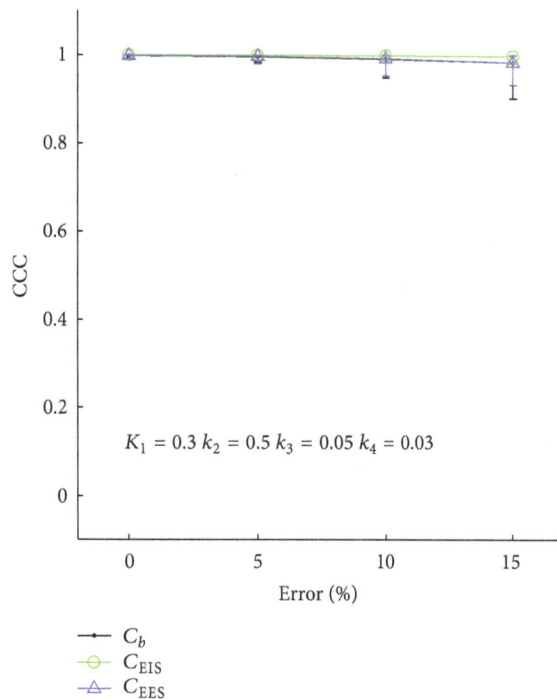

FIGURE 5: The concordance correlation coefficient between the estimated and true values for the time courses as a function of error in the DCE-MRI parameters for a single set of PET kinetic parameters. The method is able to return the time courses faithfully when the DCE-MRI parameter error is less than 5%. With higher error in the DCE-MRI parameters, the CCC remains above 0.95 on average, though some realizations returned CCC values as low as 0.9.

accuracy of the arterial input function used to estimate the parameters [18, 19]. Methods for obtaining higher accuracy in DCE-MRI parameters are an area of active research (see, e.g., [20, 21]). Recent work assessing the reproducibility of DCE-MRI parameters in preclinical models of breast cancer reported that parameter measurements for v_{EES} are repeatable between imaging sessions [22], which suggests that, with no systemic modeling errors, obtaining v_{EES} measurements with small errors is possible. The repeatability index for v_b was smaller and may be more susceptible to measurement error. Similar work in clinical applications of DCE-MRI also reported high repeatability for v_{EES} [23, 24].

The method developed by Asllani et al. [4] took advantage of the difference in spatial resolution between echo planar and arterial spin labeled MRI acquisitions to develop a system of equations similar to that given previously in (7). In that implementation, the echo planar images and arterial spin-labelled images were acquired sequentially on the same system and thus were inherently coregistered. In our method, the PET and MR images would typically be acquired on different scanners (though, as noted above, PET-MRI scanners are becoming more commonplace), and some spatial registration would be required prior to image processing. As mentioned above, our approach assumes that the TACs in each compartment are identical within a 5 × 5

window of MRI voxels, which is reasonable for MRI voxel sizes of approximately 250 μm × 250 μm in-plane resolution which is common for *in vivo* DCE-MRI studies in mice.

As noted in the Introduction, the parameters k_i used in this formulation have a fundamentally different meaning than those commonly employed in PET kinetic modeling. Typically, compartments used in dynamic PET modeling are based on biochemical compartments, whereas in dynamic MRI modeling they are based on physical compartments. One consequence of this difference is that standard metabolic rate constants cannot be calculated directly from the formalism as presented in this effort. However, even though the rate constants calculated from this model do not reflect the biochemical state of the radiotracer, they do provide information on the physical movement of radiotracers into and out of the vascular and cellular spaces. This set of parameters is potentially useful in situations where the physical location of the tracer (i.e., intra- or extracellular) may be relevant to patient diagnosis or treatment planning. For example, this model may be of potential interest in measuring the cellular uptake of glucose in dynamic FDG studies in diabetic populations. The new k_3 and k_4 parameters returned by this model reflect the rate of transport of tracer into and out of the intracellular space, respectively. These parameters may be able to report on GLUT-1 and GLUT-3 transportation in tumor cells. This model could also be of potential interest in dynamic [^{15}O]-labeled water studies. Typical modeling of [^{15}O]-labeled water utilizes a two-compartment model with one intravascular compartment and one extravascular compartment [25]. This is due to difficulty in resolving intra- and extracellular compartments due to the free diffusion of water across the cell boundary. Using DCE-MRI data to inform the fractional volume of these compartments may provide further insight into the molecular physiology. Of course, the preclinical and clinical utility of the "new" k_i parameters is left to future work.

It should also be noted that performing the analysis described in this work would, of course, not preclude any dynamic modeling with more traditional compartment definitions on the same data. Also, despite the changes in the physical interpretation of the rate constants, the arterial input function derived from the proposed method is identical to that used in more traditional dynamic PET modeling and can be used in implementing these models. Perhaps, the method proposed in this effort has value in merely providing an input function from which a standard dynamic analysis could be performed. Additionally, the input function estimated by this approach comes from the (local) tissue of interest which could potentially eliminate uncertainties related to the delay and dispersion when an input function is estimated from blood samples or ROIs in distant locations.

Future studies with this method will focus on validating the proposed method with *in vivo* data. Higher temporal resolution in the DCE-MRI data may allow for improved accuracy in the DCE-MRI parameters, but acquiring this data would cost some spatial resolution. The noise in the PET data could also be improved by effectively lowering the spatial resolution through averaging the data. The proposed method may be more effective in situations where the desire for

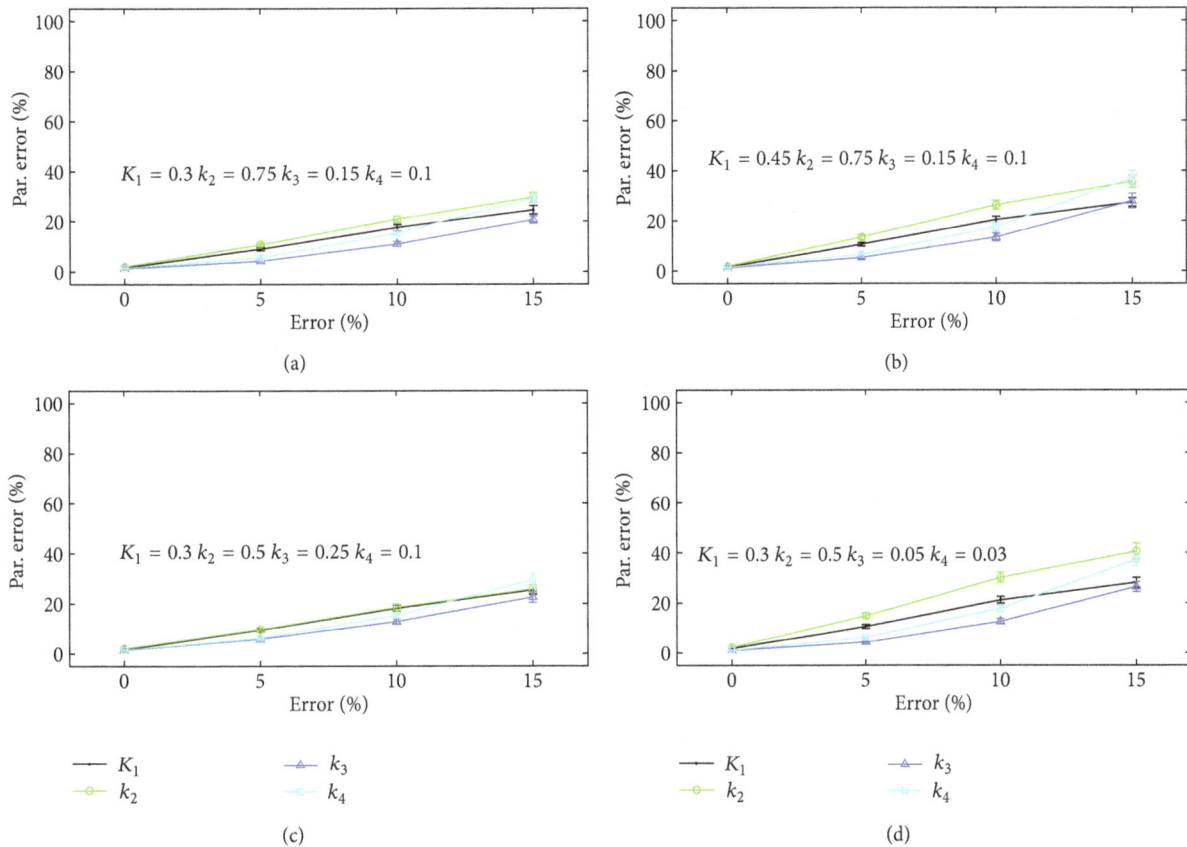

FIGURE 6: The error in the estimated PET kinetic parameters as a function of the error in the DCE-MRI parameters. Each panel corresponds to a different set of PET kinetic parameters. For each parameter combination, the error in the PET parameters is below 25% provided the error in the DCE-MRI parameters is below 10%. As the DCE-MRI parameter error increases, the error in the PET parameters exceeds 40% in some cases (see panel (d)).

quantitative information outweighs the need for high spatial resolution information.

5. Conclusion

We have presented a method that uses DCE-MRI parameters to separate the whole tissue concentration curves, C_{tissue}, into extravascular-extracellular, extravascular-intracellular, and intravascular components. These separate components are then used to initialize and constrain the model fitting for a dynamic PET compartment model. We show in simulation that this method returns PET parameters with less than 25% error provided that the noise in the tissue curves and the error in the DCE-MRI parameters are both small. In the limit of perfectly known DCE-MRI parameters and no noise in the tissue curves, the method returns parameters with no error. These preliminary (theoretical) results warrant *in vivo* experimental studies to validate or refute the method.

Acknowledgments

The authors thank the National Cancer Institute for funding through R01 CA138599, 1P50 098131, 1U01 CA142565, U24 CA126588, U01 CA174706, and P30 CA068485. The authors thank Dr. Noor Tantawy, Ph.D., and Ms. Clare Osborne, B.S., for technical assistance with the acquisition of the microPET data, and Dr. Lei Xu, Ph.D., Dr. Junzhong Xu, Ph.D., and Dr. Sepideh Shokouhi, Ph.D., for informative discussions. The authors thank Dr. Robert Doot, Ph.D., for reading and offering constructive criticism of an early version of this paper.

References

[1] Y. Ikoma, H. Watabe, M. Shidahara, M. Naganawa, and Y. Kimura, "PET kinetic analysis: error consideration of quantitative analysis in dynamic studies," *Annals of Nuclear Medicine*, vol. 22, no. 1, pp. 1–11, 2008.

[2] K. C. Schmidt and F. E. Turkheimer, "Kinetic modeling in positron emission tomography," *Quarterly Journal of Nuclear Medicine*, vol. 46, no. 1, pp. 70–85, 2002.

[3] T. E. Yankeelov and J. C. Gore, "Dynamic contrast enhanced magnetic resonance imaging in oncology: theory, data acquisition, analysis, and examples," *Current Medical Imaging Reviews*, vol. 3, no. 2, pp. 91–107, 2007.

[4] I. Asllani, A. Borogovac, and T. R. Brown, "Regression algorithm correcting for partial volume effects in arterial spin labeling MRI," *Magnetic Resonance in Medicine*, vol. 60, no. 6, pp. 1362–1371, 2008.

[5] M. Muzi, D. A. Mankoff, J. R. Grierson, J. M. Wells, H. Vesselle, and K. A. Krohn, "Kinetic modeling of 3′-deoxy-3′-fluorothymidine in somatic tumors: mathematical studies," *Journal of Nuclear Medicine*, vol. 46, no. 2, pp. 371–380, 2005.

[6] M. Muzi, A. M. Spence, F. O'Sullivan et al., "Kinetic analysis of 3′-deoxy-3′-[18F]-fluorothymidine in patients with gliomas," *Journal of Nuclear Medicine*, vol. 47, no. 10, pp. 1612–1621, 2006.

[7] W. Wang, J.-C. Georgi, S. A. Nehmeh et al., "Evaluation of a compartmental model for estimating tumor hypoxia via FMISO dynamic PET imaging," *Physics in Medicine and Biology*, vol. 54, no. 10, pp. 3083–3099, 2009.

[8] A. Radjenovic, B. J. Dall, J. P. Ridgway, and M. A. Smith, "Measurement of pharmacokinetic parameters in histologically graded invasive breast tumours using dynamic contrast-enhanced MRI," *British Journal of Radiology*, vol. 81, no. 962, pp. 120–128, 2008.

[9] R. G. P. Lopata, W. H. Backes, P. P. J. van den Bosch, and N. A. W. van Riel, "On the identifiability of pharmacokinetic parameters in dynamic contrast-enhanced imagine," *Magnetic Resonance in Medicine*, vol. 58, no. 2, pp. 425–429, 2007.

[10] G. Brix, F. Kiessling, R. Lucht et al., "Microcirculation and microvasculature in breast tumors: pharmacokinetic analysis of dynamic MR image series," *Magnetic Resonance in Medicine*, vol. 52, no. 2, pp. 420–429, 2004.

[11] L. Martí-Bonmatí, R. Sopena, P. Bartumeus, and P. Sopena, "Multimodality imaging techniques," *Contrast Media and Molecular Imaging*, vol. 5, no. 4, pp. 180–189, 2010.

[12] B. H. Hasagewa, E. L. Gingold, S. M. Reilly, S. C. Liew, and C. E. Cacc, "Description of a simultaneous emission-transmission CT system," in *Medical Imaging IV: Image Formation*, vol. 1231 of *Proceedings of SPIE*, pp. 50–60, July 1990.

[13] S. del Vecchio, A. Zannetti, R. Fonti et al., "PET/CT in cancer research: from preclinical to clinical applications," *Contrast Media and Molecular Imaging*, vol. 5, no. 4, pp. 190–200, 2010.

[14] G. Mariani, L. Bruselli, T. Kuwert et al., "A review on the clinical uses of SPECT/CT," *European Journal of Nuclear Medicine and Molecular Imaging*, vol. 37, no. 10, pp. 1959–1985, 2010.

[15] G. Antoch and A. Bockisch, "Combined PET/MRI: a new dimension in whole-body oncology imaging?" *European Journal of Nuclear Medicine and Molecular Imaging*, vol. 36, supplement 1, pp. S113–S120, 2009.

[16] B. J. Pichler, A. Kolb, T. Nägele, and H.-P. Schlemmer, "PET/MRI: paving the way for the next generation of clinical multimodality imaging applications," *Journal of Nuclear Medicine*, vol. 51, no. 3, pp. 333–336, 2010.

[17] T. E. Yankeelov, T. E. Peterson, R. G. Abramson et al., "Simultaneous PET-MRI in oncology: a solution looking for a problem?" *Magnetic Resonance Imaging*, vol. 30, no. 9, pp. 1342–1356, 2012.

[18] S. L. Barnes, J. G. Whisenant, M. E. Loveless, G. D. Ayers, and T. E. Yankeelov, "Assessing the reproducibility of dynamic contrast enhanced magnetic resonance imaging in a murine model of breast cancer," *Magnetic Resonance in Medicine*, vol. 69, no. 6, pp. 1721–1734, 2013.

[19] E. Henderson, B. K. Rutt, and T.-Y. Lee, "Temporal sampling requirements for the tracer kinetics modeling of breast disease," *Magnetic Resonance Imaging*, vol. 16, no. 9, pp. 1057–1073, 1998.

[20] J. U. Fluckiger, M. C. Schabel, and E. V. R. DiBella, "Toward local arterial input functions in dynamic contrast-enhanced MRI," *Journal of Magnetic Resonance Imaging*, vol. 32, no. 4, pp. 924–934, 2010.

[21] J. Li, Y. Yu, Y. Zhang et al., "A clinically feasible method to estimate pharmacokinetic parameters in breast cancer," *Medical Physics*, vol. 36, no. 8, pp. 3786–3794, 2009.

[22] S. L. Barnes, J. G. Whisenant, M. E. Loveless, G. D. Ayers, and T. E. Yankeelov, "Assessing the reproducibility of dynamic contrast enhanced magnetic resonance imaging in a murine model of breast cancer," *Magnetic Resonance in Medicine*, vol. 69, no. 6, pp. 1721–1734, 2013.

[23] S. M. Galbraith, M. A. Lodge, N. J. Taylor et al., "Reproducibility of dynamic contrast-enhanced MRI in human muscle and tumours: comparison of quantitative and semi-quantitative analysis," *NMR in Biomedicine*, vol. 15, no. 2, pp. 132–142, 2002.

[24] A. R. Padhani, C. Hayes, S. Landau, and M. O. Leach, "Reproducibility of quantitative dynamic MRI of normal human tissues," *NMR in Biomedicine*, vol. 15, no. 2, pp. 143–153, 2002.

[25] A. J. de Langen, M. Lubberink, R. Boellaard et al., "Reproducibility of tumor perfusion measurements using ^{15}O-labeled water and PET," *Journal of Nuclear Medicine*, vol. 49, no. 11, pp. 1763–1768, 2008.

17

Evaluation of Interpolation Effects on Upsampling and Accuracy of Cost Functions-Based Optimized Automatic Image Registration

Amir Pasha Mahmoudzadeh and Nasser H. Kashou

Biomedical Imaging Laboratory, Wright State University, Dayton, OH 45435, USA

Correspondence should be addressed to Nasser H. Kashou; nhkashou@ieee.org

Academic Editor: Yue Wang

Interpolation has become a default operation in image processing and medical imaging and is one of the important factors in the success of an intensity-based registration method. Interpolation is needed if the fractional unit of motion is not matched and located on the high resolution (HR) grid. The purpose of this work is to present a systematic evaluation of eight standard interpolation techniques (trilinear, nearest neighbor, cubic Lagrangian, quintic Lagrangian, hepatic Lagrangian, windowed Sinc, B-spline 3rd order, and B-spline 4th order) and to compare the effect of cost functions (least squares (LS), normalized mutual information (NMI), normalized cross correlation (NCC), and correlation ratio (CR)) for optimized automatic image registration (OAIR) on 3D spoiled gradient recalled (SPGR) magnetic resonance images (MRI) of the brain acquired using a 3T GE MR scanner. Subsampling was performed in the axial, sagittal, and coronal directions to emulate three low resolution datasets. Afterwards, the low resolution datasets were upsampled using different interpolation methods, and they were then compared to the high resolution data. The mean squared error, peak signal to noise, joint entropy, and cost functions were computed for quantitative assessment of the method. Magnetic resonance image scans and joint histogram were used for qualitative assessment of the method.

1. Introduction

1.1. Interpolation. One of the most important parts of designing a registration algorithm is choosing a good interpolation function in order to increase the accuracy of registration. Also, Interpolation is required if the fractional unit of the motion is not matched and located on high resolution (HR) grid. One of the ways by which we can help physicians in coming up with a better diagnosis and treatment is improving the resolution of images. One scheme for the interpolation step is shown in Figure 1. Here, a circle shows the reference HR image, and a diamond and a triangle represent a shifted HR pixel. For instance, if the image is downsampled by a factor of 4, a diamond has (0.25, 0.25) subpixel shift for the vertical and horizontal directions and a triangle has a shift that is less than (0.25, 0.25). In Figure 1, a triangle is not placed on the HR grid and it needs interpolation, but a diamond does not need interpolation.

Therefore, some interpolation approaches are proposed to overcome the problem of low resolution in medical imaging. Magnetic resonance imaging (MRI) is an invaluable modality in the medical field. Particularly, neuroimaging with MRI helps physicians to study the internal structure and functionality of the human brain. In these cases, high resolution and isotropic images are important because higher isotropic resolution could theoretically reduce partial volume artifacts, leading to better accuracy/precision in deriving volumetric measurement and decreasing considerable errors in the registration [1]. Clinically, acquiring a fully isotropic 3D image set is not feasible because of time, motion artifacts, and PSNR factors. Thus, typically, in 3D MR data, the in-plane direction has higher resolution than the slice direction (Z-axis). In this case, invaluable information will be lost in the latter direction. Our objective is to recover and fill in this missing information in order to enable the physicians to have a more accurate perspective of the underlying structure

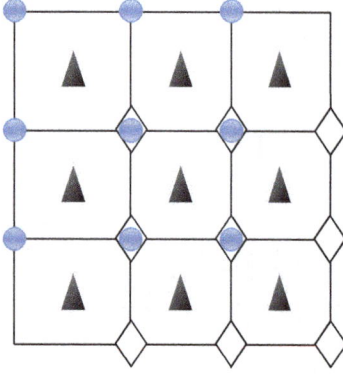

FIGURE 1: Scheme for interpolation. Straight line shows the original HR grid, circle shows the reference HR pixels, and a diamond and a triangle are shifted version of HR pixels.

available in the data by optimizing the choice of interpolation techniques.

The study of interpolation approaches dates back to the 1980s [2]. In which a great diversity of techniques can be found in the literature . For example, B-splines were sometimes referred to as cubic splines [3], whereas cubic interpolation was also known as cubic convolution [4–6] and as high resolution spline interpolation [2]. Eight interpolation algorithms are reviewed in the following sections. We first present cubic Lagrangian, quintic Lagrangian, and heptic Lagrangian. Then, we explain a nearest neighbor interpolation approach which is associated with strong aliasing and blurring effect. Next, discussions of the trilinear interpolation approach as well as B-spline 3rd order, B-spline 4th order, and windowed Sinc are explained. Finally, we discuss and evaluate the performance of these interpolation algorithms in order to find the best interpolation method for upsampling of 3D MR images. Different 2D interpolation approaches exist in medical imaging [4]. However, in this paper, we compare the performance (quality and quantity) of eight common interpolation approaches on 3D data.

1.1.1. Lagrange Interpolation. Lagrange interpolation is a famous, classical technique for interpolation. The Lagrange interpolation is a way to pass a kernel of degree $N-1$ through $N \times N$ points and is defined in X-direction (for 2D image, adds Y-direction, and for 3D image adds Y- and Z-directions) [5, 6, 8–13],

$$\text{Lagra}_{hn(x)} = \left\{ \begin{array}{ll} \displaystyle\prod_{j=0, j-(N/2)+1 \neq n}^{N-1} \frac{n-i-x}{n-i}, & n-1 \leq x < n \\ 0, & \text{elsewhere,} \end{array} \right\}, \tag{1}$$

where $i = j - (N/2) + 1$ and $n \in \{-(N/2) + 1, -(N/2) + 2, \ldots, N/2\}$ are the Lagrange kernels. The Lagrange kernel for $N = 1$ equals the nearest neighbor interpolation. In this case, $N = 2$ equals the linear interpolation. The Lagrange kernels

for $N = 4$ and $N = 5$ supporting points result in cubic and quartic polynomials, respectively, and are shown as follows

$$\text{Lagra}_{h4(x)} = \left\{ \begin{array}{ll} \dfrac{1}{2}x^3 - x^2 - \dfrac{1}{2}x + 1, & \text{for } 0 \leq x < 1, \\[2mm] \dfrac{-1}{6}x^3 + x^2 - \dfrac{11}{6}x + 1, & \text{for } 1 \leq x < 2, \\[2mm] 0, & \text{elsewhere,} \end{array} \right.$$

$$\text{Lagra}_{h5(x)}$$

$$= \left\{ \begin{array}{ll} \dfrac{1}{4}x^4 - 54x^2 + 1, & \text{for } 0 \leq x < \dfrac{1}{2}, \\[2mm] \dfrac{-1}{6}x^4 + \dfrac{5}{6}x^3 - \dfrac{5}{6}x^2 - \dfrac{5}{6}x + 1, & \text{for } \dfrac{1}{2} \leq x < \dfrac{3}{2}, \\[2mm] \dfrac{1}{24}x^4 - \dfrac{5}{12}x^3 + \dfrac{35}{24}x^2 - \dfrac{25}{12}x + 1, & \text{for } \dfrac{3}{2} \leq x < \dfrac{5}{2}, \\[2mm] 0, & \text{elsewhere.} \end{array} \right.$$

$$\tag{2}$$

1.1.2. Nearest Neighbor Interpolation. Nearest neighbor interpolation (also known as zero-order interpolation) is the simplest method, and strong aliasing and blurring effects are associated with this interpolation [14]. The local 1-point Lagrange interpolation is equivalent to the nearest neighbor interpolation, defined by

$$w(x, n) = \left\{ \begin{array}{ll} 1, & \text{for } n - \dfrac{1}{2} \leq x < n + \dfrac{1}{2}, \\[2mm] 0, & \text{otherwise.} \end{array} \right. \tag{3}$$

The images when scaled up in size may look very blocky. Likewise, the local 2-point Lagrange interpolation is equivalent to the linear interpolation, defined by

$$w(x, n) = \left\{ \begin{array}{ll} 1 - |x - n|, & \text{for } n - 1 \leq x < n + 1, \\[2mm] 0, & \text{otherwise.} \end{array} \right. \tag{4}$$

1.1.3. Trilinear Interpolation. Trilinear interpolation calculates values placed between existing *voxel* values by linearly weighting the eight closest neighboring values. In other words, trilinear is the name given to the process of linearly interpolating points within a 3D box, given the values at the vertices of the box (see Figure 2) [15].

The known values at each vertex are indicated as $V000, V100, V010, \ldots, V111$, and the unknown value is calculated by merging the known corner values weighted by their distance from the point (x, y, z) within the cube.

1.1.4. B-Spline Interpolation. B-spline interpolation uses weighted *voxel* values in a wider neighborhood compared to trilinear interpolation, but both the B-spline and trilinear kernels are symmetrical and separable. The place of the neighboring points as control points relates to B-spline interpolation and combines the intensity values at these places using a set of polynomial basis according to (5) [16].

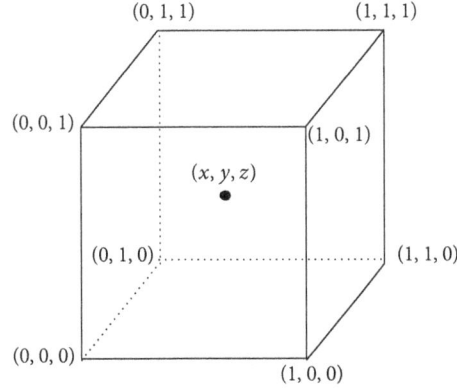

FIGURE 2: Trilinear interpolation computes values located between existing *voxel* values by linearly weighting the eight closest neighboring values (obtained from National Institutes of Health Center for Information Technology, Rockville, MD, USA).

Equation (5) shows k-order B-spline with $n + 1$ control points ($P1, P2, \ldots, Pn$),

$$P(t) = \sum_{i=1}^{n+1} N_{i,k} P_i, \quad t_{\min} \le t < t_{\max}. \quad (5)$$

In (5), $N_{i,k}$ are the polynomial functions of order k (degree $k - 1$), and n is the number of control points; k must be at least 2 (linear) and less than $n + 1$.

$P(t)$ is validly defined for $t_{\min} \le t < t_{\max}$, where $t_{\min} = t_k$ and $t_{\max} = t_{n+2}$. A knot vector ($t_1, t_2, \ldots, t_{k+(n+1)}$) must be determined. This specifies the values of t at which the pieces of curve join, like knots joining bits of string. It is important to note that the degree of the weighting polynomial (the order of the curve) is not dependent on the number of control points, n [17].

The weighting polynomial can be recursively defined by the following equation [18]:

$$N_{i,1}(t) = \begin{cases} 1, & t_i \le t < t_{i+1}, \\ 0, & \text{otherwise,} \end{cases}$$

$$N_{i,k} = \frac{t - t_i}{t_{i+k-1} - t_i} N_{i,k-1}(t) + \frac{t_{i+k} - t}{t_{i+k} - t_{i+1}} N_{i+1,k-1}(t). \quad (6)$$

In (6), $t(i)$ represents an index that refers to the control points and $t(i)$ are generally referred to as knot points (see Figure 3). The series of control point is defined as a control surface. This indexing scheme allows one to weight different control points more than other control points by using it once during the computation. Typically, the first and last control points are weighted more heavily than the internal points to give a smooth interpolating curve. Generally, the shape of the curve ($N_{i,k}$) is specified by the relative spacing between the knots ($t_0, t_1, \ldots, t_n$). The sequence ($t_0, t_1, \ldots, t_n$) is called knot vector. Knot vectors are generally placed into one of three categories: uniform, nonuniform, and open uniform. Uniform knot vectors are the vectors for which $t_{i+1} - t_i = $ const, for example, $[0, 1, 2, 3, 4, 5, 6, 7, 8, 9]$. Nonuniform knot vectors are a general case; the only constraint is the standard $t_i \le t_{i+1}$,

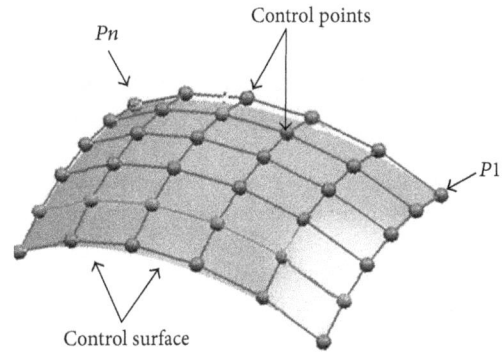

FIGURE 3: B-spline interpolation. There are n control points ($P1, P2, \ldots, Pn$). The sequence of the control point is called a *control surface* (adapted from National Institutes of Health Center for Information Technology, Rockville, MD, USA).

for example, $[0.2, 05, 0.8, 0.8, 0.8, 1.1, 1.1, 2.2, 2.7, 3.4]$. The the optimized automatic image registration (OAIR) method uses the open uniform knot vectors for computing B-spline. Open uniform knot vectors are uniform knot vectors which have k-equal knot values at each end as [3, 5, 9, 16–19]

$$t_i = t_0, \quad i < k,$$

$$t_{i+1} - t_i = \text{const}, \quad k - 1 \le i < n + 1, \quad (7)$$

$$t_i = t_{k+n}, \quad i \ge n + 1,$$

for example, $[0, 0, 0, 1, 2, 3, 4, 4, 4]$ (here $k = 3$, $n = 5$).

1.1.5. Windowed Sinc Interpolation. This interpolation function has minimum aliasing artifacts in contrast to linear interpolation. Sinc function can be windowed more generally to yield [5, 10] the following

$$\text{sinc}(x) = \begin{cases} \dfrac{\sin(x)}{x}, & \forall x \ne 0, \\ 1, & x = 0. \end{cases} \quad (8)$$

Think of an image data set comprising a 3D matrix *voxel* with intensities $I(x, y, z)$, specified by integer position coordinates (x, y, z). If one wants to calculate the intensity value at an interior point defined by noninteger coordinates (x, y, z), this can be obtained by the following equation [5]:

$$I(x, y, z) = \sum_X \sum_Y \sum_Z I(X, Y, Z) \operatorname{sinc}(\pi(x - X))$$
$$\times \operatorname{sinc}(\pi(y - Y)) \operatorname{sinc}(\pi(z - Z)). \tag{9}$$

For satisfying (9), two limiting conditions are required:

(i) $I(x, y, z)$ must be band limited. Put differently, the function must have *Fourier transform* $F\{I(x, y, z)\} = I(f) = 0$ for $|f| > B$ for some maximum frequency $B > 0$;

(ii) the sampling rate—f_s must be greater than twice the bandwidth, for example, $f_s > 2B$.

The following section discusses the registration process and explains how interpolation is involved with registration.

1.2. Image Registration Algorithms. Image registration methods in medical imaging seek to align two or more images and can be applied in the same modality on the same patient for the purpose of monitoring and quantifying disease progression over time. Registration can also be applied across different modalities, which is useful for correction of different patient positions across scans, for instance, aligning positron emission tomography (PET) data to an MRI image. Also, image registration can be used on the different patients, which is useful for studies of variability between subjects. Image registration is classified into the following categories and depends on several factors: image modalities (MRI, PET, CT, etc.), the subject of registration (a single person or different persons), the object of registration (head or heart), the image dimensionality (e.g., 2D, 3D, and 4D), and geometrical transformation (affine, rigid, projective, etc.).

This study examines 3D affine registration of brain images using *voxel* intensities similarity measures such as normalized mutual information (NMI), normalized cross correlation (NCC), least squares (LS), and correlation ratio (CR). More explicitly, if a target image is resampled to match a reference image, the image intensities at each *voxel* should be similar in the two images. In fact, when utilizing an intensity-based cost function, it is essential to repeatedly resample one of the images to match the others at several various resolutions, while searching for the min cost function. This resampling process requires interpolation during the registration process [19]. In OAIR method, interpolation involves resampling of anisotropic *voxels* in the z-direction into isotropic cubic *voxels*. Also, it is important to note that in the the optimized automatic image registration (OAIR) method, the interpolation technique utilized for registration does not necessarily need to be the same interpolation technique used during registration to compute a final image using the optimal parameters.

In this paper, we are focusing on the effect of interpolation technique and cost function used for intensity-based registration. The following sections are organized as follows, we first give some background and provide a means of defining the critical components involved in image registration and establish a theoretical framework.

1.2.1. Geometric Transformation. When registering images, one should specify a geometric transformation that specially aligns one image to another. The common transformations can be classified as rigid, affine, and projective. Rigid transformation can be defined as a simple transformation that includes only translation and rotation. The projective transformation is the most general transformation and maps lines to lines (but does not necessarily preserve parallelism). An affine transformation includes scaling, rotation, translation, shearing, and reflection. There are several scanner-produced errors that can result in skewing or scaling terms, and affine transformations are applied to overcome these problems.

An affine transformation maps straight lines to straight lines and keeps the parallelism of lines, but not their lengths or their angles. Changing scaling and shearing factors for each image dimension will extend the degree of freedom (DOF, the number of independent pieces of information that go into the estimate of a parameter) of the rigid transformation [20–27]. Figure 4 shows the five basic components of affine transformations. The following matrices constitute the basic affine transforms in 3D, addressed in homogeneous form.

Translation. Translate a point in the xyz-plane to a new place by adding a vector (t_x, t_y, t_z). $\mathbf{x}' = x + t_x$, $\mathbf{y}' = y + t_y$, and $\mathbf{z}' = z + t_z$. $\mathbf{P}'$ represents scaled matrices: $\mathbf{P}' = \mathbf{T}\mathbf{P}$, where

$$\mathbf{P}' = \begin{bmatrix} \mathbf{x}' \\ \mathbf{x}' \\ \mathbf{y}' \\ 1 \end{bmatrix}, \qquad \mathbf{P} = \begin{bmatrix} x \\ y \\ z \\ 1 \end{bmatrix}, \tag{10}$$

$$\mathbf{T}(t_x, t_y, t_z) : \begin{bmatrix} 1 & 0 & 0 & t_x \\ 0 & 1 & 0 & t_y \\ 0 & 0 & 1 & t_z \\ 0 & 0 & 0 & 1 \end{bmatrix}. \tag{11}$$

Scaling. Scaling is making the new scale of a coordinate direction p times larger. Scaling is applied to all axes, each with a different scaling factor (s_x, s_y, s_z). $\mathbf{x}' = s_x \times x$, $\mathbf{y}' = s_y \times y$ and $\mathbf{z}' = s_z \times z$. $\mathbf{P}'$ represents of scaled matrices:

$$\mathbf{P}' = \mathbf{S}\mathbf{P},$$

$$\mathbf{S}(s_x, s_y, s_z) : \begin{bmatrix} s_x & 0 & 0 & 0 \\ 0 & s_y & 0 & 0 \\ 0 & 0 & s_z & 0 \\ 0 & 0 & 0 & 1 \end{bmatrix}. \tag{12}$$

Rotation. If a point (x, y, z) is rotated an angle θ about the coordinate origin to become a new point $(\mathbf{x}', \mathbf{y}', \mathbf{z}')$, the three basic rotations in 3D can be defined as follows:

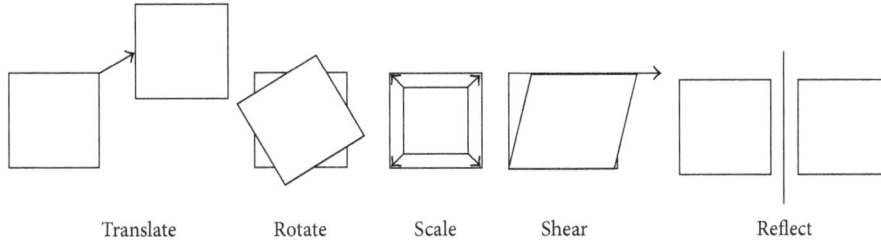

FIGURE 4: The five basic affine transformations are translate, rotate, scale, shear, and reflection. Translate moves a set of points a fixed distance in x- and y-directions, Rotate rotates a set of points about the origin, Scale scales a set of points up or down in x- and y-directions, and Shear offsets a set of points a distance proportional to their x- and y-coordinates. Reflection produces a mirror image of a set of points in x- or y-directions.

Rotation about the x-axis:

$$\begin{bmatrix} x' \\ y' \\ z' \\ 1 \end{bmatrix} = \begin{bmatrix} 1 & 0 & 0 & 0 \\ 0 & \cos\theta & -\sin\theta & 0 \\ 0 & \sin\theta & \cos\theta & 0 \\ 0 & 0 & 0 & 1 \end{bmatrix} \begin{bmatrix} x \\ y \\ z \\ 1 \end{bmatrix}. \tag{13}$$

Rotation about the y-axis:

$$\begin{bmatrix} x' \\ y' \\ z' \\ 1 \end{bmatrix} = \begin{bmatrix} \cos\theta & 0 & \sin\theta & 0 \\ 0 & 1 & 0 & 0 \\ -\sin\theta & 0 & \cos\theta & 0 \\ 0 & 0 & 0 & 1 \end{bmatrix} \begin{bmatrix} x \\ y \\ z \\ 1 \end{bmatrix}. \tag{14}$$

Rotation about the z-axis:

$$\begin{bmatrix} x' \\ y' \\ z' \\ 1 \end{bmatrix} = \begin{bmatrix} \cos\theta & -\sin\theta & 0 & 0 \\ \sin\theta & \cos\theta & 0 & 0 \\ 0 & 0 & 1 & 0 \\ 0 & 0 & 0 & 1 \end{bmatrix} \begin{bmatrix} x \\ y \\ z \\ 1 \end{bmatrix}. \tag{15}$$

There are several reasons for using homogeneous coordinates, including the ability to apply all four transformations multiplicatively. In view of the fact that transformation combinations (shearing, scaling, and rotation) are all multiplicative transforms, only translation is an additive transform.

Next, the following cost functions are defined and described: LS, NCC, CR, and NMI. Furthermore, an overview of the literature on their use in registration for medical applications is included. Among these cost functions, the NMI-based registration has become commonplace in many medical applications [28].

1.2.2. Cost Functions. The cost function or similarity measure evaluates the similarity between two images. In this section, the behaviors of four commonly used cost functions will be examined.

Least Squares (LS). The least squares method measures the average of the squared difference in image intensities [29]:

$$f = \frac{\sum_{i=1}^{N} \{R - I\}^2}{N}, \tag{16}$$

where R is the reference image, I is the input image, N is the number of values over which the sum is performed, and f is the least square. When two images differ only by Gaussian noise, the least squares will be the optimum cost function. Images of two different modalities such as MRI and PET will never differ by only Gaussian noise. Due to patient motion, even two images of the same modality, such as two MRI images, will rarely only differ by Gaussian noise. The effectiveness of LS will be extremely decreased by a small number of *voxels* having considerable intensity differences.

Correlation Ratio (CR). The main principle of the correlation ratio method is to calculate a "similarity measure" between a reference image and an input image and search for a spatial transformation T and an intensity mapping f such that by dis-replacing R and remapping its intensities, the resulting image $f(R \times T)$ can be seen as equivalent as possible to I. This can be obtained by minimizing the following CR function [30]:

$$\text{minimizing} \, (T, f) \, \text{of} \, \sum_{k} \{I(x_k) - f(R(T(x_k)))\}, \tag{17}$$

which integrates over the *voxel* positions in the image I. The minimum and maximum values for the CR are 0 and 1, respectively. The CR can be applied in multimodal image registration involving positron emission tomography (PET), MRI, and computed tomography (CT) images, providing a good tradeoff between accuracy and robustness [31].

Normalized Cross-Correlation (NCC). The cross-correlation function works very well for aligning images of the same modality. Cross-correlation function is defined by the following equation:

$$\text{CrossCorr} \, (u, v) = \sum_{x} \sum_{y} R(x, y) I(x - u, y - v), \tag{18}$$

where R is the reference image intensity, I is the input image intensity, and x and y represent the partials of images R and I in x and y-directions, respectively. The summation is taken over the region (u, v), where R and I overlap. When $I(x, y)$ best matches $R(x, y)$, CrossCorr(u, v) shows the maximum value.

Normalized Mutual Information (NMI). The algorithms of mutual information (MI) have been the most investigated measure for registration of medical image to date. The mutual information of images I and J is defined by the following [32, 33]:

$$\text{NMI}(I, J \mid T) = \sum_{i,j} P_{i,j} \log \frac{P_{i,j}}{p_i p_j}, \tag{19}$$

where $P_{i,j}$ is the joint probability distribution image of I and J and p_i and p_j are the marginal probability distribution function of I and J, respectively. The minimum and maximum values for normalized mutual information are 0 and 1, respectively.

When images are correctly registered and aligned, there is maximal dependence between the gray values of the images, meaning that the amount of mutual information would be high. Misregistration will cause a decrease in the MI measure [34]. NMI has been used with success for a wide variety of combinations, including MR, CT, SPET, PET, and also time series images [35]. NMI can be found in a large number of studies [34, 36].

1.2.3. Optimized Automatic Image Registration 3D. OAIR is a robust image registration algorithm based on FLIRT (FLIRT stands for FMRIB's Linear Registration tool 1.3) [26, 37–39]. The OAIR technique specifies a transformation that minimizes a cost function, which represents the quality of alignment between two images. The method assesses the cost function at the number of different image resolutions, starting with the lowest resolution. Each step of increasing resolution uses the previously specified optimal transformation as the starting point and further refines its values. OAIR method usually works very well with the image of the same modality (e.g., MRI-MRI, CT-CT, and PET-PET). During the OAIR registration, the resampling process will influence the computed value of the cost function; therefore, choosing the best interpolation is important.

Outline of the OAIR Method. (1) The registration algorithm specifies the minimum resolution for each dimension of the target and reference images (they are subsampled by factors two, four, and eight). (2) The reference and target images are interpolated in order to create high resolution isotropic *voxels*. (3) The centers of mass (COM) for the reference and target images are then calculated and one translation level is implemented to align the COM.

The method uses the right-hand convention in 3D coordinate systems (X, Y, Z) in order to compute the COM. The image origin is generally at the corner of the image (the upper left-hand corner of the image). The axis directions are as follows the x-axis goes left to right, the y-axis goes top to bottom, and the z-axis goes into the image. To compute the COM, the characteristics function of an object in an image is defined by the following

$$b(x, y, z) = \begin{cases} 1, & \text{for points inside of the image,} \\ 0, & \text{for points outside of image.} \end{cases} \tag{20}$$

Next, the area of the image is computed as

$$S = \iiint b(x, y, z)\, dx\, dy\, dz. \tag{21}$$

Figure 5 shows the COM.

The COM, indicated by $(x_{\text{com}}, y_{\text{com}}, z_{\text{com}})$, is given by the first moments of the object:

$$\begin{aligned} x_{\text{COM}} &= \frac{\iiint xb(x, y, z)\, dx\, dy\, dz}{\iiint b(x, y, z)\, dx\, dy\, dz}, \\[2mm] y_{\text{COM}} &= \frac{\iiint yb(x, y, z)\, dx\, dy\, dz}{\iiint b(x, y, z)\, dx\, dy\, dz}, \\[2mm] z_{\text{COM}} &= \frac{\iiint zb(x, y, z)\, dx\, dy\, dz}{\iiint b(x, y, z)\, dx\, dy\, dz}. \end{aligned} \tag{22}$$

(4) For each resampled image (which is 8, 4, 2, and 1 times) specifies the transform that minimizes the cost function.

Optimization Steps. The theoretical registration problem is completely determined by an interpolation method, a cost function, and a transformation space. However, in practice, an optimization method is needed to find the transformation that minimizes the cost function [26]. In general, all cost functions require global optimization. As a part of the transformation optimization process, the images are subsampled by several factors (e.g., eight, four, and two times) [38].

Levels Eight, Four, Two, and One Optimization. Reference and target images are interpolated and subsampled by eight, so each image is eight times smaller. The parameters corresponding to the minimum cost function are specified and used as the initial transformation. For the next level (level four) in the optimization, the reference and target images are interpolated and subsampled by four and, like in level eight, the transformation parameters corresponding to the minimum cost function are specified and used as the initial transformation for the next level (level two) in the optimization. For level two optimization, the process repeats, except that the reference and target images are first interpolated and subsampled by factor two. As mentioned above, the parameters of the transformation are systematically varied, and the cost function is assessed for each setting. For level one optimization, 1 mm interpolated images are used and the transformation is generalized to contain 12-DOF.

The merit of this multiresolution technique is that the initial optimization, at large n, has a noticeably reduced computational load, since the number of sample points is considerably less. Additionally, a large subsampling ($n = 8$) uses the lowest resolution image and coarse rotation angle, in which the large features of the image are dominate, and so the overall alignment is easier to find. The following sections explain in detail how each resampled image (which is 8, 4, 2, and 1 times) specifies the transform that minimizes the cost function.

(1) *Level Eight Optimization.* One of the most difficult tasks in image registration is finding the right orientation or rotation,

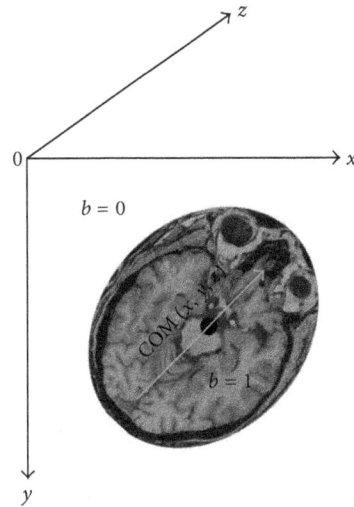

FigurE 5: Calculating the COM in the image space; the image origin is in the upper left-hand corner of the image. The x-axis goes left to right, the y-axis goes top to bottom, and the z-axis goes into image.

and most of the erroneous registrations that have been examined have happened primarily because of an incorrect orientation. Thus, the search focuses on the rotational part of the transformation.

In level eight, the reference image is directed, interpolated, and the cost function is evaluated for coarse rotations angles $(-30, -30, -30)$, $(-30, -30, -15)$, ..., $(-30, -30, 30)$, where the values represent the amount of rotation in degrees about a, y, and z axes, respectively. In this case, there would be 125 possible angle configurations, since there are three rotation angles and each angle can contain five different values. A 4-DOF local optimization is also applied to find optimal translation and global scale for each angle configuration. The best 20% of the cost values and corresponding angle configurations (candidate local minima) are stored in vector of minima that is used as starting point for a further optimization, which uses a smaller step size over a narrow range of angles. For each parameter setting related to the top 20% of the cost function minima, the algorithm performs the minima over rotation as well as global scale and translation (previously, the algorithm had not optimized over rotation). For each of these sets of parameters, a 7-DOF optimization is then performed, storing the results of the transformation and cost before and after optimization in a vector of minima. A vector of parameters and top 20% of the min cost function values are considered for the next higher resolution (level four optimization) stage, because the relative costs of each candidate solution may change at higher resolutions. The algorithm also uses interpolation to transform images to this new orientation [26, 37–39].

(2) *Level Four Optimization*. The algorithm now calls level four with the interpolated images subsampled by 4 to specify the transformation that minimizes the cost function starting with the transformations determined in level eight. The optimization specifies a 7-DOF transformation that corresponds

to minimum value of the cost function. This transformation is then perturbed and the cost function is calculated for these new settings. The perturbations correspond to six degrees for each rotation parameter and a global scaling factor of 0.8, 0.9, 1.0, 1.1, and 1.2. A vector of parameters and the top 20% of the cost function minima values are considered for the next step, which involves images subsampled by 2.

(3) *Level Two Optimization*. The algorithm uses the images interpolated and subsampled by 2 and computes the value of the cost function for each parameter setting obtained from the level four optimization. It finds the best minimum, and then optimizes it with the 7-DOF, then 9-DOF, and 12-DOF. The algorithm then returns the best minimum after optimization.

(4) *Level One Optimization*. The algorithm now level one to use the unsubsampled interpolated images and computes the value of the cost function for each parameter setting obtained from the level two optimization. In this step, one optimization run is performed, with the maximum allowable DOF, as determined by the user (max 12-DOF). The best answer is returned from level one and gives us the minimum cost of differences between the images.

2. Materials and Methods

A 3D spoiled gradient recalled (SPGR). MRI of the brain was acquired at Nationwide Children's Hospital of Columbus, Ohio, USA, using a 3T GE MR scanner from a 34-year-old participant. Interpolation techniques were performed on brain scans. Relevant imaging parameters are listed in Table 1. The first initial reference, also the HR, image dimensions were $512 \times 512 \times 120$ (this is native scanner output) with *voxel* size of $0.5 \times 0.5 \times 1.3 \, \text{mm}^3$ and with slice thickness and spacing between slices of 1.3 mm (acquiring a fully isotropic 3D scan

TABLE 1: Imaging parameters associated with 3D reference and low-resolution images.

3D images	No. of slices	Matrix size	*Voxel* size (mm^3)
Reference 1	120	512×512	$0.5 \times 0.5 \times 1.3$
Simulated reference 2	120	256×256	$1 \times 1 \times 1.3$
Low resolution 1	60	512×512	$0.5 \times 0.5 \times 2.6$
Low resolution 2	60	256×256	$1 \times 1 \times 2.6$
Low resolution 3	120	256×128	$1 \times 2 \times 1.3$
Low resolution 4	120	128×256	$2 \times 2 \times 1.3$

was not feasible because of time, motion artifact, and SNR factors). Because of interpolation and registration time, we simulated the new 3D HR images (simulated reference 2) with a resolution of $256 \times 256 \times 120$ and with a *voxel* size of $1 \times 1 \times 1.3$ mm^3 and with slice thickness and spacing between slices of 1.3 mm. In the absence of gold standards, simulations are sometimes utilized to assess registration accuracy. A common tactic is to take real data and deform it using appropriate spatial transformation model (affine, rigid, and projective) and other factors that are thought to be relevant in limiting registration accuracy such as simulating the addition of noise and blurring.

The first low resolution (LR) images were generated from the reference one, and the resolution was decreased ($512 \times 512 \times 60$ and with a *voxel* size of $0.5 \times 0.5 \times 2.6$ mm^3) along the slice direction by subsampling by a factor of 2. The second, third, and fourth LR images were generated from simulated reference 2, and they were subsampled by a factor of 2 in the x-, y-, and z directions. The second LR images were generated with a resolution of $256 \times 256 \times 60$ (axial plane) and with a *voxel* size of $1 \times 1 \times 2.6$ mm^3. The third LR images were generated with resolution $256 \times 128 \times 120$ (sagittal plane) and with *voxel* size of $1 \times 2 \times 1.3$ mm^3, and finally, the fourth LR images were generated with a resolution of $128 \times 256 \times 120$ (coronal plane) and with a *voxel* size of $2 \times 1 \times 1.3$ mm^3. We rotated the LR images in x-direction by 5 degrees. Then, we translated the rotated image above in x by 2 mm and in y by 3 mm. The LR images are corrupted by Gaussian noise (10 standard deviation) and Gaussian blurring (horizontal 5 radius).

Afterward, we used these LR images as input to our interpolation algorithms (trilinear, cubic Lagrangian, quintic Lagrangian, heptic Lagrangian, windowed Sinc, B-spline 3rd order, and B-spline 4th order) to remap to a common size. They were upsampled and back to their original dimension ($256 \times 256 \times 120$), and then we compared them to the reference images in order to find the minimum interpolation error during upsampling. Image restoration (adaptive noise reduction and blind deconvolution techniques) was implemented upon the upsampled images to reduce blurring and noise. Adaptive noise reduction algorithm reduces noise without blurring the edges by replacing a pixel value with a weighted sum of all local pixels reached by following a path with small pixel intensity values between neighboring pixels, and blind deconvolution is a method, which allows recovering of the target object from a set of blurred images

in the presence or a poorly specified or unknown point spread function (PSF) [40]. Restoration can be implemented by applying any deconvolution method that considers the presence of noise and blurring.

OAIR was applied on high resolution data set (simulated reference 2) with a resolution of $256 \times 256 \times 120$ and with a *voxel* size of $1 \times 1 \times 1.3$ mm^3, and the transformed image with a resolution of $256 \times 256 \times 120$ and with a *voxel* size of $1 \times 1 \times 1.3$ mm^3. Throughout the OAIR, when an optimal fit was achieved, the target image was reformatted using the transformation function and interpolations described above to match the reference image. For achieving a good registration (intensity-based cost function) between the fixed image (reference image) and the moving image (target image), the resampling was essential because the moving image did not necessarily have the same origin, spacing, and number of pixels as the fixed image. Therefore, the resampling process helped us to have the moving image in the grid of the fixed image.

The intensity-based registration method looked for the transformation that would give the smallest value of the cost function, which we assumed was the transformation that also gave the best alignment. During this registration for analyzing the effect of interpolation and cost function, we applied and tested various interpolations and cost functions. The cost functions which were performed in this method included

(1) normalized mutual information (NMI);

(2) normalized cross correlation (NCC);

(3) least squares (LS);

(4) correlation ratio (CR).

2.1. Image Assessment. There are various ways to evaluate the accuracy of registration technique. They can be divided into qualitative and quantitative methods. For qualitative and quantitative assessment of registered images, we proposed five ways to compare and evaluate the new transformation with the old; we needed to quantify the difference between the geometrically transformed source images with the target image.

2.1.1. Quantitative Assessment. For the quantitative assessment, we considered an a mean squared error (MSE), peak signal to noise ratio (PSNR), and entropy. The MSE and PSNR measures are estimates of the quality of registration images, and entropy is also a suitable choice for quantitative assessment of the accuracy of registration method.

(1) *Mean Square Error.* MSE was computed between the original image (reference) and reconstructed image in order to measure the average of the squared difference in image intensities:

$$\text{SE}_{ijk} = \left(R_{ijk} - I_{ijk} \right)^2, \tag{23}$$

where i, j, and k represent the direct comparison of each coordinate location, R is the reference image, and I is the

(a)

(b)

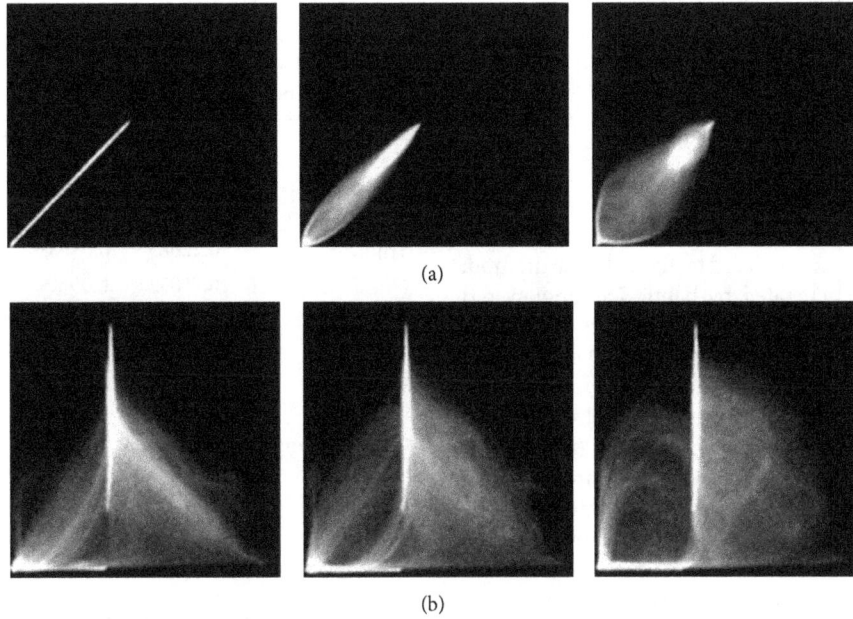

FIGURE 6: Example 2D histograms for (a) the same MR images of the head, (b) MR and CT images of the head. The left columns show two images when aligned, the middle columns show two image when translated by 2 mm, and the right columns show two images when translated by 5 mm. As can be seen, the joint histogram disperses with increasing mis-registration (obtained from Hill et al. (1994)).

reconstructed image. The MSE was computed for 3D brain image in order to assign a value and compare the results.

$$MSE = \frac{\sum_{i=1}^{n} \sum_{j=1}^{m} \sum_{k=1}^{l} SE_{ijk}}{n \cdot m \cdot l}, \quad (24)$$

where n, m, and l are the number of points in the x-, y-, z-directions, respectively, for the reconstructed volume.

(2) *Peak Signal to Noise.* PSNR in decibels (dB) between the original image and the registered image is defined by [41]

$$PSNR = 20 \times \log_{10} \left(\frac{MAX}{RMSE} \right), \quad (25)$$

where MAX is the maximum pixel value of the image and RMSE is the square root of the MSE.

(3) *Entropy.* The desire for a measure of information (commonly termed *entropy*) of a message stems from communication theory [42]. Shannon introduced an adapted measure in 1984 [43], which weights the information per outcome by the probability of that outcome occurring. Given the events occurring with the probabilities, the Shannon entropy is defined as

$$H = \sum_{i} p_i \log \frac{1}{p_i} = -\sum_{i} p_i \log p_i, \quad (26)$$

where p = (histogram count in bin)/total count. The Shannon entropy can be applied and computed for an image and be used on the distribution of the gray values of the image. An image with a low entropy value has almost a single intensity; it contains very little information. An image with a high entropy

value has more or less equal quantities of numerous different intensities; it contains a lot of information [42]. For instance, blurring an image reduces noise and high frequency and thus sharpens the images histogram, resulting in reduced entropy.

2.1.2. Qualitative Assessment. One way for qualitative assessment is the subtraction of the reference and registered images. Image subtraction techniques can be used to detect subtle changes that may reflect clinically important disease progression [21]. Another way to conduct a qualitative assessment is to create a joint histogram. The joint histogram is a functional tool for visualizing the relationship between the intensities of corresponding *voxels* in two or more images. Visual assessment is also considered for qualitative assessment.

(1) *Joint Histogram.* The joint histogram is two-dimensional for two grayscale images A and B and is created by plotting the intensity of each *voxel* in image A against the intensity of the corresponding *voxel* in image B. When two images of different modalities are produced, the spatial resolution is likely to be different (see Figure 6). Therefore, before calculating a joint histogram, it is essential to rescale the range of data of the first image to the range of data of the second image. When two images are perfectly aligned, the corresponding anatomical areas overlap, and their joint histogram is highly focused. In misaligned images, anatomical areas are not matched, and they are mixed up and their joint histogram is scattered, for example, the cerebrum region of one image overlaid onto the skull region of another image causes a more dispersed joint histogram. Note, joint histograms are commonly used for different modalities like MR-CT and PET-MR [7, 44]. We implemented the joint

histogram technique on the registered images of the same modality for checking the effect of interpolations and cost functions on the accuracy of OAIR.

3. Results and Discussion

In Figure 7, the interpolated images in axial, coronal, and sagittal views are shown for the first LR images. Part (a) illustrates the 3D image interpolated by the trilinear method; in part (b), the image generated by heptic Lagrangian and quintic Lagrangian interpolation images appears in part (c). Part (d), part (e), and part (f) show that 3D images are generated by windowed Sinc, cubic Lagrangian, and nearest neighbor interpolations, respectively. The B-spline 3rd and B-spline 4th interpolations are shown in parts (g) and (h), respectively. The 3D MSEs for 512-sized MRI images were computed in all three planes. To further test the interpolations in 3D, three typical matrix sizes were simulated, namely, 64, 128, and 256. The 3D MSEs of these matrix sizes were tabulated in Table 2. The MSE is inversely proportional to the 3D MRI images size. As a result, the trilinear method yielded more accurate (lower MSE) values than the discussed interpolations.

Also, the interpolated images were quantitatively evaluated by computing the PSNR, which is widely used in the evaluation of reconstructed images [11]. The 3D PSNRs for 64–512 sized MRI images were computed. The 3D PSNRs of these matrix sizes were tabulated in Table 3. The PSNR results for trilinear interpolation for matrix size of 64–512 were approximately 91 (dB), 100 (dB), 111 (dB), and 121 (dB), respectively. Based on Table 3, trilinear interpolation shows PSNR superiority against the other interpolation. In addition, the PSNR was found to slowly increase as the matrix size increased. The second LR images, the matrix size of $256 \times 256 \times 60$ (axial view), the third LR images, the matrix size of $256 \times 128 \times 120$ (sagittal view), and the fourth LR images, the matrix size of $128 \times 256 \times 120$ (coronal view) were simply interpolated separately, and MSE was computed. The results are tabulated in Table 4.

As a result, in Table 4, the interpolated matrix size of $256 \times 256 \times 60$ (axial view) yields more accurate (lower MSE) results than both matrix sizes of $256 \times 128 \times 120$ (sagittal view), $128 \times 256 \times 120$ (coronal view). In other words, the interpolated images in z-direction have more quality (lower MSE) than the interpolated images in x- and y-directions. However, the perceived quality of $128 \times 256 \times 120$ (coronal view) was nearly as good as that of $256 \times 128 \times 120$ (sagittal view).

3.1. Visual Quality of Interpolation Techniques. In Figure 8, we applied the trilinear algorithm on the second LR images, and the resolution in the axial view did not improve because the resolution in x- and y-directions was already high ($256 \times 256 \times 60$) with *voxel* size of $1 \times 1 \times 2.6 \, \text{mm}^3$, and the resolution in axial direction was constant. In contrast, the resolutions in sagittal and coronal views showed different results, and we saw enough improvement in both planes (interpolated images). As was mentioned before, the resolution in the slice-select direction is lower than plane direction, and

TABLE 2: 3D MSE for MR images of 64–512 for interpolations of trilinear, nearest neighbor, B-spline 3rd order, B-spline 4th order, cubic Lagrangian, quintic Lagrangian, heptic Lagrangian, and windowed Sinc.

| | MSE | | | |
| | Matrix size | | | |
Interpolation	64×64	128×128	256×256	512×512
Trilinear	0.22683	0.03088	0.00282	0.00024
Nearest neighbor	0.75852	0.09615	0.01295	0.00135
B-spline 3rd order	0.50714	0.06435	0.00706	0.00095
B-spline 4th order	0.32088	0.05742	0.00618	0.00075
Cubic Lagrangian	0.24283	0.04956	0.00554	0.00027
Quintic Lagrangian	0.24204	0.03286	0.00552	0.00026
Heptic Lagrangian	0.24181	0.03284	0.00549	0.00025
Windowed Sinc	0.24338	0.05123	0.00559	0.00027

TABLE 3: 3D PSNR for MR images of 64–512 for interpolations of trilinear, nearest neighbor, B-spline 3rd order, B-spline 4th order, cubic Lagrangian, quintic Lagrangian, heptic Lagrangian, and windowed Sinc.

| | PSNR (dB) | | | |
| | Matrix size | | | |
Interpolation	64×64	128×128	256×256	512×512
Trilinear	91.95	100.61	111.01	121.76
Nearest neighbor	86.78	95.76	104.47	114.29
B-spline 3rd order	87.62	96.57	106.17	114.73
B-spline 4th order	89.44	96.92	106.60	115.93
Cubic Lagrangian	91.73	98.63	108.14	121.29
Quintic Lagrangian	91.74	100.42	108.16	121.45
Heptic Lagrangian	91.75	100.44	108.19	121.61
Windowed Sinc	91.72	98.49	108.11	121.28

we would like to improve the resolution in the slice-selection direction. In Figure 9, we applied a trilinear algorithm on the third LR images with a resolution of $256 \times 128 \times 120$ and a *voxel* size of $1 \times 2 \times 1.3 \, \text{mm}^3$; the resolution in coronal view did not improve because the resolution in x-direction was high. However, the resolutions in sagittal and axial views were changed, and we saw enough improvement in their resolutions. The fourth LR images had a resolution of $128 \times 256 \times 120$ and a *voxel* size of $2 \times 1 \times 1.3 \, \text{mm}^3$; those results are shown in Figure 10. The resolution in the sagittal view was constant because the resolution in y was high and just the sagittal resolution in axial and coronal views was changed. The downsampled results in Figure 8 (middle row) in the sagittal and the coronal views show significant jagged-edge distortion.

TABLE 4: 3D MSE for MR image of matrix sizes of $256 \times 256 \times 60$, $256 \times 128 \times 120$, and $128 \times 256 \times 120$ for interpolations of trilinear, nearest neighbor, B-spline 3rd order, B-spline 4th order, cubic Lagrangian, quintic Lagrangian, heptic Lagrangian, and windowed Sinc (compared to 3D simulated reference 2 with resolution $256 \times 256 \times 120$).

| | MSE | | |
| | Matrix size | | |
Interpolation	256×256	256×128	128×256
Trilinear	0.002793	0.002820	0.002983
Nearest neighbor	0.014754	0.016352	0.016544
B-spline 3rd order	0.010866	0.013058	0.012870
B-spline 4th order	0.006383	0.007063	0.007319
Cubic Lagrange	0.004519	0.005546	0.005213
Quintic Lagrange	0.004504	0.005530	0.005195
Heptic Lagrange	0.004132	0.005524	0.005192
Windowed Sinc	0.004605	0.005660	0.005285

The trilinear interpolation results in Figure 8 (bottom row) and the coronal views have smoother edges but somewhat blurred appearance overall. Also, the downsampled results in Figure 9 (middle row) in the axial and sagittal views were almost equivalent to the downsampled results in the sagittal and coronal views in Figure 9, and they showed noticeable jagged-edge distortion. The trilinear interpolation results in Figure 9 (bottom row) in the axial and sagittal views had smoother edges but blurred appearance slightly. One can see enough improvement in resolution of both planes (axial and sagittal), but the resolution of the coronal view was constant. The downsampled results in Figure 10 (middle row) were similar to the downsampled results in Figures 8 and 9, but with different perspective (axial and coronal). The trilinear interpolation results in Figure 10 (bottom row) in axial and coronal views showed enough improvement in their planes, but the sagittal view was constant.

3.2. Runtime Measurement. The runtimes of the various interpolation schemes were computed on MR images with a resolution of $256 \times 256 \times 60$ (axial view). In the axial view, the nearest neighbor was the fastest interpolation, with a run time of 16.8 s, and the trilinear was a bit slower than the nearest neighbor with a runtime of 20.4 s. Cubic Lagrangian was fairly fast (35.7 s) and required less time than the quintic Lagrangian, heptic Lagrangian, and windowed Sinc, with 75.2 s, 159.6 s and 182.3 s, respectively.

Interpolation with the B-spline 3rd order and B-spline 4th order took about 48 and 185 times as long as nearest neighbor interpolation. This weak performance was caused by evaluation of the exponential function necessary to specify the weights and increasing the order of B-spline showed the interpolation drastically. The results of the run times are presented in Figure 11.

Among the interpolations techniques discussed, the trilinear method was one of the fastest techniques and had

the smallest interpolation error. The nearest neighbor had a strong point in which the original *voxel* intensities were preserved, but the resulting image was degraded significantly and had a blocky appearance. Our experiments showed that the heptic Lagrangian technique had smaller error than the quintic Lagrangian and the cubic Lagragian. The windowed Sinc had a smaller error than the nearest neighbor, B-spline 3rd order, and B-spline 4th order. The main drawback of windowed Sinc interpolation was that, it generated significant ripple artifacts in the surrounding of the images edges. The B-spline 3rd order and B-spline 4th order were the slowest techniques in this study, and B-spline 3rd order produced one of the worst results in terms of similarity to the original image. These results demonstrated that the increment of the order in B-spline will not significantly improve the interpolation quality, and this will just magnify the edge effects and the degree of blurriness, which already noticeable when compared to trilinear and Lagrangian methods. The theory and application of B-spline were analyzed by researchers [45, 46], and they found the third-order B-spline interpolator to be sufficient for some specific practical applications [47]. Currently, we believe that the trilinear can offer the best compromise between speed and accuracy in upsampling.

3.3. Analyzing the Effect of Interpolation Techniques on Accuracy of Cost Functions-Based OAIR Algorithm. We implemented OAIR 3D described in Section 1 to perform registration between images, and seven interpolation techniques using similarity measures NCC, LS, CR, and NMI. We computed MSE and PSNR of our results, and the experimental results are listed in Table 5. It is important to note that the interpolation error during upsampling (before registration) is different than the interpolation error of geometric transformation (during registration). For instance, the interpolation algorithm, which has remarkable performance in upsampling process, may have insufficient performance in geometric transformation [48]. Statistical analysis of Table 5 showed that there was insignificant difference between the sets of image registered using CR, LS, NCC, and NMI (P value > 0.9994 for all cost functions). However, the effect of interpolation was considerable, and we observed significant difference between the sets of image registered using different interpolations (P-value < 0.0001 for all interpolations). For instance, sets of images registered using windowed Sinc interpolation were significantly better than sets of images registered using B-spline 3rd-order interpolation with similar cost functions (lower MSE and higher PSNR). For qualitative assessment, we investigated the accuracy of registered results using intensity-based cost functions (CR, LS, NCC, NMI). Windowed Sinc and B-spline 3rd-order interpolations were used during registration (other interpolations schemes can also be used if more investigation is desired). Figure 12 shows axial slices from two registered 3D MRI volumes with their subtractions. The panels show axial slices from two data sets (3D simulated images with a resolution of $256 \times 256 \times 120$ and with a *voxel* size of $1 \times 1 \times 1.3 \, \text{mm}^3$) after registration of the three-dimensional volumes using an intensity-based CR (first column), LS (second column), NCC (third column),

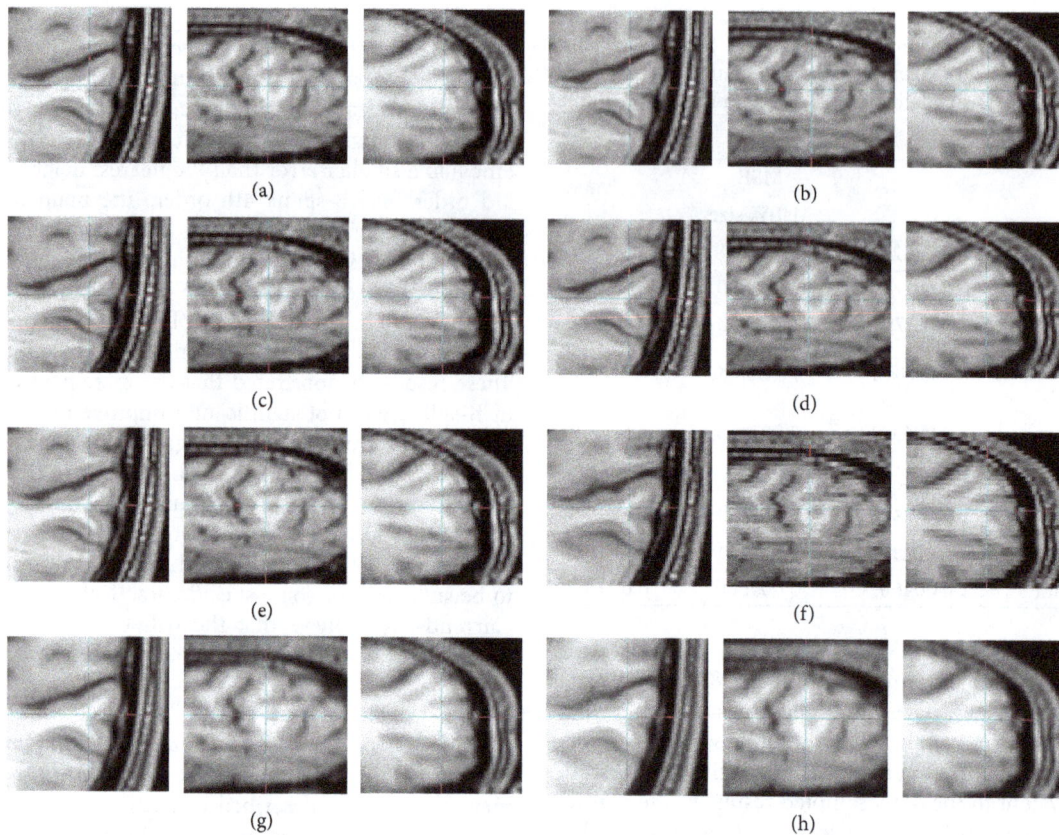

FIGURE 7: (a) Trilinear, (b) heptic Lagrange, (c) quintic Lagrange, (d) windowed Sinc, (e) cubic Lagrangian, (f) nearest neighbor, (g) B-spline 3rd order, (h) B-spline 4th order, axial view (left column), sagittal view (middle column), and coronal view (right column). These upsampled images are from images that were downsampled by a factor of two in z-direction.

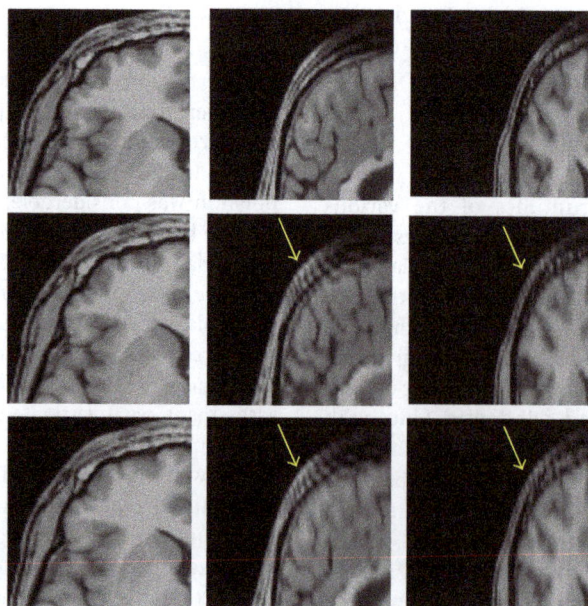

FIGURE 8: Reference with resolution $256 \times 256 \times 120$ (top row), downsampled by a factor of 2 in the Z direction with resolution $256 \times 256 \times 60$ (middle row), interpolated by trilinear (bottom row), axial view (left column), sagittal (middle column), and coronal view (right column). The yellow arrows in sagittal and coronal views show significant jagged-edge distortion.

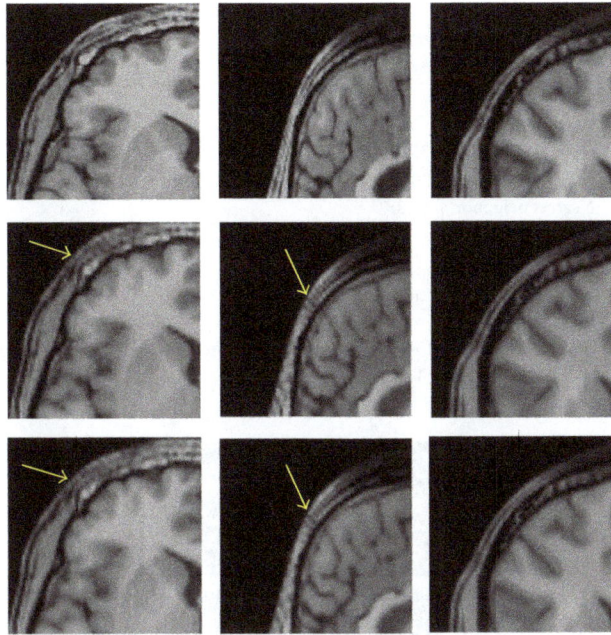

FIGURE 9: Reference with resolution $256 \times 256 \times 120$ (top row), downsampled by a factor of 2 in the Y direction with resolution $256 \times 128 \times 120$ (middle row), interpolated by trilinear (bottom row), axial view (left column), sagittal (middle column), and coronal views (right column). The yellow arrows in axial and sagittal views show significant jagged-edge distortion.

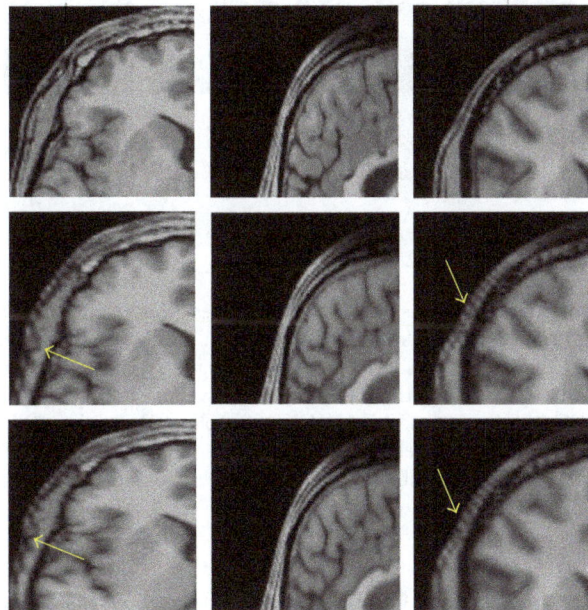

FIGURE 10: Reference with resolution $256 \times 256 \times 120$ (top row), downsampled by a factor of 2 in the X direction with resolution $128 \times 256 \times 120$ (middle row), interpolated by trilinear (bottom row), axial view (left column), sagittal (middle column), and coronal view (right column). The yellow arrows in axial and coronal views show significant jagged-edge distortion.

and NMI (fourth column). Windowed Sinc (panel one) and B-spline 3rd-order (panel two) interpolations were used as resampling. In the second row of the panels, after registration, the pixel intensities of the reference and target images were roughly identical and different images were considerably smooth. In both panels, although differences of registered 3D MRI volumes using an intensity-based CR (first column), LS (second column), NCC (third column), and NMI (fourth column) were difficult to see by visual inspection, changing the interpolation showed that significant differences between two panels exist. In panel two, where B-spline 3rd order was used during registration, the boundary of the skull, which was masked out of the images during registration, could still be observed easily in the difference images, whereas in the panel

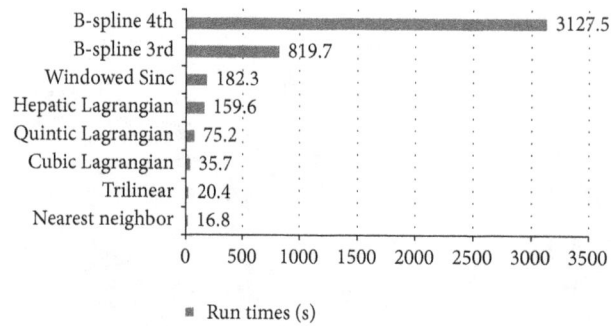

FIGURE 11: Run times measured on the Intel Xeon with 2.13 GHz 2 processor. Among the discussed interpolation techniques, the trilinear is one of the fastest interpolations and runs quickly, with 20.4 s.

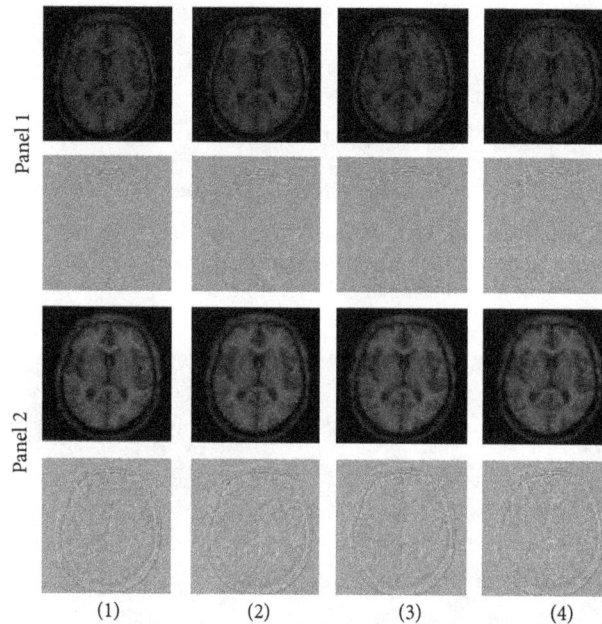

FIGURE 12: In the top panel one, axial slices from two unregistered 3D MRI volumes using an intensity-based cost function (CR (first column), LS (second column), NCC (third column), and NMI (fourth column)) are shown. Windowed Sinc interpolation was used during registration for the panel one. The second row of the panel one shows subtraction of the images (registered and reference images). The panel two shows similar axial slices from the same two data sets after registration of the full 3D volumes using the same intensity-based cost function (CR (first column), LS (second column), NCC (third column), and NMI (fourth column)). B-spline 3rd-order interpolation was used during registration for the panel two. The second row of the panel two shows subtraction of the images. Although differences of the first rows of panel one and panel two are not easily observed by eye, subtraction of the images shows that differences are present, as seen on the second rows of the panel one and panel two.

one, where windowed Sinc was used during registration, the skull in different images was not easily detected by eye. A possible reason for checking the effect of interpolations and cost functions for registration can be seen by visual inspection of the joint histogram in Figure 13, which contains several histograms of 3D MRI using an intensity-based CR (first column), LS (second column), NCC (third column), and NMI (fourth column). In the top and bottom rows, windowed Sinc and B-spline 3rd-order interpolations were used during registration, respectively. The top row in Figure 13 showed the joint histogram for 3D images at registration using windowed interpolation and with small amount of misregistration, and there was a diagonal in the distribution with the small

dispersion. However, in the bottom row, the B-spline 3rd-order interpolation led to large mis-registration of the image, and increased off-diagonal entries started to appear, and the distribution became more dispersed. The distribution of the bottom row is nonsymmetric, and so the linear relationship is not preserved. In general, the intense inhomogeneity will noticeably change for different interpolations; this is one of the reasons that will induce nonsymmetric dispersion and a nonlinear relationship between intensities. However, the change in the appearance of the histograms for these 3D MRI volumes using CR, LS, NCC, and NMI is *insignificant*. We used these joint histograms to better understand the effect of different interpolations and cost functions during

TABLE 5: The 3D MSE and PSNR for registered image of 256×256×120 using interpolations of trilinear, B-spline 3rd order, B-spline 4th order, cubic Lagrange, quintic Lagrange, heptic Lagrangian, windowed Sinc, and cost functions of CR, LS, NCC, and NMI. The affine transformation contains 12 DOF and was implemented during registration.

Interpolation	Cost function	MSE	PSNR (dB)
Trilinear	Correlation ratio	0.023505	115.32
Trilinear	Least squares	0.023591	115.16
Trilinear	Normalized cross-correlation	0.023597	115.10
Trilinear	Normalized mutual information	0.023623	115.09
B-spline 3rd order	Correlation ratio	0.065592	106.30
B-spline 3rd order	Least squares	0.065732	106.27
B-spline 3rd order	Normalized cross-correlation	0.064311	106.34
B-spline 3rd order	Normalized mutual information	0.065588	106.31
B-spline 4th order	Correlation ratio	0.037540	111.37
B-spline 4th order	Least squares	0.037597	111.36
B-spline 4th order	Normalized cross-correlation	0.037631	111.35
B-spline 4th order	Normalized mutual information	0.037604	111.36
Cubic Lagrange	Correlation ratio	0.020723	116.35
Cubic Lagrange	Least squares	0.020887	116.28
Cubic Lagrange	Normalized cross-correlation	0.020891	116.27
Cubic Lagrange	Normalized mutual information	0.020793	116.32
Quintic Lagrange	Correlation ratio	0.019982	116.76
Quintic Lagrange	Least squares	0.020108	116.71
Quintic Lagrange	Normalized cross-correlation	0.020082	116.72
Quintic Lagrange	Normalized mutual information	0.019979	116.76
Heptic Lagrange	Correlation ratio	0.019588	116.86
Heptic Lagrange	Least squares	0.019770	116.78
Heptic Lagrange	Normalized cross-correlation	0.019736	116.79
Heptic Lagrange	Normalized mutual information	0.019639	116.83
Windowed Sinc	Correlation ratio	0.019119	117.06
Windowed Sinc	Least squares	0.019190	117.02
Windowed Sinc	Normalized cross-correlation	0.019329	116.96
Windowed Sinc	Normalized mutual information	0.019160	117.04

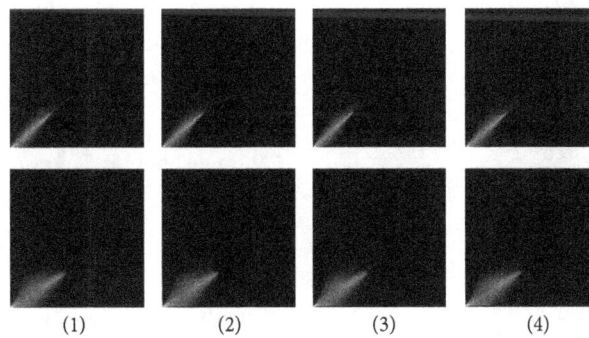

(1)   (2)   (3)   (4)

FIGURE 13: Joint histogram for registered 3D MRI volumes using an intensity-based cost function (CR (first column), LS (second column), NCC (third column), and NMI (fourth column)) are shown. The top row is generated from the images when registered using windowed Sinc interpolation, and the bottom row is generated from the images when registered using B-spline 3rd-order interpolation.

registration. We also measured joint entropy of the registered images using various interpolations and cost functions. Because joint entropy is directly related, the joint probability distribution described the statistical relationship of corresponding *voxel* intensities. Entropy increased with increasing mis-registration as can be seen in visual appearance of the joint histogram (see Figure 13). High dispersion of the joint histogram is equivalent to high joint entropy [49]. The joint entropy results are shown in Table 6, and there are no significant differences between the entropies of registered images

TABLE 6: The joint entropy for the registered images of matrix size of $256 \times 256 \times 120$ using interpolations of trilinear, B-spline 3rd order, B-spline 4th order, cubic Lagrange, quintic Lagrange, heptic Lagrange, windowed Sinc, and cost functions of CR, LS, NCC, and NMI. Their entropies were achieved using mutual information.

Interpolation	Cost function	Entropy
Trilinear	Correlation ratio	2.3723
Trilinear	Least squares	2.3718
Trilinear	Normalized cross-correlation	2.3704
Trilinear	Normalized mutual information	2.3787
B-spline 3rd order	Correlation ratio	2.4499
B-spline 3rd order	Least squares	2.4486
B-spline 3rd order	Normalized cross-correlation	2.4489
B-spline 3rd order	Normalized mutual information	2.4529
B-spline 4th order	Correlation ratio	2.3874
B-spline 4th order	Least squares	2.3889
B-spline 4th order	Normalized cross-correlation	2.3891
B-spline 4th order	Normalized mutual information	2.3881
Cubic Lagrange	Correlation ratio	2.3649
Cubic Lagrange	Least squares	2.3613
Cubic Lagrange	Normalized cross-correlation	2.3615
Cubic Lagrange	Normalized mutual information	2.3636
Quintic Lagrange	Correlation ratio	2.3527
Quintic Lagrange	Least squares	2.3559
Quintic Lagrange	Normalized cross-correlation	2.3534
Quintic Lagrange	Normalized mutual information	2.3544
Heptic Lagrange	Correlation ratio	2.3549
Heptic Lagrange	Least squares	2.3561
Heptic Lagrange	Normalized cross-correlation	2.3511
Heptic Lagrange	Normalized mutual information	2.3517
Windowed Sinc	Correlation ratio	2.3425
Windowed Sinc	Least squares	2.3452
Windowed Sinc	Normalized cross-correlation	2.3434
Windowed Sinc	Normalized mutual information	2.3443

using CR, LS, NCC, and NMI (P-value ≥ 0.9999 for all cost functions), which means that they have the similar dispersion in the joint histogram, but there were significant differences between the entropies of registered images using different interpolations (P-value < 0.0001 for all interpolations). Also, we computed costs for different *voxel* similarity cost functions

that were used in registration with different interpolations and cost functions. We used inverse cost functions; thus, the minimum cost function corresponded to better registration. The results are shown in Table 7, and the registered images using CR, LS, NCCI, and NMI yielded very close results (P-value ≥ 0.9999 for all cost functions), whereas the registered images using different interpolations yielded different results (P-value ≤ 0.0041).

Statistical analysis of Tables 5, 6, and 7 showed that interpolations had a *significant* effect on the registration accuracy, whereas cost functions had no effect on the registration accuracy.

4. Conclusion

Interpolation techniques play a critical role in the improvement and deterioration of the quality of the image as the resolution changes. Thus, the interpolation error is crucial in assessing the interpolation techniques. The interpolation error depends on features such as geometric deformation and the content of the image; therefore, only one evaluation method would not be adequate to evaluate all properties of an algorithm, and a variety of methods should be applied. The comparison is performed by visual quality assessment, quantitative interpolation error determination, and run time measurement. In this study, the results of the algorithms showed that the trilinear method had the smallest interpolation error and the highest PSNR and was one of the fastest techniques, making it appropriate for upsampling in 3D MR images and super resolution. Although super computers are able to compute a huge amount of data in real time, fast methods might be required for online resampling of image sequences or films [50]. The resulting images for trilinear interpolation were less smooth and blocky than other interpolated images. Nevertheless, trilinear interpolation has the effect of losing some high frequency information from the image [51].

Also, the effect of cost functions (LS, NMI, NCC, and CR), and interpolations (trilinear, cubic Lagrange, quintic Lagrange, heptic Lagrange, windowed Sinc, B-spline 3rd order, and B-spline 4th order) for OAIR of 3D brain images was examined, and our experimental results showed that interpolations can effectively decrease or increase the failure possibility of the registration algorithm, and the robustness of method was not due to the choice of cost function, but the choice of interpolation was critical on the robustness of registration. In addition, each component of the optimization method was also necessary to achieve the accurate registrations. Studying the precise effect of transformation on registrations is an active research area [52] but is beyond the scope of this paper.

We noted that the study presented in the tables and figures relied on the same modality (MRI); in addition, these results are not representative of different modality combinations. Perhaps other conclusions would be obtained by the use of different modality combinations or transformations, for instance, MRI-PET or CT-MRI.

TABLE 7: The CR, MI, NMI, and NCC of reference and registered images. The 3D registered images using trilinear, B-spline 3rd order, B-spline 4th order, cubic Lagrange, quintic Lagrange, heptic Lagrange, windowed Sinc interpolations, and cost functions of CR, LS, NCC, and NMI.

Registration			Pixel similarity cost functions		
Interpolation	Cost function	Correlation ration	Mutual information	Normalized mutual information	Normalized cross-correlation
Trilinear	Correlation Ratio	0.030921	0.572625	0.758732	0.016443
Trilinear	Least square	0.030943	0.575558	0.758843	0.016472
Trilinear	Normalized cross-correlation	0.030978	0.577968	0.758742	0.016498
Trilinear	Normalized mutual information	0.030874	0.571644	0.758756	0.016452
B-spline 3rd	Correlation ratio	0.091192	0.906945	0.789837	0.047106
B-spline 3rd	Least square	0.091371	0.905995	0.790105	0.047204
B-spline 3rd	Normalized cross-correlation	0.089311	0.905822	0.788936	0.046135
B-spline 3rd	Normalized mutual information	0.091554	0.906234	0.789860	0.047101
B-spline 4th	Correlation ratio	0.047523	0.645413	0.764792	0.026291
B-spline 4th	Least square	0.047664	0.647675	0.764965	0.026334
B-spline 4th	Normalized cross-correlation	0.047837	0.646529	0.764938	0.026347
B-spline 4th	Normalized mutual information	0.047741	0.646291	0.764879	0.026328
Cubic Lagrange	Correlation ratio	0.027451	0.557755	0.738121	0.014453
Cubic Lagrange	Least square	0.027678	0.559016	0.738517	0.014556
Cubic Lagrange	Normalized cross-correlation	0.027751	0.557785	0.738253	0.014558
Cubic Lagrange	Normalized mutual information	0.027632	0.558993	0.734889	0.014486
Quintic Lagrange	Correlation ratio	0.026226	0.533578	0.731717	0.013931
Quintic Lagrange	Least square	0.026307	0.538433	0.730597	0.014006
Quintic Lagrange	Normalized cross-correlation	0.026227	0.533604	0.731881	0.013986
Quintic Lagrange	Normalized mutual information	0.026234	0.532218	0.731289	0.013912
Heptic Lagrange	Correlation ratio	0.025983	0.537712	0.729622	0.013651
Heptic Lagrange	Least square	0.026274	0.532524	0.731221	0.013767
Heptic Lagrange	Normalized cross-correlation	0.026273	0.531087	0.730581	0.013741
Heptic Lagrange	Normalized mutual information	0.026162	0.531199	0.730681	0.013672
Windowed Sinc	Correlation ratio	0.024201	0.263132	0.720291	0.013392
Windowed Sinc	Least square	0.025253	0.260997	0.720884	0.013445
Windowed Sinc	Normalized cross-correlation	0.024727	0.266973	0.720306	0.013544
Windowed Sinc	Normalized mutual information	0.024819	0.262372	0.730032	0.013426

Also, OAIR was explained in detail, and it was a powerful image registration algorithm. This algorithm was a fully automated algorithm and proposed various resampling interpolation methods combined with CR, LS, NCC, and NMI as a cost function. One of the advantages of this method was using a feature detector (corners are used as the features) to automatically choose a large number of potentially matchable feature points in both images. The algorithm is able to detect identical features in all projections of the scene regardless of the particular image deformation. This method has direct potential for registering clinical MRI images. We have validated this method quantitatively and qualitatively, on the simulated and real data, respectively. Also, there are many excellent sources for more in-depth discussions of image registration that the reader may wish to read and learn [53–56].

5. Future Work

We would like to study the precise effect of transformation on registration, and we are also interested in combining the information of three MRI plane orientations using brain images in order to increase the resolution of 3D brain image based on super resolution reconstruction (SRR) technique.

References

[1] M. Sajjad, N. Khattak, and N. Jafri, "Image magnification using adaptive interpolation by pixel level data-dependent geometrical shapes," *International Journal of Computer Science and Engineering*, vol. 1, no. 2.

[2] J. A. Parker, R. V. Kenyon, and D. E. Troxel, "Comparison of interpolating methods for image resampling," *IEEE Transactions on Medical Imaging*, vol. MI-2, no. 1, pp. 31–39, 1983.

[3] H. S. Hou and H. C. Andrews, "Cubic splines for image interpolation and digital filtering," *IEEE Trans Acoust Speech Signal Process*, vol. 26, no. 6, pp. 508–517, 1978.

[4] E. Maeland, "On the comparison of interpolation methods," *IEEE Transactions on Medical Imaging*, vol. 7, no. 3, pp. 213–217, 1988.

[5] T. M. Lehmann, C. Gönner, and K. Spitzer, "Survey: interpolation methods in medical image processing," *IEEE Transactions on Medical Imaging*, vol. 18, no. 11, pp. 1049–1075, 1999.

[6] R. G. Keys, "Cubic convolution interpolation for digital image processing," *IEEE Transactions on Acoustics, Speech, and Signal Processing*, vol. 29, no. 6, pp. 1153–1160, 1981.

[7] D. L. Hill, C. Studholme, and D. J. Hawkes, "Voxel similarity measures for automated image registration," in *Visualization in Biomedical Computing*, A. Richard Robb, Ed., vol. 2359 of *Proceedings of SPIE*, pp. 205–216, 1994.

[8] E. Göçeri and N. Loménie, "Interpolation approaches and spline based resampling for MR images," in *Proceedings of the 5th International Symposium on Health Informatics and Bioinformatics (HIBIT '10)*, pp. 137–143, April 2010.

[9] D. L. G. Hill and P. Batchelor, "Medical image registration," in *Registration Methodology: Concepts and Algorithms*, V. Joseph Hajnal, L. G. Derek Hill, and J. David Hawkes, Eds., chapter 3, pp. 40–70, CRC Press, 2001.

[10] R. P. Woods, "Handbook of medical image processing and analysis," in *Within-Modality Registration Using Intensity-Based Cost Functions*, N. Isaac, Ed., chapter 33, pp. 529–553, Academic Press, 2000.

[11] F. B. Hildebrand, *Introduction to Numerical Analysis*, Dover, New York, NY, USA, 2nd edition, 1974.

[12] F. Jean-Jacques and B. Delyon, "Min-max interpolators and Lagrange interpolation formula," in *Proceedings of the IEEE International Symposium on Circuits and Systems*, pp. IV/429–IV/432, May 2002.

[13] Y. Chang and C.-D. Lee, "Algebraic decoding of a class of binary cyclic codes via Lagrange interpolation formula," *IEEE Transactions on Information Theory*, vol. 56, no. 1, pp. 130–139, 2010.

[14] P. Bourke, "Interpolation Methods," December 1999.

[15] "Trilinear interpolation," July 1997.

[16] P. Thévenaz, T. Blu, and M. Unser, "Interpolation Revisited," *IEEE Transactions on Medical Imaging*, vol. 19, no. 7, 2000.

[17] H. Du and W. Mei, "Image resizing using exponential B-spline functions," in *Proceedings of the 2nd International Congress on Image and Signal Processing (CISP '09)*, pp. 1–5, October 2009.

[18] G. Farin, *Curves and Surfaces for CAGD: A Practical Guide*, Academic Press, 5th edition.

[19] R. P. Woods, "Handbook of medical image processing and analysis," in *Within-Modality Registration Using Intensity-Based Cost Functions*, N. Isaac Bankman, Ed., chapter 33, pp. 529–536, Academic Press, 2000.

[20] P. E. Radau, P. J. Slomka, P. Julin, L. Svensson, and L.-O. Wahlund, "Evaluation of linear registration algorithms for brain SPECT and the errors due to hypoperfusion lesions," *Medical Physics*, vol. 28, no. 8, pp. 1660–1668, 2001.

[21] J. M. Blackall, D. Rueckert, C. R. Maurer Jr, G. P. Penney, D. L. G. Hill, and D. J. Hawkes, "An image registration approach to automated calibration for freehand 3D ultrasound," in *Medical Image Computing and Computer-Assisted Intervention*, vol. 1935, pp. 462–471, Springer, Berlin, Germany, 2000.

[22] Y. E. Erdi, K. Rosenzweig, A. K. Erdi et al., "Radiotherapy treatment planning for patients with non-small cell lung cancer using positron emission tomography (PET)," *Radiotherapy and Oncology*, vol. 62, no. 1, pp. 51–60, 2002.

[23] K. Van Laere, M. Koole, Y. D'Asseler et al., "Automated stereotactic standardization of brain SPECT receptor data using single-photon transmission images," *Journal of Nuclear Medicine*, vol. 42, no. 2, pp. 361–375, 2001.

[24] J. F. Mangin, C. Poupon, C. Clark, D. Le Bihan, and I. Bloch, "Eddycurrent distortion correction and robust tensor estimation for MR diffusion imaging," in *Medical Image Computing and Computer-Assisted Intervention*, W. J. Niessen and M. A. Viergever, Eds., vol. 2208 of *Lecture Notes in Computer Science*, pp. 186–194, Springer, Berlin, Germany, 2001.

[25] P. Viola and W. M. Wells III, "Alignment by maximization of mutual information," *International Journal of Computer Vision*, vol. 24, no. 2, pp. 137–154, 1997.

[26] M. Jenkinson and S. Smith, "A global optimisation method for robust affine registration of brain images," *Medical Image Analysis*, vol. 5, no. 2, pp. 143–156, 2001.

[27] J. F. Mangin, C. Poupon, C. Clark, D. Le Bihan, and I. Bloch, "Eddycurrent distortion correction and robust tensor estimation for MR diffusion imaging," in *Medical Image Computing and Computer-Assisted Intervention*, W. J. Niessen and M. A. Viergever, Eds., vol. 2208 of *Lecture Notes in Computer Science*, pp. 186–194, Springer, Berlin, Germany, 2001.

[28] D. L. G. Hill, P. G. Batchelor, M. Holden, and D. J. Hawkes, "Medical image registration," *Physics in Medicine and Biology*, vol. 46, no. 3, pp. R1–R45, 2001.

[29] R. P. Woods, "Handbook of medical image processing and analysis," in *Within-Modality Registration Using Intensity-Based Cost Functions*, N. Isaac, Ed., chapter 33, pp. 529–553, Bankman, Academic Press, 2000.

[30] A. Roche, X. Pennec, M. Rudolph et al., *Generalized Correlation Ratio for Rigid Registration of 3D Ultrasound with MR Images*, Institut National de Recherche en Informatique et en Automatique, 2000.

[31] A. Roche, G. Malandain, and N. Ayache, *The Correlation Ratio as a New Similarity Measure for Multimodal Image Registartion*, vol. 1496 of *Lecture Notes in Computer Science*, Springer, 1998.

[32] P. J. Kostelec and S. Periaswamy, *Image Registration for MRI*, vol. 46, Modern Signal Processing, MSRI Publications, 2003.

[33] C. Studholme, D. L. G. Hill, and D. J. Hawkes, "An overlap invariant entropy measure of 3D medical image alignment," *Pattern Recognition*, vol. 32, no. 1, pp. 71–86, 1999.

[34] E. R. E. Denton, M. Holden, E. Christ et al., "The identification of cerebral volume changes in treated growth hormone-deficient adults using serial 3D MR image processing," *Journal of Computer Assisted Tomography*, vol. 24, no. 1, pp. 139–145, 2000.

[35] J. P. W. Pluim, J. B. A. A. Maintz, and M. A. Viergever, "Mutual-information-based registration of medical images: a survey," *IEEE Transactions on Medical Imaging*, vol. 22, no. 8, pp. 986–1004, 2003.

[36] Y. E. Erdi, K. Rosenzweig, A. K. Erdi et al., "Radiotherapy treatment planning for patients with non-small cell lung cancer using positron emission tomography (PET)," *Radiotherapy and Oncology*, vol. 62, no. 1, pp. 51–60, 2002.

[37] M. Jenkinson, P. Bannister, M. Brady, and S. Smith, "Improved optimization for the robust and accurate linear registration and motion correction of brain images," *NeuroImage*, vol. 17, no. 2, pp. 825–841, 2002.

[38] M. Jenkinson and S. Smith, "Optimization in Robust Linear Registartion of Brain Images," FMRIB TR00MJ2.

[39] S. Smith, "BET: 'Brain Extraction Tool'," FMRIB TR00SMS2b, Oxford Centre for Functional Magnetic Resonance Imaging of the Brain), Department of Clinical Neurology, Oxford University, John Radcliffe Hospital, Headington, UK.

[40] T. J. Holmes, "Blind deconvolution of quantum-limited incoherent imagery: maximum-likelihood approach," *Journal of the Optical Society of America A*, vol. 9, no. 7, pp. 1052–1061, 1992.

[41] M.-M. Sung, H.-J. Kim, E.-K. Kim, J.-Y. Kwak, J.-K. Yoo, and H.-S. Yoo, "Clinical evaluation of JPEG2000 compression for digital mammography," *IEEE Transactions on Nuclear Science*, vol. 49, no. 3, pp. 827–832, 2002.

[42] J. P. W. Pluim, J. B. A. A. Maintz, and M. A. Viergever, "Mutual-information-based registration of medical images: a survey," *IEEE Transactions on Medical Imaging*, vol. 22, no. 8, pp. 986–1004, 2003.

[43] C. E. Shannon, "A mathematical theory of communication," *Bell System Technical Journal*, vol. 27, pp. 379–423, 1948.

[44] D. L. G. Hill, D. J. Hawkes, N. A. Harrison, and C. F. Ruff, "A strategy for automated multimodality image registration incorporating anatomical knowledge and imager characteristics," *Information Processing in Medical Imaging*, vol. 687, pp. 182–196, 1993.

[45] M. Unser, A. Aldroubi, and M. Eden, "Polynomial spline signal approximations: filter design and asymptotic equivalence with Shannon's sampling theorem," *IEEE Transactions on Information Theory*, vol. 38, no. 1, pp. 95–103, 1992.

[46] M. Unser, A. Aldroubi, and M. Eden, "B-spline signal processing. Part II. Efficient design and applications," *IEEE Transactions on Signal Processing*, vol. 41, no. 2, pp. 834–848, 1993.

[47] M. Unser, A. Aldroubi, and M. Eden, "Fast B-spline transforms for continuous image representation and interpolation," *IEEE Transactions on Pattern Analysis and Machine Intelligence*, vol. 13, no. 3, pp. 277–285, 1991.

[48] A. Amanatiadis and I. Andreadis, "A survey on evaluation methods for image interpolation," *Measurement Science and Technology*, vol. 20, no. 10, Article ID 104015, 2009.

[49] M. Holden, D. L. G. Hill, E. R. E. Denton et al., "Voxel similarity measures for 3-D serial MR brain image registration," *IEEE Transactions on Medical Imaging*, vol. 19, no. 2, pp. 94–102, 2000.

[50] O. D. Evans and Y. Kim, "Efficient implementation of image warping on a multimedia processor," *Real-Time Imaging*, vol. 4, no. 6, pp. 417–428, 1998.

[51] J. Ashburner and K. F. W. Penny, *Human Brain Function*, chapter 2, 2nd edition.

[52] P. A. Van den Elsen, E. J. D. Pol, and M. A. Viergever, "Medical image matching—a review with classification," *IEEE Engineering in Medicine and Biology Magazine*, vol. 12, no. 1, pp. 26–39, 1993.

[53] L. G. Brown, "Survey of image registration techniques," *ACM Computing Surveys*, vol. 24, no. 4, pp. 325–376, 1992.

[54] J. B. A. Maintz and M. A. Viergever, "A survey of medical image registration," *Medical Image Analysis*, vol. 2, no. 1, pp. 1–36, 1998.

[55] C. R. Maurer and J. M. Fitzpatrick, "A review of medical image registration, chapter in interactive image-guided neurosurgery," in *American Association of Neurological Surgeons*, Park Ridge, Ill, USA, 1993.

[56] F. Maes, *Segmentation and registration of multimodal medical images: from theory, implementation and validation to a useful to tool in clinical practice [Ph.D. thesis]*, Catholic University of Leuven, Leuven, Belgium, 1998.

18

Free Tools and Strategies for the Generation of 3D Finite Element Meshes: Modeling of the Cardiac Structures

E. Pavarino,[1] **L. A. Neves,**[1] **J. M. Machado,**[1] **M. F. de Godoy,**[2] **Y. Shiyou,**[3] **J. C. Momente,**[1] **G. F. D. Zafalon,**[1] **A. R. Pinto,**[1] **and C. R. Valêncio**[1]

[1] *Department of Computer Science and Statistics (DCCE), São Paulo State University (UNESP), 15054-000 São José do Rio Preto, SP, Brazil*
[2] *Department of Cardiology and Cardiovascular Surgery, São José do Rio Preto Medical School–Famerp, 15090-000 São José do Rio Preto, SP, Brazil*
[3] *College of Electrical Engineering, Zhejiang University, Hangzhou 310027, China*

Correspondence should be addressed to L. A. Neves; leandro@ibilce.unesp.br

Academic Editor: Koon-Pong Wong

The Finite Element Method is a well-known technique, being extensively applied in different areas. Studies using the Finite Element Method (FEM) are targeted to improve cardiac ablation procedures. For such simulations, the finite element meshes should consider the size and histological features of the target structures. However, it is possible to verify that some methods or tools used to generate meshes of human body structures are still limited, due to nondetailed models, nontrivial preprocessing, or mainly limitation in the use condition. In this paper, alternatives are demonstrated to solid modeling and automatic generation of highly refined tetrahedral meshes, with quality compatible with other studies focused on mesh generation. The innovations presented here are strategies to integrate Open Source Software (OSS). The chosen techniques and strategies are presented and discussed, considering cardiac structures as a first application context.

1. Introduction

The increased use of minimally invasive surgical procedures in medicine is a reality, with applications in different specialties. The small incisions ensure the patient smaller exposure to infections, as well as a quicker recovery. The radiofrequency cardiac ablation is a good example of it, being extensively used for over 10 years in the treatment of tachycardia, atrial fibrillation, and atrial flutter [1–4]. This technique is not free from complications, although it has advanced in the last decade. The esophageal injury is a common damage, characterized by the union of tissues from the left atrium and esophagus, through necrosis [1, 4]. The consequence for the patient is death caused by internal bleeding, as blood is diverted directly to the stomach, when it is not noticed by the physician.

In the literature, studies using the Finite Element Method (FEM) are targeted to improve cardiac ablation procedure and reduce possible complications, such as esophageal injury.

It is possible to highlight that the nucleus of the problem is monitoring the temperatures in the tissues involved more accurately. This approach is not simple, and the computational simulation using FEM has contributed significantly to the improvement of this technique [5–12]. For such simulations, the finite element meshes should consider the size and histological features of the target structures. Furthermore, the quality of the meshes is another fundamental property to properly simulate the desired phenomena. The techniques which are able to generate meshes with such characteristics are preferred, and when they are generated with open source codes, they make easier tests with no user restrictions. These properties can guarantee more accurate and clinically relevant simulations.

In this context, it is possible to verify that some methods or tools used to generate meshes of human body structures are still limited by providing or using nondetailed models [5–8, 10, 13–15], by the need of nontrivial preprocessing, which is a primary step applied to define, extract, or change the anatomical features (boundary domain) required by meshing generation step [7, 11, 15–18] or due to limitations of the user condition [5, 6, 8, 12, 13, 18, 19]. One of the reasons for this finding is the necessary commitment to represent the complicated geometries of the involved domains, which requires sophisticated resources being sometimes under development in specific tools for geometric modeling and mesh discretization [20, 21]. A typical integrated software tool to construct three-dimensional domains and finite element meshes may have a development time cycle of more than 10 years [22, 23] and frequently with exceptions to allow linking with other mesh generators. An alternative is integrating Open Source Software packages dedicated to solid modeling with automatic generation of tetrahedral meshes, which are available in the literature. This strategy brings obvious advantages in the context of FEM simulations.

With these findings, the present paper demonstrates alternatives to solid modeling and automatic generation of highly refined tetrahedral meshes and with quality compatible with other studies focused on mesh generation. The innovations presented here are strategies to integrate Open Source Software (OSS). The chosen tools were the Blender software [24] as solid modeler and the TetGen as automatic mesh generator [25], which uses the Delaunay tetrahedralization [25, 26]. Furthermore, in this study we demonstrate cardiac structures as a first application context, motivated by the importance that the meshes of these structures represent for studies of cardiac ablation. In the next sections a discussion concerning our strategy for software integration and performance tests in realistic application domain are presented.

2. Material and Methods

The proposed methodology for solid modeling and automatic generation of tetrahedral meshes was organized in Section 2.1, with details about the defined anatomical properties for the application context; Section 2.2, with definitions of the used packages and corresponding justifications; Section 2.3, with details about the recommendations to discretize domains; and Section 2.4, with specifications from the integration process of the models built on the solid modeler to the algorithm used in the automatic mesh generator. The proposal will be described in detail in the next subsections.

2.1. Application: Features of Cardiac Structures. The choices of cardiac structures were motivated by the complicated geometric domain and by the clinical relevance that these structures represent for the investigation of esophageal injury. Therefore, the model defined in our study was composed of cardiac regions consisting of two main parts: the right portion (venous) and the left portion (arterial). Each portion has an atrium, a ventricle, and valves: bicuspid, and tricuspid, pulmonary or aortic valve. The trunks of aorta and pulmonary artery were represented from their connections with the atriums to the beginning of their ramifications. The dimensions of these structures are presented in Table 1

TABLE 1: Values used to define the heart model. Considering the diastolic dimensions of an adult heart [27–29].

Structure	Dimension (cm)	Longest axis (cm)
Left atrium	2.1–3.0	4.6
Right atrium	1.9–4.4	5.3
Left ventricle	3.1–3.8	4.3
Right ventricle	2.1–3.7	4.2
Aorta	2.5	—
Pulmonary artery	2.5	—
Bicuspid valve	2.5	—
Tricuspid valve	3.0	—
Aortic valve	2.4	—
Pulmonary valve	2.3	—
Interventricular septum	0.8–1.2	4.0

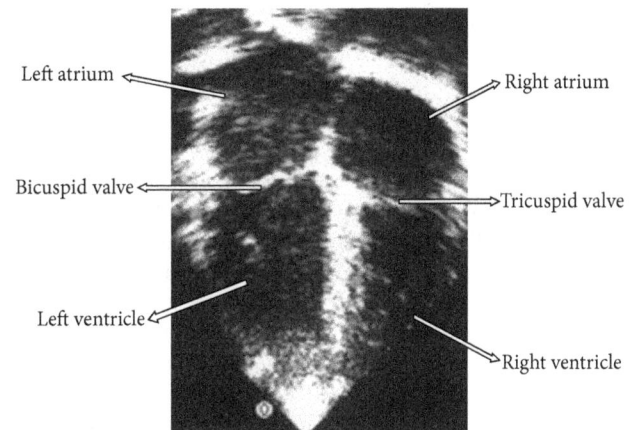

FIGURE 1: Example of echocardiography used in the modeling process. The aortic valve and the pulmonary valve do not appear in this figure.

[27–29], defined in cardiac diastole (period of heart muscle relaxation) and values present in major axes. The presence of some structures is visualized on an echocardiographic image (Figure 1), which was used as another reference during the modeling process.

2.2. Free and Open Source Packages. Creating complex three-dimensional models is not a trivial task, especially without the support of sophisticated modelers and already equipped with resources to integrate it with algorithms responsible for mesh generation. The Blender package [24] maintained by Blender Foundation was chosen. This package is an integrated system of tools, a multiplatform and contains resources to export and import objects in different formats, through scripts. Scripts are useful for automating methods, navigating and manipulating the discretized geometric domain. Moreover, Blender is available under a dual license, Blender License (BL) and GNU General Public License. With all these resources, it becomes possible to represent the domain of interest and use scripts, written in Python language, to export features required by the automatic mesh generator.

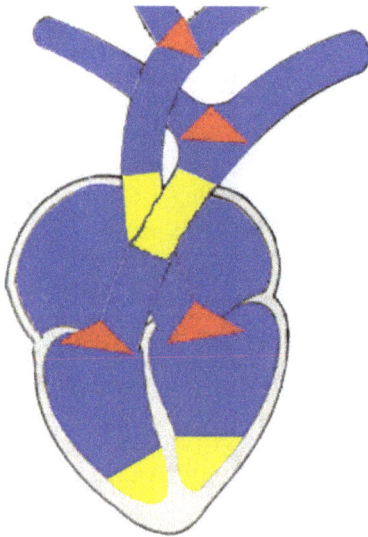

FIGURE 2: Chosen regions for quadrilateral or rectangular faces (blue), triangular faces (red), and with increased density of vertices (yellow).

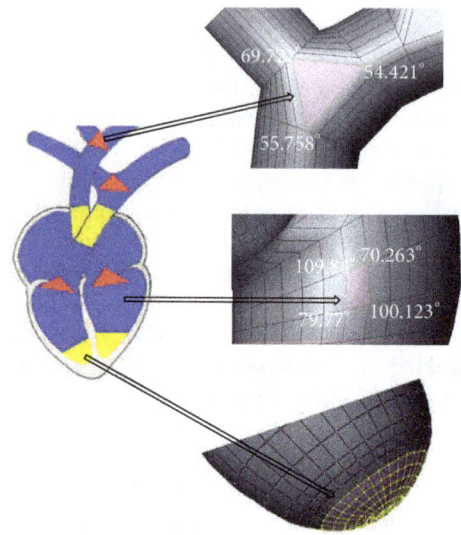

FIGURE 3: Example of regions represented with triangular faces, quadrilateral or rectangular faces, and with increased density of vertices.

The stage for automatic generation of tetrahedral meshes is not a trivial task, a fact that limits the use of a single algorithm to discretize the most different contexts. The algorithms commonly applied to generate tetrahedral meshes have good and bad points [26, 30–32], some of which require manual interference in the domain to obtain the desired discretization. Although there are different methods for generating three-dimensional meshes, we chose the Delaunay algorithm [25, 31] for being one of the most popular and one of the most efficient algorithms [30], available in the TetGen package [26]. Just as Blender, TetGen is an Open Source Software (OSS) and is available under MIT License. This package is maintained by the research group called Numerical Mathematics and Scientific Computing, Weierstrass Institute for Applied Analysis and Stochastics (WIAS), Berlin, Germany.

The selected packages for the models construction and automatic generation of meshes were explored in a computer with a 2.40 GHz quad core processor and 16 GB of RAM memory. The operating system used uses 64-bit architecture, running Blender in version 2.49b and TetGen mesh generator in version 1.4.

2.3. Definition of Strategies for Solid Construction.

The representation of solids in the Blender package must respect two strategies to ensure the integration with the automatic mesh generator. The strategies or recommendations are (1) definitions of faces and (2) density control of vertices, whereas the application of each must consider the complexity of the specific region.

The strategy definitions of faces consist of choosing the most appropriate types of faces to discretize a solid. Regular or noncomplex regions of the specific domain must be discretized with quadrilateral or rectangular faces. A quadrilateral or rectangular face can be modified to fill regions with sharp angles, since the values of the internal angles of the faces are between 30 and 160 degrees. The limits were defined on the basis of the stage of mesh generation, according to the values which propitiated intact and highly refined meshes. In the application focused on this study, quadrilateral or rectangular faces were used to discretize the atriums, the ventricles, the trunks of aorta and pulmonary artery, and the bicuspid, tricuspid, aortic, and pulmonary valves, which are regular and cylindrical regions (marked in blue in Figure 2). Regions with triangular faces were constructed where the discretization required faces with internal angles out of the predetermined range.

The triangular faces are equilateral, isosceles or scalene elements and allow more appropriated representations of regions with sharp angles, such as those occurring at bifurcations points. In the application explored in this study, that situation is commonly evidenced in the bifurcations of arteries and veins, as well as in the regions of connection between atriums, ventricles, and arteries. These regions were demarcated in red in Figure 2.

The strategy density control of vertices defines the number of nodes in a region. The increasing number of vertices allows a better representation of curved regions, by smoothing the direction transition and respecting the features defined on the first property and the orthogonality of the faces (Figure 2). In the context of cardiac structures, this strategy was applied in the construction of cardiac valves, bases of ventricles and in the change of the direction of the aorta and pulmonary artery responsible for their correct positions.

Figure 3 shows examples of regions generated with the strategies or recommendations described previously.

2.4. Application of Integration Strategies.

A domain discretized in Blender is stored in its native file format: a "blend file".

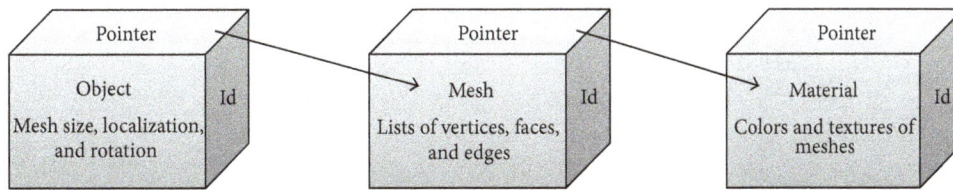

FIGURE 4: Illustration of objects, meshes, and materials data block structures in a "blend file".

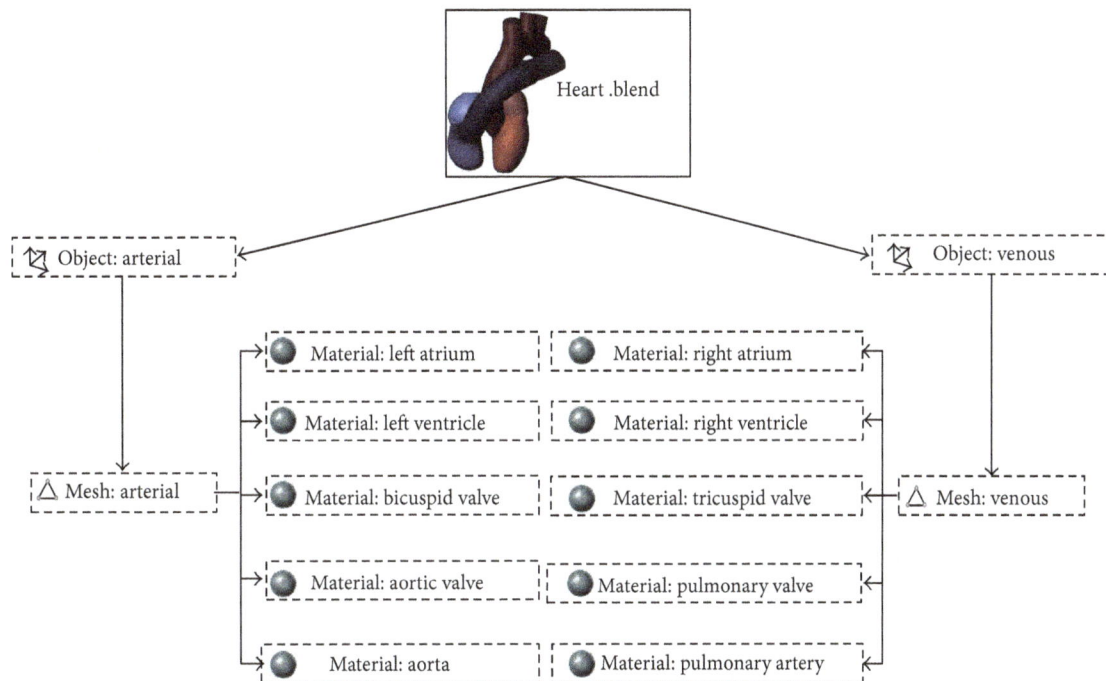

FIGURE 5: Hierarchy of the heart model determined by Blender, considering object, mesh, and material data blocks.

The data used to discretize a solid are stored in this standard file in structures named data blocks. Data blocks are data structures similar to the heterogeneous structure type. In a simple domain, several data blocks may be used. The data blocks can be made of object, mesh, material or scene type, including many others. A data block made of object type stores information about the mesh size and the linear transformations applied; a datablock made of mesh type stores information about the vertices, edges, and faces of the model; a datablock made of material type stores information about the colors assigned to a certain set of vertices, edges or faces. These colors are also called markers. Therefore, the datablocks are linked by pointers and defines a data structure of tree type (Figure 4). Figure 5 exemplifies the structures described for material, mesh, and object datablocks used to represent each cardiac structure, based on Blender Architecture, requiring a total of 14 datablocks.

The integration of the models constructed on Blender with the mesh generator TetGen was accomplished by Python script [32]. The script operates into objects generated by the Blender package through four iterative structures. These structures read the data contained in mesh and object data blocks and translate the information about vertices, faces, holes, and attributes accordingly. The processed information is an ASCII file (.poly), properly written in the formats required by TetGen. The Python script presented by [32] exports only the active solid, which limits the potential for the meshing of mixed solids. The modification performed repeats the process for the group of existing solids automatically and generates a single ASCII file (.poly). Figure 6 shows a diagram of the algorithm used for exportation, with the proposed modification.

A typical "poly file" is composed by 4 parts: an indexed list of point coordinates; a list of solid faces; a list of volume holes; and a list of attributes or boundaries (constraints), see Supplementary Material (Appendix 1) available online at http://dx.doi.org/10.1155/2013/540571.

Figure 7 represents the integration strategies of the Blender and TetGen using the Python script (Figure 6).

This process generates three files. A "node file" contains a list of three-dimensional points. Each point has three coordinates (x, y, and z) and probably includes one or several attributes and a boundary marker as well. A "ele file" contains a list of tetrahedrons. Each tetrahedron has four corners.

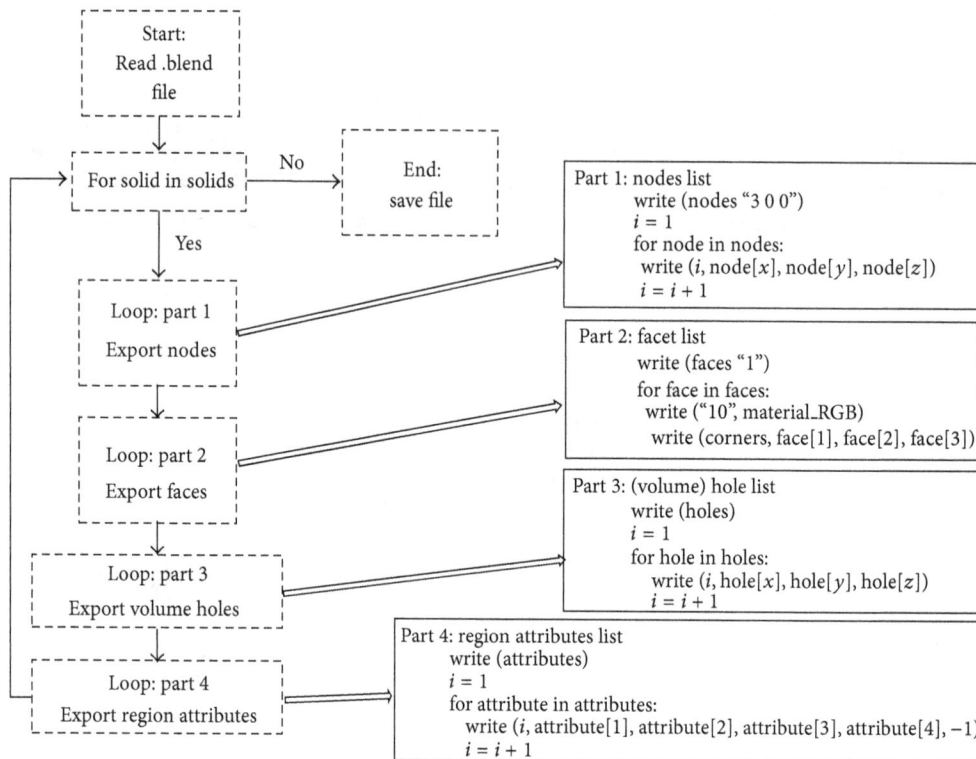

FIGURE 6: Proposed method to repeat automatically the process for the group of existing solids and generate a single ASCII file.

Nodes are indices into the corresponding "node file". The four nodes are the corner vertices. A "face file" contains a list of triangular faces, which may be boundary faces, or convex hull faces. Each face has three corners and possibly a boundary marker. Nodes are indices into the corresponding "node file" [25].

3. Results and Discussions

In this work, the cardiac structures were chosen as a first application context, since three-dimensional meshes of these structures are relevant for studies of cardiac ablation. The complicated geometric domain selected allowed to test the feasibility of the combined use of anatomical features (Section 2.1), free and Open Source Packages (Section 2.2) and apply strategies (Sections 2.3 and 2.4). The organization of the cardiac structures was represented in Blender, considering atriums, ventricles, valves (bicuspid, tricuspid, pulmonary, and aortic), and artery trunks (aorta and pulmonary artery). The model is shown in Figure 8, in different projections.

The "poly file" obtained from the strategies described above is partially shown in Supplementary Material (Appendix 2). The file stores data of 3818 vertices, 3980 faces and 10 boundary markers. Boundary markers are numerical codes such as −1000000 used to assign the blue color to the faces of left ventricle. Different colors are used to better distinguish each structure. Boundary markers are normally used to

simulations in specific regions. A preview of each structure and its boundary markers is represented in Figure 9.

A raw mesh was generated from the proposal presented, and a cut was made to better illustrate the quality of the mesh. Figure 10 shows a mesh constructed with 33875 faces, 42371 nodes, 10 boundary markers, and 223851 tetrahedral elements, a useful example to validate the concept of iteration loop described in the previous section.

Studies grounded in FEM require tools with resources to generate highly refined meshes of simple or complex domains, and in an acceptable time. The methodology proposed in this paper meets these requirements. For the chosen complicated application context, meshes were generated through successive refinements of the coarse initial mesh (Figure 10). Regions of the atriums and ventricles were used to demonstrate the number of tetrahedral elements presented in some refinements (Figure 11). It was therefore possible to estimate the processing time growth, and the number of tetrahedral elements increased. These results are shown in Figure 12 for each test performed. Just a few studies show how many elements have their meshes [16, 19]. Also, none of these studies provide information about the meshing time. This is a limitation for comparisons of our results.

The mesh quality is another important aspect that should be considered in proposals designed to generate meshes through FEM simulations. The number of meshes elements can be an important criterion for this. Another criterion commonly adopted is showing the dihedral angles obtained. The quality of a tetrahedral element is commonly measured

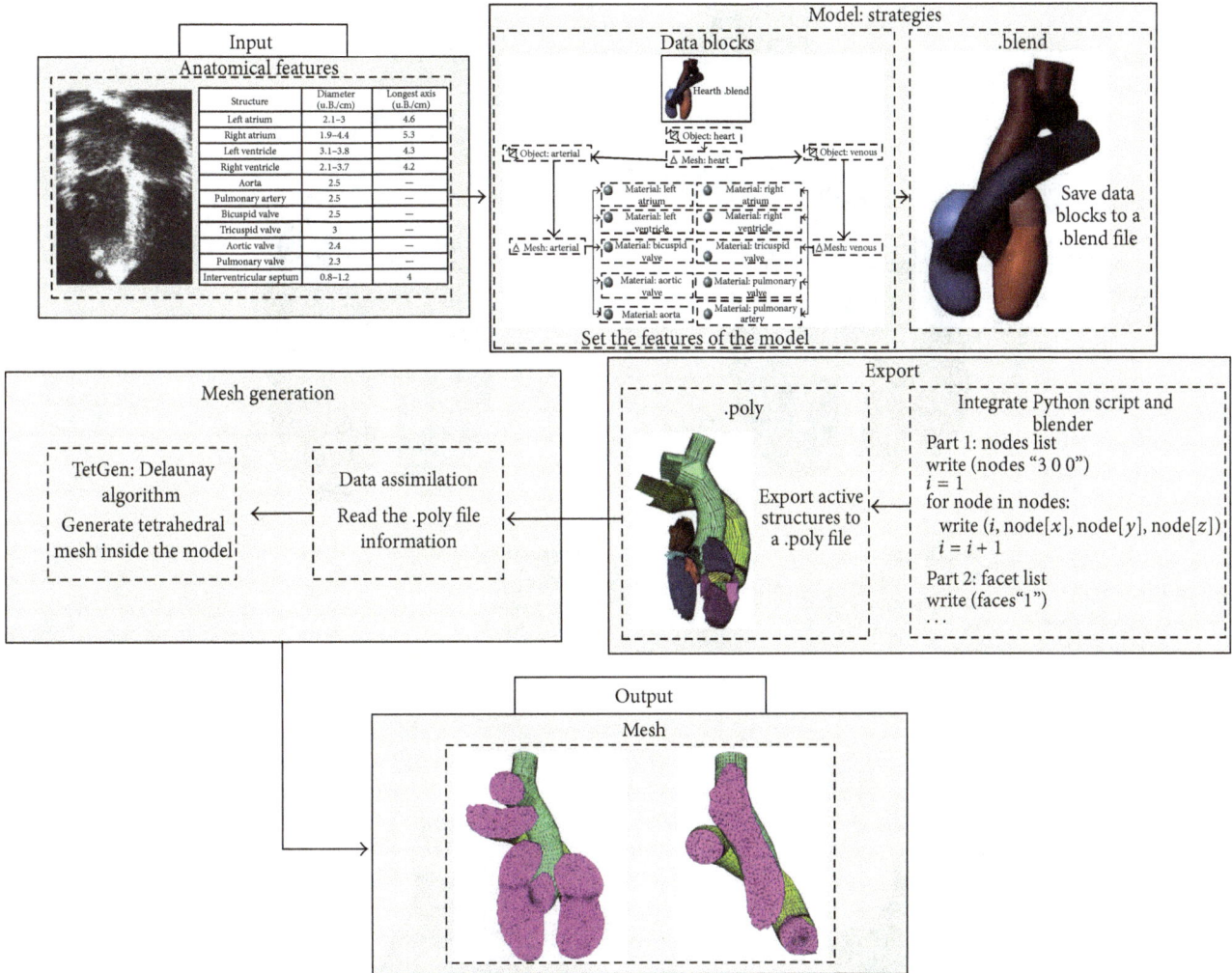

FIGURE 7: Flowchart of the steps of integration between the tools used.

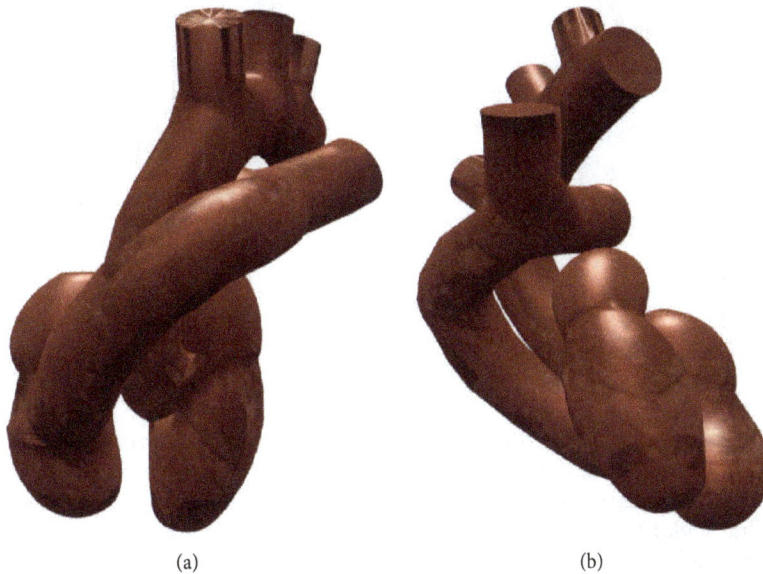

(a)   (b)

FIGURE 8: Model constructed with the approaches previously presented, of which an anterior view is in (a) and a lateral view is in (b).

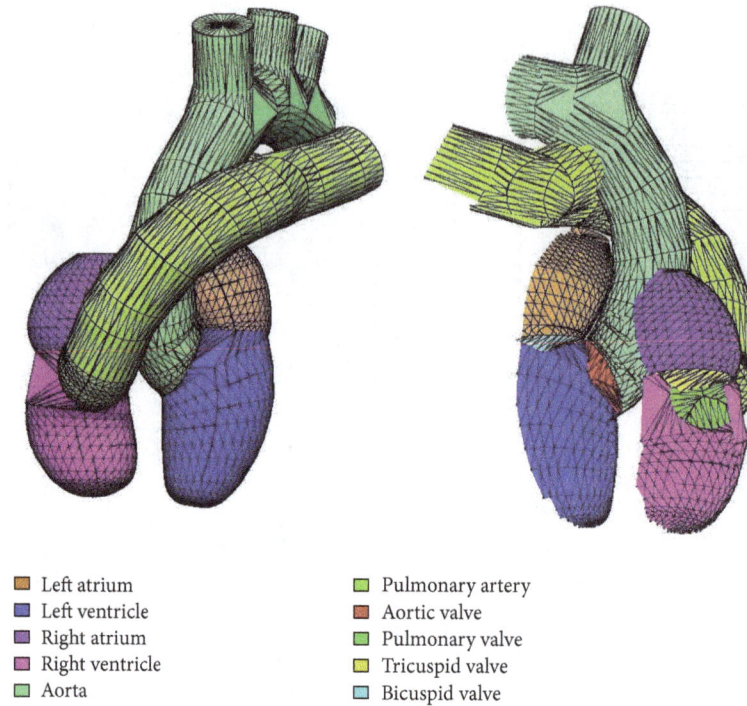

■ Left atrium	■ Pulmonary artery
■ Left ventricle	■ Aortic valve
■ Right atrium	■ Pulmonary valve
■ Right ventricle	■ Tricuspid valve
■ Aorta	■ Bicuspid valve

FIGURE 9: Structures with their corresponding boundary markers.

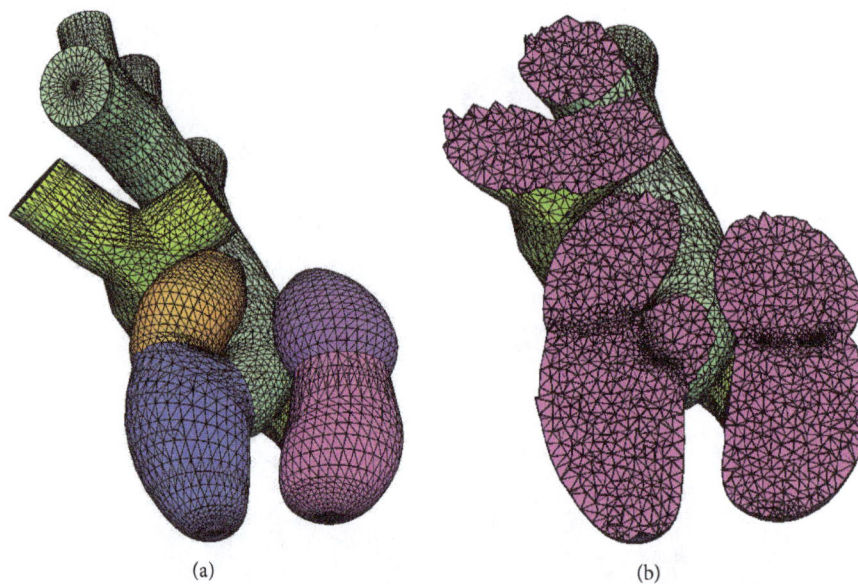

(a)   (b)

FIGURE 10: A raw mesh is shown in (a), and an x, y plane cut is shown in (b).

in terms of minimal and/or maximal dihedral angles. The success of the Finite Element Method depends on the shapes of these tetrahedra. For instance, tetrahedra constructed with too small or too large dihedral angles can cause interpolation errors and lead to numerical simulation with higher instability and less accuracy [33, 34]. The desired quality is the one in which the values of dihedral angles are close to the values set on a regular tetrahedron [26, 34, 35]. This can be verified in histograms constructed with the total of dihedral angles present in ranges of angles, as well as identification of the smallest and largest values involved [33, 34].

It is possible to verify through the presentation of the mesh constructed with 12009998 tetrahedral elements (Figure 13) and the corresponding histogram (Figure 14) that

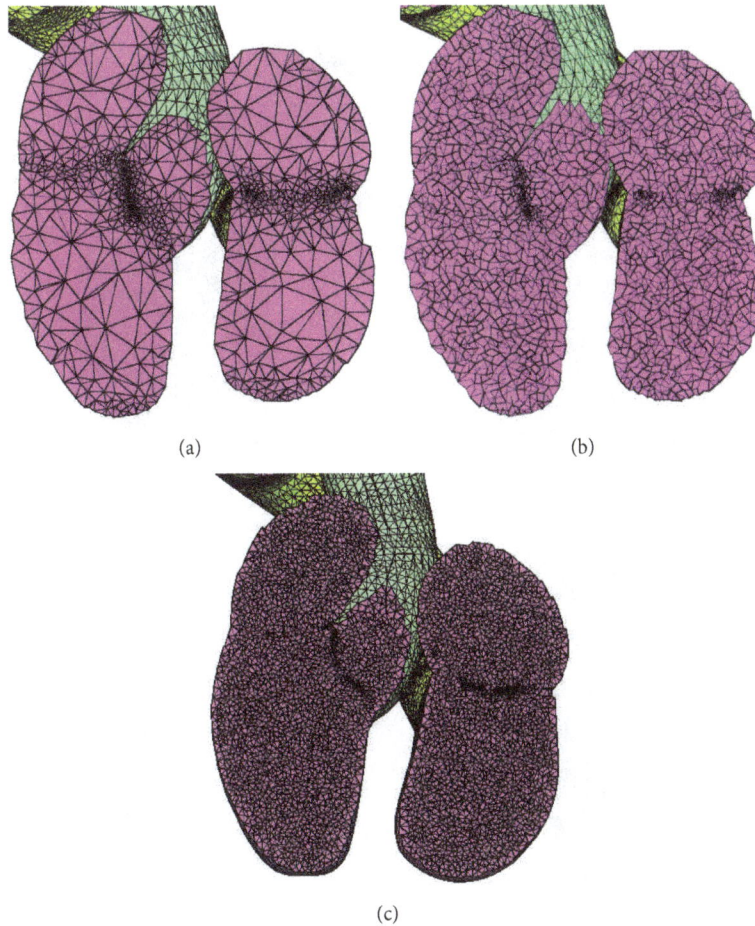

(a)

(b)

(c)

FIGURE 11: Regions of the atriums and ventricles to exemplify the increasing number of nodes in each refinement performed. The number of tetrahedral elements in each test was (a) 158610, (b) 451764, and (c) 1956490.

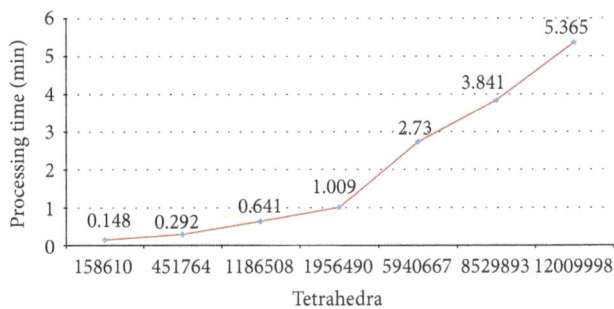

FIGURE 12: Meshing time (y-axis) as a function of the number of elements in the tetrahedral mesh (x-axis), for each refinement shown in Figure 11.

our proposal allows obtaining highly refined meshes from complex domains, in some acceptable time and quality. This number of elements may facilitate the representation of degenerated tetrahedral elements and effectively indicate the limits of the proposed approach. However, it is also possible to verify that the tetrahedral elements have dihedral angles whose values belong to the interval which varies from 5 to 170

degrees, with peak values around the condition for a regular tetrahedron. These values are close to those used to determine the mesh quality in other studies [33, 34]. For instance, the algorithm proposed by [34] is capable of producing tetrahedral meshes whose dihedral angles are bounded between 10.7 and 164.8 degrees or between 8.9 and 158.8 degrees with a change in parameters. Also, when nonuniform tetrahedra on the surface boundary are chosen, the dihedral angles are bounded between 1.66 and 174.72 degrees. In another example, tetrahedral meshes are generated with the minimal dihedral angle being guaranteed to be greater than or equal to 5.71 degrees [33].

4. Conclusion

The proposal presented in this paper considered strategies to build solid and automatic mesh generation, based on Open Source Packages. The strategies are feasible to generate highly refined mesh in some acceptable time and with the required quality for simulation using the Finite Element Method (FEM). These facts were demonstrated by considering a complex domain with some practical importance, as in the case of mesh structures for the study of cardiac ablation through

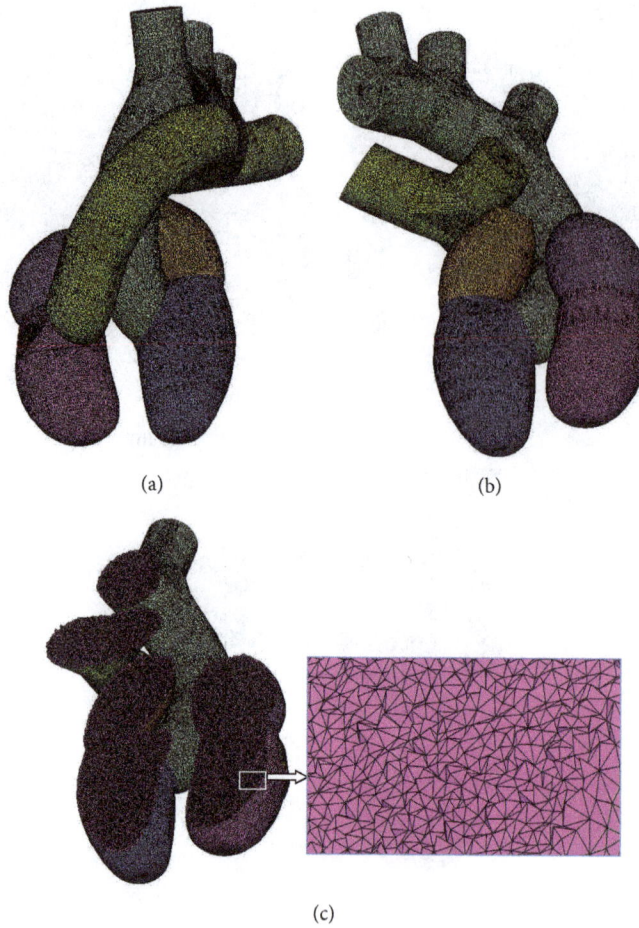

FIGURE 13: Mesh constructed with 12009998 tetrahedra in 5.36 minutes is shown in anterior (a) and posterior (b) views. A zoom view detail is given in (c), according to a transversal cut applied in the plane x, y.

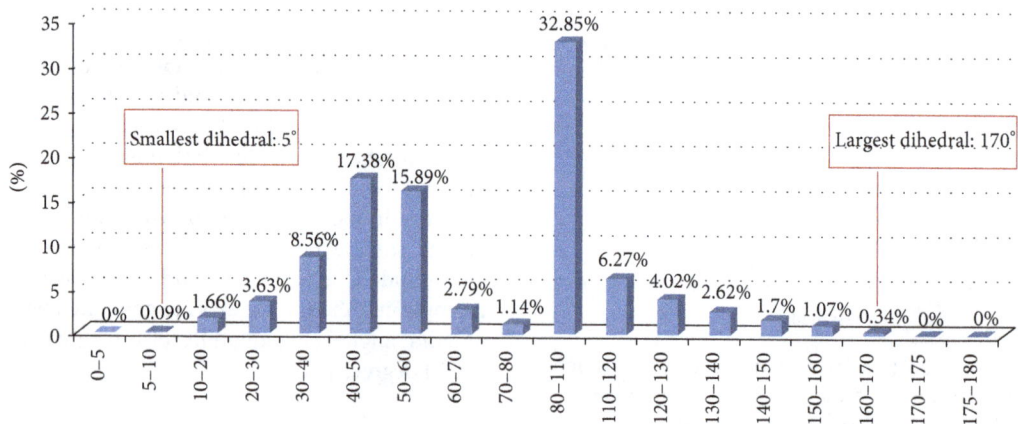

FIGURE 14: Histogram constructed with the total of dihedral angles (y-axis) inside prescribed angle intervals in degrees (x-axis). The corresponding tetrahedral mesh was shown in Figure 13.

FEM. The most refined mesh involved approximately 12 million elements and was generated in 5.35 minutes. Despite the significant number of tetrahedral elements involved, the explored example does not define the limit of possible refinements from our approach. The tetrahedral quality was also discussed and the values of dihedral angles generated are consistent with the literature. So, our proposal provides a significant contribution to the mesh generation for studies using FEM, which is a known method applied in different areas.

Acknowledgment

This work was financially supported by Pró-Reitoria de Pesquisa/UNESP (PROPe/UNESP).

References

[1] E. Sosa and M. Scanavacca, "Left atrial-esophageal fistula complicating radiofrequency catheter ablation of atrial fibrillation," *Journal of Cardiovascular Electrophysiology*, vol. 16, no. 3, pp. 249–250, 2005.

[2] S. Nath, C. Lynch, J. G. Whayne, and D. E. Haines, "Cellular electrophysiological effects of hyperthermia on isolated guinea pig papillary muscle: Implications for catheter ablation," *Circulation*, vol. 88, no. 4, pp. 1826–1831, 1993.

[3] O. J. Eick and D. Bierbaum, "Tissue temperature-controlled radiofrequency ablation," *Pacing and Clinical Electrophysiology*, vol. 26, no. 3, pp. 725–730, 2003.

[4] M. O. Siegel, D. M. Parenti, and G. L. Simon, "Atrial-esophageal fistula after atrial radiofrequency catheter ablation," *Clinical Infectious Diseases*, vol. 51, no. 1, pp. 73–76, 2010.

[5] D. Panescu, J. G. Whayne, S. D. Fleischman, M. S. Mirotznik, D. K. Swanson, and J. G. Webster, "Three-dimensional finite element analysis of current density and temperature distributions during radio-frequency ablation," *IEEE Transactions on Biomedical Engineering*, vol. 42, no. 9, pp. 879–890, 1995.

[6] S. Tungjitkusolmun, E. J. Woo, H. Cao, J. Z. Tsai, V. R. Vorperian, and J. G. Webster, "Finite element analyses of uniform current density electrodes for radio-frequency cardiac ablation," *IEEE Transactions on Biomedical Engineering*, vol. 47, no. 1, pp. 32–40, 2000.

[7] H. Cao, M. A. Speidel, J. Z. Tsai, M. S. Van Lysel, V. R. Vorperian, and J. G. Webster, "FEM analysis of predicting electrode-myocardium contact from RF cardiac catheter ablation system impedance," *IEEE Transactions on Biomedical Engineering*, vol. 49, no. 6, pp. 520–526, 2002.

[8] D. Haemmerich and J. G. Webster, "Automatic control of finite element models for temperature-controlled radiofrequency ablation," *BioMedical Engineering Online*, vol. 4, article 42, 2005.

[9] E. J. Berjano, "Theoretical modeling for radiofrequency ablation: state-of-the-art and challenges for the future," *BioMedical Engineering Online*, vol. 5, article 24, 2006.

[10] F. Hornero and E. J. Berjano, "Esophageal temperature during radiofrequency-catheter ablation of left atrium: a three-dimensional computer modeling study," *Journal of Cardiovascular Electrophysiology*, vol. 17, no. 4, pp. 405–410, 2006.

[11] R. Barauskas, A. Gulbinas, and G. Barauskas, "Investigation of radiofrequency ablation process in liver tissue by finite element modeling and experiment," *Medicina (Kaunas, Lithuania)*, vol. 43, no. 4, pp. 310–325, 2007.

[12] W. Yang, T. C. Fung, K. S. Chian, and C. K. Chong, "Finite element simulation of food transport through the esophageal body," *World Journal of Gastroenterology*, vol. 13, no. 9, pp. 1352–1359, 2007.

[13] S. F. Miller, J. D. Geiger, and A. J. Shih, "Thermal-electric finite element analysis and experimental validation of bipolar electrosurgical cautery," *Ann Arbor*, vol. 1001, Article ID 48109, 2008.

[14] C. Brock, R. E. Lontis, F. H. Lundager, P. Kunwald, A. M. Drewes, and H. Gregersen, "Model for electrical field distribution in the human esophagus during stimulation with patch and ring electrodes," *Gastroenterology Research and Practice*, vol. 2011, Article ID 562592, 8 pages, 2011.

[15] S. T. Wall, J. M. Guccione, M. B. Ratcliffe, and J. S. Sundnes, "Electromechanical feedback with reduced cellular connectivity alters electrical activity in an infarct injured left ventricle: a finite element model study," *American Journal of Physiology—Heart and Circulatory Physiology*, vol. 302, no. 1, pp. H206–H214, 2012.

[16] D. Milasinovic, M. Ivanovic, H. Tengg-Kobligk, D. Bockler, and N. Filipovic, "Software tools for generating cfd simulation models of blood ow from ct images, and for postprocessing," *Journal of the Serbian Society for Computational Mechanics*, vol. 2, no. 2, pp. 51–58, 2008.

[17] O. Ecabert, J. Peters, M. J. Walker et al., "Segmentation of the heart and great vessels in ct images using a model-based adaptation framework," *Medical Image Analysis*, vol. 15, no. 6, pp. 863–876, 2011.

[18] Z. Sun and T. Chaichana, "Fenestrated stent graft repair of abdominal aortic aneurysm: hemodynamic analysis of the effect of fenestrated stents on the renal arteries," *Korean Journal of Radiology*, vol. 11, no. 1, pp. 95–106, 2010.

[19] D. Richens, M. Field, S. Hashim, M. Neale, and C. Oakley, "A finite element model of blunt traumatic aortic rupture," *European Journal of Cardio-thoracic Surgery*, vol. 25, no. 6, pp. 1039–1047, 2004.

[20] O. Foundation, Openfoam, January 2012, http://www.openfoam.org/.

[21] "Engrid—open-source mesh generation," January 2012, http://engits.eu/en/engrid.

[22] C. Geuzaine and J. F. Remacle, "Gmsh: A 3-D finite element mesh generator with built-in pre- and post-processing facilities," *International Journal for Numerical Methods in Engineering*, vol. 79, no. 11, pp. 1309–1331, 2009.

[23] M. Botsch, S. Steinberg, S. Bischoff, and L. Kobbelt, "Openmesh-a generic and efficient polygon mesh data structure," in *Proceedings of the OpenSG Symposium*, 2002.

[24] Blender, Blender foundation, December 2011, http://www.blender.org/.

[25] H. Si, *TetGen, A Quality Tetrahedral Mesh Generator and Threedimensional Delaunay Triangulator*, Weierstrass Institute for Applied Analysis and Stochastic, Berlin, Germany, 2011.

[26] D. Gerrits, R. Gabriels, and P. Kooijmans, "A survey of mesh generation techniques," Tech. Rep., Department of Mathematics & Computer Science Technische, Universiteit Eindhoven, 2006.

[27] R. O. Bonow, D. L. Mann, D. P. Zipes, and P. Libby, Braunwald's Heart Disease: A Textbook of Cardiovascular Medicine, 2-Volume Set, Saunders, 2011.

[28] "Echocardiography in icu—left atrium dimensions," June 2012, https://www.stanford.edu/group/ccm_echocardio/cgi-bin/mediawiki/index.php/Left_atrium_dimensions.

[29] L. G. Rudski, W. W. Lai, J. Afilalo et al., "Guidelines for the Echocardiographic Assessment of the Right Heart in Adults: A Report from the American Society of Echocardiography. Endorsed by the European Association of Echocardiography, a registered branch of the European Society of Cardiology, and the Canadian Society of Echocardiography," *Journal of the American Society of Echocardiography*, vol. 23, no. 7, pp. 685–713, 2010.

[30] M. Lizier, J. Shepherd, L. Nonato, J. Comba, and C. Silva, "Comparing techniques for tetrahedral mesh generation," in *Proceedings of the Inaugural International Conference of the Engineering Mechanics Institute*, 2008.

[31] K. Ho-Le, "Finite element mesh generation methods: a review and classification," *Computer-Aided Design*, vol. 20, no. 1, pp. 27–38, 1988.

[32] D. Pedroso, Tetgen export, March 2007, http://cvs.savannah .gnu.org/viewvc/∗checkout∗/mechsys/mechsys/src/py_scripts/ blender/tetgen_export.py.

[33] J. Wang and Z. Yu, "Feature-sensitive tetrahedral mesh generation with guaranteed quality," *Computer-Aided Design*, vol. 44, no. 5, pp. 400–412, 2012.

[34] F. Labelle and J. R. Shewchuk, "Isosurface stuffing: fast tetrahedral meshes with good dihedral angles," *ACM Transactions on Graphics*, vol. 26, no. 3, Article ID 1276448, 2007.

[35] P. M. Knupp, "Algebraic mesh quality metrics," *SIAM Journal on Scientific Computing*, vol. 23, no. 1, pp. 193–218, 2002.

19

Corneal Sublayers Thickness Estimation Obtained by High-Resolution FD-OCT

Diego Alberto[1,2] **and Roberto Garello**[1]

[1] Department of Electronics and Telecommunications, Politecnico di Torino,
 Corso Duca Degli Abruzzi 24, 10129 Turin, Italy
[2] TIMA Laboratory (Grenoble INP, UJF, CNRS), 46 avenue Félix Viallet, 38031 Grenoble, France

Correspondence should be addressed to Diego Alberto; diego.alberto@to.infn.it

Academic Editor: Michael W. Vannier

This paper presents a novel processing technique which can be applied to corneal in vivo images obtained with optical coherence tomograms across the central meridian of the cornea. The method allows to estimate the thickness of the corneal sublayers (Epithelium, Bowman's layer, Stroma, Endothelium, and whole corneal thickness) at any location, including the center and the midperiphery, on both nasal and temporal sides. The analysis is carried out on both the pixel and subpixel scales to reduce the uncertainty in thickness estimations. This technique allows quick and noninvasive assessment of patients. As an example of application and validation, we present the results obtained from the analysis of 52 healthy subjects, each with 3 scans per eye, for a total of more than 300 images. Particular attention has been paid to the statistical interpretation of the obtained results to find a representative assessment of each sublayer's thickness.

1. Introduction

Optical coherence tomography (OCT) based on low coherence interferometry is a well-established imaging technique thanks to its prominent axial resolution. Since 2006, commercially available OCT systems perform visualization of tissue microstructure in the so-called Fourier Domain (FD-OCT). Differently to Time Domain OCT (TD-OCT), the whole depth structure is obtained synchronously providing higher resolution imaging with faster acquisition times. FD-OCT can be used to provide in vivo cross-sectional imaging of the eye in a noninvasive and noncontact way [1]. To date, this technique has been mostly applied to capture retinal structure and optic nerve, displaying and localizing discrete morphological changes in detail [2, 3].

In this paper we use an FD-OCT to study the anterior segment of the eye since this acquisition system can produce cross-sectional images of the cornea, which can be properly processed to analyze corneal sublayers: Epithelium, Bowman's layer, Stroma, Descemet's membrane, and Endothelium

[4–7]. The precise measurement of these sublayers thickness is very important in ophthalmics and optometrics, for therapeutic treatments, refractive surgery, and contact lens applications.

Many works have presented the thickness estimation of corneal sublayers techniques different from OCT. All these approaches have drawbacks and/or introduce some restrictions. Confocal microscopy [8] is an invasive technique that can cause lesions of corneal tissues, while electron microscopy [8, 9] deals only with histopathologic samples, and ultrasonic pachymetry [10] requires the instillation of a topical anaesthetic and well trained operators.

On the contrary, OCT has the advantage of allowing quick, noninvasive and completely safe assessment of patients [2, 3]. Unfortunately, traditional image processing techniques, such as Sobel or Canny algorithms [11], failed in boundary localization of OCT cross-sections because, in general, these images present low Signal-to-Noise Ratio (SNR) and low contrast between boundary and internal corneal regions [5–7].

In this work, a novel technique based on automated edge detection method is presented. This procedure, based on SNR enhancement and corneal sublayers segmentation, allows to accurately extract the sublayers thickness information from FD-OCT images.

2. Material and Methods

2.1. FD-OCT Corneal In vivo Images and Sublayer Thickness Estimation Problem. A FD-OCT corneal in vivo image appears as in Figure 1. Different reflectivity profile boundaries identify different corneal sublayers, as reported in histological examinations [5].

Since each image is available in grayscale format and is uploaded as a matrix of pixels [5, 6], the pixel intensity can be treated as the third coordinate. This reflectivity profile information can be considered as the amplitude of the signals to be constructed and analyzed, see Figure 1.

In more detail, the region of interest (ROI) highlighted in the Figure 1 is shown in Figure 2(a). As a reference, in Figure 2(b), a human corneal histological sample is presented and graphically compared with Figure 2(a). (The two pictures do not come from the same subject.)

Human corneas, like those of other primates, are composed of five sublayers: *Epithelium* is a layer of cells that cover the surface of the cornea; *Bowman's layer* protects the Stroma from injury; *Stroma* is the thickest layer (90% of the corneal thickness), transparent and made of collagen fibrils; *Descemet's membrane* is the thinnest layer, only one cell thick (too thin to be detected [5] and also in our study it will not be estimated); *Endothelium* is a low cuboidal monolayer of mitochondria-rich cells.

The knowledge of their thicknesses is of significant importance for ophthalmics and optometrics examinations and treatments.

To validate the proposed analysis protocol, a sample of 52 healthy patients has been considered: 25 females and 27 males, mean ± standard deviation age: 34 ± 11 years, range: 25 to 74 years. All the subjects did not present any ocular disease nor any history of ocular surgery and have been analyzed with the FD-OCT system described in Section 2.2. This group of patients can be defined as *normal* patients. In this paper, the analyses of the only right eyes are reported since no significant difference occurred in the comparison between right and left eyes, nor between male and female subgroups (for the statistical validation see Section 4).

The considered problem consists of estimating the thickness of each sublayer starting from images like that depicted in Figure 1. Unfortunately, these images are characterized by low SNR values which prevents the application of classical techniques.

Even if the algorithm is presented in general and can be applied to any starting FD-OCT image, we provide here all the details of the experimental set-up to allow reproducibility of the results and better understand the analysis scenario.

2.2. Experimental Setup and Acquisition Procedure. A FD-OCT RTVue-100 Optovue device [12] was used. The reflectivity profile (A-scan) information was acquired by a CCD

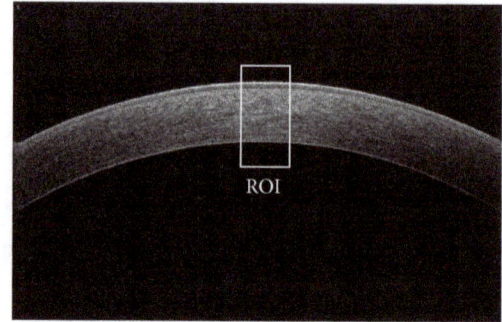

FIGURE 1: OCT grayscale corneal tomogram and the region of interest (ROI) on the corneal apex. (in this case: horizontal dimension: 6 mm, 1016 pixels; vertical dimension: 4 mm, 640 pixels.)

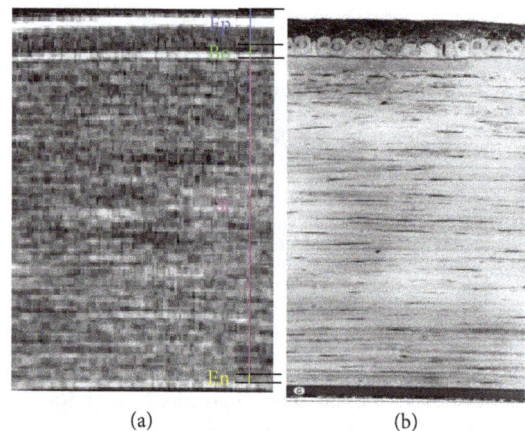

(a)   (b)

FIGURE 2: (a) Details of the ROI of Figure 1 with sublayers subdivision: Epithelium (Ep), Bowman (Bo), Stroma (St), and Endothelium (En). The Descemet's membrane is not reported. (b) Histological sample of a human cornea (the two pictures do not belong to the same patient).

camera simultaneously. Due to the fast CCD camera line transfer rate and fast Fourier transform algorithm, this FD-OCT could perform 26000 A-scan/second. Each tomogram was the average of 16 images. The Super Luminescent Diode (SLD) this device provided worked at a wavelength of 840 ± 10 nm. It was connected to a telecentric light delivery system and mounted on a standard slit-lamp. This wavelength value was adopted since it allowed higher SNR than older OCT devices [13]. Furthermore, it was already chosen to analyze retinal imaging [14] and to obtain higher axial resolutions with the same bandwidth. Corneal imaging was performed with auxiliary lens (CAM-l), helpful for corneal structures magnification.

The working distance between patients and the OCT device was 22 mm. Subjects were asked to put their chin on the slit-lamp and to watch the target in the central point of the OCT probe. The exposure power at pupil was 750 μW. This low value guaranteed no damage to analyzed eyes being below the maximum permissible exposure dictated by the American National Standards Institute (ANSI) at this wavelength [15]. The axial calibration of the OCT was performed using a set of polymethylmethacrylate (PMMA) lenses of known thickness ($546 \pm 1\,\mu m$) and constant index of refraction (1.4838 at 840 nm) [16, 17]. The PMMA lenses were measured using a Mitutoyo micrometer [18, 19]. The FD-OCT declared resolutions were: $5.0\,\mu m$ in depth (axial direction), and $15\,\mu m$ for the transverse direction [12]. The investigated corneal area was 6 mm × 4 mm, corresponding to a matrix of 1016 × 640 pixels. Simply performing the division between these correlated values, the axial resolution is equal to $6.25\,\mu m$ for and the transverse one to $5.91\,\mu m$. To find a more reliable pixel-μm conversion factor, a calibration procedure was applied. By examining 10 OCT images of a set of PMMA contact lenses with known thickness and index of refraction, the conversion factor pixel-μm has been found: 1 pixel = $4.13\,\mu m$, 1 subpixel = $0.52\,\mu m$ [16–18] for axial resolution (for the pixel-subpixel chosen ratio see Section 4). These were the mean values of the conversion factors obtained from the analysis carried on the complete set of lenses. As a simplification, it was decided to consider neither the deterministic nor the statistical errors performed both in PMMA lens thickness estimation and in their OCT acquisitions to avoid their propagations. Unfortunately, with OCT acquisitions of PMMA lenses it was not possible to estimate the transverse resolution, therefore, $5.91\,\mu m$/pixel was assumed. The difference between the chosen axial and transverse resolutions is close to the one presented in [6].

The OCT was connected to a computer to visualize and store corneal images. In a second analysis, the acquired tomograms were processed to extract the features of interest. The average time duration per patient of the medical analysis was 10 minutes, whereas the digital processing required only few seconds.

3. The Algorithm for Estimating the Sublayer Thickness: Estimation Problem

In an OCT corneal tomogram the cornea and its internal sublayers are represented by different grayscale regions since each corneal tissue presents a different reflectivity, see Figures 2(a) and 2(b). In particular, the boundary between two consecutive sublayers presents a constant reflectivity profile [5, 6]. Enhancing the SNR of each analyzed region, our algorithm quickly detects these boundaries (edges) and estimates the sublayer thicknesses evaluating the distance between two consecutive couple of edges.

As a first step, we need to identify on the tomogram the dimension and direction of the ROI to be analyzed, as in Figure 2(a). Due to the natural shape (curvature) of the cornea, particular attention must be paid to the chosen region. Taking for instance into account the central region of the cornea and working symmetrically on the apex of every meridian, it is mandatory not to consider pixels from different sublayers on the same row, see Figure 3. This kind of problem could arise if we consider too wide regions. The procedure for determining the ROI maximum dimension, denoted as the 2lag_{MAX} value, is depicted in Figure 3. As a result, this region can be assumed straight, or affected by negligible corneal curvature, and every sublayer represented on the same pixel row.

In our case study, the ROI maximum dimension chosen according to this rule has been found, on average, equal to

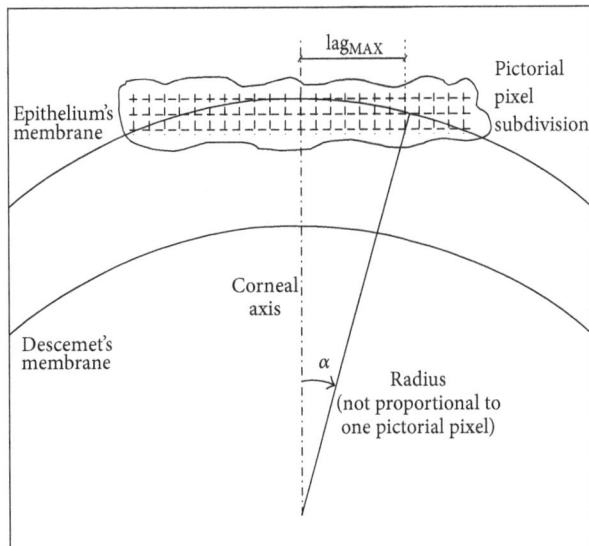

FIGURE 3: Pictorial representation of the procedure used to estimate the maximum number of columns on which the pixel intensity analysis is performed. In this sketch, the drawn Radius is not proportional to the pictorial pixel dimension.

2lag_{MAX} = 90 pixels ($\sim\!532\,\mu m$, for the transverse pixel-μm conversion see Section 2.2).

As a second step, the ROI area is divided into three slices one next to the other, see Figure 4. Each slice is composed of the same number of pixel columns (25–30 in our case study), depending on the 2lag_{MAX} value chosen in the previous step. These three slices, being adjacent, are considered not to be affected by significant differences of thickness. Note that this subdivision into three slices is essential also for the statistical validation (Section 4) of the presented approach.

With reference to the histological model (Figure 2(b)), corneal sublayers can be identified from the different reflectivity profile of the anatomical boundaries. Suppose that a slice is composed of one (central) pixel column. Different reflectivity is mapped by a proportional pixel grayscale intensity, valued between 0 and 255 [5, 6]. If the intensity depth profile is plotted as a function of pixel rows, the search of minima and maxima values leads to the localization of the beginning of corneal sublayers. In order to reduce noise (flicker, speckle, etc.), the pixel intensity reflectivity profile is linearly averaged on the number of columns composing the slice (25–30 in our case study). We will refer to this procedure as the *averaging technique*. This procedure is justified by the evidence that, inside each ROI slice, pixel rows of the same region show a Gaussian reflectivity profile distribution (Pearson's chi-square test [20], $P < 0.05$).

The same sublayer boundary shows nearly the same reflectivity index, and it is represented by a continuous line in an OCT tomogram (see Figures 2(a) and 2(b)). Conversely, regions inside two consecutive boundaries present nonconstant reflectivity values (due to the anatomy of the analyzed tissues [5]). In the current analysis, this behavior can be considered as additive noise that makes it harder to find peak values that delimit sublayer regions. The average of pixel

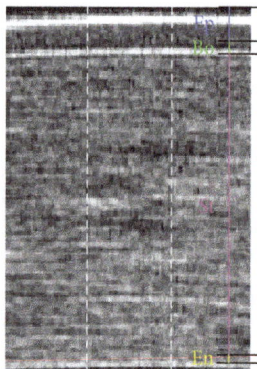

FIGURE 4: The four sublayers to be estimated with the ROI subdivision into three adjacent slides.

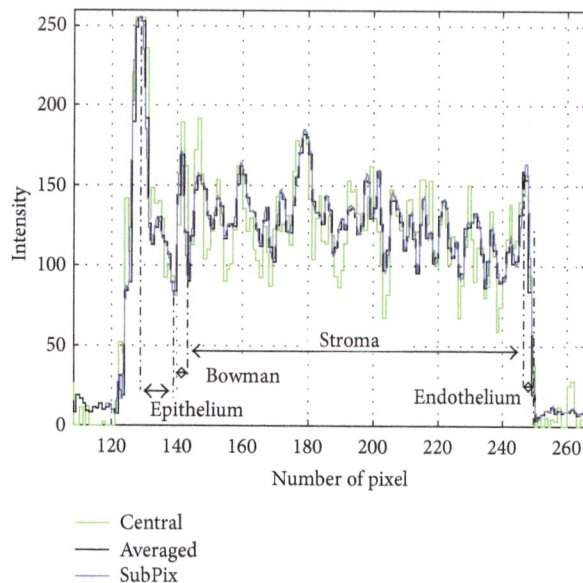

FIGURE 5: Pixel intensity profile on a 25 pixels wide slice, centred on the corneal apex. In green the intensity of the only axial column is represented, while in red and blue, the averaged intensities in pixel and subpixel elaborations, respectively.

intensity values performed on near columns can preserve the boundary pixel values and reduce the uncertainty introduced by pixels coming from inner regions. The robustness of this procedure can be estimated by comparing the SNR evaluated on a single column with the one calculated on averaged columns (see Section 4).

Figures 5 and 6 show the results of this procedure; for the pixel-subpixel chosen ratio see the following section. Epithelium, Bowman's layer, Stroma, and Endothelium sublayers can be identified. The global maximum corresponds to the anterior surface of Epithelium; the global minimum is the end of the Epithelium. The Bowman's layer starts immediately after the end of the Epithelium and it ends at the following (second) global minimum. The Stroma starts after the second minimum and ends at the last maximum on the right side of the pixel intensity profile. Endothelium starts after the last maximum and its end is assumed (approximation) where the signal goes under two RMS of pixel intensity values coming from the right region outside cornea (noise). Descemet's membrane is too thin to be detected being, if present, nearly or less than one pixel width [21].

A customized MATLAB [22] program has been developed to automatically process all the images and accurately segment the inner corneal sublayers. All analyses have been carried out using a MATLAB platform.

3.1. Subpixel Procedure. The approach described in the previous section has been carried out on three slices (see Figure 2(b)) of the same ROI to evaluate the uncertainties on the sublayer thickness estimations by means of weighted averages. It is worth noting that in using the automated procedure in pixel scale, the original image is not altered. As a further step, a subpixeling technique has been applied to reduce the uncertainty in thickness estimations when measurements were expressed in pixel scale. It was obtained with a bi-cubic interpolation [22, 23] on both image directions and was not a super-resolution technique. It simply helped in the statistical analysis to distinguish cases that presented the same thickness value estimated in pixel scale for two, or all three, slices of the same ROI. Interpolating does not increase axial/transverse resolution but can increase only digital resolution of the image. The chosen linear ratio between pixel and subpixel has

been set one to eight. For ease of elaboration it had to be a power of two [22], and the value eight was the first that highly reduced the aforementioned cases that presented the same estimated thickness. As a result, the subpixel intensity profile is smoothed if compared with the pixel averaged sample, as shown in Figure 5.

3.2. Application to Different Regions. Interpolating the air-Epithelium boundary and working orthogonally to this sublayer, the procedure described in Section 3 can be also utilized to study midperipheral corneal regions, both nasal and temporal sides, see Figure 7. For the same reason discussed in the previous section, in order not to consider pixels coming from different sublayer on the same analyzed line (orthogonal to the investigated axes, blue solid segment in Figure 7), the width of the analyzed marginal ROI must be properly chosen (about 85–90 pixels in our case study), in accordance with the estimated curvature of the considered tomogram. With this approach, a more detailed investigation of the corneal sublayers thickness behavior can be obtained.

In the literature, polynomial approximations of corneal sublayers' two dimensional profiles are widely assumed [6, 24]. In this work, however, a circumference has been preferred since this curve provides not only a good agreement with analyzed data (Pearson's chi-square goodness-of-fit test [20], $P < 0.05$), but also a reference (its center) to measure the midperipheral nasal and temporal angles at which the aforementioned method can be applied, see Figure 7.

In principle, every patient's tomogram could be analyzed on every marginal region of the corneal image. In practice, the SNR of the considered subregion limits the application of our procedure. For example, in Figure 7 the tomogram has been investigated at 23 degrees on both nasal and temporal sides.

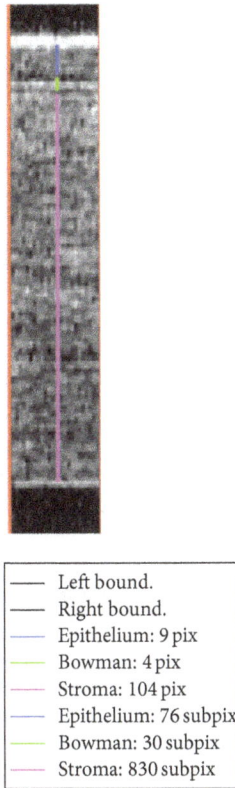

FIGURE 6: Detail of the central ROI slice. In the box, thickness estimates are reported both in pixel and subpixel scale.

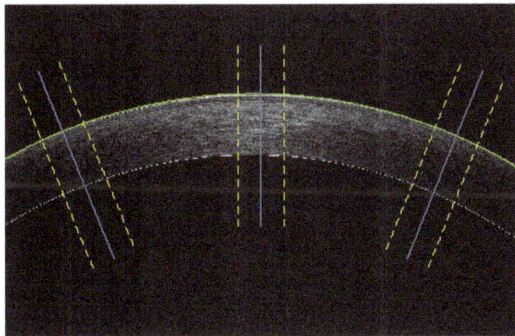

FIGURE 7: Corneal image of one of the analysed patients with the interpolated air-Epithelium boundary (green curve). Central and midperipheral (nasal and temporal) axes are represented (blue solid lines) together with the delimitations of the three ROIs (yellow dashed lines). The investigated midperipheral angle is 23 degrees in both sides.

This chosen angle represents the highest value at which the averaging technique returns signals with SNR high enough to be efficiently analyzed. The obtained results have been reported and compared in the following section.

4. Study Results

To validate our technique, the procedure described in the previous section has been applied to the sample of 52 healthy patients reported in Section 2.1.

TABLE 1: Mid-peripheral nasal, central, and mid-peripheral temporal corneal sublayers thickness estimation obtained averaging the respective evaluations performed on 156 images (right eye). The Total corneal thickness (TCT) value is calculated as the sum of all sublayers.

Sublayer	Midperiph. nasal (μm)	Central (μm)	Midperiph. temp. (μm)
Epithelium	45.3 ± 0.5	42.8 ± 0.5	45.1 ± 0.5
Bowman	17.2 ± 0.5	17.0 ± 0.5	16.9 ± 0.5
Stroma	477.0 ± 0.5	453.0 ± 0.5	473.0 ± 0.5
Endothelium	10.1 ± 0.5	9.8 ± 0.5	9.9 ± 0.5
TCT	550 ± 1	523 ± 1	545 ± 1

A statistical analysis of the proposed procedure is mandatory to validate our methodology and to build a reference of sublayer thickness values for normal patients.

For every subject, three images of each eye have been recorded on a corneal area of 6 mm × 4 mm (1016 × 640 pixels), for a total number of 312 images, see one of them in Figure 1.

Even though FD-OCT devices present very good repeatability and accuracy [25], to give an additional validation to the reported measurements, the estimated sublayers' thickness (in pixel scale) were compared, fixed the region (nasal, central or temporal), on the first and on the third acquisition of the same set of patients for the right eye. No significant differences have been identified (paired samples t-test [20], $P < 0.05$).

The complete set of images has been processed with the customized algorithm introduced in Section 3. On the apex and on the midperipheral nasal and temporal sides of the horizontal meridian, the resulting thicknesses of all sublayers and of the total cornea are reported in Table 1. It is worth recalling that the small uncertainties are due to the weighted average procedure.

The sublayer estimations of central corneal thicknesses are all in accordance with the results presented in [5] except for the Epithelium, where the difference of nearly 10 μm is clearly significant if compared with the standard deviations (unpaired samples t-test [20], $P < 0.05$). A possible explanation of this discrepancy can be found in the way the Epithelium starting point was defined in Section 3. It was assumed to be the first pixel after the global reflectivity maximum. This highest value is due to the presence of tears and can be a plateau two or three pixels wide (corresponding to 10–12 μm).

Midperipheral corneal thicknesses cannot be strictly compared with the results proposed in [5] since they refer to regions that differ by 3 degrees (angle separation). However, they remain statistically compatible (unpaired samples t-test [20], $P < 0.05$) and the difference between the Bowman's layer estimates is due to the same reason explained for the central thickness analysis. Total corneal increasing behavior is evident, as reported also in [6]. Furthermore, the contribution to the TCT increment is due to Epithelium and Stroma, while Bowman's layer remains nearly constant, in accordance with [5].

As introduced in Section 2.1, this paper reports the results of the only right eye (Table 1), since no significant difference occurred in the comparison between right and left eyes, nor between male and female subgroups (resp. paired and unpaired samples t-test [20], $P < 0.05$). These statistical results are in accordance with the previously reported study [5].

A useful feature in the processing of an OCT corneal image is represented by the SNR improvement obtained using the previously discussed averaging technique. The noise component was assumed to be studied in the only Stromal region since it is the thickest among all corneal sublayers with an average estimated thickness of the order of 100 pixels on the corneal apex.

By carrying out this analysis on the central ROI (Figure 7) in pixel scale and evaluating the SNR on the subset of images coming from the third acquisition of the right eye for all 52 patients, in every image the SNR distributions of the central pixel column and of the averaged columns composing the central slice were compared. In both cases the values were Gaussian distributed (Pearson's chi-square test [20], $P < 0.05$). The central column presented a SNR mean value equal to 6.7 dB and a RMS of 0.8 dB, while the averaged signal showed a mean value of 13.9 dB and a RMS of 1.7 dB. Taking into account the mean values of these two distributions, the improvement obtained with the averaging technique was 7.2 dB. This rise allowed an accurate and robust sublayer boundaries detection and consequent thickness estimations.

By applying the same SNR estimate procedure to midperipheral corneal regions (Figure 7) of the same subset of images, SNR values remained Gaussian distributed (Pearson's chi-square test [20], $P < 0.05$). However, central midperipheral axes presented a SNR mean value reduced to 3.7 dB and a RMS of 1.2 dB, while the signals averaged on peripheral ROIs showed a mean value of 9.4 dB and a RMS of 2.0 dB. Considering also in this case the only mean values, the improvement obtained with the averaging technique was 5.7 dB. This rise confirmed the validity of the averaging procedure but, the absolute SNR value of processed signals was the lowest able to allow an accurate and robust sublayer boundaries detection. This is the reason why more peripheral corneal regions cannot be processed with this approach on the considered tomograms. Note that these SNR evaluations on central and peripheral ROIs come from images in pixel resolution since no significant difference has been found carrying out this analysis in subpixel scale (paired samples t-test [20], $P < 0.05$).

5. Discussion

The number of patients considered in this work was more than double the ones presented in [5, 6, 21, 24]. All subjects gave the informed consent to the collection and use of recorded data and were treated according to the tenets of the Declaration of Helsinki.

Whereas the algorithm itself and the estimated results can be considered validated, the case study and its medical reliability clearly present some minor limitations. Firstly, the database was composed of 52 patients only and may be the reason why no significant age or genders differences have been identified (statistical problem). Secondly, the device returned few cases of *too dark* OCT corneal images that presented a SNR low enough to make any processing impossible, especially in midperipheral sides. In such cases new images from the same patients were acquired. Thirdly, Descemet's membrane was not distinguishable, as in the work reported in [5]. This sublayer, if present, could vary the Stroma thickness estimations of 10–15 μm for people without any ocular disease [21]. Fourthly, a precise estimate of the OCT transverse resolution was not obtained, however, it can be determined using, for example, special USAF targets [26]. To quantify the influence of this uncertainty at the considered midperipheral angle and with the procedure described in Section 3.2, a variation of ± 0.5 μm on the transverse resolution leads to a variation of $\pm 2.2\%$ in the midperipheral results reported in Table 1. Notwithstanding that, they still remain in accordance with [5].

Finally, because of this technology, the ROI regions were assumed straight or affected by negligible curvature.

6. Conclusions

A robust technique for estimating corneal sublayer thickness starting from low-SNR FD-OCT images has been presented and validated by statistical analysis. The introduced procedure allowed a significant SNR enhancement and an analysis on a wide region of the considered OCT tomograms.

The method has been utilized for the study of sublayer thickness estimations on a sample of 52 healthy patients without any optical disease on both central and peripheral regions of the horizontal meridian of the cornea by using more than 300 FD-OCT corneal images.

From this analysis, the average values for all sublayers in three different corneal regions have been provided and, fixed the corneal area, no significant difference between right and left eyes or between male and female subgroups occurred. In addition, an averaging technique has been introduced to construct reference signals to be used for thickness estimations. The improvement in SNR has been introduced and discussed. The method is very useful to provide a fast, simple but robust and noninvasive estimation of the sublayer thickness. Its advantages and limitations have been discussed in the paper.

As future work, a USAF target can be imaged to estimate OCT transverse resolution. Furthermore, the processing of corneal marginal regions can be applied to study medical cases in order to quantify the effective change in corneal sublayers produced by ophthalmological treatments. Finally, further development is in progress for studying a special class of customized contact lens thickness estimations.

Acknowledgments

The authors would like to thank Dr. Michela Greco for the useful discussions during the analysis of these images and Dr. Mauro Frisani for the acquisition of the OCT corneal tomograms and their medical interpretation.

References

[1] D. Huang, E. A. Swanson, C. P. Lin et al., "Optical coherence tomography," *Science*, vol. 254, no. 5035, pp. 1178–1181, 1991.

[2] W. Drexler and J. G. Fujimoto, "State-of-the-art retinal optical coherence tomography," *Progress in Retinal and Eye Research*, vol. 27, no. 1, pp. 45–88, 2008.

[3] N. A. Nassif, B. Cense, B. H. Park et al., "*In vivo* high-resolution video-rate spectral-domain optical coherence tomography of the human retina and optic nerve," *Optics Express*, vol. 12, no. 3, pp. 367–376, 2004.

[4] R. N. Khurana, Y. Li, M. Tang, M. M. Lai, and D. Huang, "High-speed optical coherence tomography of corneal opacities," *Ophthalmology*, vol. 114, no. 7, pp. 1278–1285, 2007.

[5] A. Tao, J. Wang, Q. Chen et al., "Topographic thickness of Bowman's layer determined by ultra-high resolution spectral domain-optical coherence tomography," *Investigative Ophthalmology & Visual Science*, vol. 52, no. 6, pp. 3901–3907, 2011.

[6] F. La Rocca, S. J. Chiu, R. P. McNabb, A. N. Kuo, J. A. Izatt, and S. Farsiu, "Robust automatic segmentation of corneal layer boundaries in SDOCT images using graph theory and dynamic programming," *Biomedical Optics Express*, vol. 2, no. 6, pp. 1524–1538, 2011.

[7] J. A. Eichel, A. K. Mishra, D. A. Clausi, P. W. Fieguth, and K. K. Bizheva, "A novel algorithm for extraction of the layers of the cornea," in *Proceedings of Canadian Conference on Computer and Robot Vision (CRV '09)*, pp. 313–320, May 2009.

[8] H. F. Li, W. M. Petroll, T. Møller-Pedersen, J. K. Maurer, H. D. Cavanagh, and J. V. Jester, "Epithelial and corneal thickness measurements by *in vivo* confocal microscopy through focusing (CMTF)," *Current Eye Research*, vol. 16, no. 3, pp. 214–221, 1997.

[9] R. W. Beuerman and L. Pedroza, "Ultrastructure of the human cornea," *Microscopy Research and Technique*, vol. 33, pp. 320–335, 1996.

[10] S. Miglior, E. Albe, M. Guareschi, G. Mandelli, S. Gomarasca, and N. Orzalesi, "Intraobserver and interobserver reproducibility in the evaluation of ultrasonic pachymetry measurements of central corneal thickness," *British Journal of Ophthalmology*, vol. 88, no. 2, pp. 174–177, 2004.

[11] R. C. Gonzalez and R. E. Woods, *Digital Image Processing*, Prentice-Hall, Upper Saddle River, NJ, USA, 2nd edition, 2002.

[12] Optovue, http://www.optovue.com/.

[13] V. Penner and G. Rocha, "Use of the Visante for anterior segment ocular coherence tomography," *Techniques in Ophthalmology*, vol. 5, no. 2, pp. 67–77, 2007.

[14] B. Cense, N. A. Nassif, T. C. Chen et al., "Ultrahigh-resolution high-speed retinal imaging using spectral-domain optical coherence tomography," *Optics Express*, vol. 12, no. 11, pp. 2435–2447, 2004.

[15] "American National Standard for the Safe Use of Lasers," Tech. Rep. ANSI Z136 1-2007, American National Standard Institute, New York, NY, USA, 2007.

[16] A. M. Moezzi, S. Sin, and T. L. Simpson, "Novel pachometry calibration," *Optometry and Vision Science*, vol. 83, no. 6, pp. E366–E371, 2006.

[17] PMMA, http://refractiveindex.info/?group=PLASTICS&material=PMMA.

[18] Mitutoyo, http://www.mitutoyo.com/home.aspx.

[19] Vogel s.r.l., Brescia, Italia,http://www.vogel.it/.

[20] J. A. Rice, *Mathematical Statistics and Data Analysis*, Duxbury Press, Pacific Grove, Calif, USA, 2nd edition, 1994.

[21] M. A. Shousha, V. L. Perez, J. Wang et al., "Use of ultra-high-resolution optical coherence tomography to detect *in vivo* characteristics of Descemet's membrane in Fuchs' dystrophy," *Ophthalmology*, vol. 117, no. 6, pp. 1220–1227, 2010.

[22] MATLAB, "The language of technical computing," http://www.mathworks.com/.

[23] R. G. Keys, "Cubic convolution interpolation for digital image processing," *IEEE Transactions on Acoustics, Speech, and Signal Processing*, vol. 29, no. 6, pp. 1153–1160, 1981.

[24] Y. Li, M. V. Netto, R. Shekhar, R. R. Krueger, and D. Huang, "A longitudinal study of LASIK flap and stromal thickness with high-speed optical coherence tomography," *Ophthalmology*, vol. 114, no. 6, pp. 1124–1132, 2007.

[25] S. Sin and T. L. Simpson, "The repeatability of corneal and corneal epithelial thickness measurements using optical coherence tomography," *Optometry and Vision Science*, vol. 83, no. 6, pp. 360–365, 2006.

[26] A. Latrive and A. C. Boccara, "*In vivo* and *in situ* cellular imaging full-field optical coherence tomography with a rigid endoscopic probe," *Biomedical Optics Express*, vol. 2, no. 10, pp. 2897–2904, 2011.

20

Localized FCM Clustering with Spatial Information for Medical Image Segmentation and Bias Field Estimation

Wenchao Cui,[1,2] **Yi Wang,**[1] **Yangyu Fan,**[1] **Yan Feng,**[1] **and Tao Lei**[1]

[1] *School of Electronics and Information, Northwestern Polytechnical University, Xi'an 710072, China*
[2] *College of Science, China Three Gorges University, Yichang 443002, China*

Correspondence should be addressed to Wenchao Cui; wenchao-cui@163.com and Yi Wang; wangyi79@nwpu.edu.cn

Academic Editor: Guowei Wei

This paper presents a novel fuzzy energy minimization method for simultaneous segmentation and bias field estimation of medical images. We first define an objective function based on a localized fuzzy c-means (FCM) clustering for the image intensities in a neighborhood around each point. Then, this objective function is integrated with respect to the neighborhood center over the entire image domain to formulate a global fuzzy energy, which depends on membership functions, a bias field that accounts for the intensity inhomogeneity, and the constants that approximate the true intensities of the corresponding tissues. Therefore, segmentation and bias field estimation are simultaneously achieved by minimizing the global fuzzy energy. Besides, to reduce the impact of noise, the proposed algorithm incorporates spatial information into the membership function using the spatial function which is the summation of the membership functions in the neighborhood of each pixel under consideration. Experimental results on synthetic and real images are given to demonstrate the desirable performance of the proposed algorithm.

1. Introduction

Medical image segmentation plays an important role in a variety of biomedical-imaging applications, such as the quantification of tissue volumes, diagnosis, localization of pathology, study of anatomical structure, treatment planning, and computer-integrated surgery [1]. However, segmentation of medical images involves three main image-related problems [2]. First, images contain noise that can alter the intensity of a pixel such that its classification becomes uncertain. Second, images exhibit intensity inhomogeneity where the intensity level of a single tissue class varies gradually over the extent of the image. Third, images have finite pixel size and are subject to partial volume averaging where individual pixel volumes contain a mixture of tissue classes so that the intensity of a pixel in the image may not be consistent with any one class. To overcome these problems, many segmentation techniques have been proposed in the past decades, such as the expectation maximization (EM) algorithm [3–5], level set method [6–9], clustering [10–17], and so on.

Clustering for image segmentation usually classifies image pixels into c-clusters such that members of the same cluster are more similar to one another than to members of other clusters, where the number, c, of clusters is usually predefined or set by some validity criterion or a priori knowledge [18]. In the clustering methods, fuzzy c-means (FCM) based algorithms have been widely used in medical image segmentation. Such a success chiefly attributes to the introduction of fuzziness for the belongingness of each image pixel. This enables the clustering methods to retain more information from the original image than the crisp or hard segmentation methods [10].

Pham and Prince proposed an adaptive FCM algorithm [10] and its extension to 3D data [11], which incorporated a spatial penalty term into the objective function to enable the estimated membership functions to be spatially smoothed. Ahmed et al. [12] modified the objective function of the standard FCM algorithm to compensate for intensity inhomogeneity and to allow the labeling of a pixel to be influenced by the labels in its immediate neighborhood. Liew and Yan [13] used a B-spline surface to model the bias field and incorporated the spatial continuity constraints into fuzzy clustering algorithm. Zhang and Chen [14] replaced the original Euclidean distance with a kernel-induced distance and supplemented the objective function with a spatial penalty term, which modeled the spatial continuity compensation. Incorporating spatial information into the membership function, Chuang et al. [15] proposed a modified FCM algorithm which was less sensitive to noise and yielded more homogeneous segmented regions. L. Szilágri et al. [16] proposed an efficient FCM clustering model for compensating intensity inhomogeneity and segmentation of magnetic resonance (MR) images, which drastically reduced the processing time without causing relevant change in terms of accuracy. Recently, local intensity information has been taken into account to deal with intensity inhomogeneity in fuzzy segmentation method. For example, Li et al. [17] proposed a new fuzzy energy minimization method based on coherent local intensity clustering (CLIC) for simultaneous tissue classification and bias field estimation of MR images. CLIC algorithm draws upon intensity information in local regions; therefore, it can be used to segment images with intensity inhomogeneity. However, spatial information is not taken into account in the CLIC algorithm; as a result, the CLIC algorithm is sensitive to noise.

Our proposed algorithm in this paper is motivated by the localized K-means clustering model proposed by Chen et al. in [6]. By introducing the fuzzy belongingness of each pixel into Chen's model, we develop a localized FCM algorithm for image segmentation. We define a fuzzy energy that depends on membership functions, a bias field that accounts for the intensity inhomogeneity, and the constants that approximate the true intensities of the corresponding tissues. Hence, image segmentation and bias field estimation are simultaneously achieved as the result of minimizing this energy. Besides, we incorporate spatial information into the membership function to suppress noise. As an important application, our proposed algorithm can effectively segment medical images with intensity inhomogeneity and noise.

The remainder of this paper is organized as follows. Section 2 reviews a relevant method. In Section 3, we represent the definition and minimization of the proposed fuzzy energy in detail. We describe how to utilize neighborhood spatial information in Section 4. The algorithm implementation and experimental results are given in Section 5. The discussion on the setting of important parameters is given in Section 6. We end this paper by the conclusion in Section 7.

2. Background

Chen et al. [6] applied a localized K-means clustering to form an objective function modeling the problem of segmentation and bias field estimation for brain MR images. The image model of intensity inhomogeneity they used is defined as

$$\log I = \log J + \log b, \qquad (1)$$

where I is the measured image intensity, J is the true image to be restored, and b is an unknown bias field. Let $\tilde{I}$, $\tilde{J}$, and $\tilde{b}$ represent $\log I$, $\log J$, and $\log b$, respectively, then (1) can be rewritten as

$$\tilde{I} = \tilde{J} + \tilde{b}. \qquad (2)$$

A generally accepted assumption on the bias field $\tilde{b}$ is that it is smooth or slowly varying [19]. Ideally, the intensity $\tilde{J}$ belonging to the ith tissue should take a specific value c_i, which represents the measured physical property [6, 8, 17].

Chen's method is based on an observation that pixel intensities in a relatively small region are separable. Let $O_y = \{x : |x - y| \leq r\}$ denote a circular neighborhood with a relatively small radius r centered on each point y in the image domain Ω. The partition $\{\Omega_i\}_{i=1}^N$ (N is the total number of segmented regions) of the entire domain Ω induces a partition of the neighborhood O_y; that is, $\{O_y \cap \Omega_i\}_{i=1}^N$ forms a partition of O_y. For example, Figure 1 presents an image consisting of three disjoint regions: Ω_1, Ω_2, and Ω_3, which divide the neighborhood O_y into three subregions: $O_y \cap \Omega_1$, $O_y \cap \Omega_2$, and $O_y \cap \Omega_3$. Chen et al. defined an objective function to classify the data $\tilde{I}(x)$ in the neighborhood O_y into N clusters using a K-means clustering method:

$$\xi_y = \sum_{i=1}^N \int_{O_y \cap \Omega_i} \omega(x - y) |\tilde{I}(x) - \tilde{b}(y) - c_i|^2 dx, \qquad (3)$$

where $\tilde{b}(y)$ is the value of bias field $\tilde{b}$ at the center of O_y, which is approximately equal to the value $\tilde{b}(x)$ for all $x \in O_y$ on account of the smoothness of the bias field [6]; that is

$$\tilde{b}(x) \approx \tilde{b}(y), \quad x \in O_y. \qquad (4)$$

Thus, $(\tilde{b}(y) + c_i)$ $(i = 1, \ldots, N)$ are considered as the approximations of the cluster centers within the neighborhood O_y, and $\omega(x - y)$ is a nonnegative weighting function such that $\omega(x - y) = 0$ for $|x - y| > r$ and $\int_{O_y} \omega(x - y)dx = 1$. Note that for each point y, $\omega(x - y)$ has the nonzero value with respect to x only in $x \in O_y$. Therefore, (3) can be rewritten as

$$\xi_y = \sum_{i=1}^N \int_{\Omega_i} \omega(x - y) |\tilde{I}(x) - \tilde{b}(y) - c_i|^2 dx. \qquad (5)$$

The ultimate goal is to find an optimal set of partitions for the entire image domain Ω, the bias field $\tilde{b}$, and the constants c_i. The minimization of a single criterion ξ_y for a point y does not accomplish this goal. The method minimizes ε_y for all $y \in \Omega$. This can be achieved by minimizing the integral of ξ_y over Ω. Therefore, the energy is written as

$$\xi = \int_\Omega \left(\sum_{i=1}^N \int_{\Omega_i} \omega(x - y) |\tilde{I}(x) - \tilde{b}(y) - c_i|^2 dx \right) dy. \qquad (6)$$

The above energy ξ is expressed in terms of the regions $\Omega_1, \ldots, \Omega_N$. It is difficult to derive a solution to the energy minimization problem from this expression of ξ. Alternatively, we can use one or multiple level set functions to represent the disjoint regions $\Omega_1, \ldots, \Omega_N$ as in [20]. Thus, this energy ξ can be converted into an equivalent level set formulation, which can be solved by using well-established variational methods [21].

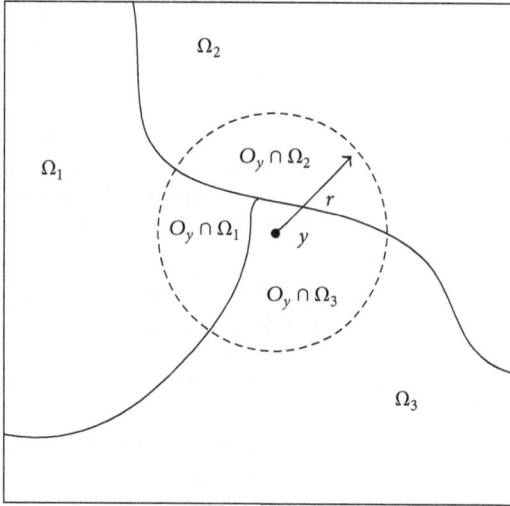

FIGURE 1: Graphical representation of $O_y \cap \Omega_i$. The dashed circle denotes the circular neighborhood O_y centered on y. The image domain Ω is divided into three disjoint regions Ω_1, Ω_2, and Ω_3, which partition the neighborhood O_y into three subregions $O_y \cap \Omega_1$, $O_y \cap \Omega_2$, and $O_y \cap \Omega_3$.

3. Localized FCM Clustering

Chen's method can be considered as a hard segmentation method in which each pixel is assigned to an exclusive cluster. However, it is more suitable for medical images that each pixel is given a membership degree of belonging to each cluster, due to the impact of intensity inhomogeneity and noise. In this paper, we introduce the fuzzy belongingness of each pixel into Chen's model and, thus, propose a localized FCM clustering algorithm to implement the task of segmentation and bias field estimation.

3.1. Energy Formulation. Similar to Chen's method, we first consider a task of classifying the data $\tilde{I}(x)$ in the neighborhood O_y into N clusters. If the K-means clustering in Chen's method is replaced by the FCM clustering, then the objective function in (3) can be converted to the following expression:

$$\varepsilon_y = \sum_{i=1}^{N} \int_{O_y} u_i^m(x)\,\omega(x-y)\left|\tilde{I}(x) - \tilde{b}(y) - c_i\right|^2 dx, \quad (7)$$

where $m > 1$ is the fuzzy coefficient, $u_i(x)$ $(0 \le u_i(x) \le 1)$ is the membership function of pixel x belonging to the region Ω_i, and $\omega(x-y)$ is the same nonnegative weight function as in (3).

Although the choice of the weighting function is flexible, it is preferable to use a weighting function $\omega(x-y)$ such that larger weights are assigned to the data $\tilde{I}(x)$ for x closer to the center y of the neighborhood O_y. In this paper, the weighting function ω is chosen as a truncated Gaussian kernel

$$\omega(d) = \begin{cases} \dfrac{1}{a} e^{-|d|^2/2\sigma^2} & |d| \le r, \\ 0 & \text{else,} \end{cases} \quad (8)$$

where σ is the standard deviation of the Gaussian kernel and a is a constant to normalize the Gaussian kernel. The above objective function ε_y can be rewritten as follows:

$$\varepsilon_y = \sum_{i=1}^{N} \int_{\Omega} u_i^m(x)\,\omega(x-y)\left|\tilde{I}(x) - \tilde{b}(y) - c_i\right|^2 dx \quad (9)$$

as $\omega(x-y) = 0$ for $x \notin O_y$.

The desired clustering on the entire image domain Ω should have a good local performance in terms of the above objective function ε_y for every neighborhood O_y. Therefore, we need to minimize ε_y for all $y \in \Omega$ like Chen's method [6]. This can be achieved by minimizing the integral of ε_y over Ω. As a result, we define the following energy for our proposed localized FCM clustering:

$$\varepsilon = \int_{\Omega} \left(\sum_{i=1}^{N} \int_{\Omega} u_i^m(x)\,\omega(x-y)\left|\tilde{I}(x) - \tilde{b}(y) - c_i\right|^2 dx \right) dy. \quad (10)$$

3.2. Energy Minimization. The above energy ε can be minimized in a fashion similar to the standard FCM algorithm. Taking the first derivatives of ε with respect to $u_i(x)$, $\tilde{b}(y)$, and c_i and setting them to zero results in three necessary but not sufficient conditions for ε to be at a local extremum. In this subsection, we will derive these three conditions.

3.2.1. Membership Functions Evaluation. The energy ε in (10) is subject to the constraint $\sum_{i=1}^{N} u_i(x) = 1$. Thus, this constrained optimization will be solved using one Lagrange multiplier

$$E = \int_{\Omega} \left(\sum_{i=1}^{N} \int_{\Omega} u_i^m(x)\,\omega(x-y)\left|\tilde{I}(x) - \tilde{b}(y) - c_i\right|^2 dx \right) dy + \lambda \left(1 - \sum_{i=1}^{N} u_i(x) \right). \quad (11)$$

Taking the derivative of E with respect to $u_i(x)$ and setting the result to zero, we have, for $m > 1$

$$\left[\frac{\partial E}{\partial u_i(x)} = \int_{\Omega} m u_i^{m-1}(x)\,\omega(x-y) \times \left|\tilde{I}(x) - \tilde{b}(y) - c_i\right|^2 dy - \lambda \right]_{u_i(x)=u_i^*(x)} = 0. \quad (12)$$

Solving for $u_i^*(x)$, we have

$$u_i^*(x) = \left(\frac{\lambda}{m \int_{\Omega} \omega(x-y)\left|\tilde{I}(x) - \tilde{b}(y) - c_i\right|^2 dy} \right)^{1/(m-1)}. \quad (13)$$

Since $\sum_{k=1}^{N} u_k(x) = 1$ for all x, we have

$$\sum_{k=1}^{N} \left(\frac{\lambda}{m \int_{\Omega} \omega(x-y) \left| \tilde{I}(x) - \tilde{b}(y) - c_k \right|^2 dy} \right)^{1/(m-1)} = 1$$

(14)

or

$$\lambda = \frac{m}{\left(\sum_{k=1}^{N} \left(1/\int_{\Omega} \omega(x-y) \left| \tilde{I}(x) - \tilde{b}(y) - c_k \right|^2 dy \right)^{1/(m-1)} \right)^{m-1}}.$$

(15)

Substituting (15) into (13), the zero-gradient condition for the membership functions can be rewritten as

$$u_i^*(x) = \frac{1}{\sum_{k=1}^{N} \left(\left(\int_{\Omega} \omega(x-y) \left| \tilde{I}(x) - \tilde{b}(y) - c_i \right|^2 dy \right) / \left(\int_{\Omega} \omega(x-y) \left| \tilde{I}(x) - \tilde{b}(y) - c_k \right|^2 dy \right) \right)^{1/(m-1)}}.$$

(16)

3.2.2. Bias Field Estimation. In a similar way, taking the derivative of E with respect to $\tilde{b}(y)$ and setting the result to zero, we have

$$\left[\sum_{i=1}^{N} \int_{\Omega} u_i^m(x) \omega(x-y) \left(\tilde{I}(x) - \tilde{b}(y) - c_i \right) dx \right]_{\tilde{b}(y) = \tilde{b}^*(y)} = 0.$$

(17)

Solving for $\tilde{b}^*(y)$, we have

$$\tilde{b}^*(y) = \frac{\sum_{i=1}^{N} \int_{\Omega} u_i^m(x) \omega(x-y) \left(\tilde{I}(x) - c_i \right) dx}{\sum_{i=1}^{N} \int_{\Omega} u_i^m(x) \omega(x-y) dx}.$$

(18)

3.2.3. Constants c_i Updating. Likewise, taking the derivative of E with respect to c_i and setting the result to zero, we have

$$\left[\iint_{\Omega} u_i^m(x) \omega(x-y) \left(\tilde{I}(x) - \tilde{b}(y) - c_i \right) dx\, dy \right]_{c_i = c_i^*} = 0.$$

(19)

Solving for c_i^*, we have

$$c_i^* = \frac{\iint_{\Omega} u_i^m(x) \omega(x-y) \left(\tilde{I}(x) - \tilde{b}(y) \right) dx\, dy}{\iint_{\Omega} u_i^m(x) \omega(x-y) dx\, dy}.$$

(20)

4. Exploiting Spatial Information

One of the important characteristics of an image is that neighborhood pixels are highly correlated. In other words, these neighborhood pixels possess similar intensity, and the probability that they belong to the same cluster is great. This spatial relationship is important in clustering, but it is not utilized in a conventional FCM algorithm. To exploit the spatial information, we refer to [15] and define a spatial function as follows:

$$h_i(x) = \sum_{s \in \mathrm{NB}(x)} u_i(s),$$

(21)

where $\mathrm{NB}(x)$ represents a square window centered on pixel x in the spatial domain. A 5×5 window was used throughout this work. Just like the membership function, the spatial function $h_i(x)$ represents the probability that pixel x belongs to the ith cluster. The spatial function of a pixel for a cluster is large if the majority of its neighborhoods belong to the same cluster. The spatial function is incorporated into membership function as follows:

$$u_i'(x) = \frac{u_i(x) h_i(x)}{\sum_{k=1}^{N} u_k(x) h_k(x)}.$$

(22)

To demonstrate the effect of removing noise by exploiting spatial information, we use a 3×3 neighborhood centered on a pixel under consideration. Without loss of generality, we assume that the image domain is divided into two regions; that is, $N = 2$. Suppose that the values of membership functions of all neighborhood pixels belonging to the first cluster are shown in Figure 2. The upper row corresponds to the original values of membership functions, while the lower row shows the new values of membership functions by using (22). If we set the threshold to 0.50 for defuzzification, then the left and right columns of Figure 2 show the variations of the membership functions of a noisy pixel and a noise-free pixel, respectively. Obviously, the value of membership function of the noisy pixel has a desired correction from 0.60 to 0.33, while the noise-free pixel still belongs to the second cluster with a larger membership function.

In general, the spatial functions simply fortify the original membership in a homogeneous region, and the clustering result remains unchanged. However, for a noisy pixel, (22) reduces the weighting of a noisy cluster by the labels of its neighborhood pixels. As a result, misclassified pixels from noisy regions or spurious blobs can be easily corrected.

5. Implementation and Experimental Results

The proposed algorithm is a two-pass process at each iteration. The first pass is to calculate the corresponding variables $u_i(x)$, $\tilde{b}(y)$, and c_i. In the second pass, the membership functions incorporated with the spatial information are updated, and the resulting new membership functions will be inserted into the next iteration. The detailed procedures can be summarized in the following steps.

0.20	0.30	0.30
0.30	0.60	0.10
0.40	0.20	0.20

↓

0.20	0.30	0.30
0.30	0.33	0.10
0.40	0.20	0.20

0.20	0.30	0.30
0.30	0.30	0.10
0.40	0.20	0.20

↓

0.20	0.30	0.30
0.30	0.13	0.10
0.40	0.20	0.20

FIGURE 2: An illustration to demonstrate the effect of removing noise by exploiting spatial information. The left and right columns show the variation of the membership functions of a noisy pixel and a noise-free pixel, respectively.

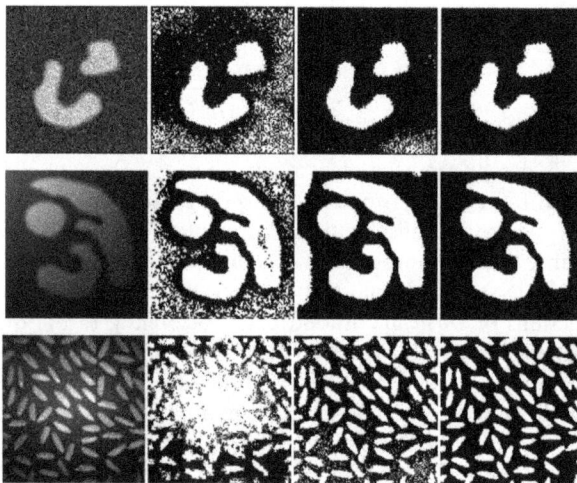

FIGURE 3: Segmentation results of the proposed algorithm on three synthetic images. Column 1: original images. Column 2-3: intermediate results. Column 4: final results.

Step 1. Initialize the number of clusters N, membership functions $u_i(x)$, constants c_i, and bias field $\widetilde{b}(y)$.

Step 2. Updating the constants c_i using (20).

Step 3. Estimating bias field $\widetilde{b}(y)$ using (18).

Step 4. Updating membership functions $u_i(x)$ using (16).

Step 5. Computing the new membership functions incorporated with spatial information using (22).

Repeat Steps 2–5 till termination. The iteration is stopped when the maximum difference between constants c_i at two successive iterations is less than a threshold (e.g., 0.001). After the convergence, defuzzification is applied to assign each pixel to a specific cluster for which the membership function is maximal.

In this section, we apply the proposed algorithm to both synthetic and clinical medical images to demonstrate its effectiveness. The parameters used in our algorithm are as follows: fuzzy coefficient $m = 2$, standard deviation of the Gaussian kernel $\sigma = 4$, and neighborhood radius of the Gaussian kernel $r = 15$. To demonstrate the robustness, the initializations of the variables $u_i(x)$, $\widetilde{b}(y)$, and c_i for the experiments in this paper are all generated as random fields or random numbers.

5.1. Segmentation of Synthetic Images. The first experiment is performed in three synthetic images, which are displayed in the first column of Figure 3. In the first image, there is strong noise in both object and background regions. The images in the middle and bottom rows are corrupted by noise and intensity inhomogeneity. The intermediate segmentation results obtained by running the proposed algorithm for different numbers of iterations are shown in the second and third columns, and the final results obtained after the convergence of our algorithm are shown in the fourth column. It is revealed from Figure 3 that the result gradually improves during the iterative segmentation process. In the final segmentation results, objects and background can be clearly differentiated despite of the impact of noise and intensity inhomogeneity.

5.2. Segmentation of Clinical Medical Images. In this subsection, we compare the proposed algorithm with the bias-corrected FCM (BCFCM) algorithm [12], the sFCM algorithm [15], and the CLIC algorithm [17] for clinical medical images.

The images in the first column of Figure 4 are two X-ray vessel images with noise and intensity inhomogeneity. It can be seen that the upper parts of the images appear brighter, while the lower parts are darker due to the intensity inhomogeneity. As a result, the intensity values of the background in the upper region may be larger than the ones of vessels in the lower region. This phenomenon can cause serious misclassification for those clustering algorithms based on global region. Both of the BCFCM algorithm and the sFCM algorithm are based on global region clustering and hence cannot overcome this problem. This can be observed from the segmentation results which contain some parts of background in the upper brighter region while losing some vessel profiles in the lower darker region. However, the aforementioned phenomenon will become unobvious in local region because intensity inhomogeneity is slowing varying. Therefore, the local region clustering-based algorithm, namely the CLIC algorithm and the proposed algorithm can handle intensity inhomogeneity to obtain the complete vessel profile. Nevertheless, the CLIC algorithm has no step to resist noise so that its results contain some spurious blobs, due to the impact of noise. By contrast, our proposed algorithm utilizes spatial information to suppress noise and thus achieves the desirable segmentation results. The two images shown in the last column of Figure 4 are the estimated bias fields obtained by the proposed algorithm.

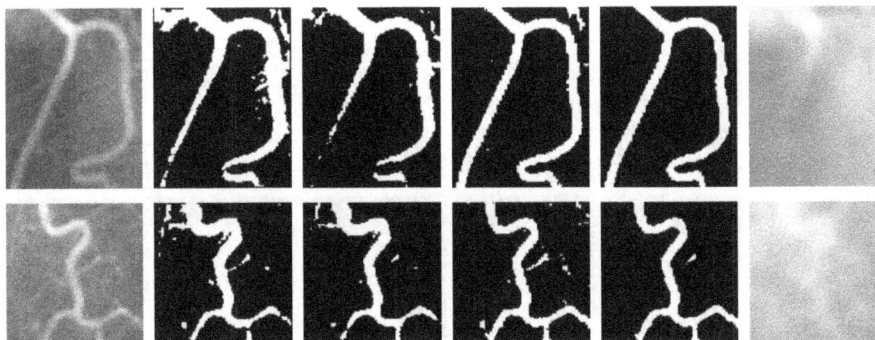

FIGURE 4: Comparison of segmentation results on two X-ray vessel images. Column 1: original images. Column 2: the BCFCM algorithm. Column 3: the sFCM algorithm. Column 4: the CLIC algorithm. Column 5: the proposed algorithm. Column 6: the estimated bias fields by the proposed algorithm.

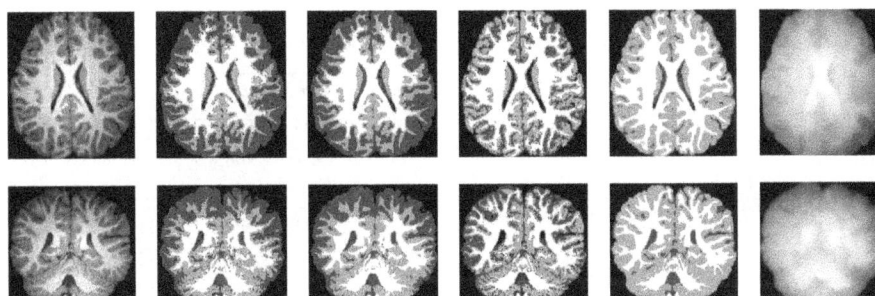

FIGURE 5: Comparison of segmentation results on two 3T brain MR images. Column 1: original images. Column 2: the BCFCM algorithm. Column 3: the sFCM algorithm. Column 4: the CLIC algorithm. Column 5: the proposed algorithm. Column 6: the estimated bias fields by the proposed algorithm.

We also apply the aforementioned four algorithms to 3T brain MR images. The original images are also corrupted by intensity inhomogeneity and noise, which makes the images brighter in the middle than in the other regions. The task of segmentation is to partition the brain MR images into four regions, that is, white matter (WM), gray matter (GM), cerebral spinal fluid (CSF), and background. The comparison of segmentation results obtained by these four algorithms is shown in Figure 5. Obviously, the BCFCM algorithm and the sFCM algorithm misclassify plentiful WM into GM in the vicinity of the skull because the WM in such region has approximate intensity values with the GM owing to the impact of the intensity inhomogeneity. The segmentation results of the CLIC algorithm show again that it is capable of dealing with the intensity inhomogeneity but unable to suppress the noise. However, our proposed algorithm gets fairly better segmentation with clear and correct classification of tissues. The estimated bias fields obtained by our proposed algorithm are shown in the sixth column of Figure 5.

5.3. Quantitative Comparison. To quantitatively compare the proposed algorithm with the above-mentioned other three algorithms, we use the T1-weighted simulated brain MR images with ground truth from Brain Web in the link http://www.bic.mni.mcgill.ca/brainweb/. The selected MR images include 40% image intensity inhomogeneity and 3% noise. The original images and the segmentation results are shown in Figure 6. We adopt Jaccard similarity (JS) [19] as a

measurement of the segmentation accuracy. The JS between two regions $S1$ and $S2$ is defined as the ratio between the areas of the intersection and the union of them, namely, $JS(S1, S2) = |S1 \cap S2|/|S1 \cup S2|$. We compute the JS between the segmented region $S1$ obtained by the algorithm and the corresponding region $S2$ given by the ground truth. The closer the JS value to 1, the better the segmentation result. The resulting JS values for the four algorithms are listed in Table 1. It can be observed from both Figure 6 and Table 1 that the segmentation results of our proposed algorithm are more accurate than the other three algorithms.

6. Discussion

The proposed algorithm suffers from manually setting of two parameters: the neighborhood radius r and the standard deviation σ of the truncated Gaussian kernel. Note that the radius r should be selected appropriately according to the degree of the intensity inhomogeneity. For more localized intensity inhomogeneity, the bias field $\tilde{b}$ varies faster, and therefore the approximation in (4) is valid only in a smaller neighborhood. In this case, a smaller r should be used as the radius of the neighborhood, and the standard deviation σ should be also selected a smaller value correspondingly.

Figure 7 shows the JS values of the segmentation results with different parameters selection. The original image is obtained from Brain Web. The upper figure shows the influence of the radius, while the lower figure shows the influence

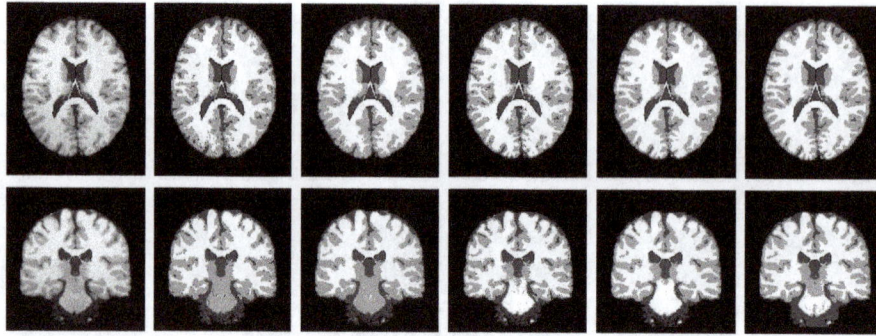

FIGURE 6: Comparison of segmentation results on two simulated brain MR images. Column 1: original images. Column 2: the BCFCM algorithm. Column 3: the sFCM algorithm. Column 4: the CLIC algorithm. Column 5: the proposed algorithm. Column 6: ground truth.

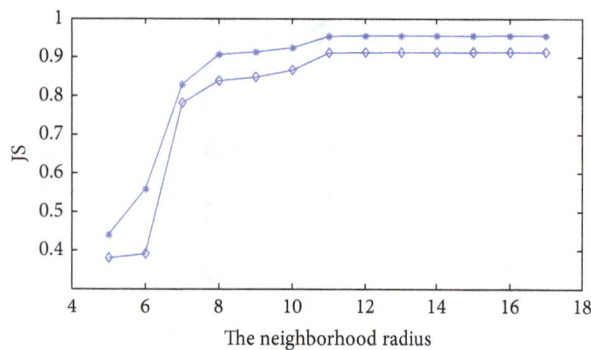

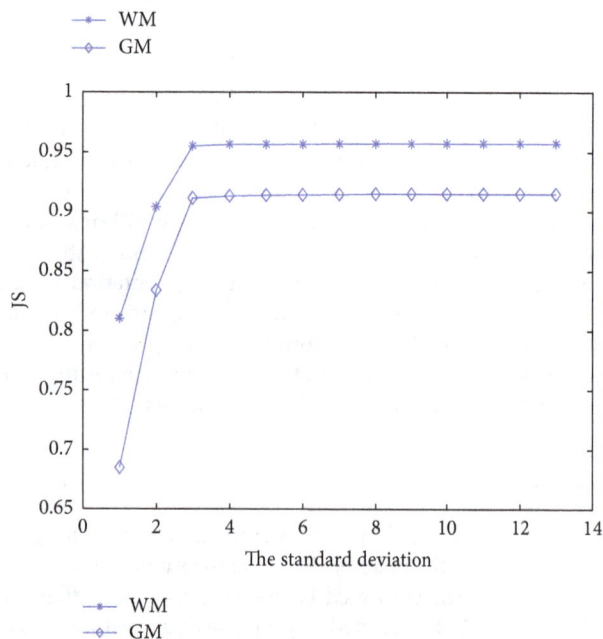

FIGURE 7: The JS values of the segmentation results obtained by using the different parameters setting of the truncated Gaussian kernel.

TABLE 1: Comparison of the JS values of the segmentation results obtained by the four algorithms.

Image	Tissue	BCFCM	sFCM	CLIC	Proposed algorithm
	WM	0.8957	0.9139	0.9321	0.9536
Brain 1	GM	0.8361	0.8598	0.8782	0.9125
	CSF	0.8847	0.8825	0.8902	0.8963
	WM	0.8152	0.8201	0.8563	0.8987
Brain 2	GM	0.7640	0.7716	0.8011	0.8376
	CSF	0.7941	0.8061	0.8128	0.8321

of the algorithm, we suggest that $9 \leq r \leq 17$ and $3 \leq \sigma \leq 6$ for this type of image. In our experiments, we set $r = 15$ and $\sigma = 4$ for all test images.

7. Conclusion

In this paper, we have proposed a localized FCM clustering algorithm for simultaneous segmentation and bias field estimation of medical images. The proposed algorithm defines a fuzzy energy that depends on the bias field, membership functions, and the constants that approximate the true signal from the corresponding tissues. Bias field estimation and image segmentation are simultaneously achieved by minimizing this energy. Besides, we also utilize the neighborhood spatial information to resist the noise interference. Moreover, the proposed algorithm is robust to initialization, thereby allowing fully automatic applications. Comparisons with other approaches demonstrate the superior performance of the proposed algorithm.

Acknowledgments

This work was supported by the National Natural Science Foundation of China (60903127, 61202314), NPU Foundation for Fundamental Research (JCY20130130, JC201108) and Ao-Xiang Star Project at Northwestern Polytechnical University (11GH0315).

References

[1] D. Pham, C. Xu, and J. Prince, "Current methods in medical image segmentation," Annual Review of Biomedical Engineering, vol. 2, pp. 315–317, 2000.

of the standard deviation. The accuracy of segmentations increases with the increasing of r and σ. When $r > 10$ or $\sigma > 3$, the JS values of WM and GM increase slightly, while the time consumption would have a significant increase. Considering the segmentation accuracy and the time consumption

[2] D. J. Withey and Z. J. Koles, "Medical image segmentation: methods and software," in *Proceedings of the Joint Meeting of the 6th International Symposium on Noninvasive Functional Source Imaging of the Brain and Heart and the International Conference on Functional Biomedical Imaging (NFSI&ICFBI '07)*, pp. 140–143, October 2007.

[3] W. M. Wells III, W. E. L. Crimson, R. Kikinis, and F. A. Jolesz, "Adaptive segmentation of mri data," *IEEE Transactions on Medical Imaging*, vol. 15, no. 4, pp. 429–442, 1996.

[4] K. van Leemput, F. Maes, D. Vandermeulen, and P. Suetens, "Automated model-based bias field correction of MR images of the brain," *IEEE Transactions on Medical Imaging*, vol. 18, no. 10, pp. 885–896, 1999.

[5] Y. Zhang, M. Brady, and S. Smith, "Segmentation of brain MR images through a hidden Markov random field model and the expectation-maximization algorithm," *IEEE Transactions on Medical Imaging*, vol. 20, no. 1, pp. 45–57, 2001.

[6] Y. Chen, J. Zhang, and J. Macione, "An improved level set method for brain MR images segmentation and bias correction," *Computerized Medical Imaging and Graphics*, vol. 33, no. 7, pp. 510–519, 2009.

[7] L. Wang, C. Li, Q. Sun, D. Xia, and C.-Y. Kao, "Active contours driven by local and global intensity fitting energy with application to brain MR image segmentation," *Computerized Medical Imaging and Graphics*, vol. 33, no. 7, pp. 520–531, 2009.

[8] C. Li, R. Huang, Z. Ding, J. C. Gatenby, D. N. Metaxas, and J. C. Gore, "A level set method for image segmentation in the presence of intensity inhomogeneities with application to MRI," *IEEE Transactions on Image Processing*, vol. 20, no. 7, pp. 2007–2016, 2011.

[9] Y. Chen, J. Zhang, A. Mishra, and J. Yang, "Image segmentation and bias correction via an improved level set method," *Neurocomputing*, vol. 74, no. 17, pp. 3520–3530, 2011.

[10] D. L. Pham and J. L. Prince, "An adaptive fuzzy C-means algorithm for image segmentation in the presence of intensity inhomogeneities," *Pattern Recognition Letters*, vol. 20, no. 1, pp. 57–68, 1999.

[11] D. L. Pham and J. L. Prince, "Adaptive fuzzy segmentation of magnetic resonance images," *IEEE Transactions on Medical Imaging*, vol. 18, no. 9, pp. 737–752, 1999.

[12] M. N. Ahmed, S. M. Yamany, N. Mohamed, A. A. Farag, and T. Moriarty, "A modified fuzzy C-means algorithm for bias field estimation and segmentation of MRI data," *IEEE Transactions on Medical Imaging*, vol. 21, no. 3, pp. 193–199, 2002.

[13] A. W.-C. Liew and H. Yan, "An adaptive spatial fuzzy clustering algorithm for 3-D MR image segmentation," *IEEE Transactions on Medical Imaging*, vol. 22, no. 9, pp. 1063–1075, 2003.

[14] D.-Q. Zhang and S.-C. Chen, "A novel kernelized fuzzy c-means algorithm with application in medical image segmentation," *Artificial Intelligence in Medicine*, vol. 32, no. 1, pp. 37–50, 2004.

[15] K.-S. Chuang, H.-L. Tzeng, S. Chen, J. Wu, and T.-J. Chen, "Fuzzy c-means clustering with spatial information for image segmentation," *Computerized Medical Imaging and Graphics*, vol. 30, no. 1, pp. 9–15, 2006.

[16] L. Szilágri, S. Szilágri, and B. Benyó, "Efficent inhomogeneity compensation using fuzzy c-means clustering models," *Computer Methods and Programs in Biomedicine*, vol. 108, no. 1, pp. 80–89, 2012.

[17] C. Li, C. Xu, A. W. Anderson, and J. C. Gore, "MRI tissue classification and bias field estimation based on coherent local intensity clustering: A unified energy minimization framework," in *Proceedings of the 21st International Conference on Information Processing in Medical Imaging (IPMI '09)*, pp. 288–299, 2009.

[18] S. Chen and D. Zhang, "Robust image segmentation using FCM with spatial constraints based on new kernel-induced distance measure," *IEEE Transactions on Systems, Man, and Cybernetics B*, vol. 34, no. 4, pp. 1907–1916, 2004.

[19] U. Vovk, F. Pernuš, and B. Likar, "A review of methods for correction of intensity inhomogeneity in MRI," *IEEE Transactions on Medical Imaging*, vol. 26, no. 3, pp. 405–421, 2007.

[20] L. A. Vese and T. F. Chan, "A multiphase level set framework for image segmentation using the Mumford and Shah model," *International Journal of Computer Vision*, vol. 50, no. 3, pp. 271–293, 2002.

[21] G. Aubert and P. Kornprobst, *Mathematical Problems in Image Processing: Partial Differential Equations and the Calculus of Variations*, Springer, New York, NY, USA, 2002.

21

An Investigation of Calibration Phantoms for CT Scanners with Tube Voltage Modulation

Jing Zou, Xiaodong Hu, Hanyu Lv, and Xiaotang Hu

State Key Laboratory of Precision Measuring Technology and Instruments, Tianjin University, Tianjin 300072, China

Correspondence should be addressed to Jing Zou; jingzoutd@tju.edu.cn

Academic Editor: Guowei Wei

The effects of calibration phantoms on the correction results of the empirical artifacts correction method (ECCU) for the case of tube modulation were investigated. To improve the validity of the ECCU method, the effect of the geometry parameter of a typical single-material calibration phantom (water calibration phantom) on the ECCU algorithm was investigated. Dual-material calibration phantoms (such as water-bone calibration phantom), geometry arrangement, and the area-ratio of dual-material calibration phantoms were also studied. Preliminary results implied that, to assure the effectiveness of the ECCU algorithm, the polychromatic projections of calibration phantoms must cover the polychromatic projection data of the scanning object. However, the projection range of a water calibration phantom is limited by the scan field of view (SFOV), thus leading to methodological limitations. A dual-material phantom of a proper size and material can overcome the limitations of a single-material phantom and achieve good correction effects.

1. Introduction

In conventional computed tomography (CT) tube voltages are fixed (constant) while CT scans are carried out. However, tube voltage modulation is helpful for at least two reasons. First, tube voltage modulation has the potential for further dose reduction [1]. In addition, tube voltage modulation can obtain satisfactory image quality avoiding detector pixel saturation. When the thickness of the scanned object varies greatly with the view angle, the constant power of the X-ray generated by traditional CT may lead to pixel saturation or at least strike a balance of quantum noise among the different views. Dynamically adjusting the X-ray tube voltage in synchrony with the CT scanning can avoid this problem. Tube voltage modulation is very helpful in CT scanning, but when the voltage is modulated at different views during a CT scan, images reconstructed through commonly used reconstruction methods may contain various artifacts leading to inaccuracy and degradation of image quality.

Ideally, monochromatic X-ray beams are required in CT scanning. However, conventionally used X-ray beams in CT are polychromatic with a moderately broad energy spectrum. In this paper, different polychromatic X-ray beams are used

through tube voltage modulating at different scanning views. As we know, X-ray attenuation processes in matter are energy dependent [2]. However, the reconstruction algorithm is based on the assumption of the monochromatic property of the X-ray beam that just computed the average attenuation coefficient and thus leads to the appearance of cupping artifacts or beam hardening artifacts within conventionally reconstructed images. Beam hardening effects in a fixed voltage are known to be one of the major sources of deterministic error. During recent decades, a number of correction methods have been developed, including physical approach, statistics approach, linearization, spectrum estimation, phantom calibration prereconstruction, threshold segmentation reprojection, and iteration method [3–9]. However, artifact correction in the case of tube modulation during a CT scan has been primarily addressed in the literature. "Water calibration for CT scanners with tube voltage modulation" in 2010, in which the ECCU algorithm for cupping artifact correction was provided, showed excellent simulation results. The typical artifact correction applied in clinical CT scanners is known as water correction, and so water phantom is used in the ECCU method [10]. To ensure the integrity of the algorithm, large water phantoms are required for routine calibrations. However, the size of the calibration phantom is limited by the scan field of view (SFOV), which may lead to methodological limitations.

In this paper, the effects of calibration phantoms for CT scanners with tube voltage modulation are investigated by a numerical simulation method. In Section 2, we provide a brief review of the ECCU algorithm, followed by a numerical implementation of the ECCU algorithm. In Section 3, we have performed two sets of simulation experiments to investigate the effect of the geometry parameter of water phantoms on the ECCU algorithm. Then, we investigate the effect of dual-material calibration phantoms on the ECCU algorithm, including the area-ratio and geometrical arrangement of different materials. Finally, conclusions and remarks are given in Section 4.

2. Principle of the ECCU Method

The log attenuation of a polychromatic X-ray spectrum, as used for CT, is given as

$$q(U, L) = -\ln \omega(U, L, E) e^{-\int \mu(E, \mathbf{r})dL} dE, \tag{1}$$

where L is the line of integration corresponding to the ray direction, $\mathbf{r}$ represents the position vector, $\mu(E, \mathbf{r})$ indicates the energy-dependent spatial distribution of the linear attenuation coefficient, E is the photon energy, and $\omega(U, L, E)$ is the normalized spectrum distribution of the emitted X-rays at tube voltage U.

Assuming the decomposition $\mu(E, \mathbf{r}) = \varphi(E)f(\mathbf{r})$, we will get the following formula:

$$q(U, p) = -\ln \int \omega(U, L, E) e^{p\varphi(E)} dE \quad \text{with } p = \int f(\mathbf{r})\, dL, \tag{2}$$

where $\varphi(E)$ is the energy dependence of the most prominent material in the object.

Let q be the polychromatic projection data and $p = D(U, q)$ the desired monochromatic material-specific projection data. The aim of the ECCU algorithm is to acquire proper p from $q(U, p)$. Let $p = D(U, q)$, which is some yet unknown decomposition function, as follows:

$$D(U, q) = \sum_{n=0}^{N-1} c_n b_n(U, q) = \mathbf{c} \cdot \mathbf{b}(U, q), \tag{3}$$

where $D(U, q)$ represents a linear combination of basis functions $b_n(U, q)$ and $b_n(U, q) = U^l q^k$ as basis functions with $k = 0, \ldots, K$ and $l = 0, \ldots, L$. A set of $(K+1)(L+1)$ basis images are defined as $f_n(\mathbf{r}) = R^{-1}b_n(U, q)$, R^{-1} represents the inverse radon transform, and f_n is the reconstruction image of the projection data q after they have been passed through the basis functions $b_n(U, q)$.

Now, the reconstruction of the material-selective projection data can be written as a linear combination of these basis images:

$$f(\mathbf{r}) = R^{-1}D(U, q) = R^{-1}\sum c_n b_n(U, q)$$
$$= \sum c_n R^{-1}b_n(U, q) = c_n f_n(\mathbf{r}) = \mathbf{c} \cdot f(\mathbf{r}). \tag{4}$$

The set of coefficients $\mathbf{c}$ is solved through minimizing the least-squares deviation:

$$E^2 = \int w(\mathbf{r}) \left(\mathbf{c}f(\mathbf{r}) - t(\mathbf{r})\right)^2 d^2r, \tag{5}$$

where $t(\mathbf{r})$ represents a given template image and $w(\mathbf{r})$ is the weight image used to suppress the contribution of unwanted structures of the calibration object.

The process of the ECCU method is calculating the coefficients $\mathbf{c}$ through calibration phantom. Furthermore, these coefficients are used to preprocess projection data acquired from ordinary scanning through formula (3). Concrete details have been shown in the literature [10]. Influence of calibration phantom material and calibration phantom size on the ECCU method is investigated in the following section.

3. Calibration Phantom Study

In this section, the effect of different calibration phantoms including single-material phantom and dual-material phantom on the ECCU method is investigated by using computer simulation data. A projection simulation based on a physical imaging model and scanning phantom simulation is introduced in Section 3.1. The investigation of single-material calibration phantom and dual-material calibration phantom is implemented in Sections 3.2 and 3.3.

3.1. Simulations. To simulate the projection data of different phantoms acquired with a polychromatic X-ray source, we utilize the same scheme as in [10]. The distribution function of a polychromatic X-ray energy spectrum emitted by X-ray tube GE Maxi Ray 125 [spectrum GUI] and the absorption attenuation coefficients were interpolated from the database of NIST (National Institute of Standards and Technology's website) [11]. We first computed the linear integral projection of every material that formed the phantom and then computed corresponding polychromatic projections using a different spectrum.

To investigate the effect of calibration phantoms on the ECCU algorithm, the well-known FORBILD head phantom as a test phantom was simulated. More detailed information about the phantom is listed in Table 1. The geometry parameters of the virtual CT system for scanning FORBILD head phantom are as follows. The distance from source to rotation center is 570 cm and the distance from source to detector is 435 cm. Detector array is 256×256 with a pixel size of 0.2067 cm. The tube voltage U as a function of the projection angle α is shown in Figure 1. Subsequently, we simulated projection data of FORBILD head phantom using voltage modulation curves shown in Figure 1, corresponding directly to the reconstructed image shown in Figure 2(a). In Figure 2(b), we show a reconstructed image from the monochromatic projection data as a contrast. In addition, all simulations were carried out using the voltage modulation profile in Figure 1.

3.2. Single-Material Calibration Phantom. In order to understand the effect of object size on the ECCU method, a series

TABLE 1: Parameters of FORBILD head phantom.

Label	Geometry	Position (cm)	Ellipsoid half-axis length (cm, cm, cm)	Elliptical cylinder/cone (radius, radius, length) (cm, cm, cm)	Φ (°)	θ (°)
1	Ellipsoid	(0, 0, 0)	(9.6, 12.0, 12.5)	N/A	0.0	0.0
2	Ellipsoid	(0, 0, 0)	(9, 11.4, 11.9)	N/A	0.0	0.0
3	Ellipsoid	(0, 8.4, 0)	(1.8, 3.0, 3.0)	N/A	0.0	0.0
4	Elliptical cylinder	(0, 3.6, 0)	N/A	(4, 1.2, 0.483)	60	90
5	Elliptical cylinder	(0, 9.6, 0)	N/A	(2, 0.525661, 0.4)	−90	−30
6	Ellipsoid	(−1.9, 5.4, 0)	(1.165, 0.406, 3)	N/A	0.0	−45
7	Ellipsoid	(1.9, 5.4, 0)	(1.165, 0.406, 3)	N/A	0.0	45
8	Elliptical cylinder	(−4.3, 6.8, −1)	N/A	(1.8, 0.24, 4)	0.0	−30
9	Elliptical cylinder	(4.3, 6.8, −1)	N/A	(1.8, 0.24, 4)	0.0	30
10	Cone	(0, −10.15, −0.2)	N/A	(0.5, 0.2, 1.5)	0.0	0.0

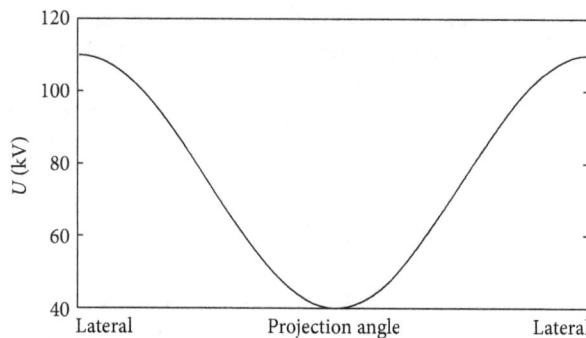

FIGURE 1: Tube voltage varied sinusoidally from 110 kV to 40 kV.

TABLE 2: Scope of projection data for different phantoms.

Phantom	Scope of projection data
Figure 2(a)	[0, 12.7046]
Figure 3(a)	[0, 29.9094]
Figure 3(b)	[0, 9.11191]

of virtual solid water phantoms with different geometry sizes were investigated. Here, two water phantoms are given as examples to illustrate the effect of geometry size on the ECCU method. The first elliptical cylinder water phantom with semiaxes 48 cm and 40 cm is shown in Figure 3(a). The second with semiaxes 28 cm and 12 cm is shown in Figure 3(b). Corresponding correction coefficients of the two calibration phantoms are computed through the ECCU method. Then, the correction coefficients are used to correct the tube voltage modulated projection of the FORBILD head phantom. The correction results through phantom Figures 3(a) and 3(b) are shown in Figures 3(c) and 3(d). To show images of a proper ratio, the SFOV of Figures 3(c) and 3(d) are simply reduced to 1/3, which is enclosed by a red square, and the corresponding zoomed images are shown in Figures 3(e) and 3(f). From Figure 3(e), we can see that the corrected image is as good as the reconstructed image from the monochromatic projection shown in Figure 2(b), which demonstrates that the ECCU method is effective when the large water phantom is used. However, severe errors appear in the corrected images when the small water calibration phantom is used, as shown in Figure 3(f). In order to analyze the reason leading to the failure of the ECCU method, we investigated the maximum and minimum values of tube voltage modulated projection data, including water phantom in Figures 3(a)

and 3(b) and FORBILD head phantom in Figure 2(a). The corresponding results are shown in Table 2. Although the size of the calibration phantom in Figure 3(b) is much the same as that of the FORBILD head phantom, we can see that the scope of the polychromatic projection data of water phantom in Figure 3(b) cannot cover the polychromatic projection data of the FORBILD head phantom in Figure 2(a), which may be the key reason leading to the failure of the ECCU method.

To verify that the above analysis is reasonable, a test phantom made of water was investigated. The semiaxes of a water elliptical cylinder are 24 cm and 22 cm. From the geometry size of Figures 3(a) and 3(b), we know that the size of Figure 3(a) is larger than that of the actual testing phantom, but Figure 3(b) is smaller than the actual testing phantom. Again, correction coefficients of water calibration phantom in Figures 3(a) and 3(b) are used to implement the ECCU method. Corrected images using calibration phantoms in Figures 3(a) and 3(b) are shown in Figures 4(a) and 4(b). The directly reconstructed image using tube voltage modulated projection data is shown in Figure 4(c) and cupping artifacts appeared. In order to quantify the accuracy of the three reconstructed images, the profiles along Figures 4(a), 4(b), and 4(c) are displayed in Figure 4(d). From these profiles, it can be observed that the profile of Figure 4(a) is a straight line, but the profiles of Figures 4(b) and 4(c) are curves, which demonstrates that when the scanning phantom to be corrected is smaller than the standard calibration phantom, cupping artifacts (see the solid line in Figure 4(d)) disappear. However, when the scanning phantom to be corrected is larger than the calibration phantom, the correction method

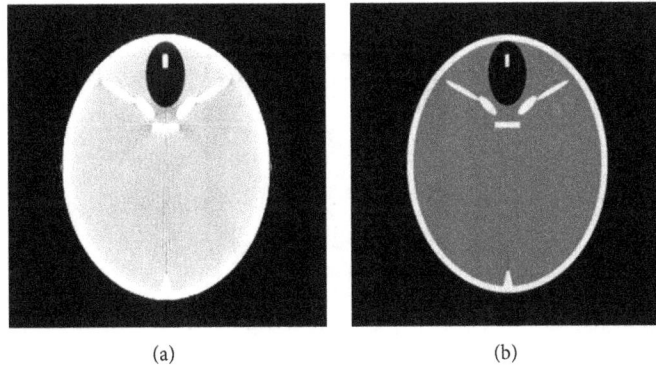

FIGURE 2: Reconstruction images of FORBILD head phantom. (a) Directly reconstructed image from tube voltage modulation projection. (b) Reconstructed image from monochromatic projection data.

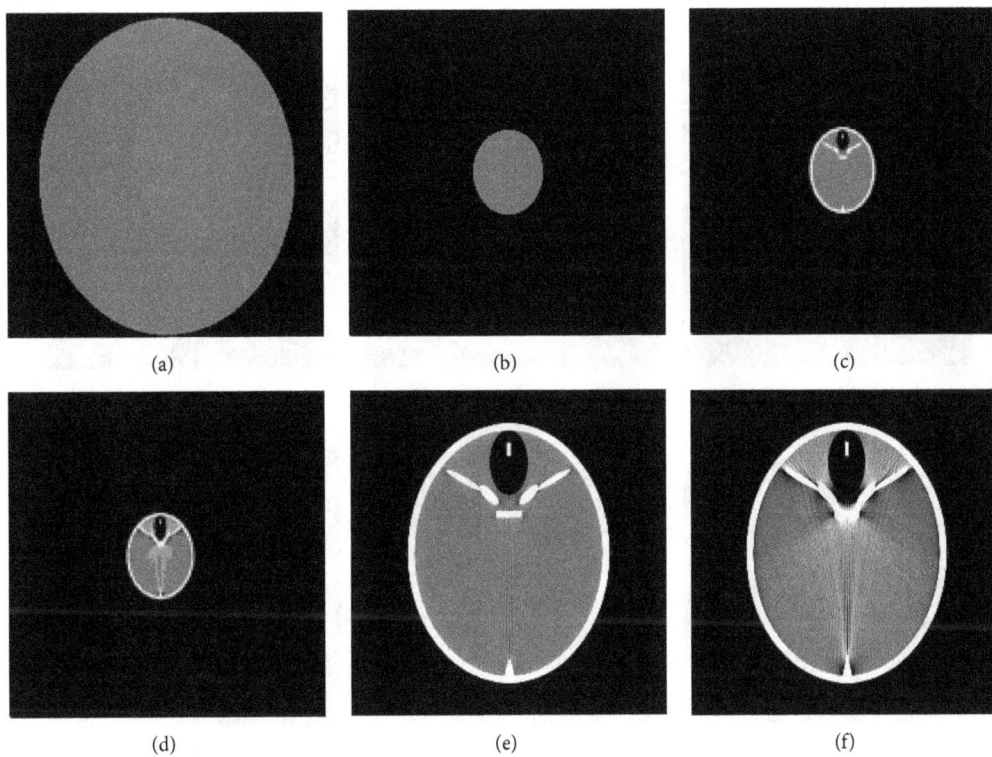

FIGURE 3: Water calibration phantoms and corresponding corrected images of FORBILD head phantom. (a) Elliptical cylinder phantom with semiaxes 48 cm and 40 cm. (b) Elliptical cylinder phantom with semiaxes 28 cm and 12 cm. (c) Corrected image using calibration phantom shown in (a). (d) Corrected image using calibration phantom shown in (b). (e) and (f) are zoomed-in images of the area enclosed by the red squares in (c) and (d). Display window is $[0, 600]$ HU.

is invalid (see the dash-dot line in Figure 4(d)). It should be reasonable to assume that the ECCU method required that the geometry of the calibration phantom be larger than that of the testing phantom when they are made of the same material. Actually, the maximum size of the calibration phantom is limited due to the actual SFOV; therefore the material and geometry design of the calibration phantom are of great importance.

3.3. Dual-Material Calibration Phantom. Actually, the maximum SFOV in the CT system is designed according to the specified parameters of the scanning objects. With high-density objects that occupy the maximum SFOV, an identically sized water calibration phantom may not be appropriate for the implementation of the ECCU method, because the polychromatic projection data of the water phantom cannot cover that of the scanning object. Inserting a high-density mass material in the water phantom is a direct way to solve this problem. Based on this idea, dual-material calibration phantoms are adopted and studied in this section. We have to mention that the polychromatic projections of dual-material calibration phantoms in this section could cover the polychromatic projection of the FORBILD head phantom,

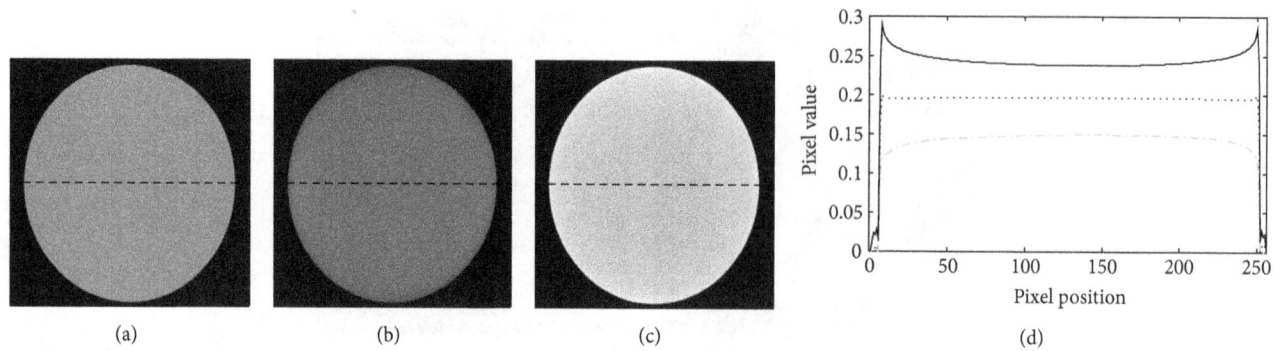

FIGURE 4: Images of water phantom. (a) Corrected image using water calibration phantom shown in Figure 3(a). (b) Corrected image using water calibration phantom shown in Figure 3(b). (c) Reconstructed image without correction. (d) Intensity plots for lines through the reconstructed images of (a), (b), and (c): the dot line, the dash-dot line, and the solid line represent intensity profiles of the central horizontal line in (a), (b), and (c), respectively.

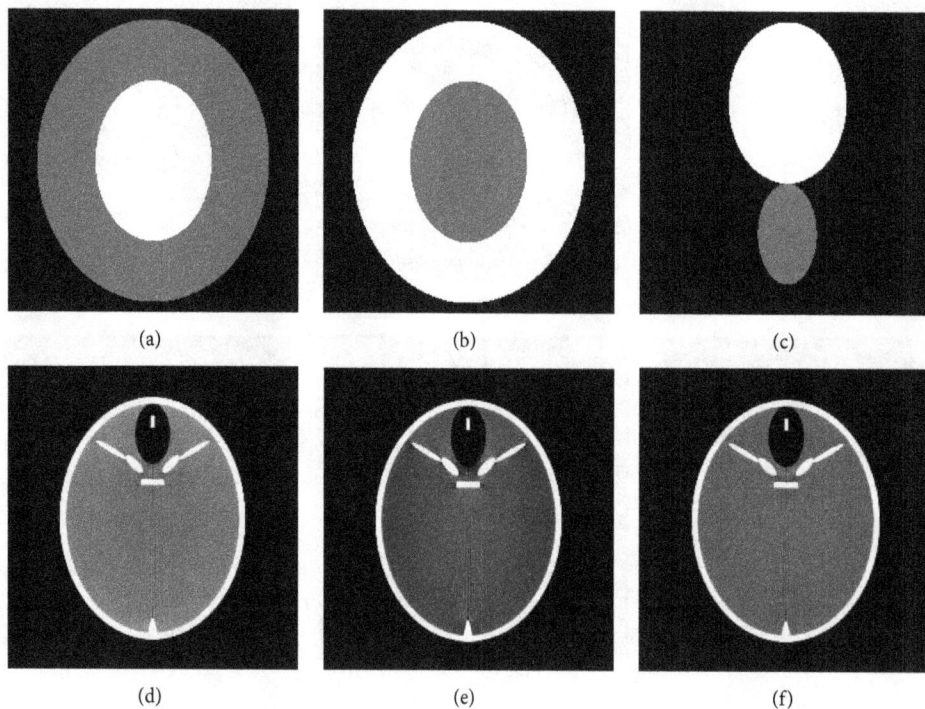

FIGURE 5: Dual-material calibration phantoms and corresponding correction images of FORBILD head phantom. The first row shows dual-material calibration phantom with different sizes. (a) A 14 × 12 cm oval water phantom with 8 × 6 cm bone insert. (b) A 14 × 12 cm oval bone phantom with 8 × 6 cm water insert. (c) A two-cylinder phantom; the upper one is an 8 × 6 cm bone cylinder and the lower one is a 5 × 3 cm water elliptical cylinder. (d), (e), and (f) are correction images of FORBILD head phantom using calibration phantoms shown in (a), (b), and (c), respectively.

which are ensured by properly adjusting the ratio of the two materials in the fixed SFOV.

Firstly, the effect of the geometrical arrangement of the dual-material phantom on the ECCU method was investigated. We conducted two cylinder-in-cylinder phantoms: one cylinder-in-cylinder phantom was a 14 × 12 cm oval water phantom with an 8 × 6 cm bone insert, as shown in Figure 5(a). The other was a 14 × 12 cm oval bone phantom with an 8 × 6 cm water insert, as shown in Figure 5(b). In addition, a two-cylinder phantom was simulated, as shown

in Figure 5(c); the upper one was an 8 × 6 cm bone cylinder and the lower one was a 5 × 3 cm water cylinder. Again, corresponding correction coefficients of the three calibration phantoms were computed through the ECCU method. These correction coefficients are then used to correct the tube voltage modulated projection of the FORBILD head phantom. The correction results through phantom Figures 5(a), 5(b), and 5(c) are shown in Figures 5(d), 5(e), and 5(f), respectively. Compared with the directly reconstructed image in Figure 2(a), the corrected images in Figures 5(d), 5(e), and

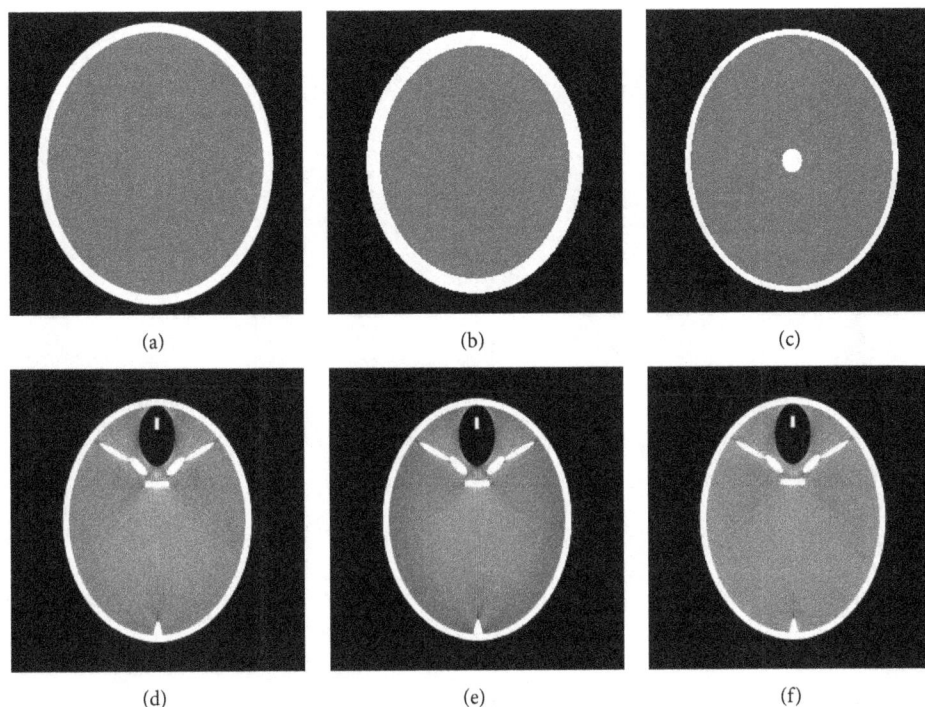

FIGURE 6: Dual-material calibration phantoms and corresponding correction images of FORBILD head phantom. The first row shows dual-material calibration phantom with different sizes. (a) A 14 × 12 cm oval bone phantom with 13 × 11 cm water insert. (b) A 13 × 11 cm oval bone phantom with 11.5 × 9.6 cm water insert. (c) A 13 × 11 cm oval bone phantom with 12.4 × 10.4 cm water insert, in which a 1.2 × 1.0 cm oval bone is inserted in the center. (d), (e), and (f) are correction images of the FORBILD head phantom using calibration phantoms shown in (a), (b), and (c), respectively.

5(f) are almost free of artifacts, although the uniformity of Figure 5(e) is not very good.

For a more detailed analysis on the influence of cylinder-in-cylinder phantoms similar to Figure 5(b) on the ECCU method, three cylinder-in-cylinder phantoms were investigated. The first one was a 14 × 12 cm oval bone phantom with a 13 × 11 cm water insert, as shown in Figure 6(a). The second one was a 13 × 11 cm oval bone phantom with a 11.5 × 9.6 cm water insert, as shown in Figure 6(b) and the last one was 13 × 11 cm oval bone phantom with a 12.4 × 10.4 cm water insert, in which a 1.2 × 1.0 cm oval bone was inserted in the center, as shown in Figure 6(c). Corresponding corrected images of the FORBILD head phantom through phantom Figures 6(a), 6(b), and 6(c) are shown in Figures 6(d), 6(e), and 6(f). We can see that bright artifacts appear in the area surrounded by the high-density materials; also streak artifacts can be observed among the higher density materials. This phenomenon shows that the geometrical arrangement of Figures 6(a), 6(b), and 6(c) is not good enough compared with calibration phantoms such as Figures 5(a) and 5(c) even though the contrast of the FORBILD image is improved to a certain degree.

Lastly, the effect of the area-ratio of the dual-material phantom on the ECCU method was investigated through cylinder-in-cylinder phantoms as in Figure 5(a). The first cylinder-in-cylinder phantom was a 14 × 12 cm oval water phantom with a 1.5 × 1.0 cm bone insert, as shown in Figure 7(a). The second one was a 14 × 12 cm oval water

TABLE 3: Scope of projection data for different phantoms.

Phantom	Scope of projection data
Figure 2(a)	[0, 12.7046]
Figure 7(a)	[0, 12.9765]
Figure 7(b)	[0, 17.6509]
Figure 7(c)	[0, 19.4019]

phantom with a 4 × 2 cm bone insert, as shown in Figure 7(b). The last one was a 14 × 12 cm oval water phantom with a 5 × 3 cm bone insert, as shown in Figure 7(c). The area-ratio of outer water phantom to inserted bone phantom for Figures 7(a), 7(b), and 7(c) is 111 : 1, 20 : 1, and 10.2 : 1, respectively. The corresponding projection ranges of these phantoms are shown in Table 3, which show that the polychromatic projections of the calibration phantom can cover the polychromatic projection data of the scanning object. Again, the ECCU method is implemented through these calibration phantoms, and the corresponding corrected images of the FORBILD head phantom through calibration phantom Figures 7(a), 7(b), and 7(c) are shown in Figures 7(d), 7(e), and 7(f). It can be observed that the corrected images agree well with the reconstructed image from the monochromatic projection data shown in Figure 2(b), which demonstrates that this kind of cylinder-in-cylinder phantom is valid for the ECCU method. Also, the area-ratio may not influence the validity of the ECCU method in case of this kind of cylinder-in-cylinder phantom.

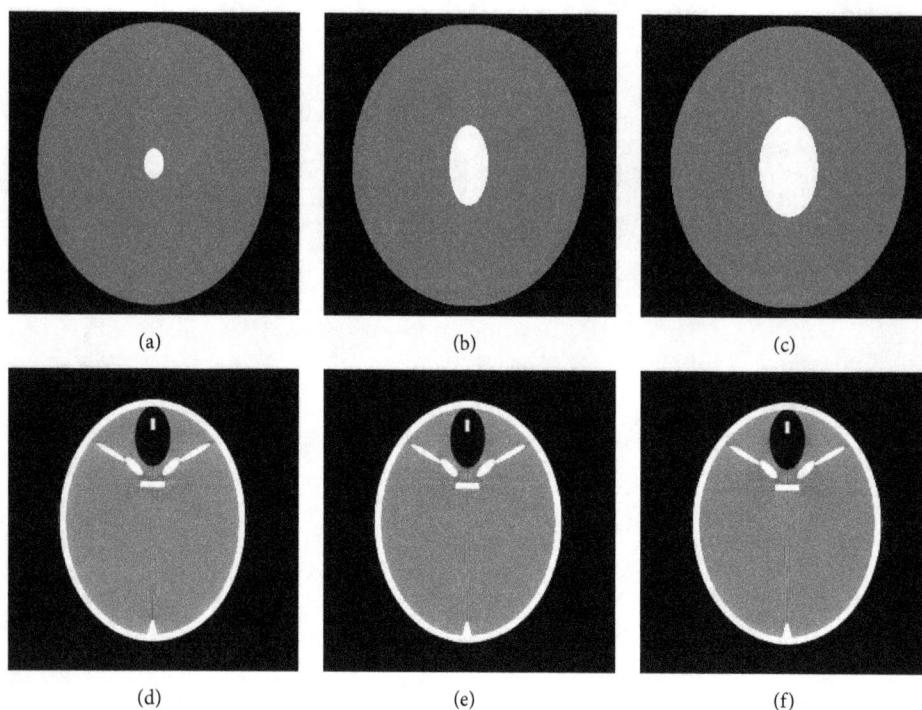

FIGURE 7: Dual-material calibration phantoms and corresponding correction images of FORBILD head phantom. The first row shows dual-material calibration phantom with different sizes. (a) A 14×12 cm oval water phantom with a 1.5×1.0 cm bone insert. (b) A 14×12 cm oval water phantom with 4×2 cm bone insert. (c) A 14×12 cm oval water phantom with 5×3 cm bone insert. (d), (e), and (f) are correction images of FORBILD head phantom using calibration phantoms shown in (a), (b), and (c).

4. Conclusions

In this paper, calibration phantoms for CT scanners with tube voltage modulation are investigated through computer simulation. We investigated the effect of the geometry parameter of the water calibration phantom on the ECCU algorithm. The simulation results show that the large water phantom can improve image quality, whilst a small water phantom may degrade image quality, because the polychromatic projection of the water phantom cannot cover the polychromatic projection of the scanning object. We find that in order to assure the effectiveness of the ECCU algorithm, the polychromatic projections of the calibration phantom must cover the polychromatic projection data of the scanning object. To assure the validity of the ECCU method, dual-material calibration phantoms are introduced. Furthermore, the geometry arrangement and the area-ratio of dual-material calibration phantoms were investigated. According to the numerical results, it can be concluded that dual-material calibration phantoms are valid in removing "cupping artifacts" and "streak artifacts".

Acknowledgments

This work was supported in part by National Key Scientific Apparatus Development of Special Item (no. 2011YQ030112), the Basic Research Program of Shenzhen City JC201005270313A, 2011 Beijing Natural Science Foundation (3112006), and the National Natural Science Foundation of China (61002041). The authors would like to thank Marc Kachelrieß of university of Erlangen-Nürnberg for his work "Water calibration for CT scanners with tube voltage modulation."

References

[1] S. V. Vollmar and W. A. Kalender, "Reduction of dose to the female breast as a result of spectral optimisation for high-contrast thoracic CT imaging: a phantom study," *British Journal of Radiology*, vol. 82, no. 983, pp. 920–929, 2009.

[2] J. A. Seibert and J. M. Boone, "X-ray imaging physics for nuclear medicine technologists—part 2: x-ray interactions and image formation," *Journal of Nuclear Medicine Technology*, vol. 33, no. 1, pp. 3–18, 2005.

[3] C. H. Yan, R. T. Whalen, G. S. Beaupré, S. Y. Yen, and S. Napel, "Reconstruction algorithm for polychromatic CT imaging: application to beam hardening correction," *IEEE Transactions on Medical Imaging*, vol. 19, no. 1, pp. 1–11, 2000.

[4] E. van de Casteele, D. van Dyck, J. Sijbers, and E. Raman, "An energy-based beam hardening model in tomography," *Physics in Medicine and Biology*, vol. 47, no. 23, pp. 4181–4190, 2002.

[5] M. Kachelrieß, K. Sourbelle, and W. A. Kalender, "Empirical cupping correction: a first-order raw data precorrection for cone-beam computed tomography," *Medical Physics*, vol. 33, no. 5, pp. 1269–1274, 2006.

[6] N. Mail, D. J. Moseley, J. H. Siewerdsen, and D. A. Jaffray, "The influence of bowtie filtration on cone-beam CT image quality," *Medical Physics*, vol. 36, no. 1, pp. 22–32, 2009.

[7] X. Q. Mou, S. J. Tang, and H. Y. Yu A Beam, "Hardening Correction Method Based on HL Consistency," vol. 6318 of *Proceedings of SPIE*, 63181U, 2006.

[8] A. E. Idris and J. A. Fessler, "Segmentation-free statistical image reconstruction for polyenergetic x-ray computed tomography with experimental validation," *Physics in Medicine and Biology*, vol. 48, no. 15, pp. 2453–2477, 2003.

[9] A. J. Coleman and M. Sinclair, "A beam-hardening correction using dual-energy computed tomography," *Physics in Medicine and Biology*, vol. 30, no. 11, pp. 1251–1256, 1985.

[10] L. Ritschl, F. Bergner, C. Fleischmann, and M. Kachelriess, "Water calibration for CT scanners with tube voltage modulation," *Physics in medicine and biology*, vol. 55, no. 14, pp. 4107–4117, 2010.

[11] http://www.nist.gov/pml/data/xraycoef/index.cfm.

22

Acoustic Angiography: A New Imaging Modality for Assessing Microvasculature Architecture

Ryan C. Gessner,[1] C. Brandon Frederick,[1] F. Stuart Foster,[2] and Paul A. Dayton[1]

[1] UNC and NCSU Joint Department of Biomedical Engineering, 304 Taylor Hall, 109 Mason Farm Road, Chapel Hill, NC 27599-6136, USA
[2] Department of Medical Biophysics, University of Toronto, Sunnybrook Health Sciences Centre, 2075 Bayview Avenue, Toronto, ON, Canada M4N 3M5

Correspondence should be addressed to Paul A. Dayton; padayton@bme.unc.edu

Academic Editor: Jun Zhao

The purpose of this paper is to provide the biomedical imaging community with details of a new high resolution contrast imaging approach referred to as "acoustic angiography." Through the use of dual-frequency ultrasound transducer technology, images acquired with this approach possess both high resolution and a high contrast-to-tissue ratio, which enables the visualization of microvascular architecture without significant contribution from background tissues. Additionally, volumetric vessel-tissue integration can be visualized by using b-mode overlays acquired with the same probe. We present a brief technical overview of how the images are acquired, followed by several examples of images of both healthy and diseased tissue volumes. 3D images from alternate modalities often used in preclinical imaging, contrast-enhanced micro-CT and photoacoustics, are also included to provide a perspective on how acoustic angiography has qualitatively similar capabilities to these other techniques. These preliminary images provide visually compelling evidence to suggest that acoustic angiography may serve as a powerful new tool in preclinical and future clinical imaging.

1. Introduction

Blood vessel structure and patency are known to be related to the state and progression of many diseases [1, 2]. Abnormal vessel and vessel network morphologies have been positively correlated to malignancy across species [3, 4]. In preclinical studies of the disease and drug research, there are several noninvasive imaging modalities that can be utilized to visualize blood vessel structure. These are magnetic resonance imaging (MRI), computed tomography (CT), ultrasound, and more recently—photoacoustic imaging. To select one of these imaging methods, researchers must compromise between the variables of system including study cost, data acquisition time, ionizing radiation dose, imaging depth, and image resolution. High-field MRI is the most expensive, requires the longest acquisition times, and requires a dedicated facility for shielding and maintenance. CT is also fairly expensive, bulky, and primarily limited by a high ionizing radiation dose. Ultrasound is the least expensive, the most

portable, and provides the fastest image acquisition. Photoacoustic imaging has similar portability to ultrasound and can provide high resolution images of the microvasculature as well as additional functional information (such as blood oxygen saturation), but is the most limited in penetration depth among these modalities.

In the past, the reputation of ultrasound has been as a modality with limited ability to assess microvasculature structure. However, recent advances in high frequency ultrasound technology have substantially improved image quality to the point that it has become a favored technique for many researchers studying small animal models. While conventional high frequency ultrasound does still lack the resolution and contrast of recently published CT [5] and MR studies [6], it has been effectively implemented to monitor disease progression and therapeutic responses in many different cancer models, including pancreatic [7], prostate [8], melanoma [9], ovarian [10], lung [11], and mammary [12] cancer models.

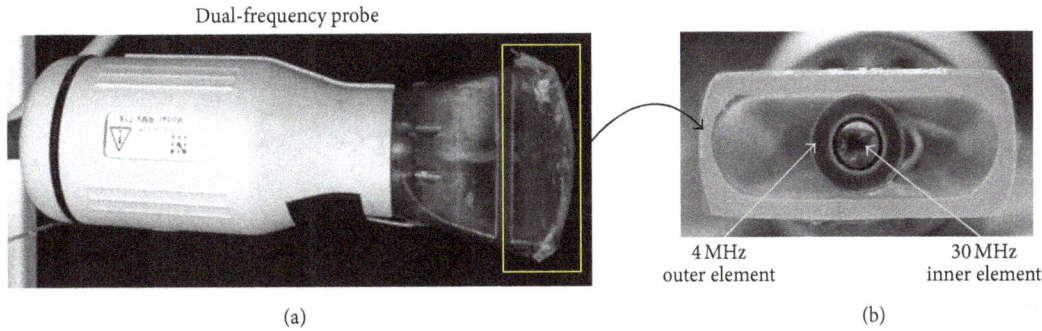

FIGURE 1: Photograph of the dual-frequency probe, illustrating the side view (a) and the bottom view (b) showing the two transducer elements. The probe housing is a modified VisualSonics "RMV" transducer housing.

Traditional noncontrast-enhanced ultrasound excels at imaging anatomical features, but is challenged when imaging blood flow in small vessels due to weak ultrasound scatter from blood components. Thus, for imaging blood flow in small vessels with high sensitivity, clinical ultrasound relies on the application of intravascular microbubble contrast agents (MCAs). Because of the nonlinear behavior of MCAs in response to an ultrasound pulse, their acoustic scatter can be detected and separated from tissue enabling image and signal processing techniques to segment blood vessels from the tissue background. Most nonlinear imaging techniques are most efficient near the resonant frequencies of microbubble contrast agents, typically less than 10 MHz, which is a good match for clinical ultrasound imaging applications. However, for the improved imaging resolution required in small-animal imaging, high frequency ultrasound systems typically utilize frequencies in the 20–60 MHz range, substantially above the resonant frequencies for most microbubbles. Typically, high frequency imaging systems have been challenged to perform nonlinear contrast imaging for this reason.

Here, we report the technique of high resolution microvascular imaging using a prototype dual-frequency transducer which enables vascular imaging with both high contrast sensitivity and imaging resolution. With this technology, the above-mentioned resolution versus contrast-sensitivity tradeoff can be partially circumvented by detecting the high frequency components from the wideband acoustic energy produced by MCAs when they are excited at low frequencies near their resonance. The potential of this technique was initially demonstrated by Kruse and Ferrara [13], where it was observed that microbubbles excited with short pulses at 2.25 MHz produced broadband energy that exceeded 45 MHz. The main challenge of this approach to date, however, has been the lack of available transducers that could transmit energy at low frequencies (such as 2–4 MHz) to excite microbubbles and, at the same time confocally detect scattered echoes in the 15–45 MHz bandwidth.

Our prototype transducer consists of both low and high frequency confocal elements, in contrast to standard ultrasound imaging transducers which typically operate within a single frequency range. The low frequency element (4 MHz) excites MCAs near their resonance, and the high frequency element (30 MHz) receives high frequency content from the excited microbubbles. The broadly separated frequency bandwidths of the two elements used in our system are what differentiate this approach from the dual-frequency probes previously presented by other groups [14–16] and are what enable its high resolution and high contrast imaging ability. This approach enables detection of signal from microbubble contrast with almost complete tissue suppression. Furthermore, because of the high frequency receive, the system is able to achieve high resolution, yet with less attenuation than systems operating with high frequency on both transmit and receive. The resulting ultrasound images illustrate high resolution depictions of the microvasculature, without background from surrounding tissue, not unlike X-ray angiography images. Furthermore, through use of traditional single-frequency pulse-echo, tissue b-mode images can be acquired for anatomical reference. Thus, we refer to images acquired with this technology as "acoustic angiography". In this paper we discuss the prototype transducer and present example of high resolution in vivo 3D images, discussing how these images could be used for diagnostics. For qualitative comparison, we also provide contrast-enhanced CT and photoacoustic images to illustrate that acoustic angiography could be considered as an alternative to these other techniques.

2. Materials and Methods

2.1. Prototype Imaging System. The custom dual-frequency transducer was fabricated by integrating a high frequency broadband 30 MHz transducer element (RMV 707, VisualSonics, Toronto, ON, Canada) with a concentric low frequency 4 MHz annulus (Figure 1), as previously described [17]. The radius of curvature for the 4 MHz element was 12.7 mm, which matched that of the 30 MHz receiver element for overlapping depth of field. The selection of the 30 MHz element was made to ensure that both rats and mice could be imaged with good spatial resolution, while the 4 MHz pulsing frequency was selected because it is near the resonance frequency of many of the contrast agents utilized by our lab. It is likely that other frequency ranges would be optimal for other contrast agents, or applications that require different depths of penetration. The electrical return path from both elements was isolated so that the transmitter could be driven by an external pulser. To drive the system, we utilized a commonly implemented high frequency preclinical Vevo770 ultrasound scanner (VisualSonics, Toronto, ON, Canada) that had been modified to work with our custom dual-frequency probe. The Vevo770 was altered by insertion of a 10 MHz high-pass filter (TTE, Los Angeles, CA, USA) after the receiver amplifier but before analog to digital conversion. This served to ensure that no tissue signal leaked into the data during dual-frequency imaging. The trigger was synchronized to an external arbitrary waveform generator (AWG 2021, Tektronix, Beaverton, OR, USA) to drive the low frequency element. Signals from the waveform generator were amplified by 55 dB through a RF amplifier (ENI, Rochester, NY, USA) before exciting the transmitter.

2.2. Characterization of the Probe. Beam-field mapping with a needle hydrophone enabled determination of the −6 dB beamwidths of the transmit and receive transducer (Figure 2). The −6 dB lateral beamwidth for the 4 MHz element was 298 μm, and the −6 dB lateral beamwidth for the 30 MHz element was 137 μm. During this procedure, it was observed that the two elements were not exactly confocal, and the lateral focal zones were actually misaligned by 90 μm. Thus, the −6 dB focal spot of the 30 MHz element was centered along the edge of the −6 dB focal spot of the 4 MHz transducer (Figure 2(c)). This misalignment was due to the challenge of the manufacturing process and will be an area for improvement in future prototypes. The axial −6 dB beamwidths of the two transducers were 7.05 mm and 1.99 mm, for 4 MHz and 30 MHz, respectively. The focal spot misalignment in the axial direction was only 0.9 mm. It is anticipated that with correction to these misalignments, future probes will be able to provide similar or improved sensitivity at reduced excitation energies.

Transmission with the high frequency (30 MHz) element allowed traditional high frequency b-mode imaging in order to obtain anatomical images, whereas transmission with the low frequency (4 MHz) element enabled Acoustic Angiography to obtain contrast only images.

Both the 4 MHz and 30 MHz transducers had approximately 100% bandwidth. A frequency domain representation approximating the probe's two transducer bandwidths, the filter cutoff, and example tissue and microbubble responses can be found in Figure 3.

Images were acquired and saved on the ultrasound system, then later exported for offline analysis. All images were acquired in 3D image using a linear translational motor stage synchronized with the frame trigger.

2.3. Animal Imaging. All animal studies were performed in rats with a protocol approved by the University of North Carolina at Chapel Hill Institutional Animal Care and Use Committee. Seven animals were imaged for this study: three animals with a flank tumor model, three healthy controls imaged in the same region, and one animal imaged for

a healthy kidney for comparison to contrast-enhanced CT imaging. The tumor model (syngeneic fibrosarcoma: "FSA"; [18]) was initiated by propagating tumor tissue through subcutaneous implant in the rodent flank. Initial tumor samples were graciously provided by the Dewhirst Lab at Duke University. The acoustic angiography strategy necessitates the use of contrast agents to provide signal from the vasculature. In these studies, microbubble contrast agent with a polydisperse diameter distribution centered at 0.9 μm with a standard deviation of 0.45 μm was prepared as previously described [19]. Microbubble contrast was diluted in saline and administered via a tail vein catheter with a syringe pump at 70 μL/min at a concentration of $3.3 \cdot 10^9$ bubbles/mL. The administration of contrast began 20 seconds prior to imaging; this waiting period would be sufficient to for the initial bolus of contrast to perfuse the tissue prior to image acquisition. Imaging pulses were 4 MHz single cycle sinusoids with a peak negative pressure of 1.23 MPa (mechanical index = 0.62). 3D ultrasound images were acquired with interplane step sizes of 150–200 μm and required fewer than 3 minutes to acquire. Since the tissues of interest were in the lower abdomen and flank, respiratory motion artifacts were limited. Acquisition of all ultrasound images was coplanar with the axial anatomical plane while the animals were in dorsal recumbency.

The CT images were acquired of the rat kidney 45 minutes after the injection of contrast. The contrast agent implemented was Fenestra VC (Advanced Research Technologies, Montreal, QC, Canada), an iodinated lipid blood pool CT contrast agent injected at a concentration of 3 mL/450 g tissue. CT images were acquired using the GE eXplore SpeCZT CT 120 SPECT/CT (GE Healthcare, London, ON, Canada) at 90 kVp using 900 views over 360 degrees with total output 576 mAs. The total dose delivered was 300 mGy. Reconstruction was performed on 100 μm isotropic grid with a standard Feldkamp-Davis-Kress algorithm.

The photoacoustic images were reproduced with permission from work by Zhang et al. [20]. That study implemented a photoacoustics system using an excitation wavelength of 590 nm, a 38 μm thick polymer ultrasound transducer with a −3 dB acoustic bandwidth of 22 MHz, and a frequency response characterized by a smooth roll-off with its zero response occurring at 58 MHz [20].

3. Results

Imaging studies with our dual-frequency transducer immediately demonstrated a new paradigm in ultrasound imaging. Images illustrated signal from contrast only, with virtually no tissue signal (Figure 4). The result was images of tissue microvascular structure; hence, we refer to this technique as "acoustic angiography."

One likely application of acoustic angiography is visualization of tumor microvascular structure with anatomical reference. Figure 5(a) illustrates the ability of the probe to acquire both vascular images and tissue images of the same in vivo sample volume. Vessels imaged in acoustic angiography mode are overlaid with the traditional high-frequency

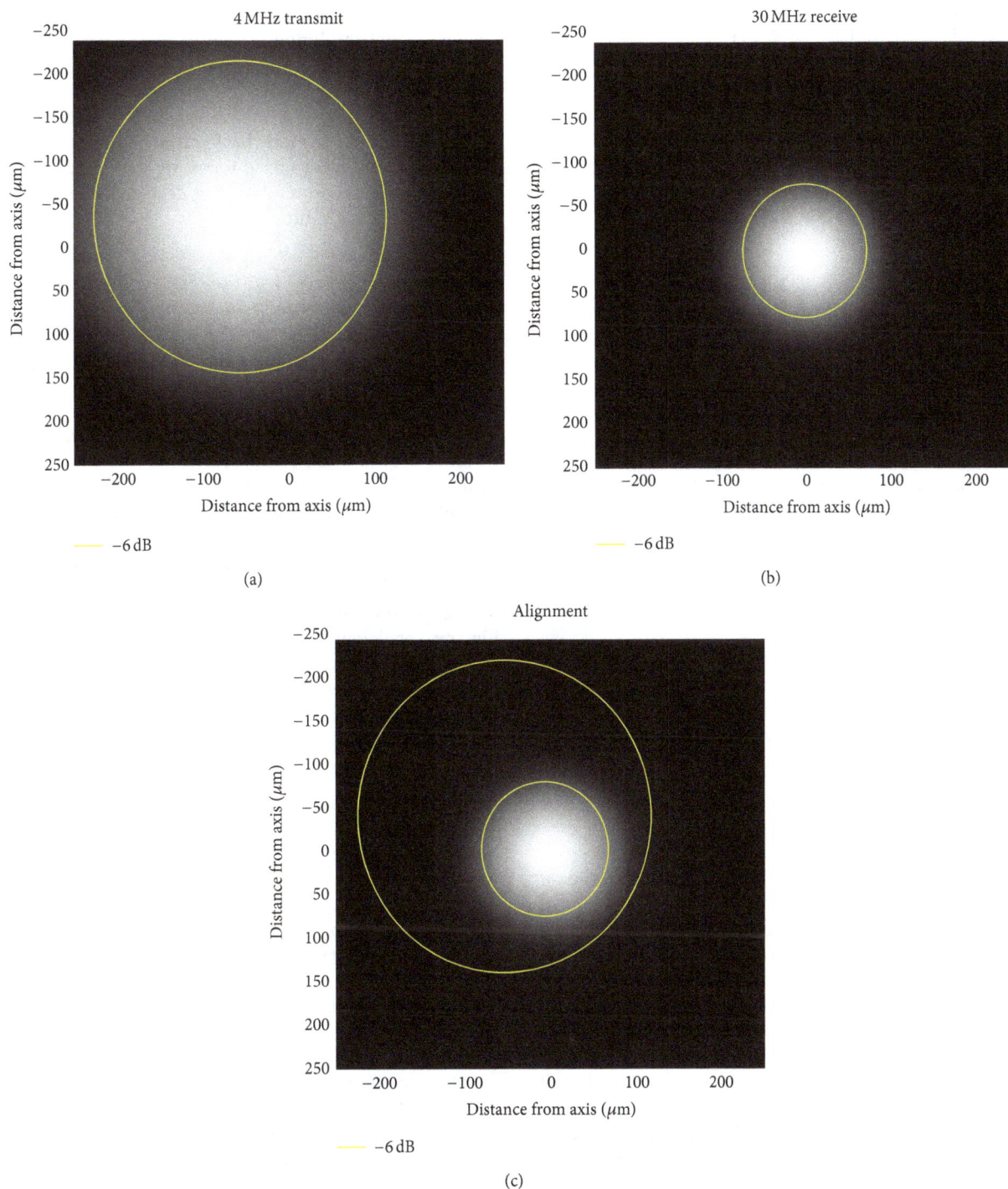

FIGURE 2: Beam plots showing the −6 dB beamwidth for the (a) 4 MHz (298 μm) and (b) 30 MHz (137 μm) elements. Panel (c) illustrates the confocal alignment of the transducers, where the circles approximate the −6 dB regions of the two transducers. There was a misalignment of approximately 90 μm of the two transducers on this prototype probe due to the challenge of the manufacturing process. Improving the element focal alignment is an obvious way to improve the performance of this system in future iterations.

b-mode image, thereby enabling the visualization and spatial characterization of vessel-tissue integration.

Figure 6 depicts both b-mode and acoustic angiography images of the microvasculature surrounding two different tumors versus microvasculature from two normal tissue volumes. Differences between the vascular architecture within these two types of tissue volumes are observable. Highly tortuous vessel structure is typical of angiogenic tumor vasculature [3, 4] and is not observed with as much frequency in the data for the healthy flank as it is in the

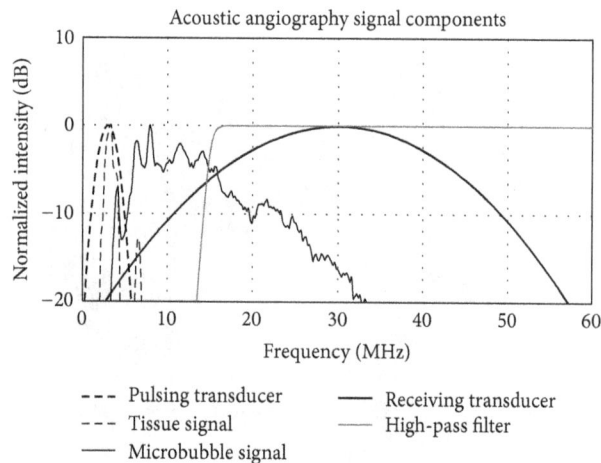

FIGURE 3: A frequency domain representation of the signals of all transmit and receive components of acoustic angiography imaging. The tissue and bubble responses were acquired using an experimental system described previously [17] and are displayed here to illustrate the relationship between the bandwidths and the two transducer elements as well as the tissue and bubble responses, for example, acoustic angiography imaging conditions.

tumor-bearing tissue volumes (Figure 6). Further analysis of microvasculature morphology is outside of the scope of this introductory paper, though these images provide compelling evidence of the possibility of applying this imaging technique toward quantitative approaches to assessing vessel architecture.

3.1. Acoustic Angiography in Comparison to Photoacoustic Imaging. Currently, photoacoustics is the gold standard noninvasive imaging technique for visualizing superficial microvascular structure. However, acoustic angiography has the potential to acquire similar images of microvessel networks. To qualitatively compare acoustic angiography images against images acquired with a photoacoustic imaging system, we present data of subcutaneous microvasculature in rodents with both imaging methods. Figure 7(a) illustrates vasculature in the lower abdomen of a rat acquired with contrast ultrasound at transmit 4 MHz and at 30 MHz receive. Figure 7(b) illustrates vasculature in the abdomen of a mouse obtained by photoacoustics as acquired by Zhang et al. [20]. In this image, the photoacoustic resolution was approximately 90 μm (depth) by 130 μm (lateral), and the imaging depth of field was 2 mm. The acoustic angiography images are of lower resolution (approximately 150 μm (depth) by 200 μm (lateral)); however, they illustrate a greater depth of penetration in this particular data set (5 mm in this case). Note that this comparison is not intended to suggest that one modality has superior resolution or penetration depth than the other; however, rather, our goal is to illustrate that acoustic angiography provides pulse-echo ultrasound with a method to achieve maps of vascular structure on a resolution and depth scale which were previously only available through photoacoustics. Although not presented

here, newer photoacoustics techniques have illustrated sub-100 μm spatial resolution at depths of almost 10 mm [21]. Similarly, we estimate that acoustic angiography could be achieved at depths up to several centimeters by reducing the receiving frequency, albeit at the expense of a reduced spatial resolution and with more background noise from tissue. Due to our transducer's fixed focus, we were unable to fully characterize limits on resolution at deeper depths, although this will be a focus of future work.

3.2. Acoustic Angiography in Comparison to Micro-CT. We also qualitatively compared acoustic angiography to contrast-enhanced CT, which has also been used for microvascular imaging. Coronal maximum intensity projections (MIPs) through the ultrasound and CT acquisitions of the same kidney were performed (Figure 8). The CT dataset was reconstructed with a 100 μm voxel grid, which resulted in an improved SNR, compared to the ultrasound image's 50 μm voxel grid. Despite the slightly lower resolution of the ultrasound, previously measured to be approximately 150 μm [17], the two imaging techniques illustrate similar anatomical microvascular features within the rat kidney. This is illustrated within the line profiles in Figure 8(c). These profiles were intensity normalized for display purposes and illustrate analogous spatial resolutions, albeit with slightly higher noise in the ultrasound signal. This increase in noise is expected, due to the 63% smaller voxel size in the ultrasound image (50 × 50 × 150 μm compared to the CT's 100 × 100 × 100 μm voxels).

4. Discussion and Summary

The new contrast imaging technology demonstrated herein, which we refer to as acoustic angiography, has the capability to obtain images of microbubbles at high frequencies traditionally not utilized for nonlinear contrast imaging. The resulting images thus illustrate high resolution (~150 μm) contrast-enhanced images of superficial microvasculature. Due to the tissue suppression achieved by detection of only harmonic energy well above the range produced by tissue, the resulting data also illustrates a high contrast-to-tissue ratio.

Our prototype transducer utilized a 4 MHz transmit, selected to take advantage of the resonant frequencies of the contrast agents utilized in our lab and 30 MHz receive for rodent imaging. It is likely that other transmit and receive combinations would be more optimal for other contrast agents, or for different depths of penetration. The tradeoff between resolution, depth of penetration, and signal separation are limitations of the acoustic angiography imaging approach. As with all high frequency ultrasound imaging methods, penetration depth is limited to a few centimeters due to the increased absorption of sound at high frequencies. One-way attenuation may be an advantage of this technique, as the high frequency components are only attenuated on receive since the bubble acts as the source. However, this is also a limitation as there is limit to how aggressively the microbubbles can be driven. In a prior study with detection of high-frequency content from microbubbles received with a

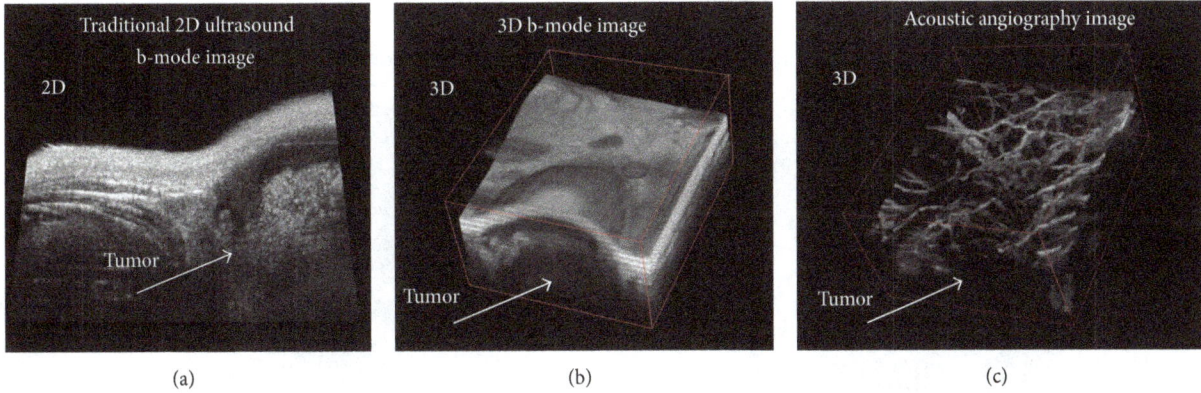

FIGURE 4: (a) 2D and (b) 3D "b-mode" ultrasound images from the same sample volume illustrating a subcutaneous tumor in a rat. (c) "acoustic angiography" image of the same sample volume as (b) acquired with dual-frequency transducer, illustrating contrast-only image, depicting microvasculature.

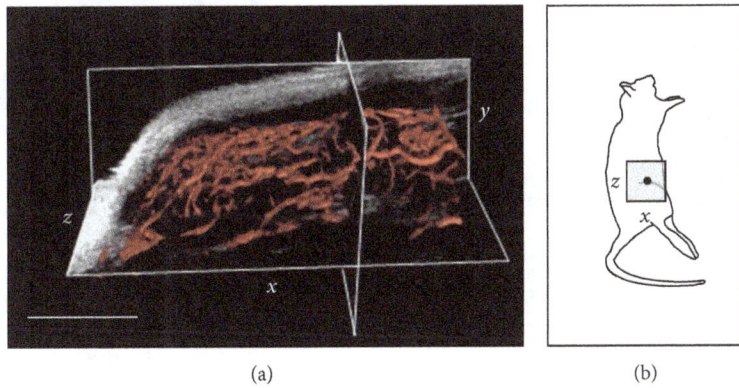

FIGURE 5: (a) An overlay of the microvasculature within a tumor provided by acoustic angiography (red) onto a tissue-only image provided by high frequency b-mode (grayscale). This figure was created using 3D slicer (National Institutes of Health) with a 3D rendering of the acoustic angiography data simultaneously displayed with a grayscale orthoslice of the b-mode data. Displaying data in this fashion illustrates microvessel and tissue morphologies, as well as vascular-tissue integration. Scale bar = 0.5 cm. (b) A cartoon illustrates the approximate location of this 3D image volume.

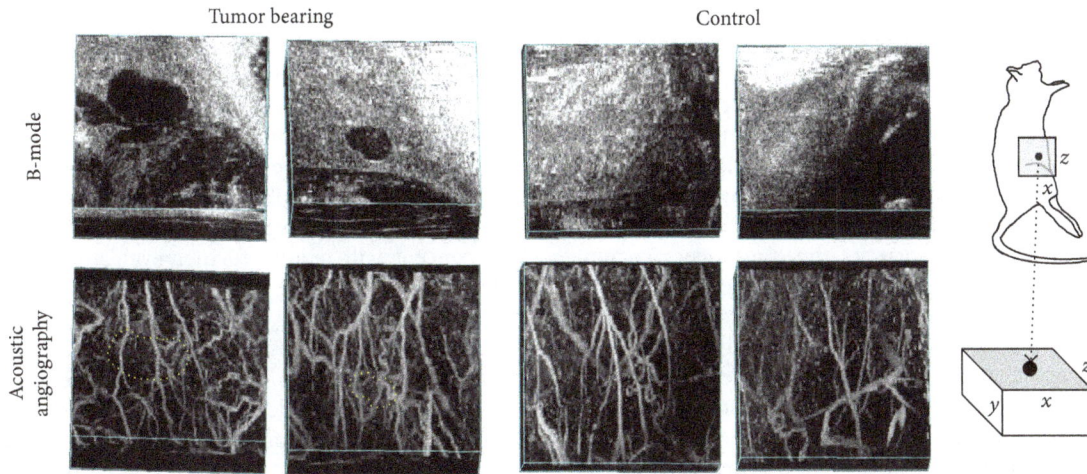

FIGURE 6: Multiple comparisons of 3D tissue volumes: two containing a tumor (left) and two healthy controls (right). The bottom images are acoustic angiography maximum intensity projections, while the top images are b-mode acquisitions of the same tissue volumes. The tortuous and chaotic morphologies of the vessels in the presence of a lesion are contrasted by the relatively homogeneous vasculature in the healthy volume (tumor boundaries delineated in acoustic angiography image with dotted line). Image volumes = ~0.75 × 1.25 × 1.5 cm (axial, lateral, and elevational). A cartoon on the right indicates the imaging location and orientations of image volumes.

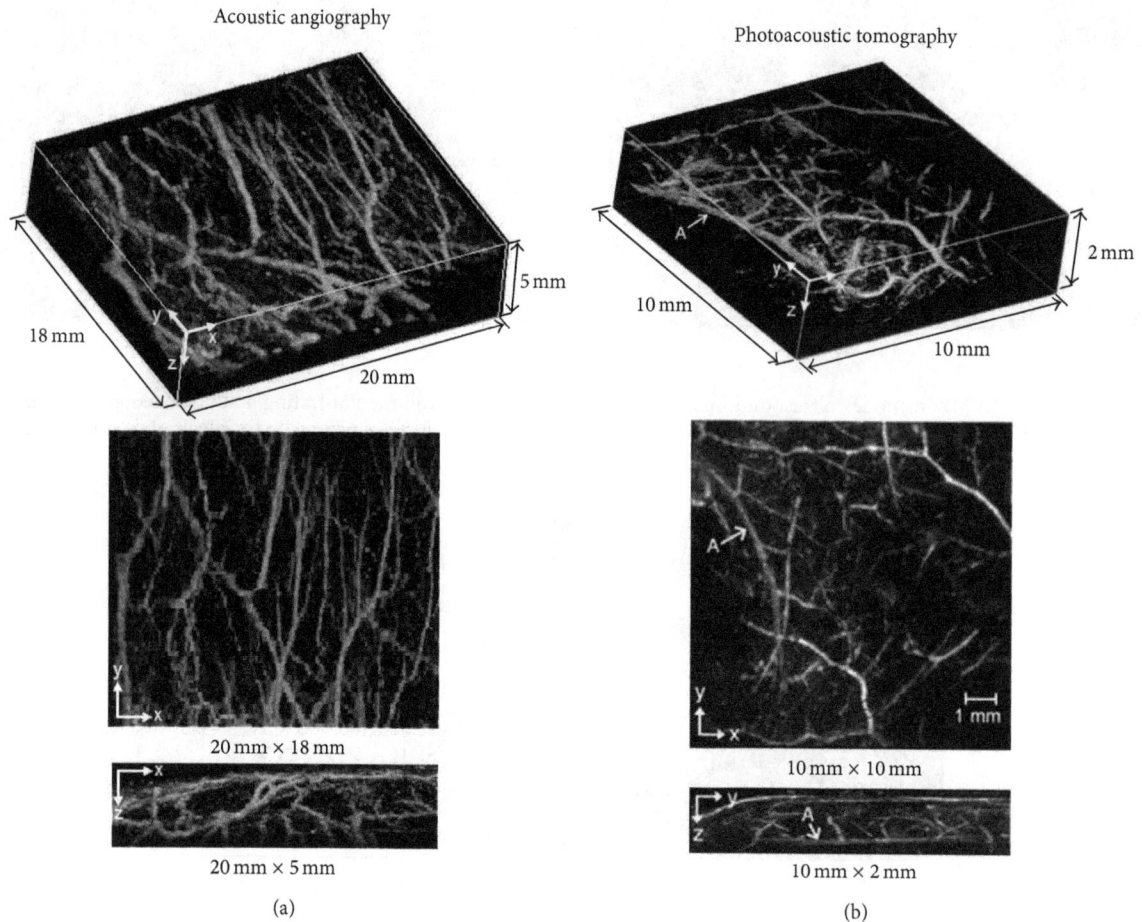

FIGURE 7: Comparison of acoustic angiography (a) to a photoacoustic imaging approach (b). The orientations of the acoustic angiography images have been purposefully arranged to mimic the photoacoustic images (adapted, with permission, from authors [20]) to allow a quick comparison between the two modalities. The imaging location of the acoustic angiography image was similar to that presented in Figure 6.

similar 30 MHz transducer, it was observed that microbubble signal in response to 2 MHz excitation increased until an MI of approximately 0.45, after which it leveled out, likely when microbubble destruction began to dominate [17]. As the receiving frequency is reduced, penetration depth increases, yet our ability to separate signal from tissue and contrast is also reduced. For our prototype probe, an additional limitation was the fixed focus of the transducer's current form factor, which also provided a fairly narrow depth of field (~1 cm). Dual or multifrequency arrays with dynamic focusing will alleviate this problem in the future.

We suggest that acoustic angiography could perform similarly to micro-CT, MRI, or photoacoustic imaging in certain scenarios. Ultrasound imaging can be low cost and high throughput and avoids some of the drawbacks of CT and MR, such as ionizing radiation dose (CT), and high cost, and long acquisition times (MR). Both photoacoustic imaging and acoustic angiography have similar tradeoffs between resolution and depth of penetration. However, photoacoustic imaging has the additional advantages that it does not require a contrast agent, and that photoacoustic data can be used

to derive other parameters about the target tissue, such as oxygen saturation. However, acoustic angiography may present an advantage of cost and simplicity over photoacoustics, since the latter requires a high power laser for signal generation. Furthermore, it might also be possible to combine acoustic angiography with targeted microbubbles for molecular imaging coregistered with microvascular features. This concept will require further evaluation to determine if acoustic angiography can be performed at low enough energies as to not destroy adherent targeted contrast agents.

The suppression of tissue signal and microvascular imaging ability demonstrated by the images within this paper provide motivation for the development of additional transducer designs to implement acoustic angiography. One obvious application of acoustic angiography is as a high throughput imaging technique for preclinical studies where there is a need for microvascular analysis, since the imaging resolution and depth are well suited to image rodents.

Preclinical arrays could be designed for larger animal models, such as for rabbit or dog imaging. It is possible that in each of these clinical and preclinical applications the

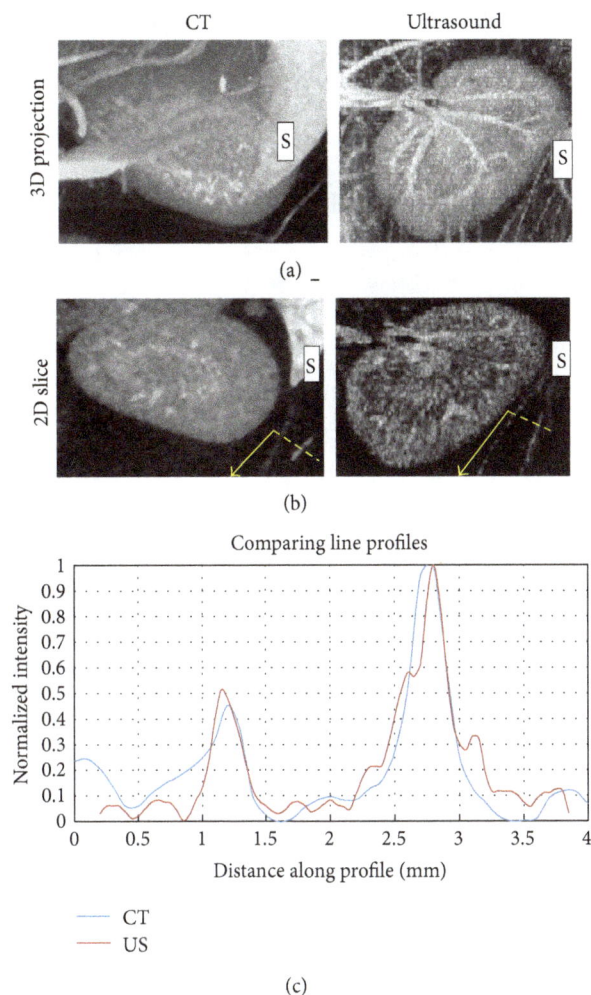

FIGURE 8: A comparison between the CT and ultrasound images acquired of the same kidney. The slight anatomical warping due to ultrasound probe contact with tissue resulted in a lack of direct one-to-one visual correspondence between the two 3D images, though the same anatomy is contained within each image. (a) Maximum intensity projections of image data. The spleen is visible in each of these images to the right of kidney (indicated with an "S"). (b) En face cuts through the 3D image. (c) Line profiles (dashed yellow lines) across two corresponding vessels near the spleen (dashed yellow lines) suggest similar feature sensitivity.

presence of disease-associated vascular abnormalities could be detected by acoustic angiography, as could the modifications to these vascular networks (such as the elimination or normalization of tumor vasculature) by effective therapeutic regimens. In the future, this technique may also find a role in clinical imaging of superficial tissues or tumors.

Clinical implementation of this technique will depend on both the commercialization of appropriate hardware, as well as the increased regulatory acceptance of ultrasound contrast. While microbubbles are utilized for several oncology applications in Europe and Asia, they are still only approved for use by the United States Food and Drug Administration for cardiac applications. Nevertheless, data suggest that ultrasound contrast agents are very safe [22, 23], and it is

likely that contrast ultrasound techniques will continue to gain increasing approval worldwide as they evolve to provide new information beyond that attainable with noncontrast techniques.

Conflict of Interests

F. Stuart Foster is a consultant and receives research funding from VisualSonics Inc. Ryan C. Gessner, F. Stuart Foster, and Paul A. Dayton are inventors on a pending patent describing the acoustic angiography technology. The authors declare that they have no conflict of interests with any other companies listed in this paper.

Acknowledgments

The authors would like to acknowledge Dr. James Tsuruta for his fabrication of the microbubble contrast agents used in this study. The authors appreciate the efforts of Marc Lukacs, Mike Lee, and Emmanuel Cherin, who contributed to the design of the prototype transducer utilized here. Funding for this work was provided by the NSF-GRFP (Ryan C. Gessner), NCI grant P30-CA016086 (C. Brandon Frederick), and NIH grants R01EB009066, R01CA170665, and R43CA165621 (Paul A. Dayton). F. Stuart Foster acknowledges the support from the Canadian Institutes of Health Research, The Ontario Research Fund, and VisualSonics.

References

[1] P. Carmeliet, "Angiogenesis in life, disease and medicine," *Nature*, vol. 438, no. 7070, pp. 932–936, 2005.

[2] M. Egeblad, E. S. Nakasone, and Z. Werb, "Tumors as organs: complex tissues that interface with the entire organism," *Developmental Cell*, vol. 18, no. 6, pp. 884–901, 2010.

[3] E. Bullitt, M. Ewend, J. Vredenburgh et al., "Computerized assessment of vessel morphological changes during treatment of glioblastoma multiforme: report of a case imaged serially by MRA over four years," *NeuroImage*, vol. 47, no. 2, pp. T143–T151, 2009.

[4] C.-Y. Li, S. Shan, Q. Huang et al., "Initial stages of tumor cell-induced angiogenesis: evaluation via skin window chambers in rodent models," *Journal of the National Cancer Institute*, vol. 92, no. 2, pp. 143–147, 2000.

[5] S. J. Schambach, S. Bag, C. Groden, L. Schilling, and M. A. Brockmann, "Vascular imaging in small rodents using micro-CT," *Methods*, vol. 50, no. 1, pp. 26–35, 2010.

[6] S. E. Ungersma, G. Pacheco, C. Ho et al., "Vessel imaging with viable tumor analysis for quantification of tumor angiogenesis," *Magnetic Resonance in Medicine*, vol. 63, no. 6, pp. 1637–1647, 2010.

[7] G. Korpanty, J. G. Carbon, P. A. Grayburn, J. B. Fleming, and R. A. Brekken, "Monitoring response to anticancer therapy by targeting microbubbles to tumor vasculature," *Clinical Cancer Research*, vol. 13, no. 1, pp. 323–330, 2007.

[8] J. W. Xuan, M. Bygrave, H. Jiang et al., "Functional neoangiogenesis imaging of genetically engineered mouse prostate cancer using three-dimensional power doppler ultrasound," *Cancer Research*, vol. 67, no. 6, pp. 2830–2839, 2007.

[9] A. M. Y. Cheung, A. S. Brown, V. Cucevic et al., "Detecting vascular changes in tumour xenografts using micro-ultrasound and micro-CT following treatment with VEGFR-2 blocking antibodies," *Ultrasound in Medicine and Biology*, vol. 33, no. 8, pp. 1259–1268, 2007.

[10] A. Barua, P. Bitterman, J. M. Bahr et al., "Detection of tumor-associated neoangiogenesis by doppler ultrasonography during early-stage ovarian cancer in laying hens: a preclinical model of human spontaneous ovarian cancer," *Journal of Ultrasound in Medicine*, vol. 29, no. 2, pp. 173–182, 2010.

[11] K. J. Niermann, A. C. Fleischer, J. Huamani et al., "Measuring tumor perfusion in control and treated murine tumors: correlation of microbubble contrast-enhanced sonography to dynamic contrast-enhanced magnetic resonance imaging and fluorodeoxyglucose positron emission tomography," *Journal of Ultrasound in Medicine*, vol. 26, no. 6, pp. 749–756, 2007.

[12] K. Hoyt, J. M. Warram, H. Umphrey et al., "Determination of breast cancer response to bevacizumab therapy using contrast-enhanced ultrasound and artificial neural networks," *Journal of Ultrasound in Medicine*, vol. 29, no. 4, pp. 577–585, 2010.

[13] D. E. Kruse and K. W. Ferrara, "A new imaging strategy using wideband transient response of ultrasound contrast agents," *IEEE Transactions on Ultrasonics, Ferroelectrics, and Frequency Control*, vol. 52, no. 8, pp. 1320–1329, 2005.

[14] A. Bouakaz, B. J. Krenning, W. B. Vletter, F. J. Ten Cate, and N. De Jong, "Contrast superharmonic imaging: A Feasibility Study," *Ultrasound in Medicine and Biology*, vol. 29, no. 4, pp. 547–553, 2003.

[15] C.-K. Yen, S.-Y. Su, C.-C. Shen, and M.-N. Li, "Dual high-frequency difference excitation for contrast detection," *IEEE Transactions on Ultrasonics, Ferroelectrics, and Frequency Control*, vol. 55, no. 10, pp. 2164–2176, 2008.

[16] D. N. Stephens, D. E. Kruse, A. S. Ergun, S. Barnes, X. M. Lu, and K. W. Ferrara, "Efficient array design for sonotherapy," *Physics in Medicine and Biology*, vol. 53, no. 14, pp. 3943–3969, 2008.

[17] R. Gessner, M. Lukacs, M. Lee, E. Cherin, F. S. Foster, and P. A. Dayton, "High-resolution, high-contrast ultrasound imaging using a prototype dual-frequency transducer: in vitro and in vivo studies," *IEEE Transactions on Ultrasonics, Ferroelectrics, and Frequency Control*, vol. 57, no. 8, pp. 1772–1781, 2010.

[18] H. Yuan, T. Schroeder, J. E. Bowsher, L. W. Hedlund, T. Wong, and M. W. Dewhirst, "Intertumoral differences in hypoxia selectivity of the PET imaging agent64Cu(II)-diacetyl-bis(N4-methylthiosemicarbazone)," *Journal of Nuclear Medicine*, vol. 47, no. 6, pp. 989–998, 2006.

[19] J. E. Streeter, R. Gessner, I. Miles, and P. A. Dayton, "Improving sensitivity in ultrasound molecular imaging by tailoring contrast agent size distribution: in vivo studies," *Molecular Imaging*, vol. 9, no. 2, pp. 87–95, 2010.

[20] E. Z. Zhang, J. G. Laufer, R. B. Pedley, and P. C. Beard, "In vivo high-resolution 3D photoacoustic imaging of superficial vascular anatomy," *Physics in Medicine and Biology*, vol. 54, no. 4, pp. 1035–1046, 2009.

[21] J. Laufer, P. Johnson, E. Zhang et al., "In vivo preclinical photoacoustic imaging of tumor vasculature development and therapy," *Journal of Biomedical Optics*, vol. 17, no. 5, article 056016, 2012.

[22] S. S. Abdelmoneim, M. Bernier, C. G. Scott et al., "Safety of contrast agent use during stress echocardiography in patients with elevated right ventricular systolic pressure: A Cohort Study," *Circulation*, vol. 3, no. 3, pp. 240–248, 2010.

[23] S. S. Abdelmoneim, M. Bernier, C. G. Scott et al., "Safety of contrast agent use during stress echocardiography. A 4-Year experience from a single-center cohort study of 26,774 Patients," *Journal of the American College of Cardiology*, vol. 2, no. 9, pp. 1048–1056, 2009.

23

Blind Deconvolution for Ultrasound Sequences Using a Noninverse Greedy Algorithm

Liviu-Teodor Chira,[1,2] **Corneliu Rusu,**[2] **Clovis Tauber,**[1] **and Jean-Marc Girault**[1]

[1] *Signal & Imaging Group, University François Rabelais of Tours, PRES Loire Valley University, UMR INSERM U930, 7 Avenue Marcel Dassault, 37200 Tours Cedex, France*
[2] *Faculty of Electronics, Telecommunications and Information Theory, Technical University of Cluj-Napoca, Cluj-Napoca 400027, Romania*

Correspondence should be addressed to Jean-Marc Girault; jean-marc.girault@univ-tours.fr

Academic Editor: Guowei Wei

The blind deconvolution of ultrasound sequences in medical ultrasound technique is still a major problem despite the efforts made. This paper presents a blind noninverse deconvolution algorithm to eliminate the blurring effect, using the envelope of the acquired radio-frequency sequences and *a priori* Laplacian distribution for deconvolved signal. The algorithm is executed in two steps. Firstly, the point spread function is automatically estimated from the measured data. Secondly, the data are reconstructed in a nonblind way using proposed algorithm. The algorithm is a nonlinear blind deconvolution which works as a greedy algorithm. The results on simulated signals and real images are compared with different state of the art methods deconvolution. Our method shows good results for scatters detection, speckle noise suppression, and execution time.

1. Introduction

Medical ultrasound imaging is considered to be one of the edge technologies in noninvasive diagnose procedures. Despite its great advantages, as cost-benefit, accessibility, portability, and safety, it has a weak resolution. This is the result of the attenuations, refractions, nonlinearities, frequency selection, or probe properties [1]. As a result, important efforts were made in the direction of image quality improvement.

Signal processing methods offer a reasonable approach for resolution improvement. From this point of view the most important methods for reconstruction are superresolution and deconvolution. If superresolution methods seem to be impractical, the deconvolution ones are more practical [2]. Supperresolution is a complex problem because of the difficulties in aproximation of reconstruction operators (e.g., motion, degradation, and subsampling operators) and the use of multiple frames which puzzles also the implementation. This was conducted on the proposition of multiple deconvolution approaches for ultrasound imaging, like methods used in system identification or Bayesian statistics based ones [3]. From these algorithms, the methods based on Bayesian

approach, especially maximum *a Posteriori* (MAP) seem to offer the most interesting results [4–10]. In these methods the point spread function (PSF) is estimated and then the information is reconstructed in a nonblind way using *a priori* information about tissue reflectivity function.

As the PSF estimation is an important problem that is complex, a lot of methods were advanced to propose an acceptable solution. Primary studies have considered a measured radio-frequency (RF) PSF [4, 11]. However, the use of only one RF PSF to deconvolve the entire image is not feasible due to the nonstationarity of the PSF along the RF line which results from the attenuations, reflections, refractions, and phase aberrations phenomena. A common solution is to estimate the PSF locally by supposing that it is a slow variant in time. This needs to divide the image in segments where one may consider that the PSF is constant and can be estimated for each segment.

Based on the local estimation of the PSF, a certain number of methods were proposed. An approach based on a 1D implementation was proposed to estimate the RF PSF using high order statistics [5].

Taxt et al. introduced a method of RF PSF estimation using the cepstrum and homomorphic deconvolution [6, 12–14]. In this approach it is considered that the PSF spectrum is a function smoother than the reflectivity function.

Another method of unidimensional RF PSF estimation from ultrasound sequences was proposed in [15]. This approach was developed for the cases when the interrogated tissues are composed by high reflectors superimposed by speckle noise, that is, the reflectivity function has Laplacian distribution. For that, it was proposed a complex homomorphic procedure, where for the elimination of the spectrum of reflectivity function a multilevel decomposition denoising technique was used [16]. This denoising technique was improved with an outlier resistant denoising procedure [17] and the phase was estimated using minimum phase assumption.

From the point of view of nonblind algorithms used for deconvolution, the proposed methods supposed that the reflectivity function has a Gaussian or a Laplacian probability of distribution function. For that it was frequently used the Wiener filter (or l_2-norm regularization) [4–6, 11–14] or l_1-norm regularization [7, 9]. If the Wiener filtering seems to smooth the information and to offer a resulted image with a small resolution improvement and speckle noise suppression, the methods based on Laplacian distribution showed a better improvement in terms of contrast and speckle noise reduction.

Other kinds of approaches were proposed in [8] or [10]. In [8] the authors proposed an expectation-maximization algorithm that solved the problem iteratively, by alternating between Wiener filtering and wavelet-based denoising. In [10], 2-steps deconvolution algorithm was proposed, where in first step the PSF is estimated using the Cepstrum technique and for deconvolution a two steps iterative shrinkage/thresholding (TwIST) is used.

However, all the previous methods suffer of difficulties in the phase approximation of the RF PSF in the algorithm robustness. To overcome these difficulties recent works were focused to extract the reflectivity function using the envelope of RF data [8–10, 18]. The most important part of algorithms based on RF envelope intends to extract the tissue reflectivity function using the idea of the inverse filtering. These methods imply matrix inversion which may produce singularities. For such reason, it was necessary to introduce regularization methods which ask for additional computation.

In this paper two major contributions are proposed. The first contribution concerns the combination of three main steps that are the envelope detection based on Hilbert transform, the PSF estimation based on a general homomorphic deconvolution approach, and the deconvolution algorithm based on greedy implementation. Knowing that each method taken alone is not novel, this combination of the above three steps constitutes a novelty. The second contribution concerns the application's field since it is the first time when it is used in ultrasound medical imaging.

Being a blind algorithm, it performs the reconstruction process automatically in two steps. Firstly, the PSF is estimated for each sequence composing the ultrasound image, and, secondly the reflectivity function is obtained using proposed algorithm with the *a priori* assumption that reflectivity

function is a sparse signal; that is, it has a Laplacian probability of density function (PDF). The proposed approach is an iterative algorithm based on the matching pursuit [19] principle that avoids the difficult *inverse problem* in signal reconstruction [20]. Finally, to take into account that PSF can be variant with depth, note that the proposed method can be used on short time subsequences derived from the analyzed sequence at different depths.

In the following, the paper is organized as follows. Section 2 describes the problem reconstruction for ultrasound imaging, Section 3 presents the proposed method, Section 4 shows the experimental results, and Section 5 provides several comments and concludes the current study.

2. Problem Formulation in Ultrasound Medical Images Restoration

In ultrasound imaging the obtained A-mode and B-mode images suppose the interaction between the acoustic beam, generated by the transducer and the scanned tissues. Usually, the phenomena are not linear but for computations simplicity the greatest part of the methods proposed in the literature suppose that the acquired signal is a quasi-linear combination between the reflectivity function and the RF pulse. This supposes that the ultrasound sequences are divided in segments and each segment is processed individually. For the sake of simplicity we reduce the analysis to singular segment. The mathematical formulation of the measured signal $y(n)$ can be described as follows:

$$y(n) = h(n) \otimes x(n) + u(n), \tag{1}$$

where $\otimes$ is the convolution operator, $h(n)$ is the PSF, $x(n)$ is reflectivity function, $u(n)$ is a Gaussian white noise, and n is the samples index. In the frequency domain, (1) can be written as

$$Y(\omega) = H(\omega) \cdot X(\omega) + U(\omega), \tag{2}$$

where the upper case letters represent the Fourier Transform (FT) of the components from (1) and ω is the angular frequency.

As previously mentioned in Section 1, the purpose of the blind reconstruction methods is to obtain the true signal $x(n)$ starting from the acquired signal $y(n)$. A natural solution from (2) is to obtain $X(\omega)$ by inverting $H(\omega)$, which is the FT of the PSF. Equation (2) can be rewritten as

$$X(\omega) = \frac{1}{H(\omega)}Y(\omega) - \frac{1}{H(\omega)}U(\omega). \tag{3}$$

The main problem is that the small values of $H(\omega)$ will amplify by its inversion the high frequencies and implicitly the noise. The most used solutions on this problem are the regularization, according to PDF of the reconstructed signals. In ultrasound imaging a part of the generated pulse is reflected when it finds an interface between two tissues with different physical properties. Therefore, we classically suppose that the reflectivity function has a Laplacian PDF [7, 9, 10, 15].

3. Envelope Based Blind Deconvolution

The acquired signal can be described like an amplitude modulated signal, where the carrier is the wave generated by the transducer and the information is located in its envelope. Based on this assumption, the proposed method starts from the acquired RF signals. From these signals, we extract the envelope and afterwards, this envelope is used in two steps blind deconvolution algorithm: in the first step, the PSF is extracted; then it is used in the greedy noninverse deconvolution algorithm. In the following sections we detail the methods implemented in this paper:

(i) hilbert transform for envelope detection;

(ii) homomorphic deconvolution and soft-thresholding denoising for PSF estimation;

(iii) noninverse greedy deconvolution.

3.1. Envelope Detection. The most popular methods for envelope detection are Hilbert transform or low-pass filtering to separate the useful information contained in envelope from the sinusoidal RF carrier wave. Since the design of low-pass filter may be critical due to the unclear signals spectrum specifications, in this work the Hilbert transform has been preferred. The envelope $y(n)$ can be extracted by applying the absolute value operator at the analytic signal as follows:

$$y(n) = |y_a(n)|, \tag{4}$$

where the $y_a(n)$ means the analytic signal, $y(n)$ means the obtained envelope, and $|\cdot|$ is the absolute value operator. The analytic signal is generated using Hilbert transform as follows:

$$y_a(n) = y_{RF}(n) + j\mathcal{H}\{y_{RF}(n)\}, \tag{5}$$

where $y_a(n)$ is the analytic signal, $y_{RF}(n)$ is the original RF signal, and $\mathcal{H}\{y_{RF}(n)\}$ is the Hilbert transform of $y_{RF}(n)$.

3.2. Point Spread Function Estimation. In ultrasound imaging it was widely assumed in many works that the PSF is a much smoother function than the tissue reflectivity function and that two composing signals of the measured signal spectrum can be separated using homomorphic deconvolution [21] and the denoising procedure as in [15]. The greatest advantage of this kind of homomorphic filters is that they may accept as input a signal composed of two components and return a signal with one of them removed.

The proposed estimation is a three steps algorithm; in the first step we assume that the noise level in (2) is quite small and we may ignore it. In this case it can be rewritten as follows [21]:

$$\ln Y(\omega) = \ln H(\omega) + \ln X(\omega), \tag{6}$$

where ln is the natural logarithm. In this way the output signal is split into two parts: a part which comes from PSF and another one, which occurs from the input signal.

This linear transformation helps us to make a distinction between the signals, under the above presented assumptions

that PSF is a smoother function. Thus, the wave separation problem could be changed in a denoising one. This is in the second step of the homomorphic deconvolution. The main idea of this technique is the use of a denoising method in the frequency domain by applying a wavelet soft thresholding and an outlier resistant denoising algorithm. The threshold was calculated as follows [22]:

$$T = \sigma\sqrt{2\ln N}, \tag{7}$$

where N is the length of the array and σ is the noise variance. The σ parameter is automatically estimated by $\sigma = M_x/0.6745$, where M_x was the median absolute value of the finest decomposition level.

Having obtained $\ln H(\omega)$, the final step of the homomorphic deconvolution is to get the PSF $h(n)$ by using the Inverse Fourier Transform (IFT) of the logarithm spectrum of the PSF, as follows:

$$h(n) = \text{IFT}\{\exp[\ln(H(\omega))]\}. \tag{8}$$

In our implementation, the Fourier Transform was evaluated using Discrete Fourier Transform (DFT).

3.3. Greedy Deconvolution Algorithm. This section describe the proposed algorithm for reflectivity function recovery. It is a greedy algorithm analogous with matching pursuit algorithm. Before describing the computational method, let us to make a short mathematical description for scanned tissues.

The ultrasound imaging is a technique based on the physical properties of acoustical wave reflection when it finds an interface of two different regions with different densities along its propagation. This allows the consideration of the acquired signal as a collection of RF echoes with different amplitude size. Using the above presented considerations, one can say that the useful information, that is, the topological function of scanned tissues can be simulated as a sparse signal superimposed by white gaussian noise. Here, the high amplitude pulses simulate the strongest reflectors and correspond to edges/details of imaging target. The white gaussian noise will correspond to the speckle noise, which according to the final objective of ultrasound sequences processing must be eliminated, reduced, or preserved.

Using the sparsity constraint, we propose an algorithm which is able to reconstruct the original signal without inverting the PSF. This helps us to avoid the inverse problem, which has been known as one of the difficult problems in signal processing.

Within this approach it is considered that the problem could be divided into subproblems. Each subproblem has the objective to eliminate the influence of the most important reflector. In this way, it extracts iteratively from the envelope of the measured signal the influence of the most important blurred scatter; then replaces it with a unit pulse in the output signal, at the same position. At the beginning, it has all positions zero. The algorithm is a greedy algorithm since it works top-down. It provides a locally optimal choice to solve the subproblem, in the hope that at the end, the final solution is

> **Input**: signal envelope $y(n)$, PSF $h(n)$, threshold k.
> **Output**: reflectivity function $x(n)$.
> **Initialisation**:
> $x(n) \leftarrow 0; R(n) \leftarrow y(n); i \leftarrow 0;$
> **Repeat**
>   (i) $n_i = \arg \max_n (R_i(n))$
>   (ii) $x(n_i) \leftarrow R_i(n_i);$
>   (iii) $R_{i+1} \leftarrow R_i - h \otimes R_i(n_i);$
>   (iv) $i \leftarrow i + 1;$
> **Until** stop criterion $(\max(R_i(n)) < k)$

ALGORITHM 1: Noninverse greedy deconvolution.

optimal [23]. For the implementation of the proposed deconvolution algorithm see Algorithm 1.

Here, $R(n)$ is so called the residual signal, $R_i(n_i)$ is the value of maximum amplitude at the position n_i at iteration i, and $\otimes$ is the convolution operator. For this study it was fixed that $k = 0$, because in this way the algorithm extracts the maximum number of possible reflectors.

Being an iterative deconvolution algorithm, its convergence must be studied. According to the condition of positiveness for the reflectivity function, the proposed algorithm iterations have sense, while the residual signal has values greater than zero. Also, the envelope of the PSF being a positive function, it results that the subtraction of a positive function from another positive one will generate a new residual function, at the iteration $i + 1$ which always satisfy the inequality $R_{i+1}(n) < R_i(n)$. This condition is enough to prove that the algorithm will always reach the exit condition. The number of iterations corresponds with the sparsity coefficient, where sparsity coefficient means the number of nonzero elements in the final result. The PSF amplitude is normalized to preserve the same amplitude as in the envelope signal for the resulted sparse signal.

4. Results

The method was tested using synthetic RF-signals and real ultrasound sequences. The experiments with simulated signals are motivated by the allowance of quantitative evaluations under controlled conditions. Then the algorithms were applied to real data to test the feasibility of algorithms in clinical applications where the original topology of tissues is unknown. In the following, these two directions of evaluation will be presented as follows: Section 4.1 presents the results for simulated data and Section 4.2 shows the results for real data.

4.1. Experiments Using Simulated Signals. The so called *reflectivity function*, which simulates the tissues topology, was generated using Laplacian PDF assumption. For the simulations we generated sparse synthetic signals for reproduction of the strongest reflectors. It is contaminated with gaussian white noise to simulate the speckle noise. The length of the signals was 512 points, the sampling frequency was 20 MHz, and the central transducer frequency was 3.2 MHz. This

corresponded to a sequence of 160 μs and an approximately 3.94 cm deep scanning (for a standard ultrasound velocity $c = 1540$ m/s). During the experiments the above mentioned added gaussian white noise was generated according to different SNR values. With this noise we intended to simulate different types of tissues. For example, we find more speckle noise and weak scatters in the soft tissues, like abdominal tissues.

This reflectivity function must be transformed into an RF signal to simulate the acquired signal of the ultrasound probe. According to (1) it can be obtained if the reflectivity function is convolved with a simulated radio-frequency PSF. For current studies the RF PSF was generated using the formula [24]:

$$\text{PSF} = A \cdot \exp\left[-\left(\frac{\omega t}{N\pi}\right)^2\right] \sin \omega t, \tag{9}$$

where A means the PSF amplitude, exp is the exponential function, ω is the angular frequency, t symbolizes time, and N is the number of the periods of the sinusoidal wave of the PSF. The use of this formula is motivated by its capability to control the number of oscillations in the simulated RF pulse. From the experiments it was observed that the sinusoidal wave had 3 or 4 periods.

Figure 1 presents an RF simulated signal example as follows: Figure 1(a) represents simulated tissue reflectivity function, Figure 1(b) represents the generated RF PSF, and Figure 1(c) represents the RF obtained after convolution and its envelope.

Wavelet decomposition and denoising were performed using Wavelab Toolbox, downloaded from http://statweb.stanford.edu/~wavelab/. For the σ parameter in (7), it was observed experimentally that using 5 levels of decomposition was enough for a good elimination of the noise. Also, the estimation of the PSF was made under assumption of minimum phase.

The second step of the algorithm was the deconvolution. The current algorithm, described in Section 3.3 was compared also with different state of the art methods used in deconvolution as follows: regularized least square using l_1-norm, Wiener filter (or l_2-norm regularization), and total variation [3, 25].

The lagrangian parameter, λ, for comparative methods was fixed empirically to obtain the best results as follows: for

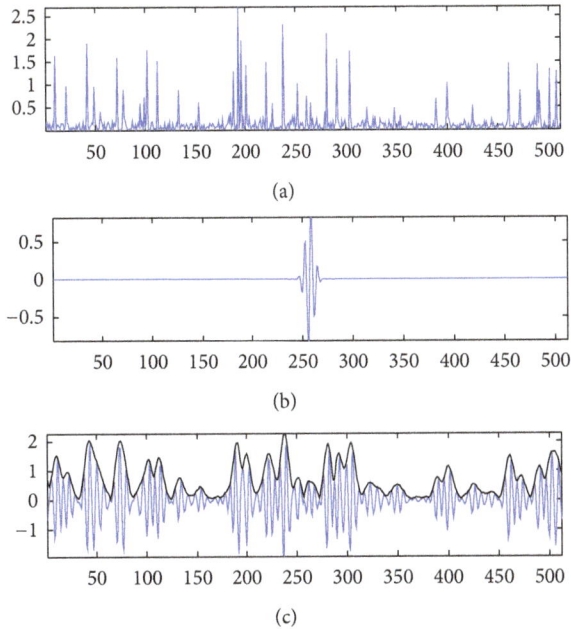

FIGURE 1: Simulated signals. (a) The generated reflectivity function. (b) The generated PSF. (c) The resulted RF signal and its envelope.

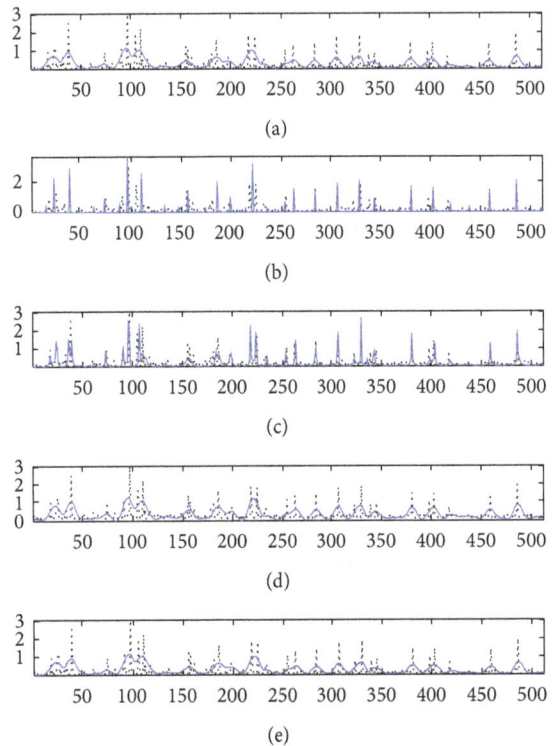

FIGURE 2: Simulated signals results. (a) Envelope of the simulated RF signal; (b) results obtained with our algorithm; (c) results obtained with l_1-norm; (d) results obtained with Wiener filter; (e) results obtained with TV-norm. All signals are superimposed over original reflectivity function (dotted signal).

l_1-norm $\lambda = 0.2$, for Wiener filter (also known as Tikhonov regularization) $\lambda = 0.08$, and for TV-norm $\lambda = 0.14$.

The results were presented in terms of visual and quantitative evaluation. For quantitative measurements, we assessed the execution time for each method and we computed the normalized Mean Square Error (nMSE) and also resolution gain (RG) parameter. RG parameter is based on the ratio between normalized autocorrelation function of the original envelope and the resulted signal higher than -3 dB [12]. The nMSE is defined as follows:

$$nMSE = E\left[\frac{\|\widehat{x} - x\|_2^2}{\|x\|_2^2}\right], \qquad (10)$$

where E is the statistical expectation, x is the original reflectivity function, and $\widehat{x}$ is the resulted reflectivity function.

Figure 2 presents the results on simulated signals. It contains in Figure 2(a) the original RF signal envelope, which was used in all deconvolution methods as input signal; then the obtained results as follows: Figure 2(b): results were obtained with our algorithm, Figure 2(c): results obtained with l_1-norm, Figure 2(d): results obtained with Wiener filter, and Figure 2(e): results obtained with TV-norm. For a better evaluation of the results, all signals were superimposed over the original reflectivity function (dotted signal). After computations, all results were normalized and then displayed to have the same dynamic ranges. It could be seen that our algorithm outperforms the comparative methods in terms of amplitude and scatters estimation. Almost all extracted peaks superimposed the original ones. l_1-norm method offered also a sparse solution for the final result, but it could be seen that the final result was more contaminated with noise, which limits the approach for clinical investigations. The last two methods, Wiener filtering and TV-norm, offered smooth

TABLE 1: Comparison of different restoration techniques according to nMSE (n-Mean Square Error) from (10) and RG (resolution gain). RG is a parameter which evaluates the level of decorrelation for speckle noise in the resulted signal.

Methods	SNR = 7 dB		SNR = 14 dB		SNR = 21 dB	
	nMSE	RG	nMSE	RG	nMSE	RG
Our method	1.36	17.56	1.17	15.48	1.05	14.28
l_1-norm	1.18	17.04	1.11	15.02	0.98	13.82
Wiener	2.82	2.15	2.62	1.68	2.69	1.52
TV-norm	2.52	0.76	2.33	0.87	2.32	0.91

solutions which did not always offer well distinct or well contoured reflectors.

To complete the qualitative evaluation, the results were assessed using some numerical criteria. Table 1 summarizes the results for the nMSE according to (10) and resolution gain. The displayed values are the results of trade off over 100 independently generated signals for all SNR values. In terms of nMSE it could be observed that the best results were offered by l_1-norm followed closely by our method, but Wiener filter and TV-norm were outperformed and in terms of resolution gain the best results are offered by our method followed by l_1-norm. Wiener filter and TV-norm had an insignificant resolution improvement.

TABLE 2: Execution time evaluation for tested algorithms.

	Our alg.	l_1-norm	Wiener	TV-norm
Time (s)	0.002	19.01	0.7	3.83

TABLE 3: Real scatters detection according to their density.

Density	Method	SNR (dB)				
		5	10	15	20	25
2%	Our. alg.	9.05	9.07	9.07	9.12	9.15
	Wiener	8.38	8.76	8.68	8.68	8.86
	l_1-norm	8.94	8.95	8.92	8.96	8.94
5%	Our. alg.	18.9	19.00	19.68	19.72	20.06
	Wiener	18.48	19.56	19.62	19.78	19.88
	l_1-norm	18.6	19.06	19.70	19.74	19.98
10%	Our. alg.	37.62	37.94	37.62	38.30	39.02
	Wiener	34.34	34.62	34.74	34.8	35.16
	l_1-norm	38.62	39.50	39.80	39.56	39.92

Also, an important feature of the proposed algorithm was its execution time. In Table 2 it could be seen that our method outperformed all the compared techniques. This was the logical consequence of the fact that it worked directly in time domain and with the most important operation being vector subtraction. It must be mentioned that for execution time, deconvolution algorithms without PSF estimation were evaluated.

Table 3 showed the results of a statistical evaluation for scatters detection for proposed algorithms (our method, Wiener filter, and l_1-norm). The evaluations were made using simulated signals using different levels of speckle noise and different number of scatters. It must be said that to make the same evaluation for Wiener filter result, we use a signal where we keep only all local maximums. The objective of this simulation was to evaluate the detection capability for each algorithm in different conditions. It could be observed that the proposed algorithm and l_1-norm offer similar results and they have a bigger detection capacity than Wiener filter. This is normal because Wiener filters smooth the information and a part of small details was lost in the reconstruction process. From the point of view of real scatters discovery, we can observe that the more the number of scatters increased, the more the number of detected ones decreased. This can be explained if we refer to Rayleigh condition of superresolution. In the case of a high number of scatters a part of them cannot be recovered, the scatters that are closer to $\lambda/2$, where λ is the wavelength of the emitted PSF. This fact is visible also in Figure 2 (at the samples 250) where a part of them is not recovered.

4.2. Experiments on Real Ultrasound Sequences. As a next step, the proposed deconvolution algorithms were compared using real ultrasound sequences composing ultrasound images. As shown in synthetic signals evaluations, the ultrasound sequences can be done in the same procedure. The envelope could be obtained using Hilbert transform;

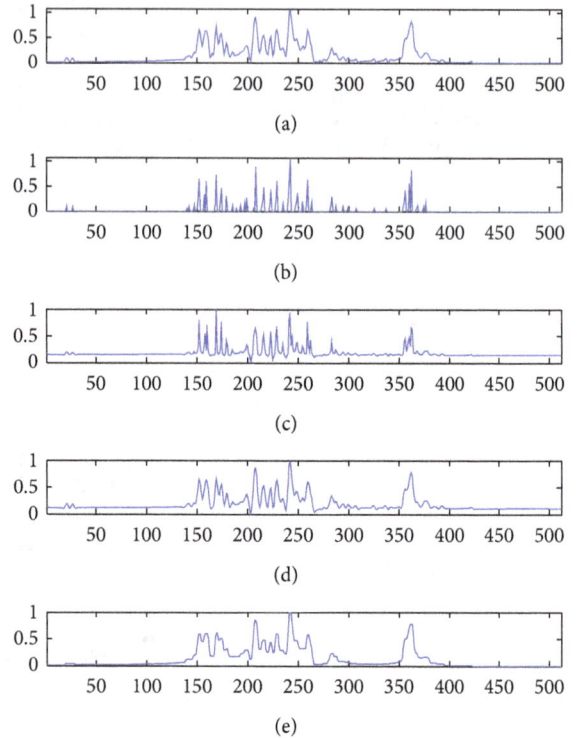

FIGURE 3: Measured signals results. (a) Envelope of measured signal; (b) results obtained with our algorithm; (c) results obtained with l_1-norm; (d) results obtained with Wiener filter; (e) results obtained with TV-norm.

TABLE 4: Resolution gain evaluation on measured signals.

Criteria	Our alg.	l_1-norm	Wiener	TV-norm
RG	15	15	3	1

then PSF was estimated for each sequence and finally the reflectivity function was estimated.

The first experiment on this section is focused on testing real independently measured signals. In the Figure 3 are shown the real measured signal in the subplot Figure 3(a) and then, the results of reconstruction for used algorithms, in the same order as in Figure 2. Because of no *a priori* information about the original reflectivity function it was impossible to evaluate the *n*MSE parameter and also to make the superimposition of the obtained results over the original reflectivity function. For that, the qualitative evaluation is completed using just the RG parameter. In Table 4 the results of quantitative evaluation for the evaluated methods using this parameter are presented. Both visual and quantitative evaluations validated the results obtained for the synthetic signals. It can be seen that our method outperforms the Wiener filter and TV-norm and offers similar results with l_1-norm.

Then, in our experiments we used multiple images obtained in our laboratory. Figure 4 is a log-compressed B-mode image of the skin obtained by an ultrasound scanner developed in-house called Ecoderm. The probe used with this imaging device is a 128 elements linear array working at

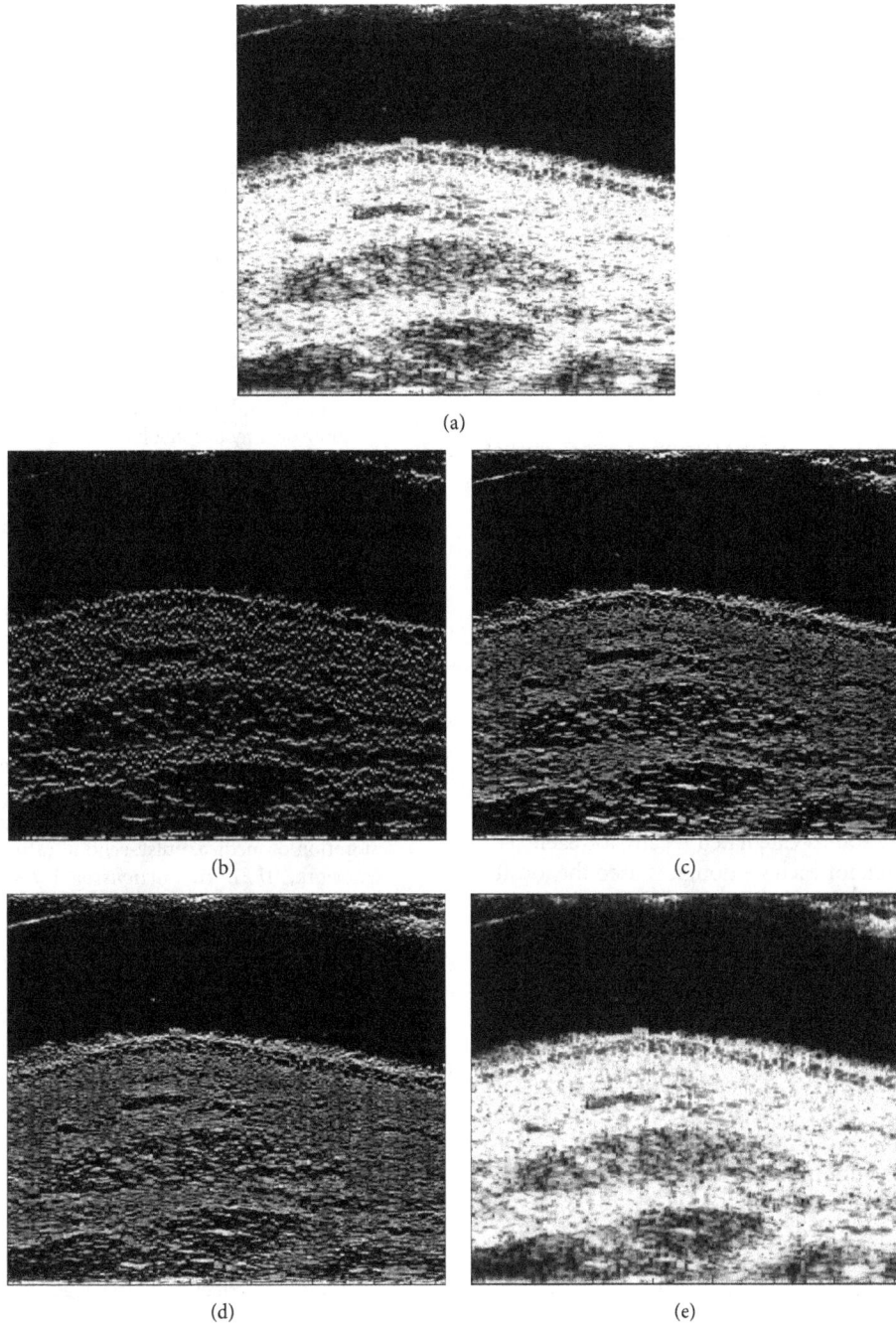

FIGURE 4: (a) Original data; (b) proposed method; (c) l_1-norm method; (d) Wiener filtering; and (e) TV-norm method.

20 MHz center frequency with 87% relative bandwidth. The linear scan is performed by the scanner through an emission aperture composed of 15 elements having focalization delays set up for 8 mm in soft tissues. For computation constraint all the sequences were zero-padded until the next 2^{power} value.

In terms of visual evaluation our method outperformed the comparative techniques. Here, the reflectors are more visible and the speckle noise, which reduces the image quality, was almost suppressed. Moreover, the contours were more visible and the regions without reflectors were better distinguished.

The proposed algorithm assumes that the signal to be recovered is sparse; that is, it has a Laplacian distribution. For that it and l_1-norm are more adapted to reconstruct ultrasound images of tissues with a small number of scatters. This means that in the final result the important details are furthermore revealed and the smaller details (i.e., the speckle noise) are reduced or eliminated. Such similar behavior is observed also in the synthetic signals and real sequences.

As expected, in some cases, the sparse reflectivity sequence is difficult to be interpreted directly because of speckle noise suppression. Some possible improvement can be made for a more realistic interpretation like convolution with an ideal PSF or superimposition of the sparse data over B-mode image.

5. Discussion and Conclusion

The present paper addresses the problem of blind deconvolution for ultrasound sequences in medical imaging by formulating a solution that is able to extract the reflectivity function avoiding the hard problem of inverse filtering. The proposed algorithm is a time domain blind deconvolution that works as a greedy algorithm. The solution estimates in a blind way the PSF, and then, it extracts iteratively the tissue reflectivity function using the estimated PSF.

Being a blind technique, it was assumed *a priori* that the reflectivity function had a sparse shape (i.e., it follows the Laplacian distribution law). Another important feature of this method is its execution time. From the accomplished experiments, it can be seen that the greedy algorithm method outperforms the most used methods in the domain. Also the algorithm works using the envelope of the acquired RF signals, which avoid the problem of the acoustic wave central frequency estimation.

It is well known that in its moving along the propagation direction the PSF shape is changing according to attenuation/nonlinear effects in the tissues. Generally, for perfect results the state of the art approaches divide the image in sections and then the PSF is calculated locally for each section. In reconstruction, for each section, it is used the locally estimated PSF with the same deconvolution algorithm. This means that the deconvolution algorithms work identically, but the results change because of the different used PSFs. The purpose of this research is to prove their feasibility for ultrasound sequences; therefore we only considered the non-variant case in the experimentations.

From the simulations it resulted as well that scatters were well identified and the speckle noise was almost suppressed. However, in some conditions the results were too sparse and this could create some difficulties in information interpretation.

Finally, a number of future works can be outlined. First, the next step will be to analyze the proposed method for different types of tissues in a clinical investigation. Also, we can try to improve the algorithm by imposing supplementary constraints for a better interfaces detection in the situations when they are very close. As discussed before, the sparsity constraint is not always well suitable and this could be improved by making a convolution of the resulted sparse signal with a PSF as in [26]. Choosing the width for PSF can be an interesting study and can offer different solutions according to desired application.

Acknowledgment

This paper was supported by the project "Improvement of the doctoral studies quality in engineering science for development of the knowledge based society-QDOC," contract no. POSDRU/107/1.5/S/78534. The project was cofunded by the European Social Fund through the Sectorial Operational Program Human Resources (2007–2013).

References

[1] T. L. Szabo, *Diagnostic Ultrasound Imaging: Inside Out*, Elsevier Academic Press, Hartford, Conn, USA, 2004.

[2] S. C. Park, M. K. Park, and M. G. Kang, "Super-resolution image reconstruction: a technical overview," *IEEE Signal Processing Magazine*, vol. 20, no. 3, pp. 21–36, 2003.

[3] P. Campisi and K. Egiazarian, Eds., *Blind Image Deconvolution: Theory and Applications*, CRC Press, Boca Raton, Fla, USA, 2007.

[4] E. E. Hundt and E. A. Trautenberg, "Digital processing of ultrasonic data by deconvolution," *IEEE Transactions on Sonics and Ultrasonics*, vol. 27, no. 5, pp. 249–252, 1980.

[5] U. R. Abeyratne, A. P. Petropulu, and J. M. Reid, "Higher order spectra based deconvolution of ultrasound images," *IEEE Transactions on Ultrasonics, Ferroelectrics, and Frequency Control*, vol. 42, no. 6, pp. 1064–1075, 1995.

[6] T. Taxt and J. Strand, "Two-dimensional dimensional blind deconvolution of ultra-sound images," *IEEE Transactions on Ultrasonics, Ferroelectrics, and Frequency Control*, vol. 51, no. 2, pp. 163–165, 2001.

[7] O. V. Michailovich and D. Adam, "A novel approach to the 2-D blind deconvolution problem in medical ultrasound," *IEEE Transactions on Medical Imaging*, vol. 24, no. 1, pp. 86–104, 2005.

[8] J. Ng, R. Prager, N. Kingsbury, G. Treece, and A. Gee, "Wavelet restoration of medical pulse-echo ultrasound images in an em framework," *IEEE Transactions on Ultrasonics, Ferroelectrics, and Frequency Control*, vol. 54, no. 3, pp. 550–568, 2007.

[9] O. Michailovich and A. Tannenbaum, "Blind deconvolution of medical ultrasound images: a parametric inverse filtering approach," *IEEE Transactions on Image Processing*, vol. 16, no. 12, pp. 3005–3019, 2007.

[10] C. Yu, C. Zhang, and L. Xie, "An envelope signal based deconvolution algorithm for ultrasound imaging," *Signal Processing*, vol. 92, no. 3, pp. 793–800, 2012.

[11] W. Vollmann, "Resolution enhancement of ultrasonic B-scan images by deconvolution," *IEEE Transactions on Sonics and Ultrasonics*, vol. 29, no. 2, pp. 78–83, 1982.

[12] T. Taxt, "Restoration of medical ultrasound images using two-dimensional homomorphic deconvolution," *IEEE Transactions on Ultrasonics, Ferroelectrics, and Frequency Control*, vol. 42, no. 4, pp. 543–554, 1995.

[13] J. Strand, T. Taxt, and A. K. Jain, "Two-dimensional phase unwrapping using a block least-squares method," *IEEE Transactions on Image Processing*, vol. 8, no. 3, pp. 375–386, 1999.

[14] T. Taxt, "Three-dimensional blind deconvolution of ultrasound images," *IEEE Transactions on Ultrasonics, Ferroelectrics, and Frequency Control*, vol. 48, no. 4, pp. 867–871, 2001.

[15] O. Michailovich and D. Adam, "Robust estimation of ultrasound pulses using outlier-resistant de-noising," *IEEE Transactions on Medical Imaging*, vol. 22, no. 3, pp. 368–381, 2003.

[16] D. L. Donoho, "De-noising by soft-thresholding," *IEEE Transactions on Information Theory*, vol. 41, no. 3, pp. 613–627, 1995.

[17] A. G. Bruce, D. L. Donoho, H. Y. Gao, and R. D. Martin, "Denoising and robust nonlinear wavelet analysis," in *The Smithsonian/NASA Astrophysics Data System*, vol. 2242 of *Proceedings of SPIE*, pp. 325–336, 1994.

[18] T. Taxt and J. Strand, "Two-dimensional noise-robust blind deconvolution of ultrasound images," *IEEE Transactions on Ultrasonics, Ferroelectrics, and Frequency Control*, vol. 48, no. 4, pp. 861–867, 2001.

[19] S. G. Mallat and Z. Zhang, "Matching pursuits with time-frequency dictionaries," *IEEE Transactions on Signal Processing*, vol. 41, no. 12, pp. 3397–3415, 1993.

[20] E. Bertero and P. Boccacci, *Introduction To Inverse Problem in Imaging*, Institute of Physics Publishing, Boca Raton, Fla, USA, 1998.

[21] A. V. Oppenheim and R. W. Schafer, *Discrete Time Signal Processing*, Prentice Hall, Upper Saddle River, NJ, USA, 3rd edition, 1989.

[22] S. Mallat, *A Wavelet Tour of Signal Processing: The Sparse Way*, Academic Press, Burlington, Mass, USA, 2009.

[23] T. H. Cormen, C. E. Leiserson, R. L. Rivest, and C. Stein, *Introduction to Algorithms*, MIT Press, Cambridge, Mass, USA, 3rd ed edition, 2009.

[24] A. Bouakaz, P. Palanchon, and N. Jong, "Dynamique de la microbulle," in *Échographie de contraste*, pp. 25–43, Springer, Paris, France, 2007.

[25] L. I. Rudin, S. Osher, and E. Fatemi, "Nonlinear total variation based noise removal algorithms," *Physica D*, vol. 60, no. 1–4, pp. 259–268, 1992.

[26] J. A. Högbom, "Aperture synthesis with a non-regular distribution of interferom baselines," *Astronomy and Astrophysics Supplement*, vol. 15, p. 417, 1974.

Permissions

The contributors of this book come from diverse backgrounds, making this book a truly international effort. This book will bring forth new frontiers with its revolutionizing research information and detailed analysis of the nascent developments around the world.

We would like to thank all the contributing authors for lending their expertise to make the book truly unique. They have played a crucial role in the development of this book. Without their invaluable contributions this book wouldn't have been possible. They have made vital efforts to compile up to date information on the varied aspects of this subject to make this book a valuable addition to the collection of many professionals and students.

This book was conceptualized with the vision of imparting up-to-date information and advanced data in this field. To ensure the same, a matchless editorial board was set up. Every individual on the board went through rigorous rounds of assessment to prove their worth. After which they invested a large part of their time researching and compiling the most relevant data for our readers.

The editorial board has been involved in producing this book since its inception. They have spent rigorous hours researching and exploring the diverse topics which have resulted in the successful publishing of this book. They have passed on their knowledge of decades through this book. To expedite this challenging task, the publisher supported the team at every step. A small team of assistant editors was also appointed to further simplify the editing procedure and attain best results for the readers.

Apart from the editorial board, the designing team has also invested a significant amount of their time in understanding the subject and creating the most relevant covers. They scrutinized every image to scout for the most suitable representation of the subject and create an appropriate cover for the book.

The publishing team has been an ardent support to the editorial, designing and production team. Their endless efforts to recruit the best for this project, has resulted in the accomplishment of this book. They are a veteran in the field of academics and their pool of knowledge is as vast as their experience in printing. Their expertise and guidance has proved useful at every step. Their uncompromising quality standards have made this book an exceptional effort. Their encouragement from time to time has been an inspiration for everyone.

The publisher and the editorial board hope that this book will prove to be a valuable piece of knowledge for researchers, students, practitioners and scholars across the globe.

List of Contributors

Paolo Bifulco, Mario Cesarelli, Maria Romano, Antonio Fratini and Mario Sansone
Department of Electrical Engineering and Information Technologies (DIETI), University of Naples "Federico II," Via Claudio 21, 80125 Naples, Italy

Alexander I. Veress
Department of Mechanical Engineering, University ofWashington, SeattleWashington, StevensWay, P.O. Box 352600, Seattle,WA 98195, USA

Gregory Klein
Synarc Inc., Newark, CA 94560, USA

Grant T. Gullberg
Lawrence Berkeley National Laboratory, Berkeley, CA 94720, USA
Department of Radiology, University of California San Francisco, San Francisco, CA 94143, USA

Colin Gilmore
TRTech Inc., Winnipeg MB, Canada R3T 6A8

Amer Zakaria and Joe Lo Vetri
Department of Electrical and Computer Engineering, University of Manitoba,Winnipeg MB, Canada R3T 5V6

Stephen Pistorius
Department of Physics and Astronomy, University of Manitoba,Winnipeg MB, Canada R3T 2N2
Medical Physics, Cancer Care Manitoba, Winnipeg MB, Canada R3E 0V9

Jason C. Crane, Marram P. Olson and Sarah J. Nelson
Surbeck Laboratory for Advanced Imaging, Department of Radiology and Biomedical Imaging, University of California, San Francisco, CA 94158-2330, USA

Ammara Masood and Adel Ali Al-Jumaily
School of Electrical, Mechanical and Mechatronic Engineering, University of Technology, Broadway Ultimo, Sydney, NSW2007, Australia

Daniel J. Tward
Department of Biomedical Engineering, Johns Hopkins University, Baltimore, MD 21218, USA

Jun Ma
Department of Biomedical Engineering, Johns Hopkins University, Baltimore, MD 21218, USA
Siemens Healthcare, Hoffman Estates, Chicago, IL 60192, USA

Michael I. Miller and Laurent Younes
Center for Imaging Science, Johns Hopkins University, Baltimore, MD 21218, USA

Du-Yih Tsai and Eri Matsuyama
Department of Radiological Technology, Graduate School of Health Sciences,Niigata University, 2-746 Asahimachi-dori, Niigata 951-8518, Japan

Hsian-Min Chen
Department of Biomedical Engineering, College of Engineering, Hungkuang University, Taichung 43302, Taiwan

Xiaojin Li, Xintao Hu, Junwei Han and Lei Guo
School of Automation, Northwestern Polytechnical University, Xi'an 710071, China

Changfeng Jin, Wei Hao and Lingjiang Li
Department of Psychiatry, The Mental Health Institute, The Second XiangyaHospital, Central South University, Changsha, China

Tianming Liu
Department of Computer Science and Bioimaging Research Center, University of Georgia, Athens, GA 30602, USA

Niranchana Manivannan and Bradley D. Clymer
Department of Electrical and Computer Engineering, The Ohio State University, Columbus, OH 43210, USA

Anna Bratasz
Small Animal Imaging Shared Resources,The Ohio State University, Columbus, OH 43210, USA

Kimerly A. Powell
Department of Biomedical Informatics, The Ohio State University, Columbus, OH 43210, USA
Small Animal Imaging Shared Resources,The Ohio State University, Columbus, OH 43210, USA

A. Budai
Pattern Recognition Lab, Friedrich-Alexander University, Erlangen-Nuremberg, 91058 Erlangen, Germany
International Max Planck Research School for Optics and Imaging (IMPRS), 91058 Erlangen, Germany
Erlangen Graduate School in Advanced Optical Technologies (SAOT), 91052 Erlangen, Germany

R. Bock, A. Maier and J. Hornegger
Pattern Recognition Lab, Friedrich-Alexander University, Erlangen-Nuremberg, 91058 Erlangen, Germany
Erlangen Graduate School in Advanced Optical Technologies (SAOT), 91052 Erlangen, Germany

G. Michelson
Erlangen Graduate School in Advanced Optical Technologies (SAOT), 91052 Erlangen, Germany
Department of Ophthalmology, Friedrich-Alexander University, Erlangen-Nuremberg, 91058 Erlangen, Germany

Interdisciplinary Center of Ophthalmic Preventive Medicine and Imaging (IZPI), 91054 Erlangen, Germany

Zangen Zhu and Khan Wahid
Department of Electrical and Computer Engineering, University of Saskatchewan, Saskatoon, SK, Canada S7N5A9

Paul Babyn
Department of Medical Imaging, University of Saskatchewan and Saskatoon Health Region, Saskatoon, SK, Canada S7N 0W8

Ran Yang
School of Information Science and Technology, Sun Yat-Sen University, Guangzhou, Guangdong 510006, China

Hong Song
School of Software, Beijing Institute of Technology, 5 South Zhongguancun Street, Haidian District, Beijing 100081, China

Xiangfei Cui and Feifei Sun
School of Computer Science & Technology, Beijing Institute of Technology, 5 South Zhongguancun Street, Haidian District, Beijing 100081, China

Fatima Sbeity and Jean-Marc Girault
Université François Rabelais de Tours, UMR-S930, 37032 Tours, France

Sébastien Ménigot
IUT Ville d'Avray, Université Paris Ouest Nanterre La Défense, 92410 Ville d'Avray, France
Université François Rabelais de Tours, UMR-S930, 37032 Tours, France

Jamal Charara
Département de Physique et d' ´Electronique, Faculté des Sciences I, Université Libanaise, Hadath, Lebanon

Andreas Fhager and Mikael Persson
Biomedical Engineering Division, Department of Signal and Systems, Chalmers University of Technology, 41296 Gothenburg, Sweden

Shantanu K. Padhi
Curtin Institute of Radio Astronomy (CIRA), ICRAR, Curtin University, Perth,WA 6102, Australia

John Howard
PRL, Research School of Physics and Engineering, Australian National University, Canberra, ACT 0200, Australia

Jacob U. Fluckiger
Department of Radiology,NorthwesternUniversity, Chicago, IL 60611, USA

Xia Li
Institute of Imaging Science, Vanderbilt University, Nashville, TN 37212, USA

Department of Radiology and Radiological Sciences, Vanderbilt University, Nashville, TN 37212, USA

Jennifer G. Whisenant
Institute of Imaging Science, Vanderbilt University, Nashville, TN 37212, USA
Program in Chemical and Physical Biology, VanderbiltUniversity, Nashville, TN 37212, USA

Todd E. Peterson
Department of Radiology and Radiological Sciences, Vanderbilt University, Nashville, TN 37212, USA
Department of Physics and Astronomy, VanderbiltUniversity, Nashville, TN 37212, USA

John C. Gore
Department of Radiology and Radiological Sciences, Vanderbilt University, Nashville, TN 37212, USA
Program in Chemical and Physical Biology, VanderbiltUniversity, Nashville, TN 37212, USA
Department of Physics and Astronomy, VanderbiltUniversity, Nashville, TN 37212, USA
Department of Biomedical Engineering, Vanderbilt University, Nashville, TN 37212, USA
Department of Molecular Physiology and Biophysics, Vanderbilt University, Nashville, TN 37212, USA

Thomas E. Yankeelov
Department of Radiology and Radiological Sciences, Vanderbilt University, Nashville, TN 37212, USA
Program in Chemical and Physical Biology, VanderbiltUniversity, Nashville, TN 37212, USA
Department of Physics and Astronomy, VanderbiltUniversity, Nashville, TN 37212, USA
Department of Biomedical Engineering, Vanderbilt University, Nashville, TN 37212, USA
Department of Cancer Biology, Vanderbilt University, Nashville, TN 37212, USA

Amir Pasha Mahmoudzadeh and Nasser H. Kashou
Biomedical Imaging Laboratory, Wright State University, Dayton, OH 45435, USA

E. Pavarino, L. A. Neves, J. C. Momente, G. F. D. Zafalon, A. R. Pinto, C. R. Valêncio and J. M. Machado
Department of Computer Science and Statistics (DCCE), São Paulo State University (UNESP), 15054-000 São José do Rio Preto, SP, Brazil

M. F. de Godoy
Department of Cardiology and Cardiovascular Surgery, São José do Rio Preto Medical School–Famerp, 15090-000 São José do Rio Preto, SP, Brazil

Diego Alberto
Department of Electronics and Telecommunications, Politecnico di Torino, Corso Duca Degli Abruzzi 24, 10129 Turin, Italy
TIMA Laboratory (Grenoble INP, UJF, CNRS), 46 avenue Félix Viallet, 38031 Grenoble, France

Roberto Garello
Department of Electronics and Telecommunications, Politecnico di Torino, Corso Duca Degli Abruzzi 24, 10129 Turin, Italy

Wenchao Cui
School of Electronics and Information, Northwestern Polytechnical University, Xi'an 710072, China
College of Science, China Three Gorges University, Yichang 443002, China

Yi Wang, Yangyu Fan, Yan Feng and Tao Lei
School of Electronics and Information, Northwestern Polytechnical University, Xi'an 710072, China

Jing Zou, Xiaodong Hu, Hanyu Lv and Xiaotang Hu
State Key Laboratory of Precision Measuring Technology and Instruments, Tianjin University, Tianjin 300072, China

Ryan C. Gessner, C. Brandon Frederick and Paul A. Dayton
UNC and NCSU Joint Department of Biomedical Engineering, 304 Taylor Hall, 109Mason Farm Road, Chapel Hill, NC 27599-6136, USA

F. Stuart Foster
Department of Medical Biophysics, University of Toronto, Sunnybrook Health Sciences Centre, 2075 Bayview Avenue, Toronto,ON, Canada M4N3M5

Liviu-Teodor Chira
Signal & Imaging Group, University Franc,ois Rabelais of Tours, PRES Loire Valley University, UMR INSERM U930, 7 Avenue Marcel Dassault, 37200 Tours Cedex, France
Faculty of Electronics, Telecommunications and Information Theory, Technical University of Cluj-Napoca, Cluj-Napoca 400027, Romania

Corneliu Rusu
Faculty of Electronics, Telecommunications and Information Theory, Technical University of Cluj-Napoca, Cluj-Napoca 400027, Romania

Clovis Tauber and Jean-Marc Girault
Signal & Imaging Group, University Franc,ois Rabelais of Tours, PRES Loire Valley University, UMR INSERM U930, 7 Avenue Marcel Dassault, 37200 Tours Cedex, France

www.ingramcontent.com/pod-product-compliance
Lightning Source LLC
Chambersburg PA
CBHW080456200326
41458CB00012B/3991